# Pregnancy, Childbirth, and the Newborn

## The Complete Guide

### FIFTH EDITION

Penny Simkin, PT

Janet Whalley, RN, IBCLC

Ann Keppler, RN, MN

Janelle Durham, MSW, ICCE, LCCE

April Bolding, PT, DPT, CD, CCE

of Parent Trust for Washington Children

Da Capo
∞
LIFE
LONG

Da Capo Press
Hachette Book Group
1290 Avenue of the Americas, New York, NY 10104
www.dacapopress.com
@DaCapoPress

Printed in the United States of America

First Edition: 1979

Fifth Edition: March 2016; color version September 2018

Published by Da Capo Lifelong Books, an imprint of Perseus Books, LLC, a subsidiary of Hachette Book Group, Inc. The Da Capo Lifelong name and logo are trademarks of the Hachette Book Group.

The publisher is not responsible for websites (or their content) that are not owned by the publisher.

Library of Congress record available at lccn.loc.gov/201504545809

ISBNs: 978-0-7382-8497-2 (paperback), 978-0-7382-8502-3 (ebook) / 978-0-7382-8501-6 (library ebook)

LSC-C

10  9  8  7  6  5  4  3  2  1

# Praise for *Pregnancy, Childbirth, and the Newborn*

"Women who use this book to prepare themselves for labor will be leagues ahead of women who don't and ahead of most of the professionals who take care of women during labor."
—Judith Rooks, CNM; author of *Midwifery in America*

"The single best book for understanding pregnancy and birth."
—Carol Jones, CNM; Director of Midwifery, Virginia Mason Clinic, Seattle, WA

"This book is authoritative without feeling overwhelming.
It keeps the woman and her family in focus and provides a range of options.
If expectant parents could have one book, this would be the one."
—Trish Booth, MA, LCCE, FACCE; childbirth education consultant, Manlius, NY

"A truly wonderful book for expectant families. It's informative, thorough,
and helpful. We give it to all our patients, and they think it's great, too!"
—Carolyn Kline, MD, MPH; perinatologist, Eastside Maternal Fetal Medicine,
Kirkland and Bellevue, WA

"The material is beautifully organized and the presentation is crystal clear."
—Sheila Kitzinger, author of *The Complete Book of Pregnancy and Childbirth*

"For the most part, pregnancy books are written for and read by women,
but if you're a caring father (or father-to-be), this is an outstanding book.
It gives the fairest and most complete descriptions of the myriad medical
options available during childbirth. It is the best of the many books available."
—Tom Seager, father of three, Potsdam, NY

# Awards

Mom's Choice Awards Gold Award Winner
iParenting Media Awards Best Products Winner
Living Now Book Awards Bronze Award Winner
National Parenting Publications Awards (NAPPA) Gold Award Winner
USABookNews.com Best Books Award Winner
ForeWord Magazine Book of the Year Awards Finalist

# Acknowledgments

This book, originally conceived as a class manual called *Becoming Parents*, was first published by the Childbirth Education Association of Seattle (CEAS) in 1976. Gillian Mitchell, Penny Simkin, Janet Whalley, and Ann Keppler wrote and edited it. In 1984 Meadowbrook Press published the first edition of *Pregnancy, Childbirth, and the Newborn* (an extensive revision of the original book) with the help of editor Tom Grady. The second edition was published in 1991 with the help of editor Kerstin Gorham. The third edition was published in 2001, with the help of editors Joseph Gredler, Nancy Campbell, and Christine Zuchora-Walske. Editors Megan McGinnis and Alicia Ester helped with the publication of the fourth edition in 2010. This fifth edition was published with the help of editors Megan McGinnis and Heidi Hogg.

Many other people have helped with the creation of this latest edition. We are most grateful to you:
- the fabulous Great Starts instructors, who provided suggestions for revisions, input on content, recommended resources, and more
- the staff of Parent Trust for Washington Children, especially Mark Buckley for his leadership, Linda McDaniels for cheerleading the project, and Audrey Miles Cherney for coordinating the Great Starts program
- the Penny Simkin, Inc. staff of Katie Rohs, Dolly Sundstrom, and Kathy Wilson for their assistance and support
- professional consultants Diana Koala, MD, and Michelle M. Grandy, RN, CNM

We also wish to thank the following people for their contributions to the artwork of this edition:
- *illustrations:* Ruth Ancheta and Shanna Alvarez; special thanks to Susan Spellman, for being so easy to work with on so many details of the illustrations.
- *photographs:* Carlos A. Arguelles; Charlotte R. Brown, Ineffable Images; Bob Cerelli; Sandra Coan; Jan Dowers; Sofia Zadra Goff; Sindea Horste; Samantha Kroop, Park Avenue Art; Willa Kveta; Spike Mafford; Katie McCollough; Medela; Marilyn Nolt; Elisha Rain; Stevens Hospital, Edmonds, WA; and Well-Rounded Maternity Center, Menomonee Falls, WI.
- *models:* Lisa Black Avolio; April Bolding; Heidi and Kate Whalley; Dina Apostlou with Kosta and Melina; Courtney, Eric, Noah, and Lucas Keppler; Michele Sonntag, Kathleen Porch, and the attendees of First Weeks in April 2010

# Dedication

To our husbands and to our children and their families:

Peter Simkin
Andy, Bess, Alfred, Arshia, Charlie, Eva Rose, and Jonathan
Linny, Peter, and Callie
Mary, Greg, Sara Jane, and Amelia
Elizabeth and Cole

Doug Whalley
Scott, Heidi, Kate, and Adelyn
Mike, Leslie, and Finn

Jerry Keppler
Eric, Courtney, Lucas, and Noah
Heidi and Paul

Peter Durham
Martin, Izzi, and Ben

Tim Hunt
Lily and Maya Rose

To the thousands of expectant and new parents whom we have taught and who have taught us so much.

And to the Great Starts Program of Parent Trust for Washington Children, which has educated, supported, and encouraged families in their transitions to parenthood since 1950.

# Contents

# Introduction

Maternity care practices are continually changing how women are cared for during pregnancy, birth, and the postpartum period. But how a woman's body functions during those times—and what she needs—hasn't changed since the beginning of humankind.

A key to having positive pregnancy, birth, and postpartum experiences is receiving care that meets the family's needs and desires. To receive such care, families must figure out just what their needs and desires *are*—and the first step is to learn all about these topics and their options for care. This is where we can help inform and guide expectant parents like you.

For this fifth edition, we've thoroughly updated the content to provide you with the latest medical information and best practices. We've used what we've learned as pregnancy and childbirth educators to most effectively present the new information and ideas so expectant parents can take full advantage of them.

## WHY READ THIS BOOK

With abundant information on maternity and newborn care available from books, blogs, podcasts, websites and TV, you may wonder if there's a need for a book like *Pregnancy, Childbirth, and the Newborn*. Our resounding response is, "Yes, more than ever!" When preparing to have a baby, you need both the "wisdom of the ages" and the latest research in a single comprehensive and balanced resource. That's what this book offers.

We have more than 150 cumulative years of experience working with expectant and new parents. We're constantly asking them what advice is—and isn't—helpful. Based on their answers, we're continuously adapting the way we teach and advise women, couples, and families. That knowledge is reflected in these pages.

We understand that "one size fits all" doesn't apply to maternity care. Our intent is to offer essential, accurate, and unbiased information—*you* decide how best to use it. Our goal is to discuss all options and help you make informed decisions that match *your* values and priorities.

## HOW TO USE THIS BOOK

Pregnancy, childbirth, and newborn care are broad topics, and we discuss each thoroughly. However, we know that expectant parents might not have the time or desire to read this book from cover to cover. To help you find the information you need when you need it, we've organized the content in the order that events typically occur. A detailed index notes where you can find information on a specific topic, and page references within the book point you to further discussion on a subject.

We first describe normal, healthy processes along with their typical variations and the usual care practices for monitoring them. We next describe comfort measures and self-help techniques that help you manage the challenges of pregnancy, birth, and the postpartum period. We then cover possible complications and the care practices and procedures for resolving them. We include information on complications for those experiencing them, as well as for those who want it on hand "just in case." (If all is going well for you, feel free to skip these chapters if reading them only makes you anxious.)

To help you recall the meanings of key words used in maternity and newborn care, we've included a glossary. We've also added a Road Map of Labor, a visual guide that helps illustrate labor as a journey to a destination (birth).

As comprehensive as this book is, we recognize that it can't fully cover every pregnancy, childbirth, or newborn topic. We refer to our companion website, http://www.PCNGuide.com, whenever we have more to say about a topic or want to provide the most up-to-date facts on medical interventions, medications, care procedures, and much more. You can also download a number of work sheets and forms to help you record important information obtained during your pregnancy, birth, and beyond.

We also recommend other reliable resources. For example, the chapters on feeding and caring for your newborn focus on key information for just the first six weeks. You'll need many other resources to help you through the next eighteen years! We suggest several books, websites, and parenting classes and support groups to help get you started on your extended parenting journey.

To present all options completely and fairly, some topics require more discussion than others. For example, we discuss breastfeeding at more length than formula-feeding simply because breastfeeding is a more complex process. We describe some nonmedical pain management options, such as self-help techniques, at more length than pain medications because these techniques require detailed instructions for use. The balance of this discussion may make you wonder if we're biased against medical maternity care. *Absolutely not!* On the contrary, we believe pain medications and interventions can benefit both parents and babies when used appropriately. We advise that you thoroughly read about *all* the available options so you can decide which ones best meet your needs and desires.

## Our Hope for This Book

It's our privilege to guide you during this life-changing journey. We hope that the following chapters will help you sift through the often overwhelming information so you can make the best decisions for you and your family. It's our wish that with the knowledge you gain from our collective wisdom, you'll have a safe, satisfying pregnancy and birth and a joyful introduction to parenting.

Penny Simkin, PT
Janet Whalley, RN, IBCLC
Ann Keppler, RN, MN
Janelle Durham, MSW, LCCE
April Bolding, PT, DPT, CD, CCE

P.S. Since the first edition of this book, we've used inclusive language to reflect various family configurations, including mother-father-children families, single-parent families, blended families formed by second marriages, families with gay and lesbian parents, and families formed by open adoption or surrogacy. We acknowledge and respect transgender men and genderqueer parents who will carry and birth their babies. Although the pregnant parent is sometimes referred to as *woman* or *mother*, most references to both expectant parents are now gender neutral. When referring to the baby, however, we've continued to alternate the use of masculine and feminine pronouns.

# Pregnancy, Childbirth,
## and the
# Newborn

# CHAPTER 1

# You're Having a Baby!

Having a baby presents some of life's greatest challenges and rewards. During pregnancy, childbirth, and your newborn's first weeks, you'll experience everything from wonder and joy to bewilderment and stress—often at the same time. You can be glad that pregnancy lasts around nine months so you have time to learn, plan, adjust, and prepare.

Day by day, your developing baby is becoming capable of thriving outside the protective environment of your body. You're becoming physically and emotionally ready to give birth, and your partner is learning how to support you during labor. Together, you'll prepare to meet your baby's needs.

This book provides reliable information and guidance for staying healthy, finding good prenatal care and support, learning about your options for maternity care, and making decisions that reflect your preferences and priorities. Your baby is getting ready to join your family, so let's turn the page and start preparing for his birth!

# Pregnancy: A Time for Change and Preparation

Like most expectant parents, you want a healthy pregnancy so you can provide a safe environment for your developing baby. Pregnancy is the time to assess your diet, fitness level, lifestyle, finances, and relationships—and make any necessary changes for optimal health. It's also the time to arrange for prenatal care and seek help to resolve or manage any medical problems or mental health challenges. Chapters 4 through 6 discuss ways to have the healthiest pregnancy possible for you and your baby.

Because pregnancy puts extra demands on your body, you may have questions about the health of your pregnancy. Chapter 3 describes common changes and concerns that can arise in pregnancy and what you can do to address them, and chapter 21 discusses what changes you can expect if this pregnancy isn't your first. During pregnancy, you'll also discover that you want to talk with other expectant parents as well as new parents so you can learn from their experiences and benefit from their support. Use this time to draw upon or develop a support system that can help you long after your baby is born.

Looking ahead to the birth, you may wonder how you'll manage labor. Will you want to use medications to reduce or eliminate pain? Will you want a natural, drug-free birth? What kind of support will you want your partner to provide? Pregnancy is the time to prepare for how you'll cope with childbirth; reading this book is a good place to start, and taking childbirth classes will enhance your knowledge of your options. Chapters 9 and 10 describe when and how labor begins and what childbirth is really like, while chapters 11, 12, and 13 provide information on the various medications and nonmedicated options for managing labor pain.

Just as most pregnancies are normal, so are most labors and births. However, just as problems can arise in pregnancy, complications can develop during childbirth, and medical interventions may become necessary for the health of the mother and baby. If your pregnancy, birth, or postpartum becomes complicated, it's helpful to be aware of the possible problems and potential solutions. Chapters 7, 14, 15, 17, and 20 describe pregnancy and childbirth complications and the options for treatment

As you anticipate parenthood, questions and deep feelings may come up about your childhood, and about your parents' relationships with each other and with you. Your partner may have the same experience. Pregnancy is a good time to strengthen bonds, mend fences, or clarify boundaries with your parents so you can enter parenthood on your own terms.

You and your partner may also spend a lot of time thinking about the amazing responsibility of physically, emotionally, and spiritually nurturing a child. Pregnancy is a good time for you and your partner to explore your expectations of parenthood and develop the qualities essential for parenting, perhaps by taking parenting classes, reading parenting books, or speaking to friends and relatives about their parenting experiences.

# Birth as a Long-Term Memory

Research shows that women vividly recall their birth experiences for many years.[1] After you give birth to your baby, you'll remember the major facts of the experience, such as how long you were in labor, the time of her birth, and her birth weight. But you'll also remember other details, such as how you knew you were in labor, how you felt during contractions, what you did to relieve the pain, and how others comforted you and helped you cope. This information will make up your unique, unforgettable story of giving birth to your child.

Some parents have positive, fulfilling, and empowering memories of childbirth. These parents feel that they were treated with kindness and their priorities and preferences for care were respected—even if labor was long and complicated. Other parents remember their birth experiences with shame, anger, remorse, or resignation. These parents feel that they were disrespected, abandoned, or powerless during childbirth, and this negative treatment tarnished their memories of the experience.

No one has complete control over pregnancy and childbirth, but the decisions you make during pregnancy will affect your memory of your birth experience. By making decisions that will help you have a satisfying birth, you increase your chances of having good memories of the experience. (See page 26 for steps to improve your chances of having a satisfying birth experience.) Conversely, if you make decisions that will hinder your ability to have a satisfying birth—or if the decisions you make aren't respected—you increase your risk of having unhappy memories of the experience.

## Your Mother's Memories of Giving Birth

Ask your mother to tell you her story of giving birth to you, and have your partner do the same with his or her mother. What does your mother remember about going into labor? What did your father do? What did her caregivers do and say? What did she feel when she first saw you and held you? How does your mother feel now about your birth? Unless she was heavily drugged during labor, she'll probably have clear and detailed memories, and the intensity of her emotions as she recalls them may surprise you.

## Different Views on Childbirth

When asked to describe their childbirth experiences to their children, parents gave a variety of responses. Here are a few examples:

- It was the best day of my life!
- I have always felt I short-changed you. I didn't welcome you the way you deserved.
- After giving birth, I knew I could do anything!
- Labor with you seemed to go on forever. But it didn't matter how tired I was or how hard it was: you were worth every minute!

# Making Decisions for a Satisfying Pregnancy and Birth

Because pregnancy and birth are normally healthy processes and highly personal, emotionally significant experiences, you typically have more choices for care than you would for a medical condition that involves disease or injury. You usually have the opportunity to make the following decisions: where you have your baby, who your caregivers are, how educated you become about pregnancy and childbirth, who provides you companionship and support in labor, how you want to manage labor pain, and to what extent you want your caregivers to manage your care.

If you're surprised by the number of decisions you'll have to make during pregnancy, you may be overwhelmed by the staggering amount of information available to you on maternity care. Some resources provide sound, reliable advice (such as this book); others don't. Chapters 2 and 8 discuss how you can find and evaluate maternity care information so you can make decisions that are right for you and your family.

This book is based on the importance of your active participation in every aspect of your care. When you're well informed of your choices and can communicate your questions, needs, and preferences, you help ensure maximum safety for you and your baby, and enhance your satisfaction with the birth experience.

# More Than the Birth of a Baby

Cultures around the world celebrate birth as a significant, joyous event marked by rituals of hope, promise, and new life. At the moment of birth, many lives are transformed. For you and your partner, your baby's birth marks your birth as parents. For your family, the birth creates their new roles as siblings, grandparents, aunts, uncles, and cousins.

When you meet your baby, you may feel that you've always known him—or you may be totally surprised by him. As you gaze at him and stroke, sniff, and snuggle him, you'll begin to fall in love as only parents and babies can. During the first few hours and days of your baby's life, you'll begin to fully appreciate the fact that this tiny person is the same mystery being you knew in the womb.

After the initial awe of new parenthood fades, you'll realize that your life has permanently changed and is more uncertain and less simple than it was before you became a parent. You may wonder how our species has ever survived when birth, breastfeeding, and baby care seem so challenging. A newborn's needs are almost constant and sometimes hard to understand. When your baby cries, you may ask yourself, "Is he hungry, wet, cold, sleepy, lonely, in pain? How do I soothe him, hold him, change him, bathe him, feed him? How do I know I'm doing a good job?" Chapters 18 and 19 describe the basics of baby care and feeding; your confidence will grow as you become more experienced with nurturing and nourishing your baby.

In the first few weeks of your newborn's life, you may have other worries, such as, "How can I get enough sleep? Can we afford a longer maternity leave? Will I ever have time to be romantic with my partner again? Will I ever *want* to be romantic again?" Chapters 16 and 17 describe what life is like for a new mother and discuss concerns, doubts, and problems that can arise in the postpartum period and what you can do to address them.

After these early challenges, the rewards will start to come. Your baby will settle down when you cuddle him. He'll gain weight. He'll smile and coo. He'll stop crying when you sing to him. His sleeping pattern will become more predictable. He won't be able to take his eyes off you, and you won't be able to take your eyes off him. At that point, you'll realize that you wouldn't return to your prebaby life, even if you could.

The time spanning pregnancy, childbirth, and your newborn's first weeks will be an unforgettable experience, one that will have a lasting impact on your life. This book will help you discover that you already know how to grow your baby, give birth to him, and nourish and nurture him. Besides good health and good care, all you really need are confidence, support, and the practical skills and knowledge provided in the following chapters.

## *Key Points to Remember*

- Pregnancy is marked by physical and emotional changes, and it's a time to prepare for childbirth and parenthood.
- Birth is an unforgettable experience. You'll remember giving birth to your baby for years to come.
- The decisions you make for your care will have a great impact on you, your family, and your baby.
- The birth of your baby will have profound emotional significance, and your journey as a new parent will be one of wonder, doubt, and self-discovery.

# CHAPTER 2

# So Many Choices

After discovering you're pregnant, you begin to make choices that will affect your entire childbearing experience. You choose how you'll gather information on pregnancy and birth. You select the kind of maternity care you'll want and decide where you'll want to give birth. You arrange for the support you'll need in the days and months after the birth and plan for your return to work. Because these choices most affect you, your baby, and your early days as a family, it's important that you play a key role in the decision-making process. Your active participation now will give you satisfaction and fulfillment for years to come, because you'll feel that your wishes were honored with kindness and respect.

# Informed Decision Making

In the United States and Canada, it's your legal right to play a central role when making decisions that affect you and your baby. To help you make an *informed decision* (or *informed choice*) about a health-care option or medical treatment (a procedure, test, intervention, or medication), you can consult with your caregiver and other knowledgeable medical professionals, as well as with supportive friends and family.

If you agree to an option or treatment after becoming informed about it, you've given your *informed consent*. By law, your caregivers can't give you medical treatment in either of the following cases:

- You're insufficiently informed about the treatment (and therefore can't give your informed consent).
- After becoming sufficiently informed about the treatment, you refuse it (*informed refusal*).

A more collaborative approach to making an informed decision is *shared decision making*, in which you and your caregiver discuss the medical risks and benefits of treatment and any possible alternatives. You also discuss any questions or concerns you may have, as well as your priorities and preferences. Shared decision making enhances trust and understanding between you and your caregiver.[1]

## YOUR CAREGIVER'S ROLE IN DECISION MAKING

Your caregiver's approach to maternity care depends on training, experience, and general perception of pregnancy and birth. If your caregiver perceives the childbearing process as usually normal and healthy, medical interventions aren't recommended unless problems develop. If your caregiver perceives the process as potentially dangerous, medical procedures, tests, and medications may be recommended more often in case they're needed later. Even though these perceptions result in different types of care, everyone's intention is to ensure a healthy mother and baby.

Sometimes, a procedure or treatment is *routine*, which means it's offered to all pregnant women or newborns. Other times, it's individualized to the current situation. Before recommending any treatment, your caregiver considers many factors, including your health; care standards set by professional organizations or government agencies; the caregiver's experience and preferences for interventions, hospital routines, and policies; the usual care practices among peers; cost; and staffing issues.

In addition, your caregiver considers whether a treatment will achieve the desired results or create problems, then weighs the treatment's benefits against its risks. This *benefit-risk analysis* sometimes shows that a relatively risk-free option is the best treatment to achieve desired results. Other times, the analysis reveals that the best treatment is the one with the greatest risk of side effects. Some caregivers always choose the treatment that best achieves results, despite any risks that come with it. Others choose a less risky option first—even if its chances of success are lower—then move to a more risky option if the first option is unsuccessful.

## *What to Do If You and Your Caregiver Disagree about Treatment*

Almost all treatment carries some risks or disadvantages, but you and your caregiver may disagree on just how risky or disadvantageous a treatment is. For example, your caregiver may believe a medical procedure is safe and low-risk, but you may feel the risks aren't worth taking. You may prefer to learn more about pros, cons, and choices regarding that procedure and to discuss them with your caregiver. If a disagreement about treatment arises, you and your caregiver can usually settle it with respectful discussion and good communication—the foundation of shared decision making.

But what if it can't be settled? Although rare, relationships between caregivers and pregnant women may fall apart because of a troubling mismatch in attitudes or opinions. When settling a disagreement is unlikely, in the United States and Canada, a pregnant woman has the legal right to change to a different caregiver, and a caregiver has the right to discontinue care if there are other care options available to the pregnant woman. See page 18 for further information on changing caregivers.

# Making Informed Decisions

This chapter covers many of the important decisions you'll make during pregnancy, during birth, and after the birth. You should make some decisions early in pregnancy (such as finding your caregiver); you can delay making other decisions until mid- to late-pregnancy. The following sections discuss topics that require you to make decisions, and they're presented roughly in the order that you should address them.

Whenever you're asked to make a choice about your or your baby's health care, ask the key questions on the right to learn more about your options. Always remember that your caregiver can provide information about treatment and recommend options, but only you can decide what's best for you and your baby.

## Key Questions for Making an Informed Decision

When you're offered a test or treatment, first ask how urgent the situation is and whether you have time to ask questions, discuss options, and consider the information you've learned. Then, ask these key questions:

**Benefits:** What's the problem we're trying to identify, prevent, or fix? Am I having that problem, or am I likely to develop it? How is the test or procedure done? How likely is it to succeed?

**Risks:** What are the possible risks or side effects for my baby or me, and how are they handled? Are there other tradeoffs or disadvantages, such as additional procedures or precautions that will be necessary to maintain safety? What's the cost (if paying out of pocket)?

**Alternatives:** What other options are available? Are there other procedures that may work? Can I delay the treatment or choose not to do it? What are the risks and benefits of the alternatives and how effective are they? (Keep in mind that low-risk options are sometimes less effective, so ask for guidance when analyzing benefits against risks.)

**Next steps:** If the procedure identifies or solves the problem, what can we expect to happen afterward? If the procedure doesn't identify or solve the problem, what will we need to do next?

# Health-Care Coverage

Having a baby can be expensive, and different kinds of maternity care have different costs. In the United States, a licensed midwife may charge as little as $3,000 for prenatal care and attendance at an uncomplicated home birth. Using a midwife for prenatal care and a birth center for the birth may cost $4,000 to $5,000. (*Note:* These estimates don't include the costs of prenatal tests, such as ultrasound scans and blood tests.) Using an obstetrician for prenatal care, having prenatal tests, and having an uncomplicated vaginal birth in a hospital cost on average $30,000. A complicated cesarean birth can cost $50,000.[2]

The Affordable Care Act requires all Americans to have health insurance or pay a tax. You have five options for obtaining insurance:

- **Through your employer:** You can get this coverage even if you're already pregnant, and you won't pay more than 9.5 percent of your income.
- **Through your spouse's employer:** Check costs carefully. It may be cheaper to choose another option.
- **Through your parents' insurance if you're younger than twenty-six:** Check to see if their plan covers pregnancy for a dependent.
- **Individual coverage from a state exchange:** Go to the Marketplace at http://www.healthcare.gov or call 800-318-2596 to check your eligibility and compare your options. (Lower- to middle-income families may qualify for tax credits, lower deductibles, or subsidies.) You must enroll during the open enrollment period, from November 15 through February 15. If you find out you're pregnant after this time, you can't obtain insurance through an exchange for that year.
- **Medicaid or the Children's Health Insurance Program (CHIP) for low-income families:** You can apply at any time by visiting http://www.healthcare.gov. *Note:* Because Medicaid doesn't reimburse providers as fully as private insurance companies do, many providers accept only a limited number of Medicaid clients.

Whether you're researching existing health insurance plans or choosing a new one, look at the detailed information about what care is covered and be sure you understand your deductibles and copays. Visit our website, http://www.PCNGuide.com, to download a work sheet that lists questions to research. If you don't understand your coverage, contact an insurance company representative for clarification.

Some insurance plans cover—but don't directly pay for—such services as midwifery care, childbirth classes, birth or postpartum doulas, home birth, and breastfeeding assistance. Instead, you pay for these services, and your insurance company reimburses you. Ask the service providers how to submit your request for reimbursement.

You may also use a flexible spending account (FSA) or health savings account (HSA). Both accounts allow you to set aside money before you pay taxes on it to use for qualified medical expenses.

When your baby is born, you can choose to add the baby to your existing health insurance, or you can apply for new insurance, even if it's outside the open enrollment period.

If you live in Canada, tax revenues pay for all citizens' health care, including maternity care (except for out-of-hospital birth or midwifery care in some provinces—check your province's regulations).

# Choosing a Birthplace

Ideally, the best place to give birth is somewhere you feel safe and comfortable. It should be somewhere you can get the help and expertise you want—not only for the birth but also during pregnancy and after the birth. That birthplace may be a hospital, a birth center, or your home.

If you can, choose your birthplace before selecting your caregiver. That way, you can select a caregiver who attends births at the place you've chosen. Since you'll begin prenatal care in early pregnancy, you may consider researching and choosing your birthplace and caregiver before conception or early in the first trimester.

## Birthing in a Hospital

Most women in the United States and Canada give birth in hospitals, and these institutions vary widely in the services they offer, their staff's attitudes toward patients, their intervention rates, and their philosophies of care. Knowing the philosophy, policies, and services of each hospital you're considering helps you choose wisely. Depending on your health-care coverage and where you live, you might or might not have a choice of hospitals. If you do, don't choose the one closest to your home just because of its location. Labor usually lasts for hours, so you'll generally have plenty of time to get to your hospital of choice. Try to learn about several hospitals, take their tours, and then choose the one that best suits your needs. If you don't have a choice of hospitals, you can at least learn what to expect when you give birth at the only available hospital.

When choosing a hospital, find out how it staffs the maternity department. Learn about its staffing policies for laboring women. Hospital administrators know the value of having continuous one-nurse-to-one-patient nursing care throughout labor, but most don't guarantee it. Because of nursing-staff shortages, many hospitals must also rely on nurses who work in several departments ("floating" nurses) and who might not have much experience in maternity nursing. Some hospitals hire temporary "traveling" nurses, who may be unfamiliar with the hospital's policies. Others use licensed practical nurses or nursing assistants, either of whom might have limited training and might not be legally allowed to perform some tasks.

### In Their Own Words

Perhaps because my first birth was at a teaching and research hospital, I felt my care was "by the book." My partner liked that the providers performed every test and asked every question for the health and safety of my baby and me.

I gave birth to my second baby at a different hospital, and from start to finish, my caregivers were experienced women, most of them mothers. I felt empowered by the calm, efficient way they took care of business. The time after the birth was more peaceful than it was for my first birth, with many fewer interruptions by staff.
—Anita

## Levels of Maternity Care

Hospitals and in-hospital birth centers vary in the services and treatment they provide mothers and babies. A birth facility's level of maternity care reflects the degree of risk for mother or baby that it's equipped to handle.

Levels of maternity care range from Level 1 (or "basic care") for uncomplicated pregnancies to Level 4 for the most complex pregnancies and critically ill pregnant people. The higher-level hospitals provide care from highly trained and experienced maternal-fetal medicine specialists, and their facilities have some or all of the following:[3]

- intensive care units for both mothers and babies
- 24-hour complete obstetrical and anesthesia services
- blood bank
- 24-hour laboratory services

If you have a difficult pregnancy or you or your baby is at risk for complications in labor, birth, or immediate postpartum, you may need to give birth in a Level 3 or 4 hospital. If your pregnancy is low risk, you can receive excellent care at a lower-level facility or an out-of-hospital birth center. Out-of-hospital birth centers are for women with very low-risk pregnancies who wish to avoid using pain medications. Care is provided by specialists in normal childbirth (usually midwives and occasionally physicians) with the ability to transfer to a higher-level hospital if necessary before or during labor.

Hospitals can't allow pregnant women to choose the staff member who administers pain medications. If you want or need epidural analgesia when laboring at the hospital, the anesthesia staff member who's on call administers it. This person may be a nurse anesthetist, an anesthesiologist, or a resident (physician-in-training). When considering a hospital, you can find out the credentials and experience of its anesthesia staff. You may also have a chance to meet with a staff member to discuss anesthesia services, especially if you have fears or a physical condition that may make anesthesia problematic.

Many hospitals provide individual birthing rooms, where women labor, give birth, and stay with their families until they're discharged—all in the same room. Other hospitals have separate postpartum rooms, where mothers and babies stay after the birth until they go home. Rooms usually have a TV, a chair-bed for the partner, and bathtubs to use during labor and afterward. Some hospitals' maternity rooms are designed to look like hotel rooms, with emergency equipment hidden in cupboards or a closet.

Some hospitals have received the World Health Organization's Baby-Friendly award, designating that the institution adheres to practices that best support and promote breastfeeding. Visit http://www .babyfriendlyusa.org for the locations of baby-friendly hospitals.

### Questions to Ask When Choosing a Hospital

To learn about a hospital's routines and policies, you can phone the hospital's labor and delivery ward or visit their website, take a hospital tour, or ask your caregiver during prenatal visits. Visit our website, http://www.PCNGuide.com, to download a list of questions to ask.

If you discover the hospital has a standard routine that you're uncomfortable with, ask your caregiver to write orders that override it, if possible. (See also chapter 8 for additional questions that may arise as you create your birth plan.)

### The Hospital Tour

For many expectant parents, seeing where they'll give birth helps boost confidence and reduce uneasiness. For this reason, most hospitals offer tours of their maternity departments. To learn details about a tour, visit the hospital's website or call the prenatal education department. Tours typically involve a visit to the triage area (see page 179), a birthing room, a postpartum room (if separate from the birthing room), and the family waiting area. Tours usually don't include the operating room where cesarean deliveries are performed. The tour guide discusses some usual routines and policies, gives practical advice (for example, which entrance to use in the middle of the night), and answers questions you may have.

# Birthing outside a Hospital

In some areas of the United States and Canada, women with low-risk pregnancies have the option of giving birth with highly qualified midwives in a *freestanding birth center* (unaffiliated with a hospital) or at home. A woman who chooses this option prefers to give birth in a relaxed, low-tech, and cozy environment. She desires the continuous personal care of her caregiver during pregnancy, birth, and the postpartum period. During labor, she wants the freedom to move and act as she wishes, surrounding herself only with people of her choosing and permitting only essential interventions.

For women who have low-risk pregnancies, good prenatal care, skilled caregivers, and hospital backup, planned out-of-hospital births are as safe for mothers and babies as planned hospital births—sometimes even safer.[4] Because planned out-of-hospital births are usually uncomplicated and normal, they require fewer routine interventions and less medical equipment. As a result, the cost of a birth-center birth or home birth is less than the cost of a hospital birth. Medicaid and many health insurance plans often cover the cost of out-of-hospital births. If a woman is transferred from a birth center or home to a hospital, however, insurance plans might not cover some costs resulting from the transfer.

You're a good candidate for out-of-hospital birth if you're physically and mentally healthy when you become pregnant and remain so throughout pregnancy. You also should have a well-trained, highly qualified midwife assess your and your baby's condition throughout pregnancy, screening for problems that make out-of-hospital birth unsafe. If a problem arises during pregnancy (such as high blood pressure, gestational diabetes, or slowed growth of the baby's body or brain), you and your midwife may decide to transfer your care to an obstetrician for the remainder of the pregnancy and plan to give birth in a hospital.

Even after careful screening, various reports have shown that at least 15 percent (one report showed 40 percent) of first-time mothers and 5 to 10 percent of second-time mothers are transferred to the hospital during labor or after the birth for problems that arise and are judged to require medical intervention.[5] Almost all transfers during labor (96 percent) are for nonemergencies, such as prolonged labor, meconium in the amniotic fluid, prolonged

## Common Q&A

Q: How do I know if I'm high-risk or low-risk?

A: A health-care provider can assess your situation with a complete medical history and exam. An example of a low-risk pregnancy may be someone who is in general good health without major medical problems or previous uterine surgery, is older than seventeen but younger than thirty-eight (older than thirty-eight may be considered low-risk if the person is otherwise in good health), is not obese, and is having an uncomplicated pregnancy with a single baby.

ruptured membranes, or desire for pain medication.[6] In these situations, procedures or medications aren't immediately necessary for the welfare of the baby or mother.

For 3 to 4 percent of home births, urgent transfers to the hospital are necessary during labor.[7] In these cases, the women were screened and had uncomplicated, normal pregnancies, but a condition arises during labor that requires immediate medical action, such as cord prolapse, hemorrhage, or concerns about the baby's heart rate and oxygen supply. After a home birth, a little more than 1 percent of mothers and a little less than 1 percent of babies require a transfer to the hospital for reasons such as bleeding in the mother, retained placenta, and respiratory problems in the baby.[8]

Qualified midwives are trained for emergencies such as these. Their immediate response is similar to the first response of medical personnel in hospitals. To handle emergencies, midwives carry oxygen tanks, IV fluids, and suctioning devices, as well as medications to stop contractions temporarily, to stop bleeding, and to lower blood pressure. When further medical care is needed, they arrange for quick transfer to the hospital.

Although emergency transfers to the hospital are rare, they can be frightening and stressful. If you're considering an out-of-hospital birth, take this possibility into account and consider how far away your home or birth center is from the hospital. (See chapter 14 for further discussion on problems that can arise during labor and how they're treated in hospital and out-of-hospital settings.) Visit our website, http://www.PCNGuide.com, to download a list of questions to ask your midwife about out-of-hospital birth.

# Choosing Your Caregiver

Since caregivers attend births only at specific birthplaces, choosing a caregiver goes hand-in-hand with choosing a birthplace. The best time to make these choices is before conceiving or in early pregnancy so you have lots of time to find the right birthplace and caregiver for you.

When you begin your search for a maternity caregiver, first ask yourself the following questions:

1. *What options do I have?* Learn what kinds of caregivers are available in your area, which ones your insurance covers, and which ones attend births at your chosen birthplace. Then, consult a trusted medical professional, local childbirth preparation group, or knowledgeable friend to further narrow your list.

2. *How does group care work? Who's in the group?* Most often when you choose a caregiver, you select a group of caregivers, not just one person. Your prenatal appointments may rotate among the group members, or you may see one or two caregivers throughout your pregnancy. The caregiver who attends your labor is the one on call at the time—and may be a stranger to you.

3. *What type of caregiver do I want? Does the gender of the caregiver matter to me? What approach to maternity care do I prefer?* The following sections provide further information to help you answer these questions.

## Types of Maternity Caregivers

Different types of providers care for women during pregnancy, birth, and after the birth. Some have extensive medical training, while others acquire much of their knowledge through hands-on training.

When choosing a caregiver, it's important to consider the state of your health. A healthy pregnant woman can safely choose among any of the following types of caregivers. If your pregnancy is complicated or if your caregiver anticipates problems in labor, your safest option is most likely an obstetrician or perinatologist, either as the sole caregiver or as a consultant with a family physician or midwife.

For any caregiver, find out the person's educational background, credentials, training, and experience. Also learn about the caregiver's backup and referral arrangements, in case you need to transfer to a specialist during pregnancy or labor.

## Physicians

*Obstetricians/gynecologists (OB-GYNs)* have graduated from medical school or a school of osteopathic medicine. They've had three or more years of additional training in obstetrics (a surgical subspecialty focused on pregnancy, birth, and the postpartum period) and gynecology (medical and surgical treatment of diseases of women). Much of their education focuses on detection and treatment of problems. To qualify for board certification, they must pass an exam administered by the American Congress of Obstetricians and Gynecologists. In the United States, obstetricians provide most maternity care (85 percent), and pregnant women in Canada commonly use their services (although many choose to use family physicians or midwives).

*Perinatologists* are OB-GYNs who have received further training and certification in managing very high-risk pregnancies and births. They often consult with other physicians and midwives or accept referrals from them. These specialists practice only in major full-service medical centers (Levels 3 and 4) in urban areas.

*Family physicians* have graduated from medical school or a school of osteopathic medicine and have completed two or more years of additional training in family medicine, including maternity and pediatric care. Their education focuses on the health-care needs of the entire family, so families may have a relationship with them before and after pregnancy. They refer to specialists if their patients develop complications. To qualify for board certification, they must pass an exam administered by the American Academy of Family Physicians.

## Midwives

Midwives are the typical maternity caregivers in most countries and are becoming increasingly popular in the United States and Canada. Their education and practice are based on the Midwifery Model of Care (see page 17), which focuses on the needs of healthy women during the childbearing year. When compared to obstetricians, midwives tend to spend more time in prenatal visits with their clients, individualizing their care; however, they refer clients to obstetricians if serious medical problems arise.

*Certified nurse-midwives (CNMs)* have graduated from nursing school, passed an exam to become registered nurses, and completed one or more years of additional training in midwifery. To become certified, CNMs must pass an exam administered by the American College of Nurse-Midwives. They deliver babies in homes, hospitals, and birth centers.

## Online Resources to Help You Make Informed Decisions

An online search for any birth-related topic will produce numerous results. The following reliable sources may help narrow your search:

- Learn more about your maternity care choices at http://www.childbirth connection.org.
- Find a birth center at http://www.birthcenters.org /birth-center-locator.
- Find an obstetrician at http://www.acog.org /About-ACOG/Find-an -Ob-Gyn.
- Learn more about family physicians at http:// familydoctor.org.
- Find a nurse-midwife at http://ourmomentof truth.com.
- Find a licensed midwife or certified professional midwife at http://www.mana.org /memberlist.html and http:// cfmidwifery.org/find.
- Find a childbirth educator at http://www.icea.org, http://www.lamaze.org, http://www.bradleybirth .com, or http://www.birthing fromwithin.com.
- Find a birth or postpartum doula at http://www.dona .org or http://www.doula match.net.

You may also search online for services in your area and visit the websites of local hospitals, birth centers, caregivers, doulas, and childbirth educators.

*Certified midwives (CMs)* have graduated from a health-related program other than nursing and must complete the same midwifery training and certification exams that CNMs do. They practice in the same settings as CNMs.

*Licensed midwives (LMs)* have completed up to three years of formal training. Their education is similar to that of CNMs, although a nursing background isn't required. To become licensed, LMs must attend a minimum number of births and pass an exam administered by their state licensing board. Twenty-eight states recognize LMs. Most LMs provide care for women planning births in homes or birth centers only.

*Certified professional midwives (CPMs)* have received training from a variety of sources, including apprenticeship, school, and self-study, and have been the primary attendant at twenty or more births. They practice outside hospitals, and their care is similar to that of LMs. CPMs must pass an exam administered by the North American Registry of Midwives. Many LMs are also CPMs.

## Other Caregivers

*Advanced practice nurse practitioners* provide prenatal and postpartum care, although they don't attend women during labor. They often work with a group of physicians or midwives.

*Naturopathic doctors (NDs)* have completed three or four years of postgraduate training in natural medicine; some take an additional year of midwifery training to be able to provide prenatal care and attend births.

*Lay or empirical midwives* have varied qualifications and standards of care—some are well trained and highly skilled; others aren't. Some are legally registered in their state or province, while others practice in states where no laws regulate their practice. Some object to certification or licensure and have chosen to practice outside the law.

## A CAREGIVER'S APPROACH TO MATERNITY CARE

Education, training, colleagues' attitudes, scientific reports, and personal experiences influence a caregiver's approach to pregnancy and birth. A caregiver's philosophy of care typically falls between the midwifery model and the medical model. Some physicians' practices closely resemble the midwifery model, and some midwives' practices lean more toward the medical model.

## Midwifery Model of Care

This model of care is based on these premises:

- Birth is a significant event in a family's life. Expectant parents need support with medical aspects of pregnancy, but also with emotional, spiritual, and physical well-being. Childbirth education is desirable because a woman's participation contributes to a healthy pregnancy, labor, and birth.
- The natural childbirth process is unpredictable but normally safe.
- A woman's state of mind influences the labor process, so individualized care is necessary.
- Caregivers monitor the mother's and baby's well-being and provide education and support. If problems arise, caregivers first use less risky and simpler interventions to restore a healthy physiological process. If unsuccessful, they try more complex and riskier interventions to solve the problem.
- Low intervention and cesarean rates are desirable.

## Medical Model of Care

This model of care is based on these premises:

- Pregnancy and birth are significant medical events. The caregiver's role is to offer wellness guidelines and to provide medical care to monitor for and treat any complications that arise. (They may encourage the family to seek emotional support from friends, other pregnant women, childbirth educators, or counselors.)
- The natural childbirth process is unpredictable and potentially unsafe.
- Routine care protocols are provided for all women and help caregivers offer reliable care.
- Caregivers use routine interventions before problems arise. If problems arise, they intervene quickly with the tool most likely to have the quickest effect.
- Medical interventions can improve labor and birth. Cesareans are no less safe for the mother or baby than natural labor and vaginal birth; in fact, they may be safer. (*Note:* Some expectant couples feel reassured with a caregiver who uses more interventions, although scientific research has shown that the routine use of technology and intervention isn't always safer for mothers and babies. In fact, this approach to maternity care sometimes causes side effects that lead to more medical problems. See chapter 14.)

# INTERVIEWING A POTENTIAL CAREGIVER

To some people, the idea of interviewing caregivers may seem daunting. They choose a caregiver or group practice based only on the recommendations of friends or another physician. Other people don't choose; they simply accept whomever is available in a particular group or clinic. However, your caregiver or group of caregivers largely determines which options you have, how you're treated during birth, how your baby is born, and how you feel about your body and your baby. An initial interview can help you decide whether a potential caregiver inspires your confidence and trust. You can learn whether a caregiver seems open and comfortable, responds thoughtfully to your questions, and is happy to provide additional explanation upon request. If a caregiver seems impatient and defensive during the interview, it's likely you'll see that behavior in your care.

When choosing a caregiver, find one who's qualified to provide the care that meets your health needs and whose approach to care appeals to you. A caregiver's or group's website can tell you their approach to pregnancy and birth. Some midwife or physician groups have open meet and greet sessions in which you can talk with the caregivers in person. Others are glad to schedule a private consultation.

Feel free to interview more than one caregiver, but schedule the appointments early. Appointments for many caregivers have long waiting periods. When scheduling an appointment, make it clear that it's only to learn more about the caregiver's practice.

## In Their Own Words

Because an interview typically lasts only ten to twenty minutes—and because most caregivers charge for office visits—prepare for it by visiting a caregiver's website or calling the office receptionist to learn about qualifications and experience, fees, backup care when off duty, and birthplaces. Also, read the questions on our website and become as knowledgeable about them as possible so you can better judge the caregiver's answers. That way, during the interview you can focus on three or four essential questions to help you decide whether the caregiver is a good fit for you.

If you're taking medications or have a medical or mental health problem, disclose that information to the caregiver during the interview. It may affect the care you're provided.

Visit our website, http://www.PCNGuide.com, to download a list of questions to ask and a work sheet to record the caregiver's responses at the interview.

## CHANGING CAREGIVERS IF YOU'RE DISSATISFIED WITH YOUR CARE

To have a satisfying birth experience, it's essential that you can trust your caregiver's recommendations and believe that your caregiver listens to you and cares about your well-being.

But what if you *don't* feel comfortable with your caregiver? Here are three ways to handle the situation:

1. Express your discomfort and explain what will make you feel more at ease, but do so calmly and without using accusatory language.

   For example: "Dr. Jones, this is hard for me to say, but I get the impression that my questions are an inconvenience to you."

   By using the pronoun *I* often, you communicate that *you* are the one experiencing a problem with the relationship. You're not directly criticizing your caregiver's behavior by saying something such as: "Dr. Jones, you're always in a rush, and you don't let me ask any questions. You don't even care about your patients." Such language will likely make your caregiver defensive and less willing to improve your relationship.

   Expressing yourself with direct but respectful language may evoke an effort to work together as equals and may improve communication. If you anticipate this conversation to be challenging, practice what you want to say ahead of time with your partner or a friend.

2. If the above approach doesn't work, consider changing caregivers. Although it's always uncomfortable to change caregivers, doing so may be better than staying with someone who makes you feel uneasy.

   Don't drop your caregiver until you've found someone who better suits you and who has agreed to become your caregiver. If your original caregiver is in a group practice, try to select a new caregiver who's not in that group. (By choosing another caregiver in the same group, you risk having your original caregiver attend you in labor.)

3. If you can't change caregivers and you can't discuss your feelings with your caregiver, consider talking with the office nurse, a childbirth educator, a doula, or others to help you cope with the relationship. Try to work with your caregiver the best you can by asserting your position reasonably and calmly. For example, you may say something such as: "I realize you don't agree with some of my choices, but I've learned that they're not unreasonable, and many caregivers allow them. Please work with me." If your caregiver continues to push for options that go against your wishes, remember that you have the right to refuse unacceptable care practices. It's unlikely you'll need to take this step, but in case you do, having the support of family, friends, and other advocates will be essential.

# Choosing Childbirth Classes

Many hospitals, colleges and universities, nonprofit community organizations, groups of caregivers, and independent childbirth educators offer childbirth classes. The programs vary in size, philosophy, cost, topics covered, and number of classes in the series. The background and training of the instructors vary (they may be registered nurses, physical therapists, teachers, psychologists, social workers, college graduates, or others), as does the quality of the classes.

Colleges and universities, community groups, and independent educators usually sponsor consumer-oriented classes, which prepare parents to take responsibility in decision making and self-care. Classes sponsored by a hospital or caregiver group are likely to be provider-oriented classes, which inform parents about the type of care provided by a hospital or caregiver group, but avoid discussion of reasonable alternatives or controversial topics in maternity care. Some classes, of course, offer a mix of consumer-oriented and provider-oriented information.

Visit the websites of organizations and institutions offering childbirth classes in your area. If possible, compare your options to determine which class best suits your needs. Visit our website, http://www.PCNGuide.com, to find a list questions you can ask to learn more about class options.

Childbirth classes on DVD or online cost less than traditional childbirth classes, and you can watch them whenever you have time and whenever you need to review topics.

But in key ways, these classes can't offer many of the features of in-person classes. They can't address local practices and incorporate up-to-date research data. They rarely provide opportunities to ask the instructor questions or to get feedback and personal advice on specific concerns or on comfort measures that aren't working for you. Lastly, they can't provide an opportunity for developing new friendships with other expectant parents.

## Different Views on Childbirth Classes

After the birth, new parents were asked to comment on how well childbirth classes prepared them for birth. Although there were many different views, the responses shared the following sentiments:

- *Childbirth classes prepared us for what to expect and do at each stage of labor and delivery. They took a lot of the "shock value" out of the process.*
- *The classes gave us a better understanding of the big picture of birth. Although the class was well taught and formatted, we discovered that some things can be learned only from experience.*
- *The class gave me confidence and a sense of security. I didn't feel scared or unsure. It gave me the chance to clarify my preferences before I went into labor.*

# All about Birth Doulas

*Birth doulas* assist families before, during, and after the birth. (Postpartum doulas help new families adjust to early parenthood; see page 23 for more information.) Trained and experienced in childbirth, birth doulas give continuous personalized care during the often-stressful and always-changing labor process. They neither perform medical tasks nor give medical advice. Instead, they provide services that are unavailable in most modern birth settings, including emotional support (such as reassurance, stress reduction, and guidance), physical comfort, and help getting needed information for decision making. Their intention is to foster both parents' well-being, self-confidence, and sense of being respected—all of which lead to positive long-term memories of birth experiences.

Numerous studies have examined the effectiveness of doula care. As of 2013, twenty-two randomized con-trolled trials from sixteen countries have been conducted and included more than fifteen thousand women. The trials compared outcomes of births in which women didn't receive continuous support ("usual care") with those in which women received continuous or nearly continuous support by a nurse, loved one, or doula.[9] All the stud-ies showed benefits from continuous support by others, especially when the support began in early labor and was given by a doula, whose only role was to provide continuous support. Support by nurses didn't achieve the same level of benefits, probably because they had many other clinical duties beyond labor support. And although the support of a loved one improved the woman's satisfaction with the birth, it didn't improve outcomes. Here are some benefits of doula support:

- shorter labors, with less need for medication to speed up labor
- more spontaneous vaginal births (births that don't require forceps, vacuum extraction, or cesarean delivery)
- fewer requests for pain medications
- less dissatisfaction with birth experiences
- fewer babies with low Apgar scores at five minutes of age

Consider hiring a birth doula if you want an additional support person with you throughout your labor and birth. In addition to bolstering your and your partner's confidence and well-being, a birth doula can guide your partner through the comfort measures to help make you more comfortable. See page 220 for more information about doulas.

## Finding a Birth Doula

To find birth doulas in your area, ask your friends, childbirth educator, or caregiver for recommendations. You can also search online (see page 15). Try to consult with several doulas by phone or e-mail to help you decide which ones you want to interview in person.

During the interview, ask the questions listed on our website, http://www.PCNGuide.com. Pay attention not only to *what* the doulas say, but also *how* they say it. Their behavior and body language will help you decide which one is a good fit for you.

Most doulas charge a fee for their services, although some doulas-in-training charge a small fee (if any) and some experienced doulas may waive or reduce their fees for clients with tight finances. A few hospitals provide doula services at low cost or no cost to the patient, and some charitable agencies or public health departments cover doulas' fees for women who can't afford the services. Given doulas' contributions to improved outcomes in maternity care, their services make financial sense; however, health insurance plans rarely cover doula services.

# Your Baby's Health Care

Your adjustment to new parenthood will be easier if you make some decisions about your baby's health care well before the birth. (See chapter 8 for more information on developing a postpartum plan.)

While you're pregnant, you can research early health-care choices, such as immediate parent-infant contact, first bath, car seats, infant feeding, circumcision, vaccinations, and more. By learning about these options before the birth, you'll be able to make informed decisions when the time comes. You can include your preferences for some of these options in your birth plan.

Learning about the types of health care available for your newborn during pregnancy gives you time to arrange for the best available care.

## Choosing a Caregiver for Your Baby

By choosing your baby's caregiver before the birth, you'll have someone to call whenever you're concerned about your newborn's health, from the moment she's born. You can also find out the schedule of well-baby checkups ahead of time.

Several types of caregivers provide health care for infants. *Pediatricians* specialize in infants' and children's health care. They've graduated from medical school and completed a pediatric residency. Their offices and waiting rooms are geared for children.

*Family physicians* provide care for the entire family. They've spent several months in pediatrics during medical school and as part of their residency training. They diagnose and treat most illnesses, but refer seriously ill children to pediatricians. If a family physician provides your care before, during, and after pregnancy, it may be a comfortable decision to extend the care to your baby.

*Pediatric and family nurse practitioners* are registered nurses who have additional training in pediatrics or family health. They provide well-child care and treat common illnesses. They usually work with a group of physicians and refer serious problems to a physician.

*Naturopathic doctors (NDs)* and other alternative practitioners provide well-child care and emphasize nonmedical or complementary treatments of illness. Their education varies but may consist of four years' training after college. Most care for the entire family. They don't have hospital privileges and refer seriously ill children to physicians.

## HEALTH-CARE COVERAGE FOR YOUR BABY

The cost of your baby's health care depends on your health insurance coverage (see page 10) and where your baby visits a caregiver. In most cases, your baby will see a caregiver for well-child visits, during which the caregiver checks your baby's growth, development, and overall health, and gives vaccinations. If you have a choice of health insurance plans, compare coverage of well-child visits. Some plans don't pay for well-child visits but cover nearly all expenses to care for an ill child.

Some caregivers practice out of private offices; others practice in clinics. Private-practice care is more expensive than clinic care, but it may be more personalized and convenient. Many health insurance plans provide a list of approved caregivers.

Children's health clinics usually cost less than private practices, but they may have longer waiting times. If the clinic is associated with a medical school, its staff may change frequently. Its caregivers are physicians or nurse practitioners who are rotating through their advanced training under the supervision of fully trained professionals. Other community-based children's clinics offer low-cost care and a consistent staff (which means you see the same caregiver at each visit). Such clinics usually also provide social services and other services to low-income families. Community health clinics or well-child clinics associated with a public health department offer free or low-cost checkups and vaccinations, but they usually don't provide care for sick children.

## FINDING A CAREGIVER FOR YOUR BABY

After choosing a type of caregiver for your baby and the setting, focus on choosing a caregiver that suits your needs. A helpful way to start your search is to ask your maternity caregiver, childbirth educator, local hospital, and family and friends to recommend pediatric caregivers. Visit these caregivers' websites or call their offices to learn information about their practices (such as their locations and office hours).

If possible before the birth, schedule an interview with one or more caregivers. Check your health insurance plan to determine whether it covers such appointments. If it doesn't, find out whether the caregiver charges a fee for the appointment, and if so, the amount.

During the interview, time may be limited, so make sure you ask the questions you most want answered. (Visit our website, http://www.PCNGuide.com, for a list of questions to ask.) Pay attention to *how* a caregiver answers your questions. Does the caregiver seem competent, caring, and considerate? Does the caregiver's style and philosophy match yours? It's important that the person who will care for your baby's health has your confidence and trust.

# Finding Help after Your Baby's Birth

For the first several weeks after the birth, you and your partner may be surprised by how time consuming baby care is, leaving you few free moments for meal preparation, basic housework, sleep, and socializing (see chapter 16). During this period, it's desirable to arrange for someone (or more than one person) to help you as you adjust to life with a newborn.

## Who Can Help You?

Family members and friends often want to help make life a little easier for the new parents. Some have a lot of time and energy to cook meals, run errands, do laundry, clean the house, walk the dog, or watch the baby. Others are able to help with just an occasional meal or service Use the key words *meal train* to search online for systems that can help you coordinate offers of help and set up sign-up sheets. The systems can be tailored to your needs, including meal preferences, chores and errands, good times to bring meals, and so on.

If family and friends don't live near you or have little time or ability to help, or relationships are strained, others can provide much-needed help. Baby nurses or nannies can take care of your baby, allowing you to do other activities. Mother's helpers cook and clean, but they don't help with baby care or give advice.

Consider the help of a *postpartum doula*, who's trained to help new parents adjust to postpartum life by teaching them about newborns' needs and abilities, feeding, sleep, and cues. A postpartum doula helps with household chores and meal preparation and focuses especially on enhancing new parents' confidence and competence and fostering their bond with their baby. As one new mother said, "It's kind of like having your favorite aunt who raised many children helping you learn the ropes of new parenthood."

Postpartum doulas and other helpers typically charge by the hour, and the potential costs may seem daunting to expectant parents. Many parents find that the help and care are well worth the price, especially years later when recalling those first few days and weeks with their newborns. The cost might be forgotten, but the doula's services are remembered clearly and positively.

To pay for these services, put money aside during pregnancy. Or if friends and relatives ask how they can help you, suggest they contribute money for this purpose or request the money as a shower gift.

## Finding a Postpartum Doula

If you decide you want a postpartum doula, try to hire one before the birth. You may have trouble finding a doula who suits your needs if you wait until after the birth to start your search. Ask your friends, childbirth educator, or caregiver for recommendations. You can also search online. Try to consult with several doulas by phone or e-mail to help you decide which ones you want to interview in person.

During the interview, ask the questions listed on our website, http://www.PCNGuide.com. Pay attention not only to *what* the doulas say, but also *how* they say it. Their behavior and body language will help you decide which one is a good fit for you.

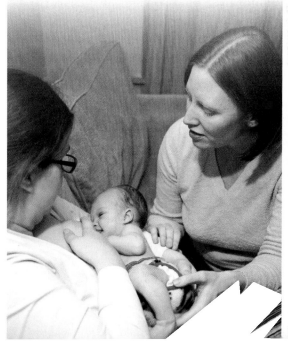

# RETURNING TO WORK

Typically before the birth, families make plans about the return to work after the baby is born. Parents may choose to work because it's essential for the family's financial well-being or for career development, or because they love their jobs. Some two-parent families may choose to have one parent return to work, letting the other parent stay at home full-time to care for the baby.

To explore the options that will work best for your family, look at the list of questions on our website, http://www.PCNGuide.com.

After you've made the best choice for you and your family, make sure you and your partner support each other to accommodate the change. Whether you stay home with your baby or work outside the home, life is more challenging with a baby—it's helpful to have an ally!

You'll also plan your parental leave before the birth. In the United States, the duration of parental-leave policies are generally short, and parents must return to work earlier than do parents in Canada and other countries. If possible, try to wait three to four months before returning to work. That way, you'll have time to recover and focus on your baby. Some couples take their parental leaves one after the other to have a longer period of time at home with the baby.

# FINDING CHILD CARE

If you (and your partner) will be returning to work or school, your first priority is finding affordable, safe, dependable child care. The best time to arrange for child care is well before the birth, but that might not be possible. When you start your search, allow at least a month to find child care that best suits your needs.

If you don't want a stranger caring for your baby, consider asking family members or friends. Or think about staggering your and your partner's work schedules so you each can provide at least some child care. In some work settings, it may be possible for you to bring your baby to work and care for him during the workday. (Some companies even offer on-site child care.)

If you decide to have someone care for your child outside your home, first visit http://families.naeyc.org and http://www.childcareaware.org for advice on evaluating child-care providers. These sites also offer directories and referrals. Your options will include licensed child-care facilities, in-home child care, or other providers, such as nannies. Ask coworkers, friends, or other working parents about their child-care arrangements to learn what works for other families. Research your options online. You'll probably be able to find online reviews of larger child-care centers but not of small in-home providers.

Visit potential child-care facilities and homes and bring a list of questions, such as these: What do you do when a baby becomes ill? How do you support breastfeeding mothers? How will you feel about my visiting when I can? What are your hours of operation and holiday schedules? (You can find additional questions to ask on the websites listed above.) Ask to see child-care licenses to ensure they're current. Pay attention to how the providers respond to you (and your baby). How do they behave with babies in their care? With gentleness and kindness or with impatience and detachment? Trust your instincts about the home or facility.

If you decide to hire a nanny or other in-home provider, interview candidates in your home. Ask the same questions you'd ask at a child-care facility. Also ask candidates how they plan to cover their duties should they become ill or go on vacation. See whether you can share a candidate's services (and the costs) with another family. Pay attention to how candidates interact with your baby and you, and trust your instincts on what you observe. Request references and contact them.

After you've chosen suitable child care, remember that you're establishing a partnership with the child-care workers. Always treat them with respect. Offer compliments and acknowledge their valuable service by giving appropriate holiday gifts.

If at any point you feel that a child-care arrangement is no longer right for your baby, find another provider so you can be assured your baby is receiving the best care.

# Ten Steps to Improve Your Chances of Having a Safe and Satisfying Birth

1. Take care of yourself during pregnancy so you begin labor in the best possible health. Exercise in moderation and eat well. (See chapters 5 and 6.) Seek prenatal care to help you detect and manage any health problems that may arise.

2. Choose a birthplace that has a low rate of cesarean birth and minimal routine interventions. (Ask the questions on our website.) If your pregnancy is low risk, consider birthing at a birth center or at home. Several studies show that women having low-risk pregnancies undergo fewer interventions in an out-of-hospital setting, and their birth outcomes are just as good as those in hospitals.[10]

3. Find a caregiver who has low intervention rates and encourages the use of self-help techniques in labor (see chapters 12). If your pregnancy is low risk, consider using a midwife (if available). Midwives typically use fewer medical interventions than physicians do. If your pregnancy is high risk because either you or your baby has a medical problem, seek the services of an appropriate specialist and learn about necessary precautions.

4. Educate yourself and prepare a birth plan (see chapter 8). Take childbirth classes that emphasize informed decision making and self-help methods to relieve pain and aid progress. Visit http://www.childbirthconnection .org to read "The Rights of Childbearing Women," which outlines a set of basic maternity rights for all childbearing women. Keep these rights in mind as you create and review your birth plan with your caregiver.[11]

5. Hire a birth doula. The continuous labor support a doula provides often leads to shorter labor, reduced need for pain medication, increased chance of normal vaginal birth, and increased satisfaction with the birth experience.[12]

6. Avoid labor induction for nonmedical reasons. If your caregiver suggests induction for reasons not clearly supported by evidence (such as a suspected big baby), ask about other alternatives (see page 280).

7. Use medical interventions only when clearly necessary, not just because they're routine. For example, avoid routine IV fluids, continuous electronic monitoring, and augmentation with Pitocin or artificial rupture of membranes (see chapter 14). In some situations, interventions may be the best option. Ask questions to ensure that you make informed decisions. That way, when you remember the birth in the years to come, you'll know you made the right choices.

8. Learn to differentiate between early labor and active labor so you can delay hospital admission until active labor (see page 177). Use labor-coping skills at home to manage pain and aid progress (see chapter 12). Eat, drink, and rest as needed to keep up your energy.

9. Use a variety of positions and activities during active labor, such as walking, dancing, rocking in a rocking chair or on a birth ball, or taking a shower or bath (see page 226).

10. Push in positions that aid descent, unless the birth is happening fast; then use positions that slow descent (see page 238). Use spontaneous pushing if you have an urge to push. Delay pushing if you don't have an urge to push (and you and baby are doing fine).

# *Key Points to Remember*

- As an expectant parent, it's your responsibility and legal right to become informed about the available options in maternity care and to communicate your preferences to your caregivers.
- To help you make informed decisions, ask key questions and consult with your caregiver and other knowledgeable medical professionals. After considering the information you've learned and weighing it against your values and concerns, you can make the best decisions.
- During pregnancy, the choices you make can help make your experiences of labor, birth, and postpartum positive and satisfying. The following choices are key to a positive experience:
  - where you want to give birth
  - who will provide your maternity care
  - what childbirth classes to take
  - whether you want a birth doula and postpartum support
  - who will provide health care for your baby
  - what child-care arrangements will best suit your needs if you return to work after the birth

# CHAPTER 3

# Common Changes and Concerns in Pregnancy

Pregnancy brings about profound physical changes in you, dynamic growth and development in your baby, and emotional adjustments for you and your partner. It's an amazing and exciting time, yet you may find yourself wondering and worrying how your pregnancy is affecting you and your baby. You may try to imagine what your baby looks like in your womb. You may be unsure how you'll react to the many changes ahead. Learning what to expect during a normal and healthy pregnancy may help put your feelings and worries into perspective and let you enjoy your pregnancy.

# Your Body's Preparation for Pregnancy

Since roughly the time you reached puberty, your body has naturally been preparing for pregnancy. The design of your body's reproductive system makes pregnancy possible.

Your reproductive anatomy includes both internal and external structures. The labia, urethra, clitoris, and vaginal opening are your external genitals, shown below. These body parts plus your anus are your *perineum*. Many pairs of muscles attached to your pelvis support the perineum and form a strong sling with openings for your urethra, vagina, and anus. These are your *pelvic floor muscles*.

The drawing on page 31 shows your internal reproductive organs. Your *uterus* (or womb) is a hollow, muscular organ the size and shape of a pear, and your *vagina* is a stretchy tube-shaped canal. The lower part of your uterus, which protrudes into your vagina, is your *cervix*. Your *fallopian tubes* provide the paths for an egg (*ovum*) to travel from your *ovaries* (sex glands) to your uterus.

Your ovaries produce the female sex hormones estrogen and progesterone (see page 34). After puberty, your ovaries undergo a cycle of changes every month (give or take a few days), unless you're pregnant. During a cycle, an egg matures in one ovary and causes increased secretion of estrogen, which along with progesterone stimulates growth of the uterine lining (endometrium). Usually only one egg ripens each cycle and is released into one of your fallopian tubes. This process is called *ovulation,* and it usually occurs about halfway through your cycle, but it can occur earlier or later. As the fine hairs in your fallopian tube propel the egg slowly toward your uterus, your ovary produces more progesterone, which stimulates the uterine lining to become a rich, nourishing home for a fertilized egg. If fertilization doesn't occur (which means you're not pregnant), your estrogen and progesterone levels diminish, and your uterus sheds its unneeded lining. This shedding process is called menstruation.

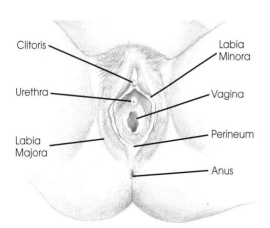

Clitoris

Urethra

Labia Majora

Labia Minora

Vagina

Perineum

Anus

Ovary

Uterus

Cervix

Bladder

Vagina

# Conceiving Your Baby

*Conception* occurs (and you become pregnant) when a sperm fertilizes (penetrates) your egg.

When a man has an orgasm, he ejaculates about 1 teaspoon of semen, which contains 150 million to 400 million sperm. If ejaculation occurs during sexual intercourse, these sperm travel from your vagina into your uterus and out to your fallopian tubes. Sperm can live inside you for up to three days, while your egg is viable for only twelve to twenty-four hours after ovulation. Conception usually happens in the part of the fallopian tube farthest from the uterus when a single sperm *fertilizes* the awaiting egg.

Occasionally, ovaries release more than one egg, and a separate sperm fertilizes each one, resulting in fraternal (nonidentical) twins, triplets, quadruplets, or higher-order multiples. Sometimes, a single fertilized egg divides into two and produces identical twins. For information on pregnancy with multiples, see page 49.

Conception
(sperm & ovum)

## Common Q & A

**Q:** If my partner and I have trouble conceiving, what can we do?

**A:** Difficulty conceiving a child can be frustrating. Visit our website, http://www.PCNGuide .com, for ways you both can improve your health before conceiving and ways to enhance fertility. If you've been trying for more than a year, you may want to consult an infertility expert who can look for possible complications with ovulation or a low sperm count. If a problem is discovered, you may choose to use assisted reproductive technology (ART). To learn more about ART, visit http://www.cdc.gov/ART or http://www.marchofdimes.com /pnhec/173_14308.asp.

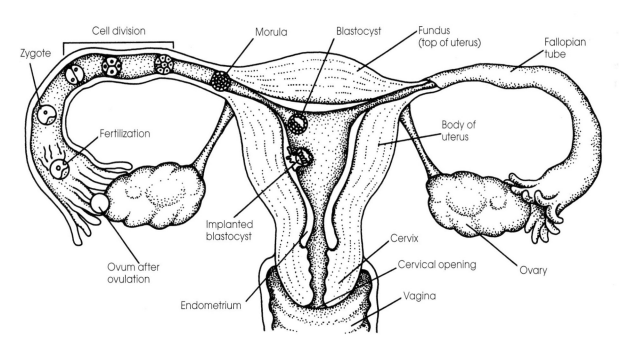

Zygote — Cell division — Morula — Blastocyst — Fundus (top of uterus) — Fallopian tube — Fertilization — Body of uterus — Implanted blastocyst — Cervix — Ovum after ovulation — Cervical opening — Ovary — Vagina — Endometrium

# Now That You're Pregnant

When you suspect that you're pregnant, you may experience some or all of the early signs of pregnancy, which are caused by hormonal changes that begin almost immediately after conception. Here are symptoms that you may notice:

- breast changes: fullness, tenderness, tingling in the nipple area, and a darkened *areola* (the area around each nipple)
- missed menstrual period
- fullness, bloating, or ache in your lower abdomen
- fatigue and drowsiness
- feeling lightheaded or faint
- nausea or vomiting at any time of the day ("morning sickness")
- frequent urination
- increased vaginal secretions

## CONFIRMING YOUR PREGNANCY

If you don't experience the above physical symptoms, you might not suspect you're pregnant until you've missed a menstrual period, at which time you may take a home pregnancy test. These do-it-yourself kits check your urine for a hormone that's produced only during pregnancy. Available in most drugstores and discount stores, they usually provide supplies for two tests. Taking one test after missing a period and another a few days later is more accurate than taking only one test.

To confirm your pregnancy, you can make an appointment for a blood test with a medical professional. If you're pregnant, you may be given basic information to help ensure a healthy pregnancy, such as taking folic acid supplements, until you have your first prenatal appointment and can learn more about prenatal health. Even before starting your prenatal visits, it's wise to begin adopting a healthy lifestyle and eating a well-balanced diet (see chapters 4, 5, and 6).

## CALCULATING YOUR DUE DATE

Pregnancy (or *gestation*) lasts an average of 280 days or forty weeks after the first day of your last menstrual period. Although conception occurs within twelve to twenty-four hours of ovulation, it's difficult to know exactly when ovulation occurred. For many women, ovulation happens about two weeks after the first day of their last period, but it can occur earlier or later in the cycle. This uncertainty makes it difficult to know exactly when someone becomes pregnant, especially if sexual intercourse has been frequent and conception can't be traced back to a particular day.

For these reasons, caregivers calculate the *due date* by using this simple formula: Subtract three months from the date of the first day of your last period (a date you can confirm), then add seven days. For example, let's say the first day of your last period was February 1. Subtracting three months from that day leads to November 1, and then adding seven days gives you a due date of November 8. Most caregivers also suggest an optional ultrasound scan in early pregnancy to help estimate your due date (see page 65).

Keep in mind that a due date is just an estimate of when your baby will be born. Generally, babies are born healthy and normal any time from three weeks before to two weeks after their due dates. In fact, most babies are born within ten days of their due dates, and only about 5 percent are born on their due dates.

If a due date is just a guess, why is it important? A due date is the basis for many assessments and decisions that help your caregiver do the following:

- determine when best to do genetic testing
- recognize whether results of specific lab tests are within the normal range
- diagnose a preterm or postdate pregnancy
- identify a baby who's growing more slowly or rapidly than normal

Because normal pregnancies vary in length, your caregiver will look at a range of normal test results when making these assessments.

# HORMONAL CHANGES DURING PREGNANCY

Changes in hormone production cause many of the physical and emotional changes in pregnancy, helping ensure a healthy pregnancy and the optimal development of your baby. The placenta is the major source of these hormones (see page 36). Here's how the various hormones affect you and your pregnancy:

- *Human chorionic gonadotropin (hCG)* is a hormone produced only during pregnancy. (Pregnancy tests check for hCG in your blood or urine.) This hormone ensures that your ovaries produce estrogen and progesterone for the first two to three months of your pregnancy until your placenta matures and produces the appropriate amount.
- *Estrogen* promotes the growth of your uterine muscles and their blood supply, encourages production of vaginal mucus, and stimulates the development of the ductal system and blood supply in your breasts. Changes in water retention, body fat buildup, and skin pigmentation are related to estrogen levels. In late pregnancy, rising estrogen levels increase the uterus's sensitivity to oxytocin and help start labor.
- *Progesterone* relaxes your uterus during pregnancy, keeping it from contracting too much. It also relaxes the walls of blood vessels (helping you maintain a healthy blood pressure) and the walls of your stomach and bowels (allowing for greater absorption of nutrients and sometimes causing constipation). In late pregnancy, progesterone has less effect on your uterus, letting contractions increase and start labor.
- *Relaxin* from your ovaries relaxes and softens your ligaments, cartilage, and cervix, making these tissues more stretchable during pregnancy and letting your pelvic joints spread during birth.
- *Prostaglandins*, produced in your amniotic membrane, increase in level during late pregnancy. Prostaglandins soften and ripen your cervix in preparation for labor and stimulate muscles in your uterus and bowels.
- *Corticotropin-releasing hormone (CRH)* comes from your baby, placenta, and tissues within your uterus. Increased levels of CRH in late pregnancy change the ratio of estrogen to progesterone.
- *Oxytocin*, produced in your pituitary gland, stimulates uterine contractions to help trigger the onset of labor and promote labor progress. Often referred to as the "love hormone," oxytocin is present during an orgasm. It's also responsible for the urge to push at the end of labor and for the let-down reflex during breastfeeding. Oxytocin improves mood and produces feelings of calmness and well-being.[1]

Pregnancy also produces greater quantities of many hormones that are present when you're not pregnant. These increased hormone levels cause other physical changes and influence your metabolism, mineral balance, tissue and organ growth, levels of still other hormones, and the onset of labor.

# YOUR PREGNANCY WEEK TO WEEK

In the next sections, we provide a comprehensive overview of pregnancy as it progresses from week to week. If you'd like weekly updates with details on your baby's development, subscribe to an e-mail newsletter that covers the subject. We recommend Lamaze International's newsletter, http://www.lamaze.org/YourPregnancy WeekByWeek, or Baby Center http://www.babycenter.com/pregnancy. The March of Dimes, http://www.march ofdimes.com, is also an excellent resource on pregnancy and a baby's development.

# First Trimester Changes for You and Your Baby

Pregnancy is divided into three *trimesters*, each one lasting about three months. The first trimester is the "formation" period, because by the end of it, all your baby's organ systems are formed and functioning. For you, the first trimester is a time of physical and emotional adjustment to being pregnant.

## THE FIRST FOUR WEEKS OF PREGNANCY

This time marks conception through the first two weeks of your baby's life (four weeks *gestational age*).

### Changes in Your Baby

At conception, your baby gets inherited characteristics from you and her father. Every normal human cell contains forty-six chromosomes of genetic material; an egg and sperm each contains half that number. When a sperm fertilizes an egg, the resulting twenty-three pairs of chromosomes combine to form a unique genetic blueprint for development. This blueprint decides at conception your baby's sex, blood type, eye and hair color, nose and ear shape, and some personality traits and mental capabilities. To a great extent, this blueprint also guides your baby's growth and development throughout her life.

Throughout pregnancy, the terms used to describe a baby change to reflect age and development. After conception, the fertilized egg quickly divides from one cell into two, then four, eight, sixteen, and so on until it becomes a multicellular structure called a *blastocyst*. Within five to nine days, the blastocyst has made its way along the fallopian tube and implants in the uterine lining, usually in the upper part of the uterus. By two weeks, the baby is called an *embryo*, and another part of the fertilized egg is developing into the placenta. This primitive placenta has tiny rootlike projections that penetrate the uterine lining and acquire nutrients for the developing embryo.

Blastocyst 6 days        23-day Embryo        28-day Embryo

### Changes in You

While these changes are taking place in your baby, you may have noticed only some breast tenderness or a slight ache in your belly. But you're about to miss your menstrual period, and the remarkable changes that you'll experience have just begun!

# THE 5TH THROUGH 14TH WEEKS OF PREGNANCY

This time marks the third through twelfth weeks of your baby's life (five to fourteen weeks gestational age).

## Changes in Your Baby

During the first few weeks of this trimester, your baby is an embryo that's developing rapidly. His nervous system and circulatory system are forming, and his heart is beating by the twenty-fifth day after conception. Your baby has simple kidneys, a liver, a digestive tract, and a developing umbilical cord. When he's only half the size of a pea, arm and leg buds appear, and his face begins to form.

Although your baby's sex is determined at conception, male and female babies appear the same until nine weeks. Then, if the embryo is male, he begins producing *androgens*, male hormones that signal the development of the scrotum and penis. If female, her external genitals and internal reproductive organs form.

By eight weeks after conception (ten weeks gestational age), your baby is structurally complete. His mouth has lips, a tongue, and teeth buds in his gums. His arms have hands with fingers and fingerprints. His legs have knees, ankles, and toes. His arms and legs move at this time, but coordinated movements don't begin until about fourteen weeks. His developing brain begins to send out impulses. His heart is beating strongly and can be seen during an ultrasound scan. Your baby grows 1 millimeter a day. When he's nine weeks old (eleven weeks gestational age), he's called a fetus.

During the first three months, your baby becomes quite active, although you're probably unaware of any movements. Legs kick and arms move. Your baby can suck his thumb, swallow amniotic fluid, and urinate drops of sterile urine into the amniotic fluid, which is completely exchanged about every three hours. Your baby makes

38-day Embryo    56-day Embryo    10-week Fetus

breathing movements (that is, his chest rises and falls); "breathing" amniotic fluid into his lungs appears to help with lung development. By ten to twelve weeks (twelve to fourteen weeks gestational age), your baby's eyelids cover his eyes, but his eyes remain closed until the sixth month.

## Development of the Placenta and Changes in the Uterus

During the early weeks of pregnancy, your uterine lining becomes thicker and provides a rich source of nourishment for your growing baby. At the end of the first month of development, projections (chorionic villi) extend into your uterine lining, becoming a primitive placenta. Your baby's blood circulates through the chorionic villi, while your blood circulates into the spaces surrounding them (intervillous spaces). A thin membrane separates the two bloodstreams, which normally don't mix.

The *membranes* (amnion and chorion) create the *amniotic sac* that surrounds your baby. The *amniotic fluid* protects your baby by absorbing bumps from the outside, maintaining an even temperature, and providing a medium for easy movement.

By twelve weeks of pregnancy, the *placenta* is completely formed and serves as an organ for producing hormones and exchanging nutrients and waste products. Most identical twins share the same placenta. Fraternal twins have separate placentas, though the placentas sometimes fuse into one.

The *umbilical cord* links the placenta to your baby's navel, and together the umbilical cord and placenta pass oxygen and nutrients from you to your baby. While the placenta provides a barrier against most (but not all) bacteria in your bloodstream, most viruses and drugs cross to your baby. The placenta also exchanges waste products from your baby, which your blood then carries to your kidneys and lungs for excretion.

By fourteen weeks of pregnancy, your uterus has grown to just above your pubic bone. The cervix is about 4 centimeters long and, though softer than before pregnancy, still fairly firm. The *mucous plug* that fills the cervical opening provides a barrier to help protect your baby.

## Changes in You

By five weeks (possibly earlier) from the first day of your last menstrual period, a pregnancy test should show a positive result. During the first trimester, you may feel unusually tired and need more sleep because of your changing metabolic rate and your increased energy needs while growing a baby. You may urinate more often as your enlarging uterus presses on your bladder. Many expectant parents experience nausea and vomiting during the early months of pregnancy (see page 113). Although usually called *morning sickness*, this symptom of pregnancy may occur at any time of the day. While the cause of morning sickness is unknown, it's thought that hormones produced by the developing placenta play a role.

Although your breasts develop in puberty, your milk glands don't fully develop until pregnancy. As hormone levels increase, your breasts change in preparation of providing milk for your baby. Your breasts enlarge, your veins appear bigger, and your nipples may be tender or have a tingling sensation. Your nipples and areolae also enlarge and become darker. Little bumps on your areolae (called *Montgomery glands*) enlarge to produce more lubricant in preparation for breastfeeding.

Although these early pregnancy changes *feel* dramatic to you, you might not *look* much different to others or to yourself.

## Your Emotions

Finding out that you're pregnant may bring about many emotions for both you and your partner. You may be proud that you conceived a child, worried about miscarriage, hesitant to focus on the baby if awaiting genetic testing results, afraid of losing your independence, fretful about changes in your relationship, doubtful of your ability to parent, and happy about becoming parents. You may cry easily or react strongly to minor inconveniences. Your mood swings seem more pronounced, which may be difficult for you and your partner to understand. Talking with your partner and sharing your thoughts and feelings can help you work through this transition together.

## Different Views on the First Trimester

Expectant parents were asked, "What emotional changes did you notice in the first trimester?" Although there were many different views, the responses shared the following sentiments:

- *I found myself crying at silly things.*
- *I was so worried all the time. I obsessively searched online for details about my baby's health.*
- *Physically, I didn't feel great. But emotionally? It feels really good to be pregnant.*

# Calendar of Pregnancy: First Trimester

| Gestational age | Six weeks | Ten weeks | Fourteen weeks |
|---|---|---|---|
| Changes in baby | About 0.1 inch long | About 1 inch long | About 3 inches long |
| | Brain and spinal column begin to form | Face is forming with simple eyes, ears, nose, mouth, and teeth buds | Weighs about 1 ounce |
| | Beginning development of gastrointestinal system, heart, and lungs | Arms and legs begin to move | Can move arms, legs, fingers, and toes |
| | Amniotic sac envelops the preliminary tissues of entire body | Fingerprints are present | Can smile, frown, suck, and swallow |
| | Is called a blastocyst from five days to two weeks, then called an embryo | Brain is forming | Sex is distinguishable |
| | | Fetal heartbeats can be seen on ultrasound scan | Bone cells begin to appear |
| | | External genitals begin to appear | Can urinate |
| | | Is called an embryo | Heartbeat can be heard with ultrasound stethoscope |
| | | | Vocal cords complete |
| | | | Is called a fetus |
| Changes in placenta and uterus | Uterus is enlarging | Uterus is size of tennis ball | Uterus is size of grapefruit and reaches just above pubic bone |
| | Uterine lining is thick, with increased blood supply | Umbilical cord has definite shape | Amniotic fluid fills uterine cavity and is continually replaced |
| | Placenta and umbilical cord are forming | Amniotic fluid cushions fetus, maintains even temperature, and allows easy movement | Placenta is small but complete, with full exchange of nutrients and waste products |
| | Human chorionic gonadotropin (hCG) is present in mother's blood and urine | | Placenta is major source of estrogen and progesterone |

**First trimester changes** (You may experience some or all of these.)

| | | | |
|---|---|---|---|
| Common physical changes in mother | No menstrual periods | Frequent urination | Fullness, bloating, or ache in pelvis or lower abdomen |
| | Breast changes: fullness, tenderness, tingling of nipples, darkened areolae | Constipation | Aversions to some foods and odors |
| | Nausea and vomiting (morning sickness) | Metallic taste | Fatigue and sleepiness |
| | Increased salivation | Feeling faint or lightheaded | Increased vaginal secretions |
| | Weight loss or gain up to 5 pounds | | |
| Common emotional changes in mother | Mood swings | Increased worries about everything | Greater interest in meaning of motherhood |
| Common emotions of father or partner | Difficulty acknowledging pregnancy | May gain weight and experience nausea as an empathetic response to her pregnancy | Difficulty seeing baby as real until proof by ultrasound scan or audible heartbeat |
| Common changes for both parents | Mixed feelings about pregnancy: happy, excited, relieved, surprised, proud, anxious, scared, and/or nervous | Examination of feelings toward own parents and their parenting techniques | Concern about mood swings and fatigue |
| | Determining parenting roles and family values | Changes in sexual relationship | Concerns about finances |
| | Fear that sexual intercourse harms baby | Concern for baby's well-being | |

# Second Trimester Changes for You and Your Baby

The second trimester is the "development" period, because your baby's organs and structures begin to enlarge and mature. For you, this trimester is a time of feeling well, energetic, creative, and emotionally sensitive.

## THE 15TH THROUGH 27TH WEEKS OF PREGNANCY

This time marks the thirteenth through the twenty-fifth weeks of your baby's life (fifteen through twenty-seven weeks gestational age).

### Changes in Your Baby

27-week Fetus

In this trimester, your baby starts to grow hair, eyelashes, and eyebrows. Fine, downy hair (called *lanugo*) develops on her arms, legs, and back. Fingernails and toenails appear. At eighteen weeks of pregnancy, your baby can do all the movements you'll see her do as a newborn.

Forming in your baby's intestines is *meconium*, a collection of digestive enzymes and residue from swallowed amniotic fluid. After birth, your baby will expel the meconium, which will appear as thick, sticky, greenish-black poop in her diaper. Her skin is wrinkled and covered with a creamy protective coating called *vernix caseosa*. During this trimester, you'll probably feel your baby move for the first time (an experience called *quickening*). You may feel a light tapping or fluttering sensation that reminds you of gas bubbles. Or you might not notice your baby's gentle movements. Although still very immature, some babies born near the end of this trimester (twenty-five weeks gestational age) survive.

### Changes in the Placenta and Uterus

Your uterus expands into your abdominal cavity to accommodate your growing baby, placenta, and level of amniotic fluid. During prenatal appointments, your caregiver measures the height of your uterus to check that your baby is growing adequately. Although a baby's size and the amount of amniotic fluid differ among pregnancies, the length of your pregnancy in weeks approximates the distance in centimeters between your pubic bone and the top of your uterus (called the *fundus*). For example, at twenty-five weeks, fundal height is about 25 centimeters.

During this trimester, your uterus normally contracts periodically, although you might not notice it. Called *Braxton-Hicks contractions*, they make your uterus feel hard or tight for about a minute but aren't painful. Different from labor contractions, Braxton-Hicks contractions don't cause changes in your cervix. If contractions do cause your cervix to change and it begins to open, you're in preterm (or premature) labor and require medical attention (see page 129).

## Different Views on the Second Trimester

Expectant parents were asked, "What emotional changes did you notice in the second trimester?" Although there were many different views, the responses shared the following sentiments:

- *I love feeling the baby move, but it's weird having a separate person inside me.*
- *Pregnancy is hard because I have no control over my emotions.*
- *I'm looking forward to having the baby, but I like being pregnant. I'll miss it.*
- *I haven't exactly "glowed" like my friends, but pregnancy has been a lot easier since I stopped having morning sickness.*

## Changes in You

During these middle months of pregnancy, you probably feel physically well, and your nausea and fatigue likely have disappeared or diminished. The milk glands in your breasts begin making small amounts of *colostrum* (a highly nutritious yellowish fluid produced before breast milk) by midpregnancy.

Just as hormonal changes make your nipples and areolae darker, they also make other skin areas more pigmented. A dark line (called "linea nigra") may appear between your pubic bone and navel. The skin around your eyes may darken, especially after sun exposure. This "mask of pregnancy" (called "chloasma") usually disappears within a few weeks after your baby's birth.

## Your Emotions

Along with these physical changes, you may experience a wide range of emotions. You may enjoy how your pregnant body looks and feels, or your growing body may make you feel unattractive, inconvenienced, and restricted. Heightened emotions may bolster your creativity and make you respond strongly and with more sensitivity to a kind word, a beautiful sunset, or a touching photo. Pregnancy may affect your sleep, and you may recall more of your dreams than you did before becoming pregnant. You also may become introspective and find yourself easily distracted by a need to examine your thoughts and feelings.

During this trimester, your swelling belly usually becomes more obvious, and your pregnancy becomes real and exciting for your partner, family, and friends. Now they can feel the baby wiggle or kick. Being able to see evidence of the growing baby, your partner typically feels more involved in your pregnancy and more interested in your baby. Like you, your partner may have a range of thoughts and feelings about your changing appearance and about becoming a parent (see pages 49–53).

Share your feelings and thoughts with your partner often, and make sure to listen when your partner shares feelings and thoughts with you. You need each other's support, now and in the months and years to come, as you adapt to parenthood. This trimester is a good time to start preparing for parenthood by reading books on parenting and newborn care, visiting websites about babies, or buying baby clothes and equipment (see page 153).

## Calendar of Pregnancy: Second Trimester

| Gestational age | Nineteen weeks | Twenty-three weeks | Twenty-seven weeks |
|---|---|---|---|
| Changes in baby | About 5–6 inches long | About 10–12 inches long (6–8 inches crown to rump) | About 11–14 inches long (9–10 inches crown to rump) |
| | Weighs about 4 ounces | Weighs ½–1 pound | Weighs 1–2 pounds |
| | Heartbeat is strong | Heartbeat is audible with ordinary stethoscope | Skin is wrinkled and covered with protective coating (vernix caseosa) |
| | Skin is thin, transparent | Hiccups | Eyes are open |
| | Downy hair (lanugo) covers body | Hair, eyelashes, eyebrows are present | Begins to hear |
| | Fingernails and toenails are forming | | Meconium is collecting in bowel |
| | Has coordinated movements; is able to roll over | | Has strong grip |
| Changes in placenta and uterus | Uterus is 3 inches above pubic bone | Uterus is at level of navel | Uterus is above level of navel |
| | Placenta performs nutritional, respiratory, excretory, and most hormonal functions for fetus | About 2–3 pints of amniotic fluid | Placenta covers less of inner surface of uterus as uterus grows |
| | Amniotic fluid volume increases | Placenta is fully developed and covers about half the inner surface of uterus | Uterus contracts periodically (Braxton-Hicks contractions), which might not be noticeable |

**Second trimester changes** (You may experience some or all of these.)

| | | | |
|---|---|---|---|
| Common physical changes in mother | Sense of well-being; increased energy | Less tenderness in breasts | Noticing movement of baby |
| | Nasal congestion | Increased appetite | Bleeding gums or nosebleeds |
| | Disappearance of nausea | Relaxation of pelvic joints | Constipation |
| | Groin pain from round-ligament contractions | Food cravings or nonfood cravings (pica) | Leg cramps |
| | Skin changes: linea nigra, mask of pregnancy (chloasma) | Weight gain averaging 0.8–1.0 pound per week | |
| Common emotional changes in mother | Feeling more dependent on others | Developing sense of growth and creativity | Introspective; have trouble concentrating |
| | Varying feelings about changing appearance | More daydreaming and dreaming at night | Increased interest in babies |
| Common emotions of father or partner | Feelings of closeness to the baby | Greater involvement in pregnancy | Evaluating readiness and ability to be a parent |
| | Varying feelings about partner's changing appearance | | |
| Common changes for both parents | Changes in sexual desire and activity | Increasing interest in and awareness of parenting styles | More enjoyment of pregnancy |
| | Eager to be prepared for baby's arrival | | |

# Third Trimester Changes for You and Your Baby

The third trimester is the "growth" period, because your baby is growing into the size and shape of a newborn. A baby born during this time usually survives, although his chances for an easy transition to life outside the womb improve the closer his birth date is to his due date. (For more information on prematurity, see pages 274–275.)

As your body continues to expand to accommodate your growing baby, you may start looking forward to the end of pregnancy and its physical discomforts and to the long-awaited joy of holding your newborn in your arms.

## THE 28TH THROUGH 38TH WEEKS OF PREGNANCY

This time marks the twenty-sixth through thirty-sixth weeks of your baby's life (twenty-eight through thirty-eight weeks gestational age).

### Changes in Your Baby

In late pregnancy, your baby's lungs mature, and your antibodies pass through the placenta to her, providing some short-term protection from the diseases to which you're immune.

Your baby's fingernails reach her fingertips and may even need to be cut at birth. The hair on her head grows, the lanugo on her body almost disappears, and fat is deposited under her skin. Buds for her permanent teeth appear behind her primary (baby) teeth buds.

Your baby has periods of sleep and wakefulness. She may move in response to bright light and loud noises. She hears and becomes familiar with your voice and your partner's voice and with other sounds, such as the placental circulation, your gurgling stomach, your heartbeat, and external sounds (for example, music or barking dogs). After birth, your baby will show a clear preference for a familiar voice by turning her head toward the speaker. In addition, sounds that mimic the placental sounds heard in the womb (such as the rhythmic sloshing of water in a dishwasher, the droning of a vacuum cleaner or a fan, or shushing sounds) often soothe a fussy newborn.

As your baby continues to grow and gain weight, she has less room to move around, and you may feel just her arms and legs move rather than her whole body. When your baby has hiccups, you feel a series of rhythmic jolts. At some point during the last trimester, your baby assumes a favorite position—usually head down. During prenatal visits, your caregiver determines the baby's position by feeling your abdomen using a technique called *Leopold's maneuvers*.

### Changes in the Placenta and Uterus

At this point in your pregnancy, changes to the system connecting you to your baby help prepare you to give birth and breastfeed. The changes also help prepare your baby for birth (see page 163). Your cervix softens, your uterus

Placenta

Umbilical cord

Baby

Uterus

Bag of waters (membranes)

Cervix

becomes more sensitive to oxytocin, and you notice more contractions. The volume of amniotic fluid decreases, from about 1½ quarts at seven months to about 1 quart around your due date.

## Changes in You

In this trimester, your uterus expands, possibly causing shortness of breath or sore lower ribs. High levels of progesterone and pressure from your uterus may cause indigestion, heartburn, varicose veins in your legs, hemorrhoids,

or swollen ankles. You may have more backaches as your pelvic ligaments relax for birth, and your heavy uterus and growing baby change your center of gravity. (See chapter 12 for ways to prevent and treat back pain.)

Small red bumps (called "vascular spiders") may appear on the skin of your upper body, along with stretch marks (striae gravidarum) on your abdomen, thighs, or breasts. These marks are reddish during pregnancy and become glistening white lines after birth. Some people attempt to prevent stretch marks by using various lotions or oils, but no evidence shows that these products effectively work.

About two weeks before the birth, your baby "drops" into your pelvic cavity. This descent is called *engagement* or *lightening*. You may feel less pressure on your diaphragm and find breathing and eating easier. The tradeoff is, however, as the baby's head presses on your bladder, you need to urinate more frequently. Some expectant parents notice that colostrum leaks from their breasts, but some don't. Either case is normal.

## Your Emotions

In the final trimester, you may think and worry more about labor, birth, and your baby. Talk to your caregiver about your thoughts and fears and take childbirth classes. Talking to other mothers about birth can be informative and reassuring; however, some of their stories may increase your fears. The same reasoning applies to surfing the Internet for information. Be aware of sources and try to avoid scare stories and alarmist websites. Aim to balance the points of view so you're accurately informed and not unduly upset.

At this point, you may feel tired most of the time. You may get more sleep if you lean on a big body pillow or use many pillows. You also may welcome a relaxing warm bath or a soothing massage. As your belly grows and you become less agile, you may depend more on your partner and others. Your sexual relationship also may require some adjustments, due to your physical limitations (see pages 49–50).

## Having Fun with Your Baby before Birth (after Thirty-Two Weeks of Pregnancy)

- Sing songs to your baby, play him your favorite music, or read the same children's book or poem aloud every day. He'll recognize it at birth.
- Talk to your baby. Have your partner "speak" to your belly. Your baby is learning to recognize your voices and may respond when he hears them.
- Press on your belly when you feel your baby's hand or foot push against your uterus. See if he responds to your touch. Try pressing twice (like double-clicking a mouse) and see if your baby mimics your action.
- Shine a flashlight on your belly. See if your baby responds to the light.

As you anticipate the responsibilities of parenthood, you may begin thinking more about how your own parents raised you. You may want to follow some of your parents' techniques to raise your child, but you may want to avoid others.

You and your partner may worry about your health or your baby's well-being, especially if you develop a condition that makes your pregnancy high risk. Know that a healthy lifestyle and early, consistent prenatal care can greatly diminish many of these conditions. If you find yourself worrying excessively or dreaming about death or harm to you or your baby, share these fears with your partner, your caregiver, a childbirth educator, a relative, or an empathetic friend. Talking about your fears doesn't make them more likely to happen. Instead, sharing your concerns with a supportive person can comfort you and help you put your fears into perspective.

## THE 39TH AND 40TH WEEKS OF PREGNANCY

This time marks the thirty-seventh and thirty-eighth weeks of your baby's life (thirty-nine and forty weeks gestational age).

### Changes in Your Baby

In this last phase of pregnancy, your baby's organs continue to mature in preparation for life outside your uterus. He also adds fat and gains about 1 pound. A newborn averages 20 inches in length, but a range of 18 to 22 inches is normal. At birth, a baby typically weighs 7 to 7½ pounds, although a normal weight for a full-term baby can vary from 5½ to 10 pounds. From the time your baby was just a fertilized egg, his weight has increased six billion times!

### Changes in the Placenta and Uterus

Depending on the size and weight of the baby, the size of the placenta varies. Once you expel the placenta after the birth, it appears round, flat, and about 1 inch thick. The side that was implanted in your uterine wall is divided into lobes and appears rough and bloody. The side that was near your baby is smooth, pale, and shiny and is covered by the amniotic membrane. The membranes (amniotic and chorionic) extending from the edge of the placenta formed the sac (bag of waters) that contained the amniotic fluid and your baby.

Cross section of placenta

Maternal side
Cotyledons

Umbilical cord
Fetal side

The moist, white umbilical cord contains two arteries and one vein. Often twisted like a corkscrew, the umbilical cord measures 12 to 39 inches when pulled straight. At birth, when your baby breathes, her circulation pattern begins to change. Blood flow through her umbilical cord shuts down and more blood flows to her lungs.

Toward the end of pregnancy, prelabor uterine contractions become more obvious and frequent. These contractions enhance circulation in your uterus, press your baby against your cervix, and work with prostaglandins to soften and thin your cervix.

## Changes in You

At this point, you may be looking forward to the end of pregnancy. You may be fed up with the light sleep, fatigue, and other typical discomforts of late pregnancy. At times, you may feel as though you'll be pregnant forever! Visits to your caregiver, childbirth classes, baby showers, nursery preparation, and other common late-pregnancy activities should help you realize that your baby is coming soon, and a new stage in your life will begin.

## BEYOND YOUR DUE DATE

This time marks the thirty-ninth week (and beyond) of your baby's life in the womb (at least forty-one weeks gestational age).

Although the average length of pregnancy is forty weeks, many pregnancies last longer and are considered *post-date*. Some post-date pregnancies are cases of mistaken due dates; however, routine ultrasound dating is making such cases less common. Other post-date pregnancies involve babies who need more time to grow and mature. Occasionally, the baby is ready to be born, but for unexplained reasons, labor doesn't begin.

After the due date, some caregivers recommend that pregnancy should continue until labor begins on its own, assuming that the mother and baby are doing well (see the next section). Some caregivers, however, follow recent recommendations from the American Congress of Obstetricians and Gynecologists and advise induction for all pregnant people at the forty-first week.[2]

### Different Views on the Third Trimester

Expectant mothers were asked, "What emotional changes did you notice in the third trimester?" Although there were many different views, the responses shared the following sentiments:

- *I'm falling in love with this little person. When she kicks, she reminds me she's there. She calms down when I play music for her.*
- *I'm more sensitive now, a little paranoid and worried—and these feelings are new and strange to me.*
- *I have trouble getting to sleep even though I'm exhausted. I just can't get comfortable in bed; sometimes I need to sleep in the recliner.*
- *I feel special carrying a new life that's a combination of my partner and me.*

## Changes in Your Baby and in the Placenta

The majority of post-date babies are doing well. They just need extra time to grow and prepare for life outside the womb. In most post-date pregnancies, the placenta continues to function well, supporting the growth and well-being of the baby.

After your due date, your caregiver determines whether your baby and the placenta are healthy by performing specific diagnostic tests (see chapter 7). If all is well, pregnancy can continue.

In rare cases, however, tests reveal that the post-date placenta is not functioning well, that the volume of amniotic fluid is dropping, and the baby is showing signs of distress. Past forty-two weeks gestation, 20 percent of babies have *post-maturity syndrome*.[3] They'll show symptoms such as no lanugo, scant vernix caseosa, long fingernails, and peeling or cracked skin. Under these circumstances, the baby's health can't wait for labor to begin on its own, and the caregiver either induces labor or performs a cesarean delivery.

## Changes in You and Your Emotions

Physically, you may continue feeling much as you did during late pregnancy. Emotionally, however, you may find waiting for labor to begin frustrating, worrisome, or depressing. Consider trying self-induction methods that may encourage labor to begin, such as sexual intercourse, nipple stimulation, or acupressure (see pages 280–281).

## Calendar of Pregnancy: Third Trimester

| Gestational age | Thirty-one weeks | Thirty-five weeks | Thirty-eight to forty-two weeks |
|---|---|---|---|
| Changes in baby | 14-17 inches long (11-12 inches crown to rump)<br>Weighs 2½-4 pounds<br>Is adding body fat<br>Is very active<br>Breathing movements are present<br>Responds to sound | 16½-18 inches long (12-13 inches crown to rump)<br>Weighs 4-6 pounds<br>Has periods of sleep and wakefulness<br>May assume birth position<br>Bones of head are soft and flexible<br>Stores iron in liver | 19-21 inches long (13-15 inches crown to rump)<br>Weighs 6-8 pounds<br>More body fat and skin is less wrinkled<br>Lanugo is mostly gone<br>Vernix caseosa is thick<br>Lungs are mature<br>Is rapidly gaining antibodies from mother<br>In birth position<br>May descend or "drop" into pelvis (engagement) |
| Changes in placenta and uterus | Uterus is three finger-breadths above navel | Uterus is just below breastbone and ribs<br>Uterine contractions (Braxton-Hicks) are more frequent | Placenta is 6-8 inches in diameter, 1 inch thick, and about 1 pound<br>More frequent uterine contractions<br>Cervix is softening (ripening) and thinning (effacing)<br>Amniotic fluid volume is decreasing |

**Third trimester changes** (You may notice some or all of these.)

| | | | |
|---|---|---|---|
| Common physical changes in mother | Heartburn or indigestion<br>Anemia<br>Light sleep or insomnia<br>Tingling or numbness in hands<br>Varicose veins<br>Increased colostrum | Backache<br>Changes in balance and agility<br>Urinary urgency and frequency (not painful urination)<br>Hemorrhoids<br>Increased perspiration and feeling warmer | Shortness of breath<br>Soreness in lower ribs<br>Vascular spiders<br>Stretch marks; abdominal itching<br>Swollen ankles<br>Total weight gain of 25-35 pounds |
| Common emotional changes in mother | Excitement and doubts about readiness for baby<br>Decreased sexual interest<br>Feelings of clumsiness<br>Difficulty in focusing attention | Increased dependency on others; desire for protection<br>Variety of feelings about body changes<br>Relief that pregnancy is almost over | Focus on labor and birth, fear of childbirth pain, anxiety about the unknown<br>Increased attention from family and friends may be enjoyable at times, tiresome at others |
| Common emotions of father or partner | Protectiveness toward family<br>Frustration about inability to "fix" partner's discomforts | Longing for relationship to return to normal<br>Fear for health of mother and baby during childbirth | Anticipation of parenthood<br>Worries when something is wrong<br>Anxiety over support role in labor |
| Common changes for both parents | Continuing changes in sexual relationship<br>Worries about labor pain and responsibilities of parenthood<br>Eagerness for pregnancy to end | Choosing names for the baby<br>Excitement about baby's arrival<br>Emotional and mental preparation for birth | Fear of harm to baby during sexual activity<br>Simultaneous feelings of anticipation, exhilaration, excitement, and apprehension |

# Common Concerns and Considerations in Pregnancy

The following are typical concerns of expectant parents. Some apply only to women in specific situations. Others are of concern to all.

## AGE OF THE MOTHER

In general, expectant parents between the ages of eighteen and thirty-five have few problems in pregnancy. Girls in their early teens and people over age forty may face more pregnancy risks; however, a healthy pregnant woman of any age is likely to have a healthy baby.

### *Teenage Pregnancy*

If you're a pregnant teenager, you have several strengths and some special needs. A teenager's body is usually fit, and your chances of a healthy pregnancy are good. Because you're young, your uterus is probably strong and your tissues are stretchy. Your labor will likely progress normally and won't need medical interventions.

Because your body is still developing, you must eat well during pregnancy to properly nourish you and your growing baby. Just like every pregnant person, you need to stay away from drugs, alcohol, and tobacco. Make sure you keep your scheduled prenatal appointments with your caregiver. Taking these steps helps prevent giving birth too early and delivering a baby with low birth weight—the main problems for teen pregnancies.

Some challenges of being a pregnant teenager can include the following:

- dealing with your parents' reactions to your pregnancy
- working with your baby's father to address his role and responsibilities
- attending school with peers who can't relate to your situation
- deciding whether to keep your baby or consider adoption
- making decisions about your health care

You can work through these challenges by talking with a school counselor, a city or county health nurse, someone at a pregnancy counseling organization or the YWCA, or understanding friends and family members.

### *Pregnancy after Age Thirty-Five*

More than ever before, people in their thirties and forties are giving birth. In 1980 about 4 percent of all births were to women thirty-five and older. In 2013 that number increased to 15 percent, and of those women, 22 percent gave birth for the first time. As an older person, you may have delayed pregnancy for various reasons, such as career or education priorities, financial considerations, infertility, or lack of a partner.

## Advice from the Authors

Pregnant teenagers have unique needs and may require resources geared toward them. Here are some great books on teenage pregnancy:

- *Life Interrupted: The Scoop on Being a Young Mom* by Tricia Goyer (2004). Practical help on juggling school and single parenthood.
- *Your Pregnancy & Newborn Journey: A Guide for Pregnant Teens* by Jeanne Warren Lindsay and Jean Brunelli (2004). Easy-to-read guide on pregnancy.
- *The Unplanned Pregnancy Book for Teens and College Students* by Dorrie Williams-Wheeler (2004). Stories by young women, helpful resources, and useful strategies.

Despite common perceptions that pregnancy after thirty-five is risky, your "advanced" age doesn't guarantee a high-risk pregnancy. If you've taken care of your health over the years, you may well have a smooth pregnancy and an easy birth.

However, when compared to a younger pregnant woman, your risk of having problems is higher: These problems include high blood pressure, gestational diabetes, growth problems or inherited disorders in the baby, preterm labor, problems with the placenta, fibroids, labor complications, and cesarean birth. It's wise to be aware of these problems and take the effort to prevent and monitor for them.

Why are you at greater risk of having these problems? The answer is simple: The longer a woman lives, the more likely poor health practices, accidents, illnesses, or environmental hazards have affected her body. Also, high blood pressure and diabetes (the two most common risks for older expectant parents) are disorders that increase with one's age.

As you age, infertility problems increase. If you used fertility drugs or treatments to get pregnant, you may be pregnant with more than one baby. If this is the case, you'll experience many of the same pregnancy risks as anyone having multiples.

Your risk of problems in pregnancy varies depending on the number of children you've borne. In one study, researchers found that first-time mothers (primiparas) who were older had increased risks of preterm labor, excessive bleeding, or cesarean birth. But pregnant mothers who had birthed before (multiparas) and were older had increased risks of diabetes and chronic or gestational hypertension.[4]

Older adults are more likely than younger people to be pregnant with a baby with a genetic disorder, such as Down syndrome. Another potential risk factor is the age of the baby's father. The risk of some genetic disorders also increases for babies whose fathers are older than thirty-five at conception.

Various screening and diagnostic tests offered in early pregnancy can detect these conditions (see pages 63 and 139). Caregivers typically recommend these tests for all women over age thirty-five.

As an older pregnant woman, your age and experiences may affect your attitude toward pregnancy. If you have a history of infertility or miscarriage, you may feel vulnerable. You may seek reassurance that your baby is normal and healthy by undergoing numerous tests and procedures designed to detect and treat problems. Be aware that some expectant parents find the testing process stressful, especially because the tests don't always give clear results and thus lead to more testing (see chapter 7).

If you're thirty-five or older, what can you do to improve your chances for a healthy pregnancy and baby? You should do what any well-informed expectant parent does: Take good care of yourself, reduce stress, and have regular prenatal visits with a caring and competent caregiver. Although some problems may arise during your pregnancy, they're almost always treatable or manageable. In fact, most expectant parents over age thirty-five give birth to healthy, full-term babies.

## EXPECTING MULTIPLES: TWINS, TRIPLETS, OR MORE

Your caregiver may suspect a multiple pregnancy if two or more heartbeats are heard or if your uterus seems to be growing faster than normal. Often, expectant parents discover they're pregnant with *multiples* when an ultrasound reveals two or more babies. Twins account for just over 3 percent of all births. One-tenth of 1 percent of births results in triplets or more.

A person pregnant with more than one baby has an increased risk of preterm birth and thus premature babies. Prematurity causes most problems for multiples. Thankfully, improved medical care for women expecting multiples has helped decrease the risk of preterm birth of extremely small and immature babies.

If you're expecting multiples, you may be both excited and stressed out. Growing more than one baby requires more energy, so you'll probably need to consume more calories and rest more often because of discomfort, fatigue, and the increased risk of preterm labor.

Because birthing multiples is often more complicated than birthing one baby, the chance of cesarean birth rises with the number of babies you're expecting. You may need the care of an obstetrician or a perinatologist. In addition to the increased medical attention, you can also expect more attention from your friends and relatives during your pregnancy. Friends and family usually offer new parents more help in the weeks after the birth of multiples. Be sure to take advantage of any such offer! In addition to this book, we recommend that you read books and other materials specific to twin pregnancies, such as *Twins! Pregnancy, Birth and the First Year of Life,* second edition by Connie L. Agnew, Alan Klein, and Jill Alison Ganon.

## SEX DURING PREGNANCY

For most couples, pregnancy changes their sexual relationship, but how it changes isn't the same for every couple. While one pregnant person may feel clumsy and fat, another may feel ripe, beautiful, and sexual. One may feel sick and uncomfortable, while another feels radiant and wonderful. One may be alone or in a difficult or abusive relationship, while another may feel secure in a loving relationship. One person's partner may find the growing belly a turnoff, while another relishes it as gorgeous.

As your pregnancy progresses, you can expect your sex life to have its ups and downs. For some people in the first trimester, hormonal changes and increased blood flow to pelvic organs (plus, no worries about getting pregnant) increase a desire for sex. For others, experiencing symptoms such as nausea, vomiting, fatigue, and breast tenderness decrease libido.

During the second trimester, many notice a stronger libido and experience more sexual pleasure than in the other trimesters. At this stage of pregnancy, many experience fewer physical discomforts, have more energy, and may be enjoying their new curvy bodies.

## Fact or Fiction?

*A woman will conceive multiples only if twins run in her family or the family of the baby's father.*
**Fiction.** The likelihood of becoming pregnant with multiples is higher for a person with the following characteristics:

- is large and tall
- is older than thirty-five
- is Caucasian or African American (Multiples are less common in Asian and Hispanic families.)
- had at least one other pregnancy
- used fertility drugs that increase the number of eggs released during ovulation
- had more than one egg implanted during procedures such as in vitro fertilization

In the last trimester, many notice a decreased desire for sexual intercourse, likely because of their bigger bellies and increasing fatigue. If you share this feeling, it's helpful to remember that sex doesn't always mean sexual intercourse. There are other ways you and your partner can stimulate and pleasure each other. Use your imagination and explore new ways to be sensual.

How safe is sex during pregnancy? In general, it's safe; however, your caregiver may suggest that you avoid intercourse for the following high-risk reasons:

- You're at risk for preterm labor (or you're expecting multiples).
- Your partner has a sexually transmitted infection (STI).
- You have placenta previa (low-lying placenta).
- You have an incompetent cervix (one that opens early).
- You have vaginal bleeding during pregnancy (though spotting after intercourse in the first month of pregnancy might not be a complication).
- You have continuing or painful cramps after intercourse. (Having a few mild contractions after orgasm is normal and doesn't harm a healthy pregnancy or baby.)
- Your membranes have ruptured.

If you're not at risk, most caregivers recommend having sex as often as you desire. Remember that the sealed, fluid-filled amniotic sac cushions and protects your baby from outside forces and elements. If you experience discomfort during sexual intercourse, try positions that don't put your partner's weight on your belly (side-lying, hands-and-knees, or pregnant person on top) or try gentle, shallow penetration.

As your feelings about sex fluctuate throughout pregnancy, your partner might or might not understand or accept them, which can create tension in your relationship. To help prevent long-term problems, keep the lines of communication open. Working through these changes in your sexual relationship can help you prepare for future challenges in your sex life after the birth.

# A Note to Expectant Fathers*

Waiting for fatherhood is a unique emotional experience that's just as meaningful as waiting for motherhood. You may have never felt so important yet so ignored, so committed yet so abandoned, and so deeply in love and sexual yet so afraid of sex. Sharing these feelings with your pregnant partner or close friends may help you through this exciting but challenging time. Consider talking with other expectant fathers (casually or in a discussion group) to help you understand and develop your unique role during the pregnancy and birth, and as a parent.

\* These notes are also relevant to nonpregnant mothers-to-be and others close to the pregnant parent who will be sharing the parenting experience. See page 54 for further discussion on nontraditional families.

## The Reality of Your Baby

During the first trimester, it's difficult to see many physical changes in your pregnant partner, and you might not yet think of your baby as real. When your partner's pregnancy is around sixteen to twenty weeks along, however, changes in her body become obvious, and you may begin to feel your baby move inside her. You may even see the bulge of a foot or elbow on her abdomen. Like many expectant fathers, you may fully comprehend your baby's existence when you see her during an ultrasound scan and hear her heartbeat. Plan to be at the appointments when these exams are done.

Although some men emotionally connect with their babies during pregnancy, many men don't begin to attach to their babies until after the birth. Some fall in love upon first seeing their newborns, while others grow to love their babies more gradually over the first months.[5]

## Excitement, Stress, and Worries of Becoming a Father

On one hand, expecting a child may bring you pride and fulfillment because you're creating another generation of your family. On the other hand, you may worry about the health of your partner and baby. It's interesting that many men find life during pregnancy more stressful than life with a newborn. This may be because seeing a healthy mother and baby reduces anxiety and makes parenthood a reality.

If you have worries during the pregnancy, use them as motivation to improve the health of your growing family. You and your partner can eat nutritious foods, avoid potentially risky activities or exposure to illness, and improve your lifestyle.

With a new life soon to come, you may begin to reflect on your own mortality. You may decide to buy more life insurance and write or update your will. One expectant father began wearing a helmet when riding his motorcycle; another quit his job in high-rise construction to take one in a safer trade. These actions show an interest in being present for the baby and providing for him as much as possible.

During pregnancy, some men experience empathy symptoms, which mimic their partners' physical symptoms or discomforts. These include weight gain, food cravings, abdominal cramps or bloating, nausea, vomiting, backaches, toothaches, loss of appetite, and insomnia. If any physical changes or problems concern you, make an appointment with your caregiver for a checkup.

## Different Views of Expectant Fathers

Expectant fathers were asked, "How did you feel when the pregnancy test was positive?" Some one-word responses included *excited, relieved, happy, anxious, surprised,* and *proud.* Many men had mixed feelings:

- *When we found out we're going to have a baby, I felt terror and excitement.*
- *Though I'm excited, I worry about money.*
- *I'm happy, but I worry about losing my freedom.*

## Resources for Expectant Fathers

*Books*

- *The Birth Partner: A Complete Guide to Childbirth for Dads, Doulas, and All Other Labor Companions* by Penny Simkin (2013). Skillfully explains what's involved in the support role during late pregnancy, birth, and afterward.
- *The Expectant Father: Facts, Tips, and Advice for Dads-to-Be* by Armin A. Brott (2010). Information-packed guide to the emotional, financial, and physical changes the father-to-be may experience during the course of his partner's pregnancy.
- *Father's First Steps: 25 Things Every New Dad Should Know* by Robert W. Sears and James M. Sears (2006). Discusses labor support, new fatherhood, bonding with baby, understanding baby talk, and being a good partner and father.

*Classes*

Classes for dads-to-be focus on learning the basic skills of baby care and fatherhood. Look for Conscious Fathering classes, Boot Camp for New Dads, or another program in your area.

# INCREASED RESPONSIBILITY OF FATHERHOOD

When contemplating fatherhood, many men fear losing their freedom and independence; some feel they've already lost both. To these men, becoming a father means becoming a responsible, mature adult. For example, earning a steady or higher income may become a priority, especially if financial concerns arise. If the duties and responsibilities of impending parenthood overwhelm you, talk to your partner about your feelings. Together you may be able to create a plan for reducing expenses or increasing your income. You can also begin developing realistic expectations of your role as a parent and provider.

# CHANGES IN YOUR RELATIONSHIP

As your partner focuses on her pregnancy and becomes more preoccupied with your baby's arrival, you may feel left out at times. You may feel displaced if others focus more on her than you, and if she turns to friends and relatives instead of you for emotional support. You may feel that you're expected to care more for her and your relationship, but that she's less available to you emotionally, physically, and sexually. To further complicate matters, you may feel guilty for any resentment or lack of enthusiasm you have about the pregnancy. One way to deal with these emotions is to talk with a friend or relative who has felt the same way. It's also important to share these feelings with your partner; she may be unaware of them and able to help put your mind at ease.

If you'd like to strengthen your relationship before the baby's birth, check out pregnancy-related workshops for couples, such as the excellent Bringing Baby Home (https://www.gottman.com/about-the-bringing-baby-home-program). Or read books and other materials on the subject, such as *And Baby Makes Three: The Six-Step Plan for Preserving Marital Intimacy and Rekindling Romance after Baby Arrives* by John Gottman and Julie Schwartz Gottman.

# YOUR ROLE DURING LABOR AND BIRTH

All expectant fathers wonder how they'll perform during labor and birth. They may think, "Will I faint at the sight of blood? Can I handle watching my partner experience pain?" To boost your confidence and prepare for your role during this exciting event, take a childbirth class, watch DVDs or read books on childbirth, and discuss any worries you may have with other fathers and your partner. Also consider having a friend, relative, or doula at the birth to offer additional guidance and help you support your partner (see page 220).

# Your Role as a Father

As the birth of your baby approaches, you may wonder what kind of father you'll be. You may wonder whether you'll act as your own father acted when you were a child. You may have already decided that you want to be more emotionally and physically involved with your baby than your father was with you.

Research shows that certain hormone levels in expectant fathers change during pregnancy. Fathers-to-be have lower levels of testosterone and cortisol and higher levels of estradiol than men who aren't expecting babies. These hormonal changes may explain why many expectant fathers have more caring and nurturing feelings than they had before learning they're to become parents.[6]

The following suggestions may help you adjust to your new role:

- Learn about the normal development and behavior of newborns by reading books on the subject and attending your baby's well-baby checkups.
- Talk with other new fathers about what to realistically expect during the first weeks after the birth.
- After the birth, be prepared for changes in your daily activities. Consider your priorities and those of your family and create strategies to care for your baby, maintain your relationship with your partner, and find time for yourself.
- Determine how you can get the help that you and your partner will need after the birth.
- Think about how you can care for your new baby (such as holding, rocking, diapering, comforting, or playing with him) and learn more about those skills.
- Plan on having the most amazing adventure in the weeks and months ahead!

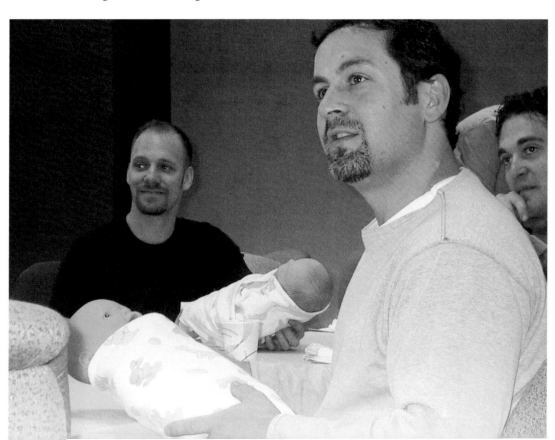

# Nontraditional Families

All kinds of relationships make up today's families. The traditional nuclear family (father, mother, and their biological offspring) is no longer the norm. Despite this fact, culture and customs have been slow to acknowledge the changing family structure, and society seems to offer little guidance and support to nontraditional families.

While parents in nontraditional families face many of the challenges that all parents face, they also may tackle puzzling or troubling situations. You can overcome them and build a strong and loving family, but it can require creativity, honesty, and support from others. See appendix C for a list of resources that offer nontraditional families support and advice.

## If You're Pregnant and Single

If you're pregnant and single, you face a different set of challenges. Although single parenthood is common today, society often offers single parents little support. For example, you may notice that not everyone reacts positively to your pregnancy.

As a single parent, you take on a role usually shared by two people. Parenting is hard work, and at times you may be relieved that you don't have to deal with the added burden of an incompatible partner. But there may be times when you doubt whether you can—or want to—parent alone. You may feel vulnerable or lonely and wish for the companionship and support of a reliable partner. At these times, it's best to reach out to others for help.

If your baby's biological father chooses not to be involved in your baby's life, you have options. You can agree to parent alone, with or without his financial help. Or you can take legal action to confirm his paternity and compel him to provide child support. If you choose this option, you need to create a plan that specifies his involvement in your baby's life.

## If Your Partner Isn't the Baby's Biological Parent

If not the baby's biological parent, your partner may feel that the pregnancy is "yours," not "ours." Your partner may question his or her role in making decisions and providing financial support for your growing family. If the baby's biological father is involved in the pregnancy, your partner may feel even less sure about this role.

If you're in a relationship with someone new since becoming pregnant, the roles and relationships between you, your partner, and the baby's father may be tense or unclear. For example, who will accompany you to prenatal appointments and who will be with you during the labor and birth?

If you conceived your baby with a donor egg or sperm, you or your partner may have difficulty coming to terms with the fact that the baby isn't the biological offspring of one or both of you.

Strangers, acquaintances, friends, relatives—and even you—likely have misplaced or unrealistic expectations and assumptions about your nontraditional family that further challenge your relationship with your partner and with the baby. Having open and honest discussions about these issues will help you reach an agreement.

# If You're in a Lesbian Relationship

The legal landscape for lesbian relationships is changing. As same-sex marriage becomes legal in all US states, other legal issues, such as adoption and custody rights, may soon be simplified. For now, though, the law in some states doesn't yet sanction married lesbian couples' roles as parents to the same extent it does for married heterosexual couples. Cultural attitudes can also be slow to change. Lesbian parents may face confusion and awkwardness from some people and outright discrimination from others.

Try to seek out the empathy and support of other lesbian parents to help define your roles as two mothers. For example, will one or both of you return to work after a maternity leave? What will your child call each of you? What role will the biological father play, if any? Discuss these questions with your partner and come to an agreement about what will happen.

# If You're Trans* or Genderqueer

You deserve a caregiver skilled in providing gender-inclusive care. Visit http://transbirth.com or http://glma.org to find a caregiver or ask for referrals from a local transgender or LGBTQI organization. Write a detailed birth plan that includes your preferred pronouns and terms such as *pregnant father*. Ask for your caregiver's support with either sharing the birth plan with hospital staff in advance or informing staff about ways to provide respectful, appropriate care for you. See http://www.PCNguide.com for more resources.

# Special Challenges in Pregnancy

For some people, past traumatic experiences can present additional challenges in pregnancy. With the proper care and support of trusted caregivers, family, and friends, these expectant parents can have positive and healthy pregnancies and childbirth experiences.

## History of Childhood Trauma

Early childhood trauma sometimes causes unexpected reactions during pregnancy, birth, or afterward. People who are physically, sexually, or emotionally abused as adults can also experience these reactions. Some are surprised by their feelings; others know the effects can continue long after the abuse stops. Someone who was abused as a child learned some long-lasting, damaging lessons about herself and others. For example, many abused adults have difficulty trusting others, especially those in authority (such as physicians or midwives).

It's estimated that 25 to 40 percent of women were sexually, physically, or emotionally abused in childhood,[7] so it's not surprising that many survivors (though not all, as it's impossible to generalize the effects of abuse) experience some of the following aftereffects during pregnancy, birth, or afterward:

* A survivor may find vaginal exams, nakedness, or the prospect of a baby coming through her vagina extremely disturbing or even intolerable.
* She may respond to the inevitable loss of control over her body that occurs in labor in the same way she had as a child, when she was helpless to stop her abuser from hurting her.
* She may equate the thought of giving another person total access to her breasts, even for breastfeeding, to her inability to prevent her abuser's violation of her body.

The extent of these problems varies and many factors influence them, including the nature of the abuse, the age at which it occurred, how long it lasted, and the presence or absence of other loving and trustworthy adults in her life. Psychotherapy and emotional support promote healing and help survivors find positive ways to deal with past childhood abuse.

Some caregivers and childbirth educators are more aware than others about the impact of child abuse in adulthood. With empathy and understanding, these professionals can help pregnant survivors have safe, satisfying childbirth experiences and a less stressful postpartum period. If you're an abuse survivor and you trust your caregiver, you may choose to disclose your history of abuse and explain how you think it's affecting your feelings about your body, your baby, the upcoming labor, and your important relationships. If experienced working with survivors, your caregiver may be able to help you address your concerns and communicate them in a birth plan. For more information, we recommend that you read *When Survivors Give Birth: Understanding and Healing the Effects of Early Sexual Abuse on Childbearing Women* by Penny Simkin and Phyllis Klaus.

## Pregnancy after a Previous Miscarriage or Stillbirth

If you've lost a baby during a previous pregnancy or at birth, becoming pregnant again can bring about a wide range of emotions. You may have trouble getting excited about your pregnancy because you fear that you may lose another baby. You may be relieved that you're pregnant again and hopeful for a healthy pregnancy. You may find that it's easier to remain emotionally detached until you have passed the point in your pregnancy when your last baby died. Or you might not want to become attached to your baby at all until after the birth, when you can see and hear your healthy newborn.

Knowing why a previous pregnancy ended in miscarriage or stillbirth may help you and your caregiver plan for a healthier pregnancy this time. Your caregiver may attempt to diminish your fears by offering more prenatal testing (see page 139), or you may request extra testing yourself to help manage your fears. Another way to help relieve your anxiety is to closely watch your baby's health. For example, you may monitor the baby's activity by counting his movements during a set time (see page 64).

Just as each person experiences grief and loss differently, each expectant parent has unique feelings about a pregnancy after a loss. Most people find it helpful to talk with family members, friends, grief counselors, and medical professionals about their feelings and fears. You may also consider talking with other parents who have lost babies to miscarriage or stillbirth. By sharing your concerns with others, you and your partner may learn how to put your grief into perspective and reduce your worries.

## Pregnancy and Disability

If you have any physical challenges, you may need extra support with adapting to the changes of pregnancy. What you will need depends on the nature of your disability. You may benefit from a consultation with a physical therapist or occupational therapist (ideally one who is a parent herself), or from connecting with other parents with your disability who have managed pregnancy and parenting. (Try searching for online discussion forums to make connections.) Take childbirth classes—although the instructor might not have worked with anyone with your disability before, she can demonstrate ideas that work for many people, and you can figure out how to adapt them to your own needs and abilities.

## *Key Points to Remember*

- Pregnancy lasts about forty weeks from the date of the first day of your last menstrual period. Normal pregnancies vary in length, so due dates are approximate. Expect your baby to be born any time from two weeks before to two weeks after your due date.
- Pregnancy is divided into three trimesters. The first trimester is your baby's "formation" period, the second is the "development" period, and the third is the "growth" period. Each trimester brings physical changes for the mother and emotional reactions for all involved.
- For better or worse, your previous experiences can affect your feelings about pregnancy and birth. Talking with someone about your circumstances can help you have a more positive and satisfying pregnancy and childbirth experience.

# CHAPTER 4

# Having a Healthy Pregnancy

To have a healthy, safe, and enjoyable pregnancy, it's important to eat well, get enough exercise and rest, and make positive lifestyle choices. It's also essential to have regular prenatal care by a maternity caregiver and to avoid hazards and situations that can harm you or your baby during pregnancy.

Ideally, you began avoiding hazards and consulting with a health-care professional *before* you became pregnant. However, getting pregnant might have been a surprise to you. Whether you've planned for this pregnancy or not, you can use the information in this chapter to improve your health and increase your chances of having a healthy pregnancy and baby.

# Caring for Yourself and Your Baby during Pregnancy

Having a healthy lifestyle during pregnancy can benefit not only your physical and mental condition, but also your baby's well-being. Here's a list of things you can do to stay healthy throughout your pregnancy:

- Attend regular prenatal care appointments with your caregiver to monitor your health and your baby's well-being (see page 61).
- Learn the warning signs of pregnancy complications to know when to get medical advice and care (see page 67).
- Maintain your general fitness to stay comfortable as your body changes (see chapter 5).
- Eat nutritious foods and gain a healthy amount of weight (see chapter 6).
- Use safe alternatives to medications to relieve symptoms of common ailments and pregnancy discomforts (see page 70).
- Avoid harmful substances and exposure to hazards (see pages 72–78).
- Treat harmful conditions and illnesses before pregnancy and those that develop during pregnancy (see chapter 7).
- Reduce harmful stresses in your life (see pages 68–69) and practice relaxation skills (see chapter 12).

## A NOTE TO FATHERS AND PARTNERS

Your compassion, care, and encouragement are critical to your pregnant partner's well-being during pregnancy. You can help your partner by encouraging her to have a healthy lifestyle. Support her efforts by making healthy changes to your lifestyle as well. For example, if you smoke, you can quit so your partner (and your baby) avoids the harmful effects of secondhand smoke. You can also strive to exercise regularly and avoid consuming unsafe foods and substances.

Get involved in your partner's pregnancy. Attend some or all prenatal appointments, show an interest in prenatal tests and their results, and learn the warnings signs of pregnancy complications (see page 67). Help reduce your partner's pregnancy discomforts by doing the strenuous household chores and assisting her with comfort measures (see pages 98–101). If she's upset or distressed, discover what's bothering her and help alleviate anxiety. Review the stress-coping skills discussed on page 68 for ways to decrease your own stress. Because pregnancy can strain a couple's relationship, you may need counseling to help resolve any family problems before the birth.

# Prenatal Care

When you know (or strongly suspect) you're pregnant, schedule a visit with your caregiver. (See page 14 for information on the different types of maternity caregivers.) The wait to get an appointment with some caregivers can be several weeks, so call promptly.

Before your first prenatal visit, start making healthy lifestyle changes, such as quitting smoking, avoiding alcohol, eating nutritious foods, and taking folic acid. Consider having your partner accompany you to prenatal appointments so you both can discuss your partner's role at the birth with your caregiver. Visit our website, http://www.PCNGuide.com, to download a work sheet to bring to appointments.

At your first or second prenatal visit, your caregiver will likely give you a complete physical examination and administer numerous tests. Your caregiver (or an office nurse) will also ask questions about your current life situation and family medical history. At each prenatal appointment, your caregiver will monitor your health and your baby's growth. In midpregnancy, you'll usually have an appointment scheduled for every month. Toward the end of your pregnancy, you'll have an appointment every two weeks, then every week as your due date approaches.

Some caregivers schedule brief appointments; others schedule longer visits so you have time to build a relationship and discuss concerns and questions you may have. If you want a longer appointment than usual, request one in advance.

Toward the end of your pregnancy, schedule a long visit to talk about your birth plan with your caregiver (see chapter 8). Also, if your caregiver is part of a group, try to meet the others in the practice in case one of them is on call when you're in labor. If meeting the others isn't possible, a written birth plan can communicate your specific birth preferences and help introduce you to unfamiliar care providers.

## PRENATAL TESTS

Throughout your pregnancy, your caregiver will offer you routine screening tests and diagnostic tests to detect possible problems with your health or your baby's.

A *screening test* is a quick, easy, and inexpensive way to rule out a particular condition. (See page 63 for a list of routine screening tests.) If the results of your test are negative, you don't have the condition. For inclusion in standard practice, screening tests must have a minimal "false negative" rate; that is, they must be unlikely to *miss* detecting when someone has the condition. If screening results are positive, you may need further testing to confirm a diagnosis of the condition. A *diagnostic test* is more specific and more reliable than a screening test in identifying women with a pregnancy complication or a baby with a problem. Sometimes, diagnostic testing determines you don't actually have the condition, which means your screening test gave a "false positive" reading (see page 66 for more information).

Diagnostic tests are often more invasive, more expensive, and usually have more side effects than routine screening tests. As a result, most caregivers use diagnostic tests only if indicated by a positive screening test or other pertinent factors. (See pages 139–141 for more information on diagnostic tests.)

## What Information Should I Include in My Medical History?

Your caregiver can provide better prenatal care when aware of any of the following potentially troubling health or social problems concerning you, your partner, and your families (all may influence your medical care or your responses to care or medical procedures).

- prior surgeries or illnesses that required medical treatment
- hereditary conditions or illnesses, including birth defects, developmental delays, blindness, deafness, stillbirths, and miscarriages
- prior or current behavioral or mental health conditions, such as depression or eating disorders
- ethnic or cultural traditions that may affect prenatal care, birth procedures, and postpartum care
- gender identity or family structure (for example, same-sex parents, three-parent family, or single parent)
- current prescription medications, drug allergies, and drug reactions
- prior negative experience with a hospitalization, caregiver, or illness
- prior sexual abuse, domestic violence, or any other significant mistreatment
- heavy use of alcohol, tobacco, recreational drugs, or other harmful substances

When your caregiver suggests a prenatal test, ask the following key questions to help you make an informed decision about whether to have the test. These questions are particularly important if the test carries potential risks:

- **What is the procedure?** How is the test done?
- **What are the benefits?** Is this a screening or diagnostic test? What condition are we looking for? How reliable or accurate are the results—that is, are false positives or false negatives likely? How will the results affect my prenatal care?
- **What are the risks?** Are there risks to me or my baby? How much does the test cost? Will my insurance cover it?
- **What are the alternatives?** Are there other tests for this condition? What are their benefits and risks? What are the consequences of not having the test?

You also have questions to ask yourself before having a prenatal test. What will you do with the results? How will you feel and what will you do if the results are positive? Negative?

Some prenatal tests reveal certain conditions that can improve with self-care or medical treatment. For example, tests that measure the amount of glucose (sugar) in your blood show whether you have gestational diabetes (see page 63). To treat the condition, you can make changes to your diet, get physical activity, and perhaps take medications.

Other prenatal tests reveal conditions that can't be treated or cured. For example, screening tests can show how likely it is that a baby has Down syndrome, and amniocentesis can diagnose the presence of the condition. However, these tests can't predict how seriously the condition will affect a baby or her family.

Before testing for birth defects, families should know how they'll respond if the results are positive. Some families will consider whether to terminate the pregnancy. Others believe abortion isn't an option for them, and they'll choose to prepare for the baby by learning about the condition, understanding what to expect, and gathering the resources they'll need.

Some families choose not to test for untreatable or incurable conditions. They may believe testing is unnecessary because their risk of the conditions is low. Or they would rather handle a diagnosis of a condition after the baby is born than spend the pregnancy worrying about challenges that might not come.

To learn more information about prenatal testing, visit http://www.marchofdimes.com. You can also visit our website, http://www.PCNGuide.com.

# Routine Exams and Screening Tests

Your caregiver will perform some exams and tests at just one prenatal visit and will perform others periodically throughout your pregnancy. Caregivers typically perform the following assessments at every prenatal visit:

- **urine test** to detect bacteria, protein, and sugar (At first visit, a urine test may be used to confirm pregnancy.)
- **blood pressure check** to screen for high blood pressure
- **weight check** to monitor nutritional status and detect sudden weight gain (which can indicate preeclampsia—see page 134)
- **abdominal exam** to measure uterine growth or fundal height (which indicates the baby's growth) and estimate the baby's position
- **listening to fetal heart tones (FHT)** to help confirm the baby's well-being

Caregivers perform the following assessments only at specific visits:
- **pelvic exam** to help confirm pregnancy, estimate the size of the mother's pelvis, check for infection, or perform a Pap smear. In late pregnancy, a pelvic exam reveals cervical changes.
- **blood test** (at first visit) to confirm pregnancy, determine blood type, test for anemia, and assess exposure to infection. For women with diabetes, caregivers check blood glucose levels periodically throughout pregnancy.
- **breast exam** to help screen for breast cancer and assess breasts for conditions affecting breastfeeding

For more information on routine exams and screening tests, visit our website, http://www.PCNGuide.com.

# Other Exams and Screening Tests

Caregivers often perform the following exams and tests, but not routinely. Some caregivers don't offer certain tests. If a specific test interests you, talk to your caregiver about your wishes and concerns.
- **Dental exam** (performed by dentist) to check for tooth decay and repair if needed, clean teeth, and check for gum infection. Gum infection is associated with preterm labor.
- **Fetal movement counts** (kick counts) to help assess your baby's well-being by detecting changes in his normal pattern of movements. This test is performed by you, not your caregiver (see page 64).
- **Ultrasound** to help confirm pregnancy, estimate due date, and estimate your baby's size. Ultrasounds also help detect or rule out complications (see page 65).
- **Integrated prenatal screening** to assess risk of Down syndrome and neural tube defects. See page 63 for more information on tests that screen for birth defects. See pages 139–141 for information on diagnostic tests that are performed if screening results are positive.
- **Genetic screening** to check for diseases such as cystic fibrosis, Tay-Sachs, thalassemia, and sickle cell anemia. Depending on your family's medical history and ethnicity, your caregiver may offer carrier-screening tests. If these blood or saliva tests reveal a risk, your caregiver may recommend further diagnostic testing.
- **Glucose screening** for gestational diabetes (see page 127), between the twenty-fourth and twenty-eighth weeks of pregnancy. After you've had a sugary drink or snack, your blood is drawn. If your blood sugar is high, your caregiver will recommend a glucose tolerance test.
- **Group B streptococcus (GBS) screening** to detect the presence of GBS bacteria in secretions swabbed from the vagina and anus and cultured in a laboratory. See also page 125.

## Fetal Movement Counting

During late pregnancy, keeping track of your baby's movements for a short time helps you learn more about your baby and his health. The method below explains how to count a baby's movements. You can do it anytime if you're curious about your baby's patterns. If you have a high-risk pregnancy, knowing your baby's patterns can be especially helpful, because your caregiver may ask you to monitor the movements for any changes.

### The Count-to-Ten Method

Any time after the twenty-eighth week of pregnancy, count your baby's movements at roughly the same time of day when he's normally active, such as after lunch or dinner. You don't need to count movements every day, just when convenient.

Find a comfortable position and avoid doing anything distracting, then time how long it takes your baby to move ten times. A movement may be short (a kick or a wiggle) or long (a continuous squirming motion). Don't count hiccups. Count it as a movement when it's followed by a clear (but brief) pause. Record movements on a chart, such as the one below. Visit our website, http://www .PCNGuide.com, to download a template of this chart.

The length of time it takes to complete ten movements varies among babies. Focus not on how your baby's movements compare with other babies', but on whether his activity has slowed down compared to his usual pattern.

Babies who are doing well in the uterus have several active, wakeful periods during the day. They also have quiet periods, when they're sleeping. Healthy babies move slightly less often toward the end of the pregnancy because there's less space to move around.

If your baby doesn't move at all during the chosen time, he may be asleep. Try waking him with a loud noise, or eat or drink something sugary. Wait until you feel him move and then begin counting his movements (it may take only a few minutes if you've chosen a time when your baby is usually active). Call your caregiver if your baby clearly takes a longer time than usual to make ten movements or if he doesn't move at least ten times or have an active period within the next twelve hours.

## Sample Fetal Movement Counting Chart

| Date | Starting Time | Record of Movements | Time of 10th Movement | Total Time |
|------|--------------|---------------------|----------------------|-----------|
| 8/24 | 7:30 pm | ℍℍ ℍℍ | 7:53 pm | 23 min |
| 8/25 | 6:00 pm | ℍℍ ℍℍ | 6:15 pm | 15 min |
| 8/26 | 6:30 pm | ℍℍ ℍℍ | 6:35 pm | 5 min |
| 8/27 | 7:00 pm | ℍℍ ℍℍ | 7:25 pm | 25 min |
| 8/28 | 7:15 pm | ℍℍ ℍℍ | 7:33 pm | 18 min |
| 8/29 | 6:30 pm | ℍℍ ℍℍ | 6:47 pm | 17 min |
| 8/30 | 9:00 pm | ℍℍ ℍℍ | 10:05 pm | 65 min |

## Understanding Ultrasound

Many caregivers rely heavily on ultrasound to check the baby's heart rate, observe her development within the uterus, and make clinical decisions. Most pregnant women have at least one ultrasound at some point in their pregnancies.

There are two forms of ultrasound: Doppler ultrasound and diagnostic ultrasound scans. *Doppler ultrasound* (or simply Doppler), which monitors the baby's heart rate, uses continuous transmission of sound waves to detect motion of the baby's heart as it beats. Women receive Doppler from a hand-held device at prenatal visits. (See page 182 for more information on monitoring your baby's heart rate.)

*Diagnostic ultrasound scans,* which help caregivers "see" inside the uterus, use intermittent transmission of sound waves for less than 1 percent of the time during the test. For the rest of the test, the equipment receives the echoes of the sound waves, which indicate differences in tissue density. The echoes are converted into a video image that shows the baby's skeleton and organs, amniotic fluid, umbilical cord, placenta, and the mother's womb. Diagnostic ultrasound scans at twenty weeks is standard in many maternity-care practices.

The accuracy of ultrasound depends on the quality of the equipment, the skill and experience of the technician and caregiver, and the purpose of the test. In addition, some tests are less reliable than others. For example, using ultrasound scans to estimate the baby's gestational age and weight are less accurate in late pregnancy than in early pregnancy.

Many expectant parents like ultrasound because it allows them to see their babies' faces, fingers, toes, beating hearts, and wriggling bodies. This first sight of their babies inspires many parents to make an effort to have a healthy pregnancy and birth.

Although studies haven't found evidence that ultrasound harms the mother or baby, health-care experts recommend that pregnant women avoid frequent ultrasound scans. For example, if you had a nuchal translucency scan (see page 66) at eleven weeks or a standard diagnostic ultrasound at twenty weeks, you may consider asking your caregiver what additional information would be gained by having additional scans later in pregnancy. Visit our website, http://www.PCNGuide .com, for more information on diagnostic ultrasound scans.

## Fact or Fiction?

*Nonmedical use of ultrasound, such as at-home Doppler heartbeat monitors and 4-D ultrasound videos or photos, are completely safe.* **Fiction.** The US Food and Drug Administration (FDA) and the American Institute of Ultrasound in Medicine acknowledge that the medical use of ultrasound by a well-trained technician poses no known risks to babies. However, ultrasound can affect the body, and the long-term effects of repeated or prolonged exposure are unknown.

To be safe, health-care experts recommend that ultrasound be performed only by a trained provider and only when medically indicated.

## Screening for Birth Defects

Your caregiver may recommend screening for chromosomal abnormalities, such as Down syndrome, and neural tube defects, such as spina bifida. Screening is typically recommended for expectant parents older than thirty-five, especially those with a personal or family history of birth defects. There are many options for such testing:

- **First trimester screening**—This blood test, done between ten and thirteen weeks, assesses the risk of chromosomal defects.
- **Nuchal translucency**—This ultrasound scan, done around eleven weeks, measures a space at the back of the baby's neck, where fluid tends to accumulate in babies with chromosomal defects.
- **Cell-free fetal DNA testing***—This blood test, done between ten and thirteen weeks, checks for fetal DNA to assess the risk of chromosomal defects. It can also identify the baby's sex.[1]
- **Second trimester quad screen**—This blood test, done between sixteen and eighteen weeks, tests for chromosomal defects and for neural tube defects.
- **Second trimester ultrasound scan**—This scan, done between eighteen and twenty weeks, checks for signs of neural tube defects and other anatomical defects.

\* The American Congress of Obstetricians and Gynecologists (ACOG) recommends that women have this test only if first trimester screening and nuchal translucency scan show increased risk of chromosomal abnormalities.[2]

Sometimes the results of screening tests are combined for greater accuracy. *Integrated prenatal screening* combines the first and second trimester blood tests and nuchal translucency screening into one result, which is reported after the second trimester quad screen is done. In *sequential screening*, the results are given after each test; families can then decide whether to have additional screening or diagnostic tests.

Screening tests can show only *how likely* it is that a baby has a condition. A *screen-negative* result means that it's very unlikely the child has the defect—although there's some risk of a false negative result. A *false negative* means the test didn't detect a condition that the baby actually has.

A *screen-positive* result does *not* mean a baby has that defect. Instead, it means that the chances of having the condition are high enough that a caregiver recommends further testing to confirm a diagnosis. (See diagnostic tests on page 139.) Caregivers should explain each test's false positive rate. A *false positive* means that although the result of a screening test is positive, the baby doesn't actually have that defect. For example, in one study of cell-free fetal DNA testing, almost two thousand people were tested. Eleven people screened positive for Down syndrome, but only five babies actually had the condition. In other words, six of the eleven people who screened positive really had a false positive result because their babies did *not* have Down syndrome.[3]

Don't make choices you can't change later (such as termination) based on the result of only one screening test. Discuss your options with your caregiver before taking any actions.

# Warning Signs of Pregnancy Complications

Although most pregnancies are healthy, it's extremely important to know the following warning signs and immediately call your caregiver for an early diagnosis and prompt treatment. See chapter 7 for more information on complications in pregnancy.

| Warning signs | Possible problems |
|---|---|
| Vaginal bleeding (even a small amount) | Miscarriage (see page 122); placenta previa (see page 132); placental abruption (see page 133); preterm labor (see page 129) |
| Abdominal pain | Ectopic pregnancy (see page 121); miscarriage (see page 122); placental abruption (see page 133); preterm labor contractions (see page 129). May indicate a medical problem, such as appendicitis or gallbladder disease. |
| Continuing, intermittent abdominal cramping or uterine tightening (contractions) | Preterm labor (see page 129) |
| Constant and severe abdominal pain and a hard abdomen, with or without vaginal bleeding | Placental abruption (see page 133) |
| Leaking or gushing of fluid from your vagina | Rupture of the membranes (see page 165) |
| Sudden swelling of your face, hands, or fingers | Preeclampsia (see page 134) |
| Severe, persistent headache | Gestational hypertension or preeclampsia (see page 134) |
| Problems with your vision (seeing spots or flashes, blurring, or blind spots) | Preeclampsia (see page 134) |
| Severe and persistent dizziness, lightheadedness | Preeclampsia (see page 134); supine hypotension (see page 83) |
| Noticeable reduction or change in your baby's movement or activity after the 28th week of pregnancy | Fetal distress (see page 64 for fetal movement counting) |
| Painful area in leg, swelling or redness over affected area, or pain in leg when standing or walking | Blood clot in leg or inflammation of vein (venous thrombosis—see page 124) |
| Severe pain in pubic area and hips, with trouble moving your legs | Strain or separation of pubic symphysis joint or sciatica (pain in the lower back from pelvic joint stress) |
| Painful urination or burning sensation, with or without the urgent and frequent need to urinate | Urinary tract infection or UTI (see page 126); sexually transmitted infection or STI (see page 125) |
| Irritating vaginal discharge, genital sores, or vaginal itching | Vaginal infection or STI (see page 125) |
| Fever (temperature over 102°F or 38.9°C) when feeling sick | Infection (see page 124) |
| Persistent nausea or vomiting | Hyperemesis gravidarum (see page 123); infection (see page 124) |
| Feeling depressed or overwhelmed with worries | Perinatal mood and anxiety disorder (see page 351) |

# Reducing Stress during Pregnancy

Your emotions affect your body and your baby. Throughout pregnancy, you'll experience times when you feel anxious, times when a situation stresses you out, or moments when a loud noise or other unexpected event startles you. During these times, your body produces adrenaline and cortisol, stress hormones that signal a "fight or flight" response, causing tight muscles, constricted blood vessels, and elevated heart and breathing rates. In the short term, this response to stress doesn't harm you or your baby and can be beneficial. For example, it may boost your energy level or encourage you to prepare for an upcoming event.

In the long term, however, chronic (continual) stress can constrict blood vessels to the placenta and within it, reducing the amount of blood and nutrients to your growing baby. Constant severe stress may increase your chances of preterm labor or decrease your baby's birth weight even if she's not preterm.[4] High anxiety levels throughout pregnancy can also affect your baby later in life by increasing her chances of developing behavioral and neurodevelopmental problems, such as attention deficit disorder/hyperactivity, anxiety disorders, and language delays.[5]

Stress can make you feel overwhelmed, out of control, and less productive. Typically, following the self-care steps on page 69 can help you manage these effects. Stress, however, becomes detrimental when it makes you extremely anxious or depressed, affects your sleeping and eating schedules, or causes health problems. If you experience any of these harmful effects, contact your caregiver for help immediately. See page 351 for warning signs of perinatal mood and anxiety disorders (PMAD) that can also occur during pregnancy. If diagnosed with depression or a mood disorder, you may need the care of a mental health counselor or need to take medications to manage your stress. You may also want to contact a counselor or an organization that's devoted to the emotional support of pregnant women and new mothers.

## WHAT CAUSES CHRONIC STRESS?

Any situation or event that upsets you can cause chronic stress if left unmanaged. Examples include a demanding job, financial worries, an unstable home life, problems with your partner, pregnancy complications, a loved one's illness, or violence or danger in your life. (If your partner or your home environment is violent or abusive, see page 76 for more information.)

Other ongoing conditions may trigger an excessive stress response to every challenging experience. For example, you may have an extreme reaction to everyday pressures because of unresolved or untreated anxiety from a previous traumatic event (including emotional, physical, or sexual abuse), a chemical imbalance that causes your brain to interpret minor stresses as major ones, or hormonal changes (such as those that occur during pregnancy) that can intensify emotional problems.

## COPING WITH CHRONIC STRESS

To help cope with chronic stress, take these steps:

1. Recognize your stress response. Notice how you feel when you're anxious or stressed; for example, you may feel overwhelmed, have trouble sleeping, or have frequent headaches or bowel problems.
2. Identify the source of your stress. Try to discover which person, situation, or experience is triggering the stress.
3. Try to eliminate that source, if possible. For example, you may decide to quit a stressful job or transfer to another work setting, or you may leave an abusive home environment.
4. Learn better ways to cope with a stressful condition when eliminating the source is difficult or impossible. The following are steps to help reduce the tension and pressure of stressful situations:
   - Think of ways to modify the situation. For example, you can stay away from people who trigger a stress response.
   - Take action to reduce your stress. Sometimes, simply attempting to solve the problem diminishes the stress to a manageable level.
   - Try to get enough sleep at night and nap during the day. If you can't sleep, sit or lie down and rest. Remember that fatigue makes everything seem worse.
   - Use the relaxation skills described on pages 234–237. Also use slow breathing (see page 243) while resting, meditating, or listening to soothing music.
   - Eat nourishing foods and drink plenty of water and other fluids.
   - Exercise regularly to help relieve stress, promote sleep, keep you fit, and improve your health (see chapter 5).
   - Discuss your problems and worries with someone you trust, such as your partner, a friend, a relative, your caregiver, or another professional. Sharing your concerns at a support group also may help.
   - Nurture yourself by doing something you enjoy. Have a massage, manicure, or facial. Go to a movie. Take a walk through a park. Spend time with people who comfort you.

If these steps don't ease your stress or you're unable to use them, you may need to live with the stress—at least for a while. If you're concerned the stress will harm your baby, many counselors suggest regularly talking to your baby to express your love and to reassure him that your troubles aren't his fault and that he's safe. Your baby, of course, won't understand your words, but saying them can lower your stress level and give you a chance to connect with your baby.

## In Their Own Words

During my pregnancy, I had a very demanding job as a nurse and was on my feet for most of every twelve-hour shift. I'd come home at the end of a shift, slump into my chair, and watch reruns of my favorite TV show. After my baby was born, that show's theme song would calm her when she was fussy, just as it had calmed me when she was in utero!
—Amy

# Treating Illness and Discomforts during Pregnancy

If you're in discomfort or feel sick, you may be tempted to take over-the-counter or prescription medications to feel better. If possible, try some of these home remedies first. Before taking any medication, talk to your caregiver.

## Home Remedies to Help Relieve Common Discomforts

These nonmedicinal treatments of common ailments may help you, but if discomforts persist or worsen, consult your caregiver.

### Headache

Instead of taking aspirin, acetaminophen (Tylenol), or ibuprofen to relieve a headache, try taking a warm bath, having a massage, or doing tension-reducing exercises (such as shoulder circles). (See pages 234–237.) Try laying a hot pack across your shoulders or on the back of your neck, or try placing a cool cloth on your forehead. Hunger, dehydration, and fatigue can cause headaches. Make sure to eat frequently, drink enough fluids, get more sleep, and arrange for periods of rest and relaxation in your daily routine. Report a severe, persistent headache to your caregiver; it may be a warning sign of a pregnancy complication (see page 67).

### Cold, hay fever, runny nose, or cough

Safe ways to relieve these ailments include getting additional sleep and rest, using a cool-mist vaporizer or spending time in a steamy bathroom, drinking plenty of liquids, and swallowing a mixture of honey and lemon juice. For nasal congestion, you can purchase saline nose drops at a drugstore or make your own with 1 cup warm water, ½ teaspoon salt, and a small pinch of baking soda. Administer the drops by using a dropper or a neti pot. If using a neti pot, make sure to use water that's free of dangerous bacteria. You can use distilled or sterile water, or you can boil tap water for three to five minutes, then let it cool to lukewarm.

### Nausea, heartburn, and constipation

See page 113 for nonmedicinal treatments.

### Back pain

Upper and lower back pain is common in pregnancy, but you can help prevent it by maintaining good posture, using good body mechanics, and doing exercises that strengthen your abdominal muscles and decrease the curve in your lower back (see chapter 5). Treat back pain with rest, massage, warm baths, and hot or cold packs. Avoid taking aspirin, ibuprofen, and muscle relaxants unless your back pain is severe and your caregiver approves or prescribes these drugs.

### Sleeplessness

Sleeplessness is especially common in late pregnancy because of frequent trips to the bathroom, an active baby, light sleeping, or difficulty finding a comfortable sleep position. (See page 83 for sleep positions.) To help release stress and tension, try exercising or taking a brisk walk each day (but not just before bedtime). At bedtime, try taking a warm bath, drinking warm milk, having a massage, or listening to soothing music. If you awaken at night, try reading, writing your thoughts in a journal, or using the relaxation techniques described in chapter 12. Avoid watching TV or using your computer or mobile device, which tends to stimulate your brain and make you feel more awake.

## Medications

If home remedies don't make you feel better and your symptoms are troubling, check with your caregiver about over-the-counter medications, which may relieve symptoms but don't treat or cure an illness. If you have a chronic condition or current disease during pregnancy, your caregiver may prescribe medications (such as antibiotics, insulin, antidepressants, antiseizure drugs, and steroids).

When deciding whether to use a medication, consider the seriousness of your symptoms or condition, the relief the medication may provide, and its possible side effects. To help make an informed decision, ask the following questions:

1. What are the medication's benefits, risks, and alternatives (see page 9)?
2. If the benefits clearly outweigh the risks and you decide to take the medication, ask your caregiver or a pharmacist the following questions:
   - What dose should I take, and how often should I take it?
   - What's the maximum dose in a 24-hour period?
   - Should I avoid any foods or other drugs while taking it?
   - How long should I take it? Should I stop taking it at any specific time in pregnancy?
3. If the benefits don't clearly outweigh the risks, avoid taking the medication and seek a safer alternative.

## Over-the-Counter (OTC) Medications

When buying any OTC medication, look at its ingredients. Many medications include more than one drug in their pills or capsules. You'll need to learn the benefits, side effects, and possible risks for every drug in the medication. Visit our website, http://www.PCNGuide.com, or use the resources listed on page 77 to learn current information on some common OTC medications.

## Prescription Medications

Some prescription medications are safe to use in pregnancy; others aren't (see below). The safety of many drugs is yet unknown. Some caregivers may feel these medications are safe to take at certain times in pregnancy but dangerous at other times. They may prescribe them only if the benefits clearly outweigh the known risks. Or they may closely supervise their use in certain circumstances when the risks are unclear. When talking to your caregiver about a prescription medication whose safety isn't completely known, discuss other available treatments and their benefits and risks.

## Medications to Avoid

During pregnancy, a few medications are extremely harmful to your baby. Many are teratogens, which are substances that can cause birth defects, deformities, or even death. Some (such as thalidomide and diethylstilbestrol or DES) were prescribed for pregnant women before their severe side effects were known. Now their use has almost disappeared. Research will undoubtedly find more medications that can harm unborn babies. When considering any medication, make sure that all health-care professionals working with you know that you're pregnant.

The following are medications known to be harmful during pregnancy:
- chemotherapy drugs (methotrexate and aminopterin)
- oral drugs to treat severe acne, such as isotretinoin (Accutane) and vitamin A derivatives (the vitamin A in acne medications differs from the vitamin A found in vitamin pills; vitamin A in prenatal vitamins is safe to take in pregnancy)
- radioactive isotopes (used in nuclear imaging studies such as bone scans )

The following drugs are potentially harmful if taken during pregnancy, but their benefits may outweigh the risks:
- some medications used to treat hyperthyroidism (such as propylthiouracil, methimazole, or iodide)
- certain medications used to treat seizure disorders (phenytoin, valproic acid or Depakote, and others), bipolar disorder (lithium), and other conditions—unless your caregiver closely supervises their use

## Common Questions about Alcohol and Pregnancy

**What if I drank before I knew I was pregnant?**

If you had only a few drinks, the risk of long-term harm to your baby is low. If you drank heavily, talk to your caregiver to assess the risk to your baby.

**What if I drink just a little only occasionally while pregnant?**

Current studies show that moderate drinking (one standard drink per day) has minimal effect on a baby's risk of birth defects. However, research hasn't determined a safe amount of alcohol, because blood alcohol levels vary depending on physical size, genetic factors, the amount of food eaten while drinking, and the amount of time between drinks. For that reason, it's best to avoid alcohol.

**How can I easily avoid drinking alcohol?**

At any occasion where alcohol is available, choose a nonalcoholic beverage such as mineral water with a lemon twist, fruit or vegetable juice, a refreshing seltzer, or a "virgin" (nonalcoholic) mixed drink. If offered an alcoholic drink, request something else. You can say that you're pregnant and want to avoid alcohol. Or if you don't want to announce your pregnancy, you can say that you'll be driving home and are already tired.

# Substances and Hazards to Avoid during Pregnancy

Just about everything you consume or are exposed to during pregnancy affects your baby. Some substances and situations are more harmful than others. When you begin learning about these hazards, it's easy to worry constantly about possible harm to your baby. Don't panic! Babies can be remarkably resilient and can do well despite multiple exposures to harmful substances or situations. We encourage you to use the information in this section to reduce your exposure to hazards *as much as possible*, but try not to become too anxious about minimal or infrequent exposure.

With any harmful substance or situation, its effect on your baby and pregnancy depends on the amount and frequency of exposure as well as what trimester of pregnancy you're in when exposed. (Some substances can also affect the reproductive health of men and nonpregnant women.) For example, exposure to a hazardous substance in the first trimester can increase your risk of miscarriage or birth defects; exposure in the second and third trimesters can increase your risk of slowed growth of your baby's body or brain (intrauterine growth restriction, or IUGR) or preterm labor.

In general, the more you're exposed to a harmful substance or situation, the higher your risk of serious problems for your baby or pregnancy—and the less your exposure, the lower the risk.

## DRINKING, SMOKING, AND DRUG USE

When you're pregnant, be extremely cautious about using alcohol or other drugs. Substance abuse can severely harm your baby or pregnancy.

### *Alcohol*

Any alcohol you drink while pregnant crosses the placenta and enters your baby's blood in the same concentration as in your blood. The extent that alcohol can harm your baby depends on the amount you drink, how often you drink, and when in pregnancy you drink.[6]

Babies whose mothers drink heavily at any time during pregnancy are at high risk of developing severe problems. In the first trimester, when a baby's organs are forming, excessive alcohol can cause organ defects, facial abnormalities, or miscarriage. Alcohol abuse in the second trimester can affect nerve formation in the brain, and in the third trimester it may interfere with the development of the nervous system. It may also cause preterm labor. Of the babies whose mothers drank heavily while pregnant, 4 percent develop fetal alcohol syndrome (FAS), a cluster of physical, mental, and behavioral disabilities that include growth problems, heart defects, mental retardation, facial abnormalities, and problems with muscle and nerve development.

What's the definition of *heavy drinking*? Some researchers define it as having more than four drinks a day. Other researchers define it as having two or more drinks per day or binge drinking more than three drinks on one occasion. A standard drink is ½ ounce of distilled alcohol (by itself or in a mixed drink), one can of beer, or a 4-ounce glass of wine.

Even light to moderate drinking (one standard drink per day) during pregnancy increases a baby's risk of fetal alcohol effects (FAE), characterized by problems that are less severe than FAS but still have subtle, long-lasting neurological and behavioral consequences. When compared to a child whose mother didn't drink any alcohol during pregnancy, a child exposed to alcohol before birth may have a slightly lower IQ, may be less agile or athletic, or may have more trouble with concentration, organizational skills, or impulse control.

It's best to avoid alcohol during pregnancy—the earlier the better. In fact, avoiding alcohol *before* becoming pregnant may help you conceive; drinking, especially heavy drinking, may contribute to infertility problems.

If you find it difficult to quit drinking alcohol, try to avoid occasions, locations (such as bars), and friendships that focus on drinking alcohol. Seek people who support your decision not to drink and consider attending Alcoholics Anonymous (AA) meetings.

## Smoking

Cigarette smoke contains numerous toxins that can harm you and directly affect the growth and development of your baby and placenta. These toxins include nicotine, tar, carbon monoxide, lead, and other substances. During pregnancy, the risks of complications from smoking and exposure to second-hand smoke increase with the amount and frequency of exposure.

When compared to pregnant nonsmokers, pregnant smokers have a greater risk of miscarriage, stillbirth, infant death, or having a baby with birth defects. The more a woman smokes while pregnant, the greater the risk is that she may develop placenta previa or placental abruption or have an ectopic pregnancy. Pregnant smokers also often give birth to babies with low birth weight (who tend to have health problems) and have a higher risk of preterm birth.

Smoking may harm a baby after birth. If a mother smokes during pregnancy or if she or her baby are exposed to secondhand smoke during pregnancy or after birth, the baby's risk of respiratory problems (such as asthma) later in life is increased, and the risk of sudden infant death syndrome or SIDS (see page 385) is considerably increased.[7]

If you smoke, try to quit (or at least significantly cut back) before pregnancy or as soon as possible during pregnancy.[8] The withdrawal symptoms you'll experience (physical discomfort and psychological stress that last for several days or a few weeks) are difficult. But it takes just a day or so for your baby to begin to benefit from a smoke-free environment. To reduce your exposure to secondhand smoke, stay away from smoky areas and ask friends, colleagues, and relatives not to smoke near you or your baby.

## Marijuana[10]

Some states have legalized the recreational use of marijuana, and several states have legalized marijuana for medicinal purposes. However, marijuana use is still a *federal* crime. For example, federal laws on child abuse and neglect may consider marijuana use to be the same as illegal drug use.

## Common Q&A

**Q:** I know I shouldn't smoke during pregnancy, but what can I do to quit? Are e-cigarettes are safer than regular cigarettes?

**A:** Ask your caregiver for information about quitting. You may also be given a list of local smoking cessation programs. In addition, you can visit http://smokefree.gov and http://www.cancer.org for helpful tips, as well as other websites of organizations that help people stop smoking.

One thing not to do is use smoking substitutes (nicotine patch, gum, or nasal spray) during the first trimester. They can increase the risk of malformations in your baby if used when his organs and structures are forming.[9]

Although it's possible that e-cigarettes are safer because they contain fewer chemicals and no smoke is produced, their effects in pregnancy haven't been studied. Regardless, e-cigarettes still contain nicotine, which is known to be harmful to babies, and should be avoided.

Some studies show that marijuana use in pregnancy doesn't increase the risk of birth defects. Other studies indicate that babies born to mothers who regularly used marijuana had a higher risk of premature birth, low birth weight, small head circumference, and attention deficit disorder and developmental delays. These studies, however, may have been influenced by two factors. First, they were generally done before states began legalizing marijuana use, which likely limited the number of women included in the studies (because many didn't want their marijuana use known). Second, women who regularly used marijuana were also more likely to use alcohol, tobacco, and other drugs and less likely to have access to prenatal care—situations that can raise a baby's risk of harm.

Until more research is done, avoid recreational marijuana use and use it medicinally only with the supervision of your caregiver.

## Illegal Drugs and Prescription Drug Abuse

The most commonly abused drugs are illegal, and most have no accepted medical use. Illegal drugs are often sold on the street, come from unregulated sources, and lack medical supervision. Because most illegal drugs readily cross the placenta to your baby, taking these substances while pregnant can harm not only you, but also your growing baby, depending on the drug you took, how much you of it you took, when in pregnancy you took it, and how often you took it.

If you take an illegal drug in the first trimester, your baby may develop a defect or deformity or you may have a miscarriage. If you take an illegal drug in the second or third trimester, your baby may have intrauterine growth restriction or IUGR (that is, grow slowly) or suffer the effects of prematurity because of a preterm birth. Each drug has its own harmful effects, and taking a combination of two or more drugs may increase the damage. Visit our website, http://www.PCNGuide.com, for more information.

Instead of taking illegal drugs—or in addition to taking them—some pregnant women abuse prescription drugs by using them without medical supervision. These women mistakenly believe these substances are safer than illegal drugs and are therefore okay to use during pregnancy. But the effects of prescription drugs can be just as dangerous to babies as the effects of illegal drugs (see page 71). Try to stop using *all* drugs before you're pregnant or as soon as you know you're pregnant, to improve your baby's chances of a healthy life.

# POTENTIALLY HARMFUL SUBSTANCES AND HERBS IN FOODS

Some substances and herbs that are in several common foods and beverages may be potentially harmful to consume when pregnant. During your pregnancy, be careful about consuming the following items.

## Caffeine

Caffeine is a stimulant that can raise your heart rate and blood pressure, constrict blood vessels, affect your ability to sleep, and make you jittery. It's also a diuretic (a substance that makes you urinate more fluid, more often) and increases the amount of calcium you expel in your urine.

Coffee, tea, energy drinks, colas, and other soft drinks contain significant amounts of caffeine. To learn the amount of caffeine in packaged products, read the labels. Companies aren't required by law to list amounts, but many choose to do so. For brewed beverages (such as coffee and tea), the amount of caffeine in a serving depends on how it's made and the number of ounces in a serving. For example, an 8-ounce serving of brewed coffee may have 65 to 120 milligrams of caffeine. An 8-ounce serving of black or green tea has 20 to 90 milligrams of caffeine.[11] A 12-ounce serving of caffeinated soda typically has 34 to 54 milligrams of caffeine. In addition, several over-the-counter medications include caffeine, and chocolate contains a small amount of a caffeine-like chemical.

Before getting pregnant, consuming more than 300 milligrams per day may increase the time it takes to conceive. During pregnancy, most experts agree that moderate consumption of caffeine (less than 200 milligrams per day) is fine for the mother and baby. A few studies, however, show that consuming even a moderate amount during the first trimester can increase the risk of miscarriage,[12] especially if the expectant parent also uses alcohol or tobacco.

Consuming caffeine throughout pregnancy also can reduce the baby's birth weight. One study found that drinking 100 milligrams of caffeine a day can reduce birth weight by up to 1 ounce. (*Note:* Although lower birth weights may sound appealing to some mothers, babies who are small for gestational age often have additional health problems.) The study also showed that coffee (but not other sources of caffeine) prolonged pregnancy. Pregnancy lasted eight hours longer for every 100 milligrams of caffeinated coffee that the mother drank each day.[13]

Given the potentially harmful effects of caffeine, consider switching to a decaffeinated version of your favorite drink whenever available.

## Herbal Teas, Tinctures, and Capsules

Traditional healers have used herbal remedies for centuries to help treat or cure various ailments. Pharmacies and specialty shops sell hundreds of herbs and dietary supplements, although little is known about their ingredients. The US Food and Drug Administration (FDA) hasn't tested or approved most of these herbs and botanicals, and their safety is often uncertain. When and how an herb was harvested and processed influence a product's potency, which may range widely from one brand to another and even among different batches of the same brand.

It's key to remember that just because herbs are considered "natural," they're not necessarily safe. Some herbal preparations and dietary supplements contain potentially harmful ingredients that may cross the placenta and affect your baby.

### Teas

Some expectant parents switch to herbal teas to minimize caffeine consumption. Many packaged teas are fine in moderation, but be aware of the ingredients. Some herbs may cause undesirable side effects. For example, if you're allergic to ragweed and related plants, you may develop allergic symptoms after drinking chamomile tea. In addition, certain herbs have specific side effects when consumed in large amounts. For example, drinking licorice root tea can increase water retention, raise blood pressure, and decrease potassium. Drinking tea with ginseng can cause swollen and painful breasts.

### Herbal products

During pregnancy, research suggests the potential harm of herbal products on the baby's health stems more from hormonal effects (for example, herbs containing estrogen-like substances) and drug interactions (increasing or decreasing the effect of a prescription medication) than from toxic effects. However, some Chinese herbal medicines, specifically An-Tai-Yin and huanglian, may cause congenital malformations.[14] It's important to consult with your caregiver about any herbal remedies or dietary supplements that you've taken or are considering taking.

### Herbs used in maternity care

For the mother, caregivers sometimes recommend red raspberry leaf to tone uterine muscles. At the end of pregnancy, some caregivers may recommend herbs that can start labor (such as blue cohosh, evening primrose, and black cohosh); however, women should avoid these uterine stimulants in early pregnancy because they may cause miscarriage. Uterine stimulants can also have potentially dangerous side effects. For example, blue cohosh may cause elevated blood pressure, irritated mucous membranes, and multiorgan injury from lack of oxygen. It should be used only under the guidance of a naturopathic doctor or other expert.

## Mercury and Other Substances in Food That May Cause Harm

For information on mercury, food-borne bacteria (such as listeriosis and salmonella), and other substances that can cause harmful illnesses when consumed during pregnancy, see page 114.

# ENVIRONMENTAL HAZARDS AND HARMFUL SITUATIONS

The following sections discuss hazardous substances that are present in many homes and workplaces, as well as harmful situations that can affect the health of your pregnancy and baby, such as being in an abusive relationship or having workplace stress.

## Abuse and Domestic Violence

Abuse and domestic violence (any combination of verbal, psychological, emotional, sexual, economic, or physical abuse) can happen to any woman regardless of her age, physical ability, lifestyle, religion, ethnicity, or socioeconomic and educational backgrounds. When you're pregnant, abuse increases your risk of serious pregnancy problems, such as high blood pressure, vaginal bleeding, severe nausea or vomiting, urinary tract infections (UTIs), preterm birth, a baby with low birth weight, or a baby who needs intensive medical care.[15] In addition, your risk of being killed by an abusive partner increases during pregnancy.[16]

If you're in an abusive relationship, you are *not* at fault. The goal of abuse is to leave you feeling confused, ashamed, powerless, hopeless, and out of control. Living with abuse is painful, confusing, and stressful. The suggestions for coping with stress on page 69 may be useful. Talking with a trusted friend or relative also may help you cope. You may choose to call your caregiver for information on counselors and local agencies that offer support or resources for abused women. If you decide to leave the relationship, you may require their help. Your caregiver also may suggest further testing to detect any sexually transmitted infections (STIs) or to evaluate you for stress-related pregnancy complications. Childhood sexual, emotional, and physical abuse can also have troubling long-term effects that interfere with your joy in pregnancy (see page 56).

National agencies can help you as well. Memorize the phone number for the National Domestic Violence Hotline, 800-799-SAFE (7233), and call if you need to talk to someone or need resources, including help making an escape plan. See also page 356 for more information on abuse and domestic violence.

## Insecticides, Herbicides, and Pesticides

During pregnancy, avoid frequent, sustained exposure to chemicals that kill insects (insecticides), weeds (herbicides), or unwanted insects, bugs, or animals (pesticides). The presence of these chemicals in the air and on food may cause miscarriage, poor growth in the baby, birth defects, and childhood neurobehavioral problems. Because some of these chemicals haven't been tested for their effects on pregnant women and young children, their safety is unknown; however, many governments have banned the use of chemicals that have been proven harmful, such as Glyphosate, which is still a widely used herbicide in the United States. In March 2015, the World Health Organization (WHO) classified glyphosate as "probably carcinogenic in humans."

To avoid exposure to these chemicals, wash fruits and vegetables well or consider buying organic food. If you need to use a pesticide to remove household pests, plan on leaving your home for at least a day to allow the chemicals to dissipate from the air. Before using the pesticide, close all drawers, cupboards, and other doors to food-storage areas. When you return home, wash counters, tables, and food-preparation surfaces thoroughly.

## Occupational Hazards

Some occupations and workplaces may be more hazardous than others during pregnancy. Studies have shown the potential harm of some workplace chemicals, including anesthetic agents, benzene, cancer treatment (cytotoxic) drugs, carbon monoxide, ethylene oxide, ethylene glycol ethers, formaldehyde, ionizing radiation (x-ray), lead, methyl mercury, organic solvents, polybrominated biphenyls (PBBs), polychlorinated biphenyls (PCBs), and the medications listed on page 71. Some chemicals can cause severe problems such as miscarriage, birth defects, low birth weight, preterm birth, developmental delays, and childhood cancers.

People who may encounter these chemicals include health-care workers (including dental and veterinary offices), pharmacists, battery makers, solderers, welders, radiator repairers, industrial painters, home remodelers, and atomic and electronic workers.[17] In addition, farm workers may be exposed to pesticides.

Researchers are constantly revising the list of substances that are harmful in pregnancy, so ask your caregiver about potentially dangerous chemicals. If you work with any dangerous chemicals, talk with your employer about limiting your exposure to them. Visit the websites at right for information about occupational hazards.

## Chemicals Used for Hobbies

Many people enjoy hands-on hobbies such as arts-and-crafts projects, furniture refinishing, and auto repair. Several of these hobbies aren't risky during pregnancy, but some (such as furniture refinishing) may involve exposure to dangerous chemicals. If you plan to continue a hobby that uses a potentially toxic product, learn about risks of exposure during pregnancy by contacting the manufacturer or a poison control center, or by getting the product's Material Safety Data Sheets (MSDS) from a store that sells it.

## House Paint

Many people prepare for parenthood by repairing or renovating their homes, which often includes painting. Caregivers generally discourage pregnant women from spray painting (because they can inhale the paint particles), but rolling or brushing house paint onto surfaces is probably safe during pregnancy. However, many brands of paint contain potentially dangerous chemicals (such as ethylene glycol ethers, mercury, formaldehyde, and hydrocarbon solvents) that you may inhale or absorb through touch. Try to avoid using paints that have these chemicals; instead look for less-toxic, low-VOC or no-VOC paints.

When painting, wear gloves, make sure there's ample ventilation, and consider using a face mask to reduce inhalation of chemical fumes. (Better yet, have someone else do the painting!)

If your home contains lead-based paint (which is often found in homes built before 1978), don't try to remove it or paint over it yourself. There is no known safe level of exposure to lead. Look for a professional painter who is certified to handle lead-paint issues, stay away from home while the work is being done, and wait until the job has been completed and your home is well-cleaned before returning.

## Hair Treatments

Women who have their hair colored or chemically treated may worry whether these treatments will harm their babies during pregnancy. During treatments, a small amount of chemicals can penetrate your skin, but the exposure is unlikely to harm your baby. To minimize the risk of exposure, treat your hair in a well-ventilated area, use gloves to apply chemicals, leave them in no longer than recommended, and rinse your hair thoroughly. Also, consider waiting until the second trimester to treat your hair, when babies are more developed and less vulnerable.

## Saunas, Hot Tubs, and Heat

During pregnancy, exposure to the extreme heat of saunas, hot tubs, or even a hot day outside may raise your baby's temperature along with your own. Once overheated, your baby takes much longer than you to cool down. In early pregnancy, high temperatures can cause birth defects or even miscarriage if the exposure is frequent and prolonged or if it occurs at a critical point in your baby's development. For your baby's safety, keep your body temperature below 102°F (38.9°C) during pregnancy. Avoid using saunas and heat wraps. If you find soaking in a

## Internet Resources about Hazards in Pregnancy

Fact sheets for consumers on many common hazards are available from the Organization of Teratology Information Specialists on its **MotherToBaby** website, http://www.mothertobaby.org/otis-fact-sheets-s13037. Here are some other helpful resources:

**Environmental Working Group**
http://www.ewg.org
**March of Dimes**
http://www.marchofdimes.org
**US Food and Drug Administration (FDA)**
http://www.fda.gov
**LactMed: Drugs and Lactation Database**
http://toxnet.nlm.nih.gov/newtoxnet/lactmed.htm
**US Centers for Disease Control and Prevention (CDC)**
http://www.cdc.gov/pregnancy

hot tub relaxing, turn down the temperature on the hot tub to 99°F (37.2°C), limit use to ten minutes, and keep your shoulders and arms out of the water. Monitor your temperature with a thermometer, if possible. You can also take a warm bath instead.

## Electric Blankets

Consider using a down comforter or wool blankets to keep warm. If you use an electric blanket, make sure you won't get overheated. Set the temperature to low or use the blanket just to warm your sheets and turn it off when you get into bed.

## Ionizing Radiation (X-rays)

High doses of radiation—such as for cancer treatment or ongoing exposure in a workplace with high radiation levels—will harm a developing baby. The level of radiation in diagnostic x-rays, however, is lower. If you're advised to have an x-ray to diagnose a potential health problem, be sure the caregiver knows you're pregnant so the benefits of diagnosing and treating the problem can be weighed against the risk of the radiation.

## Wi-Fi and Radio Frequency Radiation

The prevalence of wireless devices and Wi-Fi hotspots, which emit electromagnetic field radiation (EMF), have increased exponentially over recent years. Long-term studies about the effects during human pregnancy do not yet exist (and will not exist for several decades). Scientists and public health experts recommend that pregnant women take a precautionary approach until more is known. Here are a number of ways you can decrease your exposure to EMF. In general, the farther away you are from EMF-emitting technologies while they are turned on, the lower your exposure. Use a wired headset or the speaker function while speaking on a cell phone. Carry your phone in your purse (held away from your belly) rather than in a pocket. Turn off Wi-Fi routers and Wi-Fi functions on devices when they are not in use. Use wired land lines and Internet connections when possible.

## Infectious Diseases

Several infectious diseases may harm your baby before and after birth. See pages 125–126 for more information.

# THE FATHER'S EXPOSURE TO HAZARDS AND DRUGS

Although little is known about the effects of drugs, environmental and occupational hazards, and other potential dangers on male reproductive health, increasing evidence suggests that a man's exposure to certain hazards during the months before conception may increase the risk of miscarriage, childhood brain tumors, and other problems.[18] Exposure to hazards also may affect a man's fertility. Before conception, men should limit their exposure to the same hazards that are harmful to women in pregnancy, to increase the chances of producing a healthy baby.

In addition, fathers and partners can create an environment that supports a healthy pregnancy by controlling their alcohol, tobacco, or drug use. Before and during pregnancy, a woman is more likely to control her use of alcohol, tobacco, or drugs if her partner (male or female) does so as well.

# Traveling during Pregnancy

Being pregnant doesn't mean you can't take a trip, but you may have some restrictions depending on when, where, and how you'll be traveling. In general, traveling during your second trimester may be an ideal time. Why? If you had low energy and morning sickness in your first trimester, both may have disappeared. Although your belly has grown, you may still be physically comfortable most of the time. In addition, traveling in the second trimester has the least risk of complications such as miscarriage or preterm labor. Traveling during pregnancy may be more enjoyable if you follow some common precautions.

When planning a trip, consult with your caregiver for travel suggestions and any precautions specific to your pregnancy. If you have pregnancy complications, your caregiver may recommend against travel. In the last month of pregnancy, your caregiver may suggest staying within an hour's travel time from home. Even if your pregnancy is healthy, get a copy of your medical history to take with you while traveling.

If you're planning to fly, especially in late pregnancy, find out if your airline has restrictions for pregnant passengers. Some airlines limit travel on domestic flights in the week before a due date, and many have restrictions for international trips. You may be required to provide a note from your caregiver that verifies your due date. Throughout pregnancy, avoid flying at altitudes above 7,000 feet in small planes without pressurized cabins; the oxygen available to your baby may be reduced.

If you're planning to take a cruise, be aware that some cruise-ship companies also have restrictions for passengers in late pregnancy.

If planning a trip to an international destination, check for any special health concerns or travel warnings. If certain vaccinations are recommended before entering a country, check with your caregiver to learn if you can receive them when pregnant. For more information, contact the US Centers for Disease Control's international travel line at 877-394-8747 or visit http://www.cdc.gov/travel. For information about travel warnings, contact the US Department of State at 202-647-5225 or visit http://www.travel.state.gov.

During pregnancy, long trips by car, bus, plane, or train may limit your movement, which can affect your circulation, increase swelling in your legs, and thereby increase your risk of developing a blood clot in a leg vein. Walking every hour or so and stretching as much as possible can eliminate or minimize this risk. In an airplane, try to sit in an aisle seat or one at the bulkhead to allow for more legroom and an easy exit. Do simple exercises while in your seat to help increase circulation to your legs and arms (see chapter 5). If you have varicose veins, consider wearing support stockings (available at medical supply stores).

In vehicles and airplanes, always wear your seat belt to protect you and your baby in a collision. Fasten the belt low on your hip and below your belly. Use the shoulder strap if available; don't tuck it behind you. If an accident occurs, the seat belt will keep you in your seat, while your muscles and pelvic bones protect your uterus and the amniotic fluid cushions your baby.

Pregnancy discomforts may seem worse while traveling. The constant motion may aggravate morning sickness or nausea. Hours of sightseeing or long business meetings may increase fatigue. Back pain may become more noticeable when your usual comfort measures aren't available. The change in routine may disrupt when you eat, as well as what you eat. Air travel, hot climates, and places with forced air ventilation may increase dehydration if your availability to fluids is limited.

To help minimize pregnancy discomforts when traveling, try to drink lots of fluids, eat well, walk around, and get plenty of rest. Try to use your typical comfort measures as best as you can, or adapt them if possible.

## *Key Points to Remember*

- Throughout your pregnancy, you'll have opportunities to improve your health. By learning about healthy lifestyle choices, knowing potential pregnancy hazards to avoid, and recognizing the warning signs of pregnancy problems, you can make the best choices for you and your baby.
- You can improve your chances of having a healthy, safe, and enjoyable pregnancy by actively participating in your prenatal care. Ask key questions about prenatal tests or procedures so you can make informed decisions about whether to have them.
- Eliminating or reducing your exposure to harmful substances and situations will increase your chances of having a healthy pregnancy and baby.

# Feeling Good and Staying Fit

To have a healthy pregnancy, it's important to eat well, get enough rest, and avoid hazards. As your body changes to meet your growing baby's needs, it's also essential to exercise regularly, maintain good posture, and move your body with care. Regular exercise helps improve and maintain your overall health and well-being, and it can help prepare you for the physical challenges of childbirth and postpartum recovery. Maintaining good posture helps prevent back pain and reduce fatigue. Moving comfortably and safely reduces the likelihood of becoming injured or worsening any existing discomforts.

# Maintaining Good Posture and Moving with Care

As your belly grows and your center of gravity shifts forward, maintaining good posture is essential for keeping your balance, preventing back pain, and reducing fatigue. When you're standing, sitting, or lying down, gravity exerts a force on your joints, ligaments, and muscles. Good posture distributes that force evenly throughout your body, preventing excess stress to one or more parts. When someone has good posture, her body is in alignment. When viewing her from the side as she stands, you see that her ears, shoulders, hips, and ankles are in a straight line. (See illustration below.)

As you move your changing body, you protect your muscles, joints, and bones by adjusting how you stand, sit, lie down, lift objects, and so on. Moving with care can reduce fatigue, prevent strain, and minimize common pregnancy discomforts.

## STANDING

To stand with good posture, begin by imagining you're wearing a crown. To keep it in place, position your head so the crown is parallel with the floor. Then use your neck muscles to pull your head back until your ears are in line with your shoulders. Lengthen your spine and let your hips and ankles align with your ears and shoulders. Remind yourself throughout the day to keep the crown on your head.

During late pregnancy, avoid standing for long periods. Prolonged standing may slow blood flow from your legs to your heart and head, making you feel faint or lightheaded and stressing any swollen veins you may have in your legs, vulva, or anus (hemorrhoids). If you must stand for a long time, shift your weight from leg to leg, march in place, rotate your ankles, or rock back and forth.

To help prevent back pain while standing, place one foot on a stool, chair rung, or opened drawer. After a while, switch to your other foot.

## SITTING

When sitting, follow the same directions for standing with good posture to align your ears, shoulders, and hips.

As your belly grows, you may find that sitting in a straight-back chair is more comfortable (and easier to get out of) than sitting in a low, deep chair. For additional comfort, place a small, firm pillow at the small of your back and a low stool under your feet. To prevent straining your back when rising from a chair, move to the seat edge, lean forward, then push against the arm rests or seat and push through your heels to raise your body.

During late pregnancy, avoid sitting for long periods. Prolonged sitting can affect blood circulation in your legs. If you must stay seated for a long time, shift your position often, rotate your ankles, and avoid crossing your legs at the knees. To help decrease swelling, sit with your feet propped up and calves supported on another chair or ottoman.

## Lying Down

As your pregnancy progresses, staying comfortable while lying down can become more challenging. For example, you may experience heartburn or shortness of breath while lying on your back, especially near the end of pregnancy. To help alleviate  these discomforts, lie on your side or use pillows to prop yourself in a semireclined position. You can also place pillows or a long body pillow under one shoulder, hip, and leg to tilt your body from the back to one side.

Lying on your back can make you feel dizzy or lightheaded. If this happens, roll to your left side or sit up. For some people, lying on their backs in late pregnancy causes *supine hypotension*, in which the uterus presses on the abdominal vein (inferior vena cava) that carries blood from the legs to the heart and causes a drop in blood pressure. Extended supine hypotension can reduce blood flow to the placenta and restrict oxygen to the baby. For this reason, health-care providers recommend that pregnant clients lie on their sides after the twenty-sixth week of pregnancy.

When lying on your side, place a pillow between your knees and another under your head to keep your body in alignment. In late pregnancy, you may need to support your abdomen with a small pillow, a wedge-shaped pad, or a long body pillow.

Some people find lying on their sides more comfortable when they roll their bodies slightly forward. To get into this position, place a firm pillow on the side you'll roll toward. As you roll to this side, keep your lower leg straight and bend the knee of your top leg to rest on the pillow. Rest your lower arm behind you and bend your upper arm at the elbow, setting it in front of you so your hand is near your face.

Lying on your side can cause sore hips. To help manage any pain or swelling, apply an ice pack on the sore area. Also consider supplementing your mattress with a deep foam pad or a pillow-top mattress cover.

## Getting Up after Lying Down

Getting up from lying on the floor or in bed also becomes more difficult as your pregnancy advances. Before your belly started to grow, you got up by sitting straight up, then rising. As your pregnancy progresses, however, this movement may strain your abdominal and lower back muscles.

To get out of bed safely, roll onto your side, put your lower legs over the edge of the bed, push yourself to a sitting position, and stand up.

To get up from the floor, follow these steps:

1. Bend your knees and roll onto your side. Use your arms to raise your upper body.
2. Get onto your hands and knees. Place one foot on the floor in front of you, while keeping the opposite knee on the floor.
3. Use your legs to stand up. For balance, place your hand on your knee or a stable object.

# LIFTING OBJECTS

During pregnancy, hormones cause your ligaments to relax and soften, and the muscles supporting your posture and core (abdominal, pelvic floor, and back muscles) adapt to your changing shape. As a result of these changes, lifting heavy objects while pregnant increases the likelihood of back injury. To help prevent back injury, avoid heavy lifting whenever possible. For example, teach your toddler to climb into his car seat or onto your lap instead of picking him up.

When lifting any object from a low surface (even a sheet of paper), protect your back by following these guidelines:

- Get as close to the object as possible.
- With your feet shoulder-width apart, squat while keeping your back straight and sticking out your buttocks for balance.
- Grasp the object and hold it close to you. Try not to twist at your waist.
- As you rise, tighten your abdominal muscles, and squeeze your pelvic floor muscles upward and exhale (instead of holding your breath) to prevent straining your perineum. Use your legs instead of your lower back to raise your body. Keep your back straight.
- Avoid twisting your spine to turn or set down the object. Instead, move your feet in the direction you want to go.

## General Guidelines for Safe, Effective Exercise

- Exercise three to seven days per week. Try to do a variety of activities. Always include a warm-up and a cool-down.
- Build your strength and endurance gradually. In the beginning, keep the intensity of your workout low to moderate. As your strength and stamina increase, so can the intensity. Toward the end of pregnancy, the intensity should naturally decrease. Late pregnancy is not the time to push your limits.
- Modify exercises so you can do them safely. If taking an exercise class, let the instructor know you're pregnant and request pertinent exercise modifications.
- Lying flat on your back in pregnancy can cause supine hypotension (see page 83). If you feel dizzy, short of breath, or lightheaded while on your back, roll onto your left side until you've recovered.
- To prevent dizziness and to avoid increased pressure on your pelvic floor and abdominal muscles, don't hold your breath while exercising.
- Use the "talk test" (see page 87) to ensure you're not exercising too vigorously.
- Eat enough to meet the caloric needs of pregnancy as well as your exercise regimen. Not eating enough can put you and your baby at risk for complications (see page 111).
- Drink water before, during, and after exercising to replace fluids lost through perspiration and respiration. Keep a water bottle with you.
- Don't exercise vigorously in hot, humid weather or when you have a fever. Your body temperature shouldn't exceed 101°F (38.3°C).
- Stop exercising if you experience pain, headache, nausea, severe breathlessness, dizziness, blurred vision (or you see spots), vaginal bleeding, or continuing strong uterine contractions. (See When *Not* to Exercise on page 85.)
- Be flexible and patient as you work to meet your fitness goals. Pay attention to how your body feels and adapt your exercise regimen accordingly.
- Consult your caregiver or physical therapist if you have questions about exercise.

# Exercise in Pregnancy

When pregnancy makes you feel overwhelmingly tired, uncomfortable, and moody, the last thing you want to do is exercise. But exercise can be just what you need to feel energized and healthy.

Regular, moderate physical activity during pregnancy improves or maintains your muscle tone, strength, and endurance. Exercise also protects against back pain, reduces the intensity of common pregnancy discomforts, and boosts your energy level, mood, and self-image. During the last trimester, regular exercise increases your body's production of endorphins (natural pain relievers), which can help you cope with labor.

## HOLISTIC BENEFITS OF EXERCISE

During the childbearing year (from pregnancy through three months after the birth) and beyond, regular physical activity does more than keep your body fit. Exercise also benefits your mental, emotional, spiritual, and social well-being. All these benefits help you meet the demands of pregnancy, childbirth, and motherhood.

### Physical benefits

Appropriate exercise strengthens the muscles most affected by pregnancy and childbirth, including those in the pelvic floor, abdomen, and lower back. Exercise during pregnancy helps maintain good respiration, circulation, and posture. It can also ease common discomforts of pregnancy, such as constipation, heartburn, shortness of breath, leg cramps, fatigue, swollen ankles, and insomnia.

In addition, maintaining your fitness during pregnancy and the postpartum period more easily helps you recover your energy level, strength, and pre-pregnancy size after the birth.

### Mental and emotional benefits

Regular exercise helps decrease mental stress and fatigue. Aerobic activities release pain-relieving endorphins that improve your sense of well-being, help stabilize hormone-driven mood swings, and can decrease the risk or severity of depression and mood disorders during pregnancy and afterward.

### Spiritual benefits

Whatever your spiritual beliefs, regularly finding time to meditate, relax, or pray lets you quiet your mind and connect to something greater than you (such as nature or a higher power). During this quiet time, let what's most important to you come to mind. Honor the changes you're experiencing and connect and communicate with your baby. An ideal opportunity for this quiet time is during a bath, a walk in nature, or after aerobic exercise, when your body experiences a natural physiologic calmness.

### Social benefits

During the childbearing year, you increasingly need others to offer you support and validate your feelings. Taking prenatal exercise classes lets you connect with other expectant parents, and you may learn about pregnancy, birth, the postpartum period, and newborn care through shared experiences.

## When *Not* to Exercise

Avoid or stop exercising if you have the following conditions:

- vaginal bleeding
- persistent Braxton-Hicks contractions
- increased risk for preterm labor
- preeclampsia
- premature rupture of membranes (loss of fluid from your vagina)
- placenta previa diagnosed after the twenty-sixth week of pregnancy
- a baby with intrauterine growth restriction (IUGR)
- a baby whose movements have noticeably decreased

Consult with your caregiver about exercising if you are pregnant with multiples, are on bed rest, or have high blood pressure, diabetes, chronic heart problems, thyroid disease, or joint disease or injury.

# FINDING YOUR MOTIVATION TO EXERCISE

Throughout pregnancy, your motivation to exercise may ebb and flow as your energy level rises and falls. At times, you know you *should* exercise, but find any excuse not to. When you can't motivate yourself to exercise, reminding yourself of the benefits of physical activity can give you the push you need to keep a regular exercise regimen.

If you need additional help getting your body moving, there are other tricks to try. For example, you're much more likely to do an activity if it's something you enjoy. If you love to dance, consider taking a dance class or dancing at home to some energizing music.

Find what time of day works best to exercise and schedule that time for physical activity. Depending on what trimester you're in, you may need to work around certain physical symptoms. For example, if you have intense heartburn after eating, choose another time to exercise (or eat a lighter meal and bring antacids with you when you exercise).

Sometimes hearing or reading encouraging words or listening to your favorite music can motivate you. Even an activity you might not enjoy, such as housecleaning, can be fun exercise if you play your favorite music. Perhaps warm up with some light dusting, then mop and vacuum vigorously before ending with some gentle stretching. If encouraging words or music motivate you, consider sharing this information with your labor-support team to give them ideas for motivating you during labor.

If you don't want to exercise because you're feeling down or your back aches, remind yourself that exercise can help relieve these and other emotional and physical problems. If you have trouble making time to exercise regularly on your own, consider signing up for a class, hiring a personal trainer, or scheduling a regular appointment to do a physical activity with someone. The extra commitment may prompt you to make the time to exercise.

Visit our website, http://www.PCNGuide.com, to download a work sheet to record your fitness goals. If you try every trick to get yourself to exercise but are unsuccessful, be kind to yourself and try again the next day.

# EXERCISE OPTIONS

Aerobic exercise is physical activity that increases your heart rate for an extended time, which improves endurance and strengthens your heart and lungs. Anaerobic exercise focuses on strengthening certain muscles and improving balance and flexibility. Both kinds of exercise benefit your health.

How much you should exercise and what kind of activities you should do depend on your general health, the health of your pregnancy, your fitness level, and your usual activity level. Physical changes during pregnancy directly affect your tolerance for exercise. Hormonal changes cause your ligaments to relax and your joints to become more mobile. Your growing belly shifts your center of gravity forward. Changes in your cardiovascular system increase your heart rate more quickly, and your body temperature and metabolic rate (the rate at which you burn calories) are higher.

As you become more aware of these changes, you can better sense when something doesn't feel right and can fix the problem. For example, if an activity leaves you excessively tired, do it more slowly next time or do a less demanding activity instead. If your pelvis feels unstable or painful because of pelvic joint problems, avoid asymmetrical movements with your legs (such as taking the stairs or doing pigeon pose in yoga). Responding to your body's signals when exercising also prepares you to respond to physical cues in labor and after the birth.

To ensure that an exercise regimen is appropriate for you, consult with your caregiver before starting or continuing to exercise. You may also want to consult with a physical therapist who specializes in pregnancy. This professional can assess any discomforts you have and customize exercises that will benefit you most.

## Aerobic Exercise

In general, low-impact aerobic exercise is best for pregnant women because it doesn't involve movements that can strain joints and the pelvic floor, such as jumping and running. Low-impact activities include brisk walking, cycling, low-impact aerobics, and even cross-country skiing. Dance classes—including belly dancing, Nia, and Zumba—can also provide appropriate total-body workouts. Elliptical machines and stationary bikes offer safe workouts as well; however, be aware that spinning classes can quickly elevate your heart rate and body temperature.

Swimming or taking a water aerobics class provides a total-body workout with the lowest possible impact, because the water reduces the force of gravity on your body. In addition, standing or sitting in water that reaches your shoulders reduces swelling (edema) by pushing tissue fluid into your circulation (and eventually out of your body through urination).

Ideally, you should do some kind of aerobic exercise at least three times per week. Aerobic exercise regimens for pregnant women should include the following:

- at least a five-minute warm-up, consisting of slow, smooth movements and stretching
- about thirty minutes of aerobic exercise of moderate to vigorous intensity
- at least a five-minute cool-down (until your heart rate returns to what it was before you began the workout), consisting of mild activity and possibly exercises for strength, flexibility, and relaxation

If you're just beginning an exercise regimen, start slowly and gently. To determine whether you're exercising too hard, take the "talk test."[1] If you can talk without gasping while exercising, your heart rate is at an acceptable level. If you can't talk without gasping, slow down until you can.

## Anaerobic Exercise

The following exercise practices don't increase your heart rate as much as aerobic exercise does, but offer other health benefits.

### Yoga

This practice promotes self-nurturing and harmony of the mind, body, and spirit. Yoga also strengthens core muscles (abdominal, pelvic floor, and back) and postural muscles, and improves flexibility, balance, breathing, and mental focus (see page 95).

### Pilates

Pilates is a system of conditioning exercises that strengthens core and postural muscles and improves flexibility and mental focus. During the childbearing year, avoid doing advanced abdominal exercises. They can aggravate or cause abdominal separation (see page 334).

### Tai Chi

This system of exercises emphasizes balance, focus, meditation, and smooth, fluid movement.

### Weightlifting

Weightlifting strengthens the targeted muscles and core muscles (when you contract them to stabilize your body). If you lifted weights regularly before becoming pregnant, you can continue working with light weights. If you didn't lift weights before pregnancy and want to begin a regimen, do so only under the direction of a professional trainer knowledgeable about pregnancy. Vigorous weightlifting workouts, such as CrossFit, can strain the abdominals and pelvic floor if not significantly modified.

Gyms, community centers, and even some hospitals offer beginning or prenatal yoga, Pilates, tai chi, and weightlifting classes. You can also find many excellent classes online or on DVD.

## Sports and High-Intensity Activities

Pregnancy isn't the time to take up a new sport or activity that requires good balance or sudden movements, or puts you at risk for falling. If before becoming pregnant you played sports such as tennis or softball, or engaged in activities such as vigorous swimming or cycling, you may continue doing them while pregnant for as long as you feel comfortable and if your pregnancy remains low risk.

In late pregnancy, avoid downhill skiing, water-skiing, snowmobiling, and horseback riding, regardless of your skill level. These activities require excellent balance (which you might not have), and your likelihood of falling increases if you participate in them.

Throughout your pregnancy, avoid potentially dangerous activities, such as skydiving, scuba diving, springboard diving, surfing, rock or mountain climbing (especially at elevations higher than 6,000 feet).

To decide whether the benefits of a particular athletic activity outweigh the possible risks, ask yourself the key questions on page 9. If you have further questions about an activity's safety, talk with your caregiver.

# Core Exercises to Prepare You for Labor

Core muscles include the abdominal and deep back muscles, pelvic floor muscles, and diaphragm (breathing muscle). All of these muscles work together to provide stability, balance, and proper posture. Giving birth relies on these muscles, and conditioning them during pregnancy prepares them for labor and promotes their speedy recovery afterward.

## CONDITIONING YOUR PELVIC FLOOR MUSCLES

Your *pelvic floor muscles* comprise three layers of muscles that have varying functions. The innermost layer is connected to the base of your pelvis and acts like a sling to support the pelvic organs. During pregnancy, the increased weight of your uterus and the relaxing effect of hormones put an increased demand on these muscles. Learning how to work with your pelvic floor muscles through strengthening exercises, down-training, or perineal massage (see page 252) can benefit you during pregnancy, birth, and the postpartum period. Strengthening the pelvic floor muscles during pregnancy can reduce the heavy, throbbing feeling you may experience in the area and can help prevent incontinence (leaking urine or feces) and control flatulence (gas).

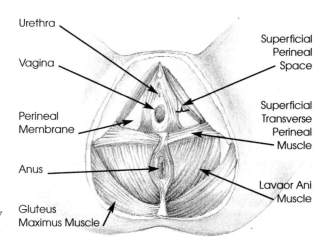

Pelvic floor exercises can prepare you for labor by letting you work with these muscles as they stretch in preparation for pushing your baby out. When these muscles are healthy, they can more easily return to their original length after being stretched, which helps with postpartum recovery. As an added benefit, having normally functioning pelvic floor muscles can make sex more enjoyable and satisfying throughout your lifetime.

For proper functioning, pelvic floor muscles must have good muscle length, tone, symmetry, coordination, strength, responsiveness, and endurance. All of these variables show that pelvic floor exercises are not "one size fits all." For most women, regularly doing exercises that strengthen and support pelvic floor muscles help maintain their function and improve circulation in the area during the childbearing year and beyond.

To check the strength of your pelvic floor muscles, try these exercises:

- While urinating, partially empty your bladder, then stop the flow. If you can't, your muscles aren't performing well and are probably weak. Do this test only once or twice—any more often and you may interrupt the complex neuropathways of your urinary system (that is, how your brain and urinary system communicate).
- Insert one or two fingers into your vagina and tighten your pelvic floor muscles until you feel them squeeze your fingers. The tighter the squeeze is, the stronger your muscles are.
- During intercourse, you can ask for your partner's feedback about the strength of your pelvic muscles as you tighten around the penis or fingers.

If the muscles seem weak, pelvic floor contractions can help (see page 90). If the muscles are very tense, they may need to be "down-trained" to help them relax when at rest. Down-training tight muscles can help you more successfully push your baby out. The following problems may point to a pelvic floor with high muscular tension:

- pain in vagina, rectum, tailbone, sacrum, lower back, or hips
- straining or difficulty with bowel movements

- pain or discomfort during intercourse or orgasm
- urinary issues (trouble starting to urinate, stopping and starting while urinating, not completely emptying the bladder, or pain while urinating)

A pelvic floor with any of these problems may benefit from pelvic floor relaxation or bulging (see below and page 91). When first testing your pelvic floor muscles, don't worry if they seem weak or too tense. Muscles are dynamic and will respond to strengthening or relaxing exercises.

You may wonder which exercises are right for you and how to do them correctly. You're not alone. For example, women are often advised to do pelvic floor contractions, but many report that they don't know if they're doing them right. The best way to know what you need to do to prepare your pelvic floor muscles for birth (and beyond) is to have them evaluated by a specialist trained in internal pelvic floor techniques, such as a women's health physical therapist. A specialist can give you feedback on muscle function and teach you how to properly do the exercises that are most effective for you.

## Pelvic Floor Contractions (Kegels)

**Aim:** To strengthen your pelvic floor muscles, improve blood circulation in them, decrease the incidence and severity of hemorrhoids and incontinence, and support your uterus and other pelvic organs.

**Starting position:** Lying on your back or side is easiest. You can progress to sitting and standing positions and use gravity to further strengthen the muscles.

**Exercise:** Without holding your breath, tighten the muscles around your urethra and vaginal opening as if you're stopping the flow of urine. (Try not to tighten the muscles in your buttocks, thighs, or abdomen.) You should feel your pelvic floor lift slightly and become tense. Hold tightly for ten seconds. You can put your hand on your pelvic floor to feel if it's lifting.

At first, you may notice the muscle tension diminishing or fading without your control before ten seconds has passed. If so, tighten the muscles again until time is up, then relax for five seconds before doing another contraction. Do up to ten repetitions. If you're unable to hold the contraction for ten seconds, hold it for as long as you can and remember that Kegels are more challenging during pregnancy. You'll strengthen your pelvic floor more effectively in the postpartum period.

**Repetition:** Try to do several sets of ten Kegels throughout the day.

## Pelvic Floor Relaxation

**Aim:** To reduce muscular tension in your pelvic floor, to improve your mind-body connection to this area, and to prepare you for pushing your baby out. Make sure your bladder is empty when practicing this exercise.

**Starting position:** In a relaxed environment, lie down in a comfortable position with your body fully supported.

**Exercise:** Relax your whole body by doing the relaxation countdown (see page 236). Bring your attention to your pelvic floor. Visualize these muscles letting go, melting, or becoming heavy. Then bring your attention to your breath. Notice that when you inhale deeply, your pelvic floor naturally bulges downward. When you exhale, your pelvic floor naturally lifts back up. Inhale and exhale several times, paying attention to the sensation in your pelvic floor. Be patient if you don't feel it at first—it's subtle, and recognizing it is part of the process.

**Repetition:** Try to practice this exercise daily. Progress to practicing it while sitting.

## *Pelvic Floor Bulging*

**Aim:** To prepare for pushing your baby out (the second stage of labor). Make sure your bladder is empty when practicing this exercise

**Starting position:** Tailor-sit (sit cross-legged on the floor) or get into any birthing position (see pages 240).

**Exercise:** Consciously relax your pelvic floor muscles. Hold your breath and bear down gently as you do when having a bowel movement, letting your pelvic floor muscles further relax and bulge outward. Don't bear down or strain forcefully. (Put your hand on your perineum to help you feel the bulge.) Hold for three to five seconds, then stop bearing down. Inhale, contract your pelvic floor muscles, then exhale and rest. After you can do this exercise while holding your breath, try it while exhaling. Notice how your breathing changes the effectiveness of the bulge.

**Repetition:** Do this exercise one to two times per week.

# CONDITIONING YOUR ABDOMINAL MUSCLES

Conditioning your abdominal muscles during pregnancy helps you maintain good posture, keep your core stable, avoid pain in your back or pelvis, push your baby out more easily, and recover your abdominal strength after the birth. The four layers of your abdominal muscles work together with other core muscles to bend your body forward or sideways, rotate your trunk, tilt your pelvis, help with breathing, and stabilize your body when you lift objects.

Because your growing uterus already stretches your abdominal muscles, doing traditional exercises that work these muscles puts you at risk for back and abdominal strains. In late pregnancy, avoid doing double leg lifts or abdominal crunches (traditional sit-ups). The following exercises condition your abdominal muscles without causing excessive strain.

## *Transverse Abdominal Contractions*

**Aim:** To strengthen your innermost abdominal layer (transverse abdominis), which provides core stability and helps you actively push your baby out. After the birth, this exercise begins flattening your abdomen and closing any muscle separation (see page 334).

**Starting position:** Sit upright with your back supported against a straight-back chair or a wall.

**Exercise:** Inhale deeply, letting your abdomen expand. Slowly exhale, bringing your belly button toward your spine. (Put your hand on your belly to ensure you're doing this movement.) Hold the contraction for ten to twenty seconds without holding your breath.

**Variation:** Pulse the contraction by releasing it slightly as you inhale and tightening it as you exhale. Pulse ten to twenty times.

**Repetition:** Begin with two sets of ten repetitions and add repetitions as you become stronger. Expect this exercise to become more difficult in late pregnancy, and remember it's also good to do after the birth.

## Pelvic Tilts I, II, and III

**Aim:** To strengthen your abdominal muscles, improve posture, and relieve back pain.
**Starting position:** Lie on your back, get on your hands and knees, or stand. (See following sections for further directions.)

**Exercise:** With an exhalation, tighten your abdominal muscles and hold the contraction for five to ten seconds. Imagine that these muscles are hugging your baby. Contract your lower abdominals to tilt the front of your pelvis upward. Return to starting position, then repeat.

**Repetition:** Do ten pelvic tilts each day.

### I. Pelvic tilt on your back

**Starting position:** Lie on your back with knees bent and feet flat on the floor. When contracting your abdominal muscles, the small of your back flattens onto the floor. Don't push with your feet or tighten your buttocks. Placing a hand under your lower back may make it easier to feel that the small of your back is flattening. *Note:* If you feel dizzy or lightheaded while on your back, roll onto your left side and try pelvic tilt II or III instead.

### II. Pelvic tilt on hands and knees

**Starting position:** Get on your hands and knees. Keep your back in a neutral position (neither sagging nor arched) and your knees hip-width apart. As you tighten your abdominal muscles, your pelvis curls under and your lower back arches. Your upper back may arch as well.

### III. Pelvic tilt when standing

**Starting position:** Lean against a wall with knees slightly bent and feet apart and 12 to 15 inches away from the wall. Let your buttocks and shoulders touch the wall. As you contract your abdominal muscles, your back presses against the wall.

After you've mastered the pelvic tilt while leaning against a wall, try it while standing upright. As you tighten your abdominal muscles in this starting position, your pubic bone tilts upward, tilting the top of your pelvis backward. To feel this movement, put your hands on your hips.

## PREPARING FOR THE SECOND STAGE OF LABOR WITH SQUATS

During the second stage of labor (pushing phase), positions that use gravity can help the baby descend through the pelvis. Squatting not only works with gravity, but it also lets the pelvic joints be mobile while the inner thighs pull open the pelvic outlet.

*Caution:* If you have problems with your hips, knees, ankles, pelvis, or have hemorrhoids, avoid squatting.
**Aim:** To become more comfortable in this position, increase the flexibility of your pelvic joints, and stretch the muscles of your inner thighs and calves.
**Starting position:** Stand with your feet about 24 inches apart.

**Exercise:** Keeping your heels on the floor, squat by lowering your buttocks toward the floor and letting your lower back curve. For better stability and more of a curve in your lower back, distribute your weight evenly between your heels and toes. Hold the position for as long as is comfortable, then use your legs to rise slowly. As you become stronger, increase the amount of time you hold the position to ninety seconds, which is roughly the length of a long labor contraction.

If you have trouble squatting, try stretching the muscles of your inner thighs by tailor-sitting with your soles touching. If you can't maintain your balance when squatting, hold on to a stable piece of furniture, the door-knobs on either side of a door, or your partner's hands. You can also try this alternative position if squatting causes pain in your legs or pubic area: Have your partner sit on a chair. Facing away from your partner, stand between your partner's knees. Then squat, leaning back with your arms over the knees.

If it's difficult to keep your heels on the floor when squatting or if your feet roll inward, your calf muscles are tight. Try squatting with your feet farther apart, wearing shoes with heels of moderate height, putting a book under each heel, or placing a rolled-up mat or towel under your heels. Many birthing beds in hospitals have squat bars to grip while squatting.

**Repetition:** Getting and staying in a full squatting position takes practice. Starting at about the thirty-fifth week of pregnancy, squat for thirty seconds ten times each day. Try to relax your pelvic floor as you squat.

## Common Q & A

**Q:** I know it's good to squat during pregnancy, but I'm having trouble getting up from the position. What can I do?

**A:** To rise from a squat more easily, add an exercise to strengthen your thighs and buttocks, such as wall-sitting. Stand with your back resting against a wall and your feet 12 inches away from the wall. Bend your knees so they're directly above your feet, letting your back slide down the wall. Remain in this position for up to one minute. Try to rise by pushing through your heels. Repeat this exercise five to ten times each day. As you become stronger, place your feet farther from the wall, until you can bend your knees 90 degrees and your thighs are parallel with the floor.

# Postural Exercises to Align Your Body

Your postural muscles keep your body in proper alignment. Having good posture throughout your lifetime allows your body to function optimally. During pregnancy, your center of gravity shifts forward as your baby and uterus grow, requiring you to make an extra effort to maintain good posture (see page 82).

The normal changes of pregnancy also stretch your abdominal and upper back muscles and tighten your pectoral (chest) muscles and hip flexors (the muscles in the front of your hips). Strengthening and stretching these muscles helps relieve lower back pain and other discomforts that can arise when your body is out of alignment.

## POSTURE CHECK

To maintain correct postural alignment, prevent back pain, reduce fatigue, and allow optimal body function, it's important to check your posture several times throughout the day. Follow the instructions on page 82 to ensure good posture when standing or sitting.

## *Shoulder Circles*

**Aim:** To release tension and put your shoulders into correct postural alignment.
**Starting position:** Stand or sit with your back straight. Keep your arms relaxed and your chin level.
**Exercise:** Raise your shoulders toward your ears, then slowly roll them back and down, then forward and up. Feel the tension release. End with your shoulders in a relaxed back-and-down position.
**Repetition:** Circle your shoulders as many times throughout the day as feels comfortable.

## PECTORAL STRETCH

**Aim:** To lengthen your pectoral muscles, which naturally shorten during pregnancy or with poor posture. This exercise also may help you breathe more deeply.
**Starting position:** Stand with good posture in a doorway.
**Exercise:** With your elbow at shoulder level, rest your forearm on the doorframe. While pulling your shoulder blades down your spine, turn your body away from the doorframe until you feel your chest stretch. Breathe deeply, letting your ribs expand with each inhalation. Hold the stretch for fifteen to thirty seconds. Relax, then repeat on your other side.
**Repetition:** Stretch your pectoral muscles twice on each side.

## HIP FLEXOR STRETCH

**Aim:** To stretch the muscles in the front of your hips that naturally tighten in pregnancy and from too much sitting.
**Starting position:** Stand with your right leg forward (knee slightly bent) and your left leg back (knee straight). Keep both feet flat on the floor and about hip-width apart. You can hold on to a stable chair for support.
**Exercise:** Contract your left buttock and pull the front of your pelvis upward (as you do with the pelvic tilt—see page 92) until you feel a stretch in the front of your left hip. Hold the stretch for fifteen to thirty seconds. Relax, then repeat with your left leg forward and your right leg back.
**Repetition:** Stretch your hip flexors twice on each side.

# Yoga Poses to Align Your Body, Mind, and Spirit

Yoga builds strength and stamina, improves flexibility and balance, encourages mindfulness, increases energy, and promotes meditation (which calms the mind and nourishes the spirit).

Unlike many other forms of exercise, yoga focuses on *practicing* movements, not *mastering* them. Even if you practice yoga regularly, you may feel flexible and strong one day and less so the next—and that's okay. Letting go of expectations and self-criticism is essential to the practice of yoga.

This section features yoga poses that especially benefit you during pregnancy and birth. It also includes a sequence of poses that mimics the rhythm of labor by alternating poses that require exertion with those that call for relaxation. Because your joints are more relaxed in pregnancy, the goal is to promote muscle flexibility, while protecting your joints by not pushing your range of motion too far.

While doing these poses, make sure you control your movements and pay attention to your body position, mental activity, and emotional reactions. What you learn may help you work with your body in labor. For more guidance, consider taking a prenatal yoga class or following a class on DVD.

Whenever you feel dizzy in a pose, lie on your left side to recover.

## Cat Pose

**Aim:** To strengthen your abdominal muscles and stretch your back. This pose may help your baby assume a head-down position for birth.

**Starting position:** Get on your hands and knees.

**Exercise:** Inhale and relax the muscles in your back while lifting your tailbone and breastbone. As you exhale, round your mid-back, letting your head, tailbone, and breastbone sink toward the floor. Flatten your mid-back with your next inhalation, making sure your belly doesn't sag.

**Repetition:** Do this pose for five inhalations and exhalations, keeping the movements smooth.

## Opposite-Limb Extensions

**Aim:** To strengthen your core and postural muscles and help you coordinate your breathing with muscle exertion.

**Starting position:** Get on your hands and knees. In early pregnancy or after the birth, you can lie on your stomach.

**Exercise:** Extend one leg back, with your toes on the floor. Tighten your abdominal muscles to pull your belly button toward your spine. Inhale and tuck your tailbone as you lift your straight leg behind you,

then exhale and reach the opposite arm out in front of you. Breathing evenly, lengthen the stretch by reaching toward the wall behind you with your heel and the wall in front of you with your fingertips. Keep your gaze on the floor and your back in a neutral position. Lower your arm and leg after a few breaths, and repeat with the opposite arm and leg. If you have trouble extending an arm and leg at the same time, extend them one at a time.

**Repetition:** Do this pose five times for each side.

## Yoga Practice for Labor Preparation

This sequence of poses mimics the rhythm of labor (contractions followed by periods of rest) by alternating poses that require exertion with those that call for rest.

- Tailor-sit with eyes closed while focusing on your breathing, quieting mental distractions, and concentrating on being with your baby.
- Cat pose
- Child's pose
- Opposite-limb extensions
- Child's pose
- Downward-facing dog
- Child's pose
- Half-dog pose
- Final pose for relaxation or meditation: Choose corpse pose, side-lying, legs-up-the-wall pose (see page 100), or tailor-sitting.

*Note:* Adapt your yoga practice to accommodate how you're feeling. If at any time you become dizzy or fatigued, rest in child's pose or lie on your left side.

# CHILD'S POSE

**Aim:** To widen your pelvis, stretch your groin and torso, and provide active relaxation between more challenging poses.

**Starting position:** Kneel on the floor with your knees in a wide V, then rest your bottom on your heels.

**Exercise:** Keeping your torso straight, slowly bend forward from the hips, using your arms to guide yourself forward onto the floor. Fold your arms on the floor and rest your head on your forearms. (If this position causes too deep of a stretch, prop yourself up on bent elbows.) If your buttocks have risen, try to return them to your heels. Rest your forehead on the floor and breathe deeply and evenly.

For more of a stretch, rest your forehead on the floor and extend your arms out in front of your head. Use your fingers to pull and lengthen your torso.

**Duration:** Remain in this position for five full breaths, or for as long as it takes to relax.

# DOWNWARD-FACING DOG

**Aim:** To stretch your calf and hamstring muscles (which become tighter as pregnancy progresses), reduce fatigue, and improve circulation in your legs. This pose also helps relieve tension in your shoulders and spine, and helps improve upper body strength while stretching your chest.

**Starting position:** Get on your hands and knees.

**Exercise:** Spread your fingers wide with the middle finger of each hand pointing straight ahead of you. Tuck your toes under and inhale deeply. As you exhale, make an inverted V with your body by lifting your tailbone toward the ceiling, straightening your legs, and lengthening your spine. Let your head hang and breathe evenly. Position your feet so they're hip-width apart and your toes are facing forward. Try to rest your heels on the floor. To release the pose, lower your knees or get into child's pose to rest completely.

**Duration:** Hold this pose for five full breaths.

# HALF-DOG POSE

**Aim:** To stretch your back, release tension in your shoulders, and stretch your hamstrings. You can use this pose as an alternative to downward-facing dog.

**Starting position:** Stand facing a wall, then lean forward and place your hands shoulder-width apart on the wall. Walk your feet backward as you bend forward from the hips, sliding your hands down the wall until your back and arms are parallel with the floor. Keep your head in line with your arms and gaze at the floor.

**Exercise:** Inhale and push your hands into the wall. As you exhale, elongate your spine by stretching your tailbone straight out behind you. To keep the natural curve of your spine, rotate your sit bones (the bones you sit on) upward to keep your lower back from flattening.

**Duration:** Hold this pose for five to ten full breaths.

## Corpse Pose

**Aim:** To completely relax while remaining awake and attentive. This restorative pose nurtures the mind-body-spirit connection and helps you connect to your baby.

**Starting position:** Lie on your back with your legs extended, your arms by your side (but not touching you), and your palms up.

**Exercise:** Actively lengthen your body from your heels, through your arms and head. Then relax all your muscles. End the pose by rolling onto your side and into a fetal position. Stay in this position for a few moments, until you feel ready to sit up.

If you become lightheaded, dizzy, or short of breath while on your back (common in late pregnancy), do this pose by lying on your left side and cradling your head with your arms or placing pillows under your head and between your legs.

**Duration:** Stay in this pose for five to ten minutes.

## Five-Minute Meditation

**Aim:** To nurture your mind-body-spirit connection as well as your connection to your baby, and create time to release tension and focus on what's important to you. This exercise lets you release your need for control and embrace "going with the flow"—an important mind-set for pregnancy, childbirth, and parenthood. This exercise can follow or be integrated into corpse pose.

**Starting position:** Because you can do this exercise anywhere, choose a position that works in the moment and one that you can comfortably maintain for five minutes. Options include tailor-sitting, lying on your back or left side, legs-up-the-wall pose (see page 100), sitting in a chair, or lying in a warm bath.

**Exercise:** Quiet any distracting thoughts by focusing on your breathing. With each breath, let your body and mind release any tension and expectations so you can completely relax. Take this time to thank your hardworking body, send your baby loving energy, and honor yourself as well as your partner and family. This exercise can clarify your hopes and fears, and can reveal any gaps in your childbirth preparation or support system. You can also use this time to practice the visualization techniques discussed on page 226.

**Duration:** As the birth approaches, you may want to meditate for longer than five minutes, and you may want to meditate more often.

# Comfort Measures for
# Common Discomforts in Pregnancy

Even if you consistently maintain good posture, move with care, and exercise moderately, you may still experience discomforts during pregnancy. This section explains the causes of some common discomforts, offers ways you can prevent or minimize them, and suggests treatments to relieve them.

## LOWER BACK PAIN

Over the course of your pregnancy, your abdominal muscles lengthen up to 120 percent. To maintain your balance and alignment, your lower back muscles and hip flexors shorten and tighten, which may cause lower back pain. Here are ways to help prevent lower back pain:

- Maintain good posture. (Poor posture often contributes to back pain.)
- Move with care to prevent straining joints, ligaments, and tendons (which soften and relax from hormonal changes).
- Use positions and exercises that stretch tight muscles and strengthen abdominal muscles.

To relieve pain from muscular tension, use a heating pad or hot-water bottle, or take a warm bath or shower. Use an ice pack to decrease inflammation and relieve pain. For enjoyable relief, get a professional massage or have your partner give you a soothing back rub.

Here are exercises that can relieve lower back pain:
- half-dog pose, cat pose, or child's pose (see pages 96–97)
- pelvic tilt on hands and knees (see page 92)
- tailor-sitting (sitting in this position can keep your lower back relaxed)
- squatting (see page 92)

Another good exercise to try is the **knee-to-shoulder exercise**. Here's how to do it: Lie on your back. Draw one knee toward your chest and hold that leg behind your thigh with one hand, then do the same for your other leg. Keep your knees apart to avoid putting pressure on your belly. Keeping your head on the floor, gently pull your knees toward your shoulders until you feel a slight stretch in your lower back. Hold for a slow count of five, then release without letting go of your knees. Stretch your lower back this way five times. Then lower your feet one at a time. Roll onto your side after you've finished the exercise.

*Note:* In late pregnancy, you may wish to pull only one leg at a time. If this exercise makes you dizzy or lightheaded, don't do it.

## UPPER BACK PAIN

As your pregnancy progresses, your breasts become heavier and your pectoral (chest) muscles shorten as your upper back muscles lengthen. Your shoulder and neck muscles may try to compensate for these changes by working harder. To prevent or relieve upper back pain, try to maintain proper posture, stretch your pectoral muscles regularly, and do movements to reduce tension in your shoulders, neck, and jaw. Several times a day, take a deep breath, relax your jaw, and roll your shoulders back and down. Massage and the relaxation exercises described in chapter 12 can also help ease upper back pain.

Shoulder circles (see page 94) and half-dog pose (see page 96) help increase circulation, stretch tense muscles, and decrease back pain. An **upper body stretch** can also help. Here's how to do this exercise: Sit in a chair, tailor-sit on the floor, or stand. Raise your arms (palms down) in front of you to shoulder height. Cross them at the elbows; feel your upper back stretch. While inhaling slowly, raise your hands toward the ceiling and gradually uncross your arms (as if pulling a shirt over your head). Reach upward to feel the stretch in your entire upper body. Keeping your arms extended, exhale as you lower them in an arc along each side of your body until your hands are about 12 inches from each hip. Point your thumbs behind you and tilt your head to look up. Feel the stretch across your chest and upper arms. Maintain this stretch as you breathe deeply, allowing your rib cage to expand. Release your arms to your sides and relax without slumping. Repeat this entire sequence five times.

## Relieving Severe Back Pain

If you have severe back pain, ask your caregiver to refer you to a physical therapist or chiropractor who specializes in perinatal issues. This expert can provide treatment that may include ice packs, heat, hydrotherapy, massage, techniques to mobilize joints, and an exercise regimen designed to address your specific problem. Your caregiver may recommend that you wear a special garment or belt to support your abdomen and lower back.

## TINGLING OR NUMBNESS IN YOUR ARMS OR HANDS

Especially during the night or in the morning after awakening, excess tissue fluid during pregnancy puts pressure on the nerves and blood vessels, causing tingling or numbness in the arms or hands. If the symptoms are confined to the hands, the condition is called "carpal tunnel syndrome." If symptoms involve the entire arm, it's called "thoracic outlet syndrome."

To prevent or treat the problem, try the following suggestions:

- Lie on your side in a position that supports you without lying on your arm. Or use pillows to support you (see page 83).
- Try doing shoulder circles and the upper body stretch (see pages 94 and above).
- Several times a day, stretch one arm upward. Wiggle your fingers for a slow count of five. Lower your arm and repeat with your other arm.
- If you have severe carpal tunnel syndrome, wear a wrist splint (available at pharmacies) to hold your wrist in the best position to prevent tingling and numbness.
- For thoracic outlet syndrome, try raising your arms to shoulder height, then bending your elbows and placing one hand on top of the other on your forehead. *Note:* Wearing a wrist splint doesn't relieve thoracic outlet syndrome.

# ACHING LEGS, SWOLLEN FEET AND ANKLES, OR VARICOSE VEINS

Hormonal changes and increased body weight often affect the blood circulation in pregnant women, causing aching legs, swollen feet and ankles, or varicose veins. To promote better circulation and ease or prevent these discomforts, try these suggestions:

- As soon as you start to notice these discomforts, do something that relieves them (for example, change position).
- Prolonged standing, walking, and sitting can aggravate these discomforts. Try not to stay in any position too long.
- When sitting, avoid crossing your legs at the knees and instead elevate your legs. If you plan to sit for a while, try rocking in a rocking chair to exercise the muscles in your legs and feet.
- These discomforts are often worse at the end of the day. Consider doing more strenuous activities earlier in the day.
- Do pelvic tilts on your hands and knees (see page 92). This exercise reduces the weight of your uterus on the blood vessels in the pelvis and abdomen. The rocking movement promotes blood flow.
- Walk (or play) in deep water for an hour every other day. The weight of the water presses on your swollen tissues, reducing swelling and promoting urination to get rid of the excess fluid. These benefits last for about forty-eight hours. If you use a hot tub, make sure the water temperature doesn't exceed 99°F (37.2°C).
- Wear support stockings, especially if your job requires a lot of standing. The best time to put on the stockings is before you get out of bed in the morning, because the swelling is at its minimum after you've been lying down for an extended time. Standing for long hours may also lead to heaviness or pressure on the vulva. You can purchase specialty compression garments to help relieve the pressure.

To decrease swelling while relaxing, you may want to try the **legs-up-the-wall pose**. To do this yoga exercise, place a folded blanket 6 inches from a wall. Sit on the edge of the blanket so your side is parallel with the wall

and your hip is touching it. Bend your knees. As you lean backward, bring your knees to your chest, then extend your legs up the wall as you rotate your body 90 degrees. Your buttocks now should be on the blanket, and your legs should be relatively straight. Hold this pose for five minutes. If you like, instead of having your legs straight up the wall, stretch your inner thighs by separating your legs into a V shape. Or you can bend your knees, plant your feet on the wall, and lift your hips (but only if your membranes, or bag of waters, haven't yet ruptured).

To get out of this pose, bend your knees, then roll onto your side. Stay on your side for a few breaths before sitting up. *Note:* If you feel dizzy, short of breath, or uncomfortable in this pose, roll onto your left side and remain there until the symptoms disappear.

# LOWER LEG AND FOOT CRAMPS

Cramps in the calves or feet commonly occur when women are resting or asleep. Several things can cause cramps, including pressure on leg nerves, dehydration, impaired circulation, fatigue in calf muscles, or a mineral imbalance in the blood (that is, too little calcium or magnesium, or too much phosphorus, which is found in foods such as soft drinks and processed foods).

To prevent cramps, eat well, drink plenty of water, and avoid pointing your toes or standing on your tiptoes. Right before going to bed, try the following exercises to stretch your calves or hamstrings.

## Relieving Lower Leg Cramps

Stand with your weight on the cramped leg. Step forward with your other foot and bend the knee of that leg. Keeping the knee of your cramped leg straight and the heel on the floor, lean forward to stretch the cramped muscle.

If the cramp is severe, you may need help from your partner. Sit on a chair or bed and have your partner hold the knee of your cramped leg steady with one hand and, while gripping your heel with the other hand, use the forearm to gently press your foot and toes up toward your knee.

## Relieving Foot Cramps

A cramp in your foot tightens the muscles of the arch and curls the toes. To relieve the cramp, stretch your toes up and back toward your shin.

## SUDDEN GROIN PAIN

Round ligaments connect the front of your uterus to each groin, the crease or hollow that connects your inner thigh to your trunk. These ligaments contract and relax like muscles, but much more slowly. When you're in labor, this design is beneficial. As your uterus contracts, these ligaments contract and pull the uterus forward, aligning it and your baby with the vagina for efficient birthing.

Because these ligaments stretch and contract slowly, they work to prevent sudden overstretching. When you stand up quickly or when you sneeze or cough, you may stretch the ligaments too quickly, causing them to contract rapidly (stretch reflex) and causing pain in your lower abdomen or groin.

You can prevent this pain by moving slowly, letting the ligaments stretch gradually. Before sneezing or coughing, try to flex your hips to bring your thighs near your belly to reduce the pull on the ligaments.

# *Key Points to Remember*

- Maintaining good posture and moving with care increase your comfort during pregnancy and promote a faster recovery from birth.
- Regular exercise during pregnancy improves or maintains your muscle tone, strength, and endurance. It also protects against back pain, reduces the intensity of common pregnancy discomforts, and boosts your energy level, mood, and self-image.
- Most pregnant women should do various physical activities three to seven days per week to reap the benefits of moderate exercise.
- Exercises for your core and posture are essential during the childbearing year to condition your muscles for effective birthing and promote a speedier postpartum recovery.
- Align your mind, body, and spirit and connect with your baby through yoga and meditation.
- It's never too late to start an exercise regimen. Set reasonable fitness expectations and celebrate your successes.

# CHAPTER 6

# Eating Well

The quality of the foods you eat before and during pregnancy has a huge impact on your health and on your baby's development and long-term well-being. But which foods should you eat to ensure the best possible pregnancy? How much should you eat? How much weight should you gain? What about salt, food cravings, and morning sickness? Over the years, health-care professionals have given different answers to these and other nutrition questions. Some advice is based on accurate information; some isn't. This chapter provides the most accurate, up-to-date recommendations so you can make choices that best fit your lifestyle and food preferences.

# Good Nutrition during Pregnancy

For good nutrition during pregnancy, your daily diet should be varied and include plenty of fresh fruits and vegetables, whole grains, dairy products, foods that contain protein, and about 2 quarts of liquids. By eating small, frequent meals each day (for example, three small main meals and three light snacks), you help keep your blood sugar level stable throughout the day, reduce morning sickness in the first trimester, and reduce heartburn in the third trimester.

During the first trimester, you don't need to eat more than you did before you became pregnant. Beginning in the second trimester, however, you need to consume about 200 extra calories each day (assuming you exercise daily for thirty to sixty minutes). Two hundred calories isn't a lot—just two glasses of milk, one chicken drumstick without skin, or 2 tablespoons of peanut butter.

In the third trimester, you need to consume about 400 more calories than you did before pregnancy. Ideally, these additional calories should come from high-protein, high-calcium, and iron-rich whole foods—not from foods lacking in nutrition, such as chips, cookies, candy, and soft drinks.

Whenever you consider what to eat, make the best possible choice at the time. Don't feel that your diet must always be perfect. Some days, it may be hard to get the healthful food you need. Just be aware of what you eat and try to eat healthfully whenever possible.

Always keep in mind that your baby benefits from any healthy changes you make to your diet. To analyze your diet, visit our website, http://www.PCNGuide.com, to download a food diary so you can keep track of what you're eating. After recording what you ate for a week, look at the nutritional balance of your food choices and make plans to improve your nutrition for the next week.

## A NOTE TO FATHERS AND PARTNERS

You may be surprised to learn that most of the information in this chapter also applies to you. Even though you're not growing a baby, you can still use these forty weeks to begin eating a well-balanced diet and maintaining a healthy weight and activity level. By making these positive lifestyle changes, you increase the likelihood that you'll have a longer, healthier life to share with your child. You'll also model the healthful choices you want your partner and child to make.

Although recommendations for specific amounts of nutrients are for pregnant women, this chapter directs you where to find information specific to your needs.

## MYPLATE: RECOMMENDED FOOD GROUPS

In 2011 the US Department of Agriculture (USDA) developed MyPlate (http://www.choosemyplate.gov), a food guidance system designed to provide customized information for specific audiences—including pregnant and breastfeeding women—based on current dietary and physical activity recommendations known to promote health.

MyPlate describes five food groups and suggests what to eat each day; for example, "Make half your plate fruits and vegetables." Visit our website, http://www.PCNGuide.com, to download our food diary so you can track your consumption of foods from each of these groups.

## Grains

This group includes any food made of wheat, rice, oats, cornmeal, barley, or rye. Grains contain iron, B vitamins, minerals, and fiber; some are fortified with folic acid. **Try to make at least half your grains whole.** Whole grains contain the entire grain and all its nutrients. They include brown rice, oatmeal, barley, millet, quinoa, spelt, buckwheat, bulgur, and wild rice. For prepared foods, check the ingredients list for whole-wheat flour, whole oats, and so on.

**Try to limit refined grains**; these grains have been processed, which removes nutrients. Often, they have vitamins and minerals added back in (*enriched*) but not fiber. Refined grains include white rice, white flour, and most prepared grain-based foods (such as bread, tortillas, noodles, crackers, cereal, and pastries).

*If you have a gluten sensitivity or celiac disease*—Continue to avoid wheat, barley, rye, and triticale. To learn more, visit http://celiac.org/live-gluten-free.

## Vegetables

Vegetables are rich sources of fiber, vitamins, and minerals. **Try to vary your veggies.** Different vegetables have different nutrients, so eating a variety of vegetables ensures that you and your baby get the nutrients you need. Here are examples of the different types of vegetables:

*Dark green vegetables*—Bok choy, broccoli, greens (collard, mustard, turnip, chard, and kale), lettuce (dark green leafy lettuce and romaine), spinach, and watercress

*Orange vegetables*—Carrots, pumpkin, squash, sweet potatoes, and yams

*Dried beans and peas (legumes)*—Black beans, black-eyed peas, garbanzo beans (chickpeas), kidney beans, lentils, pinto beans, soybeans and soy products, split peas, and white beans (these foods also belong in the Meats and Beans category because they are a good source of protein; see page 106.)

*Starchy vegetables*—Corn, green peas, and potatoes

*Other vegetables*—Artichokes, asparagus, beets, Brussels sprouts, cabbage, cauliflower, celery, cucumbers, eggplant, green beans, mushrooms, okra, onions, peppers, tomatoes, vegetable juice, turnips, and zucchini

## Fruits

Apples, pears, peaches, plums, bananas, citrus fruits (such as oranges, grapefruit, lemons, and limes), tropical fruits (such as papaya, mango, and guava), melons, berries, and more are rich in fiber, potassium, vitamin C, and folate. **Eat a variety of fruits.**

## Milk and Dairy Products

Dairy products are a good source of calcium, protein, potassium, and vitamins A, B, and D. Full-fat dairy products may be the best choice. Research shows, paradoxically, that people who consume full-fat dairy are less likely to become obese than those who consume low-fat or nonfat dairy.[1] When possible, choose organic dairy products, which come from the milk of cows that haven't been exposed to antibiotics, bovine growth formula, or

## Tips for Choosing and Preparing Fruits and Vegetables

Eating fruits and vegetables is very important during pregnancy. To minimize the amount of chemicals you consume, choose organically grown varieties when possible. Unfortunately, organic produce may not be readily available and may stretch your budget. Some produce is more important to buy organically than others. These conventionally grown produce items are most likely to contain pesticide residue: apples, strawberries, grapes, celery, peaches, spinach, sweet bell peppers, nectarines, cucumbers, and cherry tomatoes.[2] If only conventionally grown varieties are available, wash them well or peel before eating.

Choose fresh local produce that's in season, when it's cheapest and at its peak flavor. The more recently produce was picked, the more nutrients it has. If you can't get fresh produce, frozen is the next best option. Avoid dried produce that has added sugar or salt. Canned produce should be considered a last option (to avoid BPA).

When you cook produce, the following methods are ordered from best to worst for preserving nutrients: steaming, microwave cooking, stir-frying, roasting, baking, then boiling.

## Sample Daily Menu during Pregnancy

**When you get up for the day**
- Peppermint tea (1 cup)
- 6 whole-grain crackers (that include 2 grams protein)

**Breakfast**
- Oatmeal (1 cup cooked oatmeal with ¼ cup berries, ¼ cup chopped walnuts, a sprinkle of cinnamon)
- Milk (1 cup)

**Morning snack**
- Broccoli florets and humus
- Water

**Lunch**
- Southwestern salad (¾ cup black beans, ½ avocado, ½ cup corn, ½ cup tomato, 1 tablespoon chopped onion, sprinkle of cumin, and cilantro, with 1 tablespoon lime juice and olive oil dressing) served over 1 cup romaine lettuce
- 2 flour tortillas
- Milk (1 cup)

**Afternoon snack**
- Apple with peanut butter
- Water

**Dinner**
- Stir-fry (4-ounce chicken breast, 1 carrot, ½ cup broccoli, ¼ red pepper, 6 snap peas, and five-spice), cooked in 1 tablespoon olive oil with garlic and ginger
- White rice (1 cup)
- Green tea (1 cup)

**Evening snack**
- Smoothie (8-ounce yogurt, 1 banana, 6 frozen strawberries)

To analyze your own daily diet, visit https://www.supertracker.usda.gov. Enter the foods you've eaten in a day, and the program calculates how many servings you've had in each food group and how much of each nutrient you've consumed.

pesticide-heavy feed. Organic, grass-fed dairy products are also higher in beneficial omega-3 fatty acids.

*If you don't like milk*—Try yogurt and cheese.

*If you're lactose intolerant*—Try lactose-free milk, or take a lactase enzyme before eating dairy products.

Try cultured forms of milk, such as cheese, yogurt, or acidophilus milk. Your body may tolerate digesting several small servings of dairy instead of a few large servings.

*If you choose not to consume milk products*—Other sources of calcium include canned fish with bones; dark green leafy vegetables; dried beans; nuts and seeds; tofu with calcium sulfate; and calcium-fortified juice, nut milk, coconut milk, soymilk, flax milk, or rice milk. Your caregiver may recommend supplements such as calcium, vitamin D, potassium, and magnesium.

## Meats and Beans

Meats and beans contain protein, which builds muscles, skin, enzymes, hormones, and antibodies. They also contain B vitamins, vitamin E, iron, zinc, and magnesium.

*Making healthy choices about meat and fish*—Use food safety practices (see page 114). To minimize your intake of saturated fat, choose the leanest cuts of meat, trim away extra fat, and drain off grease after cooking. When buying prepared meats, check the ingredients label on the package and choose meats that don't include excess salt and fat. If possible, choose organic and/or grass-fed meats to minimize your exposure to chemicals, medications, and hormones. Grass-fed meat may also contain more omega-3 fatty acids. Eat fish twice a week. Choose seafood that's low in mercury and high in omega-3 fatty acids (see page 114).

*If you choose not to eat meat or fish*—Get the protein you need from eggs, dairy, beans, nuts, seeds, and tofu. You might not get enough iron, calcium, vitamin $B_{12}$, or zinc unless you closely monitor your intake of those nutrients. If you're vegan, health-care professionals typically recommend that you take a daily supplement of at least 1 microgram of vitamin $B_{12}$.

## Empty Calories

Some foods, such as candy and soda, provide calories but no nutrients. Other foods, such as sweetened applesauce, fried chicken, or sugary cereals, contain some nutrients but also contain empty calories from solid fats and added sugars. Minimize your intake, or choose naturally lower-fat, lower-sugar options. Artificial sweeteners are not recommended (see page 109).

## MyPlate Food Groups and Servings[3]

| Food Group | What Equals a Serving? | Recommended Daily Servings* |
|---|---|---|
| Grains | 1 slice bread; 1 cup dry cereal; ½ cup cooked cereal, rice, or pasta; ½ bagel; 1 pita; 1 tortilla; 1 potato | 9 servings |
| Vegetables | 1 cup raw or cooked vegetables; 2 cups raw leafy vegetables; 1 cup 100 percent vegetable juice | 3½ servings |
| Fruits | 1 cup chopped fruit; 1 orange; 1 apple; 1 banana; ½ grapefruit; ⅛ cantaloupe; 1 handful grapes; 1 cup 100-percent fruit juice | 2 servings |
| Milk | 1 cup milk, cottage cheese, or yogurt; 1½-inch cube hard cheese | 3 servings |
| Meat and beans | 1 ounce meat, poultry, or fish; 1 egg; ½ cup tofu; ¼ cup cooked beans; ¼ cup nuts or seeds; 1 tablespoon peanut butter | 6½ servings |

These serving sizes are based on the assumption that you're choosing only foods that are naturally low fat and without added sugar. You may also consume up to 360 "discretionary" calories per day from foods that contain added **oils, fats, or sugars.**

\* Amounts are for a 2,600-calorie diet, appropriate for the second trimester of a 25-year-old, 5-foot 4-inch woman who weighed 160 pounds before pregnancy and exercises 30 to 60 minutes each day. For recommendations customized to you, visit http://choosemyplate.gov.

# Nutrients

Certain nutrients are particularly important for ensuring a healthy pregnancy. The following sections discuss these nutrients.

For a complete summary of the functions and sources of all major nutrients, along with recommendations for daily intakes, visit our website, http://www.PCNGuide.com.

## *Protein*

Protein builds all your body's cells. During pregnancy, your protein requirement increases to 70 to 80 grams (about 20 grams more than your pre-pregnancy requirement). Your growing volume of blood and amniotic fluid, plus the rapid growth of your placenta, uterus, and baby, are the reasons for the increased requirement.

You should get protein only from food sources. Prenatal vitamins don't supply protein, and protein supplements can lead to nutritional imbalances.

## Fact or Fiction?

*To ensure you get the best nutrition, you should eat fortified food products that have been scientifically designed to meet all your nutritional needs.*

**Fiction.** Nutrition is an inexact science, and researchers are still learning about the components of a healthy diet. If you consider all the advice that nutritionists have given over the last fifty years, it's amazing to see how much of it was based on faulty reasoning or incomplete information!

The best advice for optimal health is to eat a wide variety of real food that has been processed as little as possible. To learn more about the importance of eating whole foods, read the books *In Defense of Food: An Eater's Manifesto* (2008) or *Food Rules: An Eater's Manual* (2009) by Michael Pollan.

## *Fats*

Healthy fats are essential for your baby's brain growth, nervous system development, and aiding the absorption of vitamins A, D, E, and K. The healthiest fats are omega-3 fatty acids. Sufficient levels of these essential fatty acids in a pregnant woman's diet may help reduce preterm labor, hypertension, and depression. You can get omega-3 fatty acids only from your diet; your body can't synthesize them. The major sources are flaxseed oil and fish (see page 106). You can also find them in soybeans; walnuts; pumpkin seeds; pecans; hazelnuts; organic grass-fed dairy products; and omega-3 eggs. Omega-3 supplements from fish oil or flaxseed oil are also good sources.

After omega-3 fatty acids, the next best fats are unsaturated fats from plants, such as nuts and vegetable oils like safflower, sunflower, olive, and coconut. You can eat these fats in moderation.

Whether you're pregnant or not, your total fat intake each day shouldn't make up more than 30 percent of your diet and shouldn't exceed 85 grams. Limit your intake of saturated fats from animal food sources (such as bacon and other fatty meats) to no more than 28 grams, and avoid hydrogenated fats and trans fat. These bad fats can elevate cholesterol levels, and they may be linked to other health problems (such as obesity, diabetes, and heart disease).

## *Fluids*

During pregnancy, fluids help deliver nutrients to your baby. They also help prevent constipation and urinary tract infections (UTIs). Drinking plenty of fluids doesn't cause swollen ankles; in fact, it helps keep you from retaining too much fluid in your tissues.

Try to drink at least 64 ounces of fluids each day. You know you're drinking enough fluids when your urine is pale yellow.

The healthiest fluid to drink is water, but some of your fluid intake can come from milk, juices, soups, and decaffeinated teas and coffees. Caffeine is a diuretic, which means it increases the amount of fluid in your urine (and decreases fluid retention in your body). As a result, don't count caffeinated beverages as part of your 64-ounce daily goal. For more information on caffeine intake during pregnancy, see page 74.

You may find it difficult to drink enough fluids if doing so isn't a habit. To help make fluids (especially water) enjoyable to drink, find some favorite ways to prepare them. Here are some options to try: over ice cubes, at room temperature, warmed, or with a squeeze of lemon or lime juice. You may also try different ways to drink fluids, such as through a straw or from a water bottle, to discover which ways help you drink more.

## *Carbohydrates and Sugars*

Carbohydrates (also called "carbs" or starches) are your main source of energy. The 200 grams (or more) of carbohydrates you consume each day make up 45 to 70 percent of your total calories. The majority of your carbohydrate intake should come from foods containing complex carbohydrates. Examples include whole grains, legumes, starchy vegetables, citrus fruits, and nuts. Some of the carbohydrate intake can come from foods containing simple carbohydrates, such as fruit, dairy products, and unsweetened but refined cereal, bread, and pasta.

Minimize your consumption of sugars. Excess sugar may lead to tooth decay, obesity, decreased immune function, diabetes, and osteoporosis. Sugars that are lower on the *glycemic index* won't rapidly raise your blood sugar level (causing a "sugar rush"). Here's a list of sugars that range from low (1) to high (5) on the glycemic index:

1. Fructose (fruit) and sugar alcohols (sorbitol, xylitol, erythritol, and mannitol)
2. Lactose (milk products)
3. Less refined sugars (honey, molasses, maple syrup, date sugar, and fruit juice concentrate)
4. Refined sugar (table sugar, brown sugar, turbinado sugar, corn syrup, and glucose syrup)
5. High-fructose corn syrup

***Sugar substitutes (artificial sweeteners)***—Low-calorie sugar substitutes are found in diet soft drinks, chewing gum, desserts, and individualized packets on restaurant tables. The most common ones are aspartame (Equal and NutraSweet), saccharin (Sweet'N Low), sucralose (SPLENDA), acesulfame-K, neotame, and purified stevia (Truvia).

Several studies have shown that artificial sweeteners are safe for consumption by pregnant and breastfeeding women; however, other studies question the short- and long-term effects. Anyone who has phenylketonuria (PKU) should avoid aspartame because it may cause severe health problems.[4] Whole stevia leaves and stevia extracts haven't been tested or approved for safe consumption.

Although caregivers may prescribe sugar substitutes for women who have diabetes, most advise pregnant women to minimize their intake of sugar substitutes.

## Salt

For years, caregivers told pregnant women to limit salt, based on a mistaken belief that salt and water retention caused high blood pressure. We now know that moderate water retention in pregnancy is normal. To help maintain a healthy fluid balance during pregnancy, salt your food to taste.

Table salt is also supplemented with iodine, which is essential for thyroid function and your baby's brain development. The salt in prepared foods generally isn't supplemented with iodine. If you consume salt mostly from eating ready-made foods, the American Academy of Pediatrics recommends taking an iodine supplement of 150 micrograms a day during pregnancy and while breastfeeding.

## Folate and Folic Acid (Vitamin B₉)

Folate is a B vitamin that's found naturally in foods such as leafy green vegetables and some fruits. It's essential for your baby's normal growth, and it's especially important in early pregnancy to prevent certain birth defects. Folate helps form blood cells and promotes the normal development of your baby's brain and spine. Folate that's produced synthetically is called folic acid. Caregivers recommend a daily folic acid supplement of 400 micrograms (0.4 milligram) for all women of childbearing age and 600 micrograms (0.6 milligram) for pregnant women.

## Common Q & A

**Q:** I've heard that bottled water is safer than tap water for me and my baby. Is this true?

**A:** This isn't generally true. In the United States, municipal water systems are tightly regulated and monitored, making their water supplies safe for consumption. Bottled water may lack healthful minerals, which were filtered out before the water was bottled. Unless you're opposed to additives (such as fluoride) or dislike the taste, you may benefit (and save money) from drinking tap water.

In addition, there's some concern over whether plastic bottles leach harmful chemicals into the water. If you want to drink bottled water, a better alternative is buying water packaged in glass bottles.

## What about Prenatal Vitamins?

Eating a varied, high-quality diet is the best way to ensure you get all the vitamins and minerals you need. If your diet is excellent, you might not need prenatal multivitamin and mineral supplements. However, most caregivers recommend that pregnant women take a daily multivitamin and mineral supplement to help ensure they get the required nutrients. This recommendation may be especially important for women who are underweight, have poor eating habits, or avoid many kinds of food.

Talk to your caregiver about prenatal vitamins. If they're recommended, choose one that meets all your nutritional needs. Don't take several different kinds of multivitamins—doing so may lead to an accidental overdose of one or more nutrients. During pregnancy, avoid taking more than 100 percent of the recommended daily allowance (RDA) of any nutrient, unless your caregiver specifically recommends you do so.

Visit our website, http://www.PCNGuide.com, for more information on recommended nutrients.

## Calcium

Calcium is important for the growth of your baby's bones and teeth. It's especially vital in the third trimester, when your baby requires about two-thirds more calcium than he did earlier in his development. Calcium is also stored in your bones as a reserve for breast milk production. Caregivers recommend that pregnant women consume 1,000 milligrams of calcium each day (1,300 milligrams if you're younger than eighteen).

## Iron

Iron is required for the production of hemoglobin, which carries oxygen through your bloodstream to your baby and your cells. During the last six weeks of pregnancy, your baby stores enough iron to supplement her needs for the first three to six months after the birth. Caregivers often recommend that pregnant women take a daily iron supplement of 30 to 60 milligrams. Foods rich in vitamin C (such as citrus fruits and tomatoes) enhance iron absorption, while some antacids and caffeine interfere with it.

Iron supplements can cause nausea or constipation in some women. To relieve these unpleasant side effects, try taking the supplements with food, or try a different brand of supplement that doesn't cause constipation. You may also want to try reducing the dosage of the supplements and taking them more often throughout the day.

## Vitamin A

Vitamin A helps form and maintain healthy teeth and bones, soft tissue, mucous membranes, and skin. It also promotes good vision.

During pregnancy, getting too little vitamin A (less than about 770 micrograms per day) can lead to preterm birth and an underdeveloped baby. However, getting too much vitamin A (more than 3,000 micrograms per day) in the first seven weeks of pregnancy can lead to a higher incidence of birth defects.

## Vitamin D

Vitamin D helps with bone growth and cellular metabolism. A minimum of 600 international units (IU), or 15 micrograms, per day is recommended, and getting up to 4,000 IU (100 micrograms) per day may be beneficial. Although you can make vitamin D by exposing your skin to the sun, or get it by consuming foods supplemented with vitamin D, your caregiver may recommend a vitamin and mineral supplement to help you get the amount that's right for you.

# Weight Gain during Pregnancy

A common question women ask during pregnancy is how much weight they should gain. The answer varies because no single amount is appropriate for every woman. The proper amount of weight to gain depends on a woman's pre-pregnancy weight and height, the quality of her diet before and during pregnancy, her ethnic background, and the number of previous pregnancies she has had.

## RECOMMENDATIONS FOR YOUR WEIGHT GAIN[5]

How can you determine the proper amount of weight to gain during pregnancy? First look at the chart on page 112 to figure out your pre-pregnancy *Body Mass Index (BMI)*, which takes into account your height and pre-pregnancy weight to gauge your total body fat. For example, let's say your height is 5-feet 4-inches, and your pre-pregnancy weight was 160 pounds. By looking at the chart, you can see that your pre-pregnancy BMI is 28. The chart shows the results of a mathematical formula (rounded to the nearest whole number), in which BMI equals weight multiplied by 703 and divided by height in inches squared.

After you've figured out your pre-pregnancy BMI, look at the table to determine the amount of weight you should gain.

These recommendations are guidelines. Many women gain more or less weight during pregnancy, and they and their babies are fine. Some women feel pressured to gain a certain amount weight; others feel they're being judged about how much or little weight they've gained. Remember that your caregiver is monitoring your weight with your baby's well-being in mind. Women who gain too little weight increase their risk of having a premature baby or one with low birth weight. Women who gain too much weight increase their risk of developing preterm labor, gestational diabetes, high blood pressure, or macrosomia (large baby that can be difficult to deliver vaginally). These women also find it harder than usual to lose the extra weight after the birth.

Your caregiver will likely monitor your weight gain at each prenatal visit. In early pregnancy, you'll gain weight slowly, typically just 1 to 5 pounds by the end of the first trimester. Beginning in the second trimester, as your baby grows and your amniotic fluid and blood volume increases, you'll gain weight more rapidly—up to 1 pound per week.

An obese woman may not need to gain weight until mid-pregnancy; at that point, she may need to gain just ½ pound a week. Gaining less than the recommended amount is fine as long as the baby is growing well, and it may reduce the risk of weight-related complications.[6]

## Where Does That Extra Weight Go?

Here's a breakdown of the weight distribution in a pregnancy with an average weight gain:

| | |
|---|---|
| Baby | 7 to 8½ pounds |
| Placenta | 1 to 1½ pounds |
| Uterus | 2 pounds |
| Amniotic fluid | 2 pounds |
| Breasts | 1 pound |
| Blood volume | 2½ pounds |
| Fat | 5 to 8 pounds |
| Tissue fluid | 6 pounds |
| **Total** | **27 to 31½ pounds** |

## Body Mass Index (BMI)

| | Prepregnancy BMI | Total Weight Gain |
|---|---|---|
| Underweight | Less than 18.5 | 28 to 40 pounds |
| Normal Weight | 18.5 to 24.9 | 25 to 35 pounds |
| Overweight | 25 to 29.9 | 15 to 25 pounds |
| Obese | 30 to 39.9 | 11 to 20 pounds |
| Morbidly Obese | More than 40 | Less than 15 pounds |

ARE YOU AT A HEALTHY WEIGHT?
WHAT IS YOUR BODY MASS INDEX?

Weight in Pounds

| Height in Feet and Inches | 120 | 130 | 140 | 150 | 160 | 170 | 180 | 190 | 200 | 210 | 220 | 230 | 240 | 250 |
|---|---|---|---|---|---|---|---|---|---|---|---|---|---|---|
| 4'6 | 29 | 31 | 34 | 36 | 39 | 41 | 43 | 46 | 48 | 51 | 53 | 56 | 58 | 60 |
| 4'8 | 27 | 29 | 31 | 34 | 36 | 38 | 40 | 43 | 45 | 47 | 49 | 52 | 54 | 56 |
| 4'10 | 25 | 27 | 29 | 31 | 34 | 36 | 38 | 40 | 42 | 44 | 46 | 48 | 50 | 52 |
| 5'0 | 23 | 25 | 27 | 29 | 31 | 33 | 35 | 37 | 39 | 41 | 43 | 45 | 47 | 49 |
| 5'2 | 22 | 24 | 26 | 27 | 29 | 31 | 33 | 35 | 37 | 38 | 40 | 42 | 44 | 46 |
| 5'4 | 21 | 22 | 24 | 26 | 28 | 29 | 31 | 33 | 34 | 36 | 38 | 40 | 41 | 43 |
| 5'6 | 19 | 21 | 23 | 24 | 26 | 27 | 29 | 31 | 32 | 34 | 36 | 37 | 39 | 40 |
| 5'8 | 18 | 20 | 21 | 23 | 24 | 26 | 27 | 29 | 30 | 32 | 34 | 35 | 37 | 38 |
| 5'10 | 17 | 19 | 20 | 22 | 23 | 24 | 26 | 27 | 29 | 30 | 32 | 33 | 35 | 36 |
| 6'0 | 16 | 18 | 19 | 20 | 22 | 23 | 24 | 26 | 27 | 28 | 30 | 31 | 33 | 34 |
| 6'2 | 15 | 17 | 18 | 19 | 21 | 22 | 23 | 24 | 26 | 27 | 28 | 30 | 31 | 32 |
| 6'4 | 15 | 16 | 17 | 18 | 20 | 21 | 22 | 23 | 24 | 26 | 27 | 28 | 29 | 30 |
| 6'6 | 14 | 15 | 16 | 17 | 19 | 20 | 21 | 22 | 23 | 24 | 25 | 27 | 28 | 29 |
| 6'8 | 13 | 14 | 15 | 17 | 18 | 19 | 20 | 21 | 22 | 23 | 24 | 25 | 26 | 28 |

Healthy Weight     Overweight     Obese

Note: This chart is for adults (aged 20 years and older).

Source: U.S. Surgeon General

Although a minor increase or decrease in your weight may be a sign that you've eaten more or less than usual, a sudden, excessive change can be a sign of illness or preeclampsia (see page 134), especially if accompanied by other symptoms (such as sudden swelling).

Health-care professionals stress that pregnant women should worry less about gaining a specific amount of weight and focus more on eating a high-quality diet in appropriate amounts and maintaining an active lifestyle that includes moderate exercise.

## WEIGHT LOSS AFTER THE BIRTH

You'll lose some of the weight you gain during pregnancy within a few weeks after the birth. By eating sensibly and exercising adequately, some women can lose most of the remaining weight over the following months. For other women, losing the extra weight takes longer.

Breastfeeding promotes weight loss because milk production burns calories. The fat stored during pregnancy provides some of these calories; the food you eat provides the rest. Until your breastfed baby weans, your body may naturally hang on to a few pounds of fat as a way to ensure your baby is well nourished should you experience a food crisis. This extra weight is typically easy to lose after weaning.

# Common Concerns

During pregnancy, normal changes in hormone production, plus the increased size and weight of the uterus, can cause digestive and other problems. The following sections discuss these problems, their causes, and treatments.

## NAUSEA AND VOMITING

During pregnancy, nausea is also called "morning sickness." But for many women, morning sickness isn't limited to the morning; they experience nausea at any time throughout the day.

What causes nausea? As production of the hormones that support pregnancy increases, you may feel nauseated until your body adjusts to the increased levels. (Some women also experience diarrhea in early pregnancy, which may be due to hormones or dietary changes.) In the first trimester, nausea is common in women who haven't eaten for several hours, who smell certain odors, or who encounter other triggers. Nausea is neither abnormal nor a sign that you're unconsciously rejecting your baby. See above for tips on managing nausea.

If your nausea leads to vomiting, you may worry about your baby's health. But unless severe and unusually frequent, vomiting doesn't harm your baby. Studies show that a woman who's healthy when she conceives has sufficient reserves to nourish her growing baby, even if she can't eat well for the first several months of pregnancy.

## HEARTBURN

Heartburn is a condition in which you burp up stomach acid, causing a burning feeling in your chest or throat. In late pregnancy, many women experience heartburn. Its cause is a combination of increased pressure from the growing uterus and hormonal effects that relax the muscular opening at the top of the stomach and cause the stomach to empty more slowly. To help ease or prevent heartburn, follow these tips:

- Avoid eating fatty foods, spicy foods, and foods that produce gas or heartburn.
- Eat several small meals a day. Drink only a small amount of fluid with meals.
- Eat slowly and avoid eating just before bedtime.
- To decrease discomfort when in bed, semi-sit rather than lying flat on your back.

## Tips for Managing Nausea

- Eat several small meals a day to prevent an empty stomach and to keep your blood sugar level stable. Include a protein-rich food with each meal.
- Don't drink a lot of fluids with meals. Instead, drink between meals.
- Keep a bland food (such as crackers) by your bed and eat some just before getting up.
- Trust your food preferences. If something sounds good to eat, you'll probably tolerate it.
- Identify and avoid odors that make nausea worse. Try smelling peppermint oil or fresh lemon slices to ease nausea. (Drinking peppermint tea may also help.)
- Caregivers often recommend ginger (but not supplements of dried, powdered ginger root). You can eat ginger in foods, eat candied or pickled ginger, or drink ginger tea or natural ginger ale.
- Increase your intake of foods rich in vitamin $B_6$ (pyridoxine), such as whole grains and cereals, nuts, seeds, and legumes. Vitamin $B_6$ supplements may reduce nausea. Your daily intake should never exceed 100 milligrams; discuss safe amounts with your caregiver.
- Use acupressure wristbands, which are marketed to relieve motion sickness.
- Know that the nausea and vomiting usually passes within three to four months.
- On rare occasions, nausea and vomiting are severe and a woman becomes dehydrated, loses a lot of weight, and can't keep down any food. This condition (called "hyperemesis gravidarum") may require medications (such as Zofran) or even hospitalization (see page 123). Because these medications cross the placenta and their safety for the baby hasn't been established, take them only if your caregiver prescribes them.

- Taking antacids or other medications sometimes controls heartburn, but you should take them only if necessary. Ask your caregiver for recommendations.

## CONSTIPATION

During pregnancy, food moves through your intestines more slowly to let your body absorb more nutrients and water. This slowdown sometimes causes constipation, and pressure from your growing uterus on the large intestine magnifies the problem. Constipation can also aggravate hemorrhoids. Some tips to avoid constipation include the following:

- Exercise regularly and consume plenty of fluids and high-fiber foods, such as fruits and vegetables, whole grains, bran, and prune juice. An easy way to increase your fiber intake is to add a tablespoon of flax meal to your food.
- If proper diet and exercise don't prevent constipation, try an over-the-counter high-fiber product such as Metamucil or Fiberall. Such products are safe and effective; however, avoid taking intestinal stimulants (laxatives). Your body may become dependent on them.
- If you're taking an iron supplement and you think it's causing the problem, ask your caregiver about changing to one that causes less constipation.

## FOOD CRAVINGS AND PICA

Pregnant women frequently crave specific foods in large quantities. Sometimes women eat foods they rarely ate before pregnancy, such as hot peppers or other spicy foods, one flavor of ice cream, potatoes, or pickles. Although health-care professionals don't know why pregnant women crave certain foods, the cravings are usually harmless unless they interfere with good nutrition.

Also common during pregnancy is pica (craving and eating nonfood items). Pregnant women have reported craving ice, baking soda, flour, cornstarch, dirt, clay, cigarette ashes, and other nonfood substances. They've also described cravings to smell such substances as gasoline, fingernail polish remover, bleach, and ammonia.

Eating nonfood products and smelling substances can cause mild to severe side effects in both the mother and baby. While many women worry about these side effects, they're reluctant to share their concerns with their caregivers. They may be confused or ashamed by their behavior, or they may worry that their caregivers will advise them not to satisfy the craving.

If you have nonfood cravings, have your caregiver or a counselor help you determine whether satisfying them is harmful to you or your baby. If it is, you can learn ways to cope with the cravings and avoid the harmful substances.

# Food Safety

Some forms of bacteria and environmental contaminants can harm babies' development in the womb. Although the risk of harm is small, pregnant women should take precautions to prevent exposure. The following sections discuss ways you can limit your exposure. For more information on food safety, visit http://www.fda.gov/Food/ResourcesForYou/HealthEducators/ucm081785.htm.

## MERCURY

Mercury is a metallic element that can harm your baby's developing brain and nervous system. It's found in large, long-lived fish, which is regrettable because fish are a great source of essential nutrients, including omega-3 fatty acids. As long as the fish has low levels of mercury, it's better to eat it in moderation than to stop eating fish entirely.

Here are amounts of fish that pregnant women can safely eat, based on mercury levels. The asterisked items are highest in omega-3 fatty acids.

- **Up to 12 ounces per week**—Anchovies*, catfish, clams, cod, crab, flounder, herring*, oysters, pollock, salmon*, sardines*, scallops, shrimp, sole, tilapia, and trout*
- **Up to 6 ounces per week**—Halibut, snapper, lobster, tuna, and mahi-mahi
- **Avoid completely**—Shark, tilefish, king mackerel, swordfish, grouper, marlin, and orange roughy[7]

## FOOD-BORNE BACTERIA

Pregnant women are more susceptible to listeriosis, salmonella, and toxoplasmosis bacteria than other people are. These bacteria can sicken pregnant women and cause miscarriage, preterm labor, and stillbirth. These bacteria live in undercooked meat, fish, and eggs; unpasteurized milk and cheeses; and unwashed fruits and vegetables. Although the chance of exposure is small, the effects can be grave. Use the following food safety practices to decrease risk of exposure. (See our website, http://www.PCNGuide.com, for more information on infections in pregnancy.)

- **Keep things clean**—Before and after handling food, wash your hands thoroughly with warm soapy water. Rinse raw fruits and vegetables thoroughly. Separate raw meat, poultry, and seafood from ready-to-eat foods. After using cutting boards, knives, and plates to prepare raw meat, poultry, or seafood, wash the items thoroughly in hot soapy water before using them to prepare other foods.
- **Cook meat, fish, and eggs thoroughly**—In addition, before eating hot dogs and luncheon meats (such as ham, turkey, bologna, salami), heat them until they're steaming. Cook refrigerated smoked seafood (such as Nova-style lox salmon) before eating.
- **Store foods well**—Set your refrigerator to 35°F to 40°F (2°C to 4.4°C) and your freezer to 0°F to 4°F (–18°C to –16°C). Regularly clean the interior of your refrigerator, and discard all food that's past its expiration date.
- **Use the two-hour rule**—Discard any food that's prone to spoilage if it's been left out at room temperature for more than two hours.
- **Be smart about takeout foods, delivered foods, and restaurant leftovers**—Eat hot foods as soon as possible after purchasing. Eat cold foods within two hours. Refrigerate restaurant leftovers within an hour and eat within two days. Eat delivered foods within two hours.
- **Avoid eating unpasteurized foods and some raw foods**—It's fine to eat foods that contain pasteurized milk, cooked fish, shelf-stable smoked seafood, and canned pâtés and meat spreads. But it's best to avoid eating the following foods:
  - unpasteurized milk products, including soft cheeses made from unpasteurized milk (such as Brie, Camembert, blue cheese, feta, and Mexican fresh cheese)
  - raw fish, especially raw shellfish
  - refrigerated pâtés or meat spreads
  - raw vegetable sprouts (such as alfalfa sprouts and bean sprouts)

# Nutrition for Special Circumstances

In certain cases, having good nutrition is especially important during pregnancy. If one or more of the following sections describe your situation, be particularly conscientious about eating nutritious foods. Seek nutritional counseling from your caregiver or a nutritionist.

## PREGNANT WITH MULTIPLES

If you're pregnant with twins, increase your prenatal vitamin dosages by 50 percent and consume an extra 600 calories each day. You should try to gain 35 to 50 pounds. If you're pregnant with triplets or more, ask your caregiver for nutrition advice.

When pregnant with multiples, it's important to gain at least 24 pounds by the twenty-fourth week of pregnancy to help reduce the risk of preterm birth and babies with low birth weight.

## TEENAGE PREGNANCY

A pregnant teenager needs to eat particularly well to promote her own growth while nourishing her baby. If you're a pregnant teenager, make sure to consume enough calcium, phosphorus, and magnesium.

## PREGNANT WITHIN A YEAR OF GIVING BIRTH

Pregnancy can temporarily deplete your reserves of certain nutrients, such as calcium and iron. If you become pregnant within a year of your last birth, you may need extra calories and nutrients. The time needed between pregnancies to correct deficiencies depends on your overall nutritional status and the quality of your diet. Talk with your caregiver about your needs.

## PREGNANT AND CONSIDERED OBESE

If you were considered obese when you became pregnant, learn more about the impact of maternal obesity on pregnancy and maternity care by visiting http://www.wellroundedmama.blogspot.com or reading the series "Maternal Obesity: A View from All Sides" on http://www.scienceandsensibility.org.

## FOOD ALLERGIES

If you have significant food allergies, eliminating problem foods can lead to an inadequate diet. You may need a nutritionist to help you plan a healthful pregnancy diet.

## ANOREXIA AND BULIMIA

If you have a history of anorexia or bulimia, you may have difficulty accepting the weight gain and body changes that occur with pregnancy. In addition, your low weight and poor nutritional status may harm your and your baby's health during pregnancy. Psychological and nutrition counseling may help you, as may anorexia and bulimia support groups.

# HIGH BLOOD PRESSURE

Developing high blood pressure during pregnancy—or gestational hypertension—isn't always preventable. But by eating a healthful diet, drinking plenty of fluids, exercising regularly, and avoiding alcohol and caffeine, you may reduce your risk of severe complications. Although research hasn't yet found a single nutrient that prevents gestational hypertension, several nutrients may reduce the risk, including protein, calcium, magnesium, zinc, vitamins C and E, and omega-3 fatty acids. Make sure your diet includes healthy amounts of these key nutrients. (See page 133 for more on high blood pressure.)

# DIABETES IN PREGNANCY

Whether you have diabetes or are at high risk for developing diabetes, carbohydrates shouldn't make up more than 40 percent of your daily caloric intake. Avoid eating more than 30 to 45 grams of carbohydrates at one meal. Complex carbohydrates are much better for you than simple carbohydrates.

Keep your fat intake to less than 30 percent of your daily caloric intake, and increase your protein intake to 75 to 100 grams. Eat at the same times every day, and eat several small meals each day to keep your blood sugar level stable. (See page 127 for more on diabetes.)

# LOW INCOME

If you're pregnant and have a low income, you may find it difficult to obtain the proper nutritious foods. Here's a list of resources that can help you:

- WIC (Women, Infants, and Children) provides supplemental food and nutrition education to low-income families. To find out if you're eligible for these services, visit http://www.fns.usda.gov/wic.
- You can use government food stamps to purchase food. To find out if you're eligible, visit http://www.fns .usda.gov/fsp.
- Food banks provide supplemental foods. Check a phone book or search online to find a local food bank.

## *Key Points to Remember*

- Eat a well-balanced diet that includes lots of whole grains, vegetables, and fruits. Include plenty of protein from milk products, low-fat meat, fish, nuts, beans, and legumes. Drink plenty of liquids, and salt your food to taste. Don't try to achieve perfection—just make the best choices you can each day.
- Talk with your caregiver about supplementing your diet with a prenatal vitamin or specific nutrients. (Visit our website, http://www.PCNGuide.com, for a chart of recommended nutrients.)
- Gain an amount of weight that's appropriate for you by considering your pre-pregnancy weight and height, and the quality of your diet before and during pregnancy.
- Normal changes in hormone production, plus the increased size and weight of the uterus, can cause nausea, vomiting, constipation, and other problems that can be treated.
- You can reduce the risk of food safety problems by following the sensible guidelines we've provided.

# CHAPTER 7

# When Pregnancy Becomes Complicated

Most women have normal and healthy pregnancies. Some women, however, begin pregnancy with a chronic (preexisting) health problem that can make pregnancy more challenging, and some women develop a condition during pregnancy that can be alarming or stressful. Having good prenatal care and prompt treatment may minimize complications and maximize your chances of having a healthy baby. In this chapter, you'll learn about complications in the order in which they may appear in pregnancy, beginning with conditions that may affect your pregnancy from conception and ending with complications that can arise in the days before the birth.

*Note:* If you're in good health at this time and find it troubling to read about possible complications, you may choose not to read this chapter in its entirety. It's important, though, for you to know the warning signs on page 130 so you can detect and report a problem early on.

# Chronic Conditions That May Affect Your Pregnancy

If you have a chronic condition or illness before becoming pregnant, it might or might not cause problems in pregnancy. With good prenatal care, most people with chronic health problems have healthy babies.

The following is a list of conditions and illnesses that may affect prenatal care:

- cardiovascular disease (high blood pressure, heart disease, or sickle cell anemia)
- gastrointestinal illness or nutrition problems (inflammatory bowel disease, phenylketonuria or PKU, Crohn's disease, eating disorders, or gastric bypass surgery)
- respiratory or lung disease (asthma)
- hormonal imbalance or disease (diabetes, thyroid disease, polycystic ovarian syndrome or PCOS, or pituitary disorder)
- autoimmune disorder, in which the immune system harms instead of protects the body (rheumatoid arthritis, lupus erythematosus, and antiphospholipid antibody syndrome or APS)
- other condition or illness (kidney disease, epilepsy, or physical disability)

If you have one or more of these conditions or illnesses, you improve your chances of having a healthy baby by controlling the symptoms *before* becoming pregnant. Once you're pregnant, talk with both your regular physician or specialist and your maternity caregiver to create a plan for maintaining your health and to learn what you can expect during pregnancy, labor, and the months after the birth.

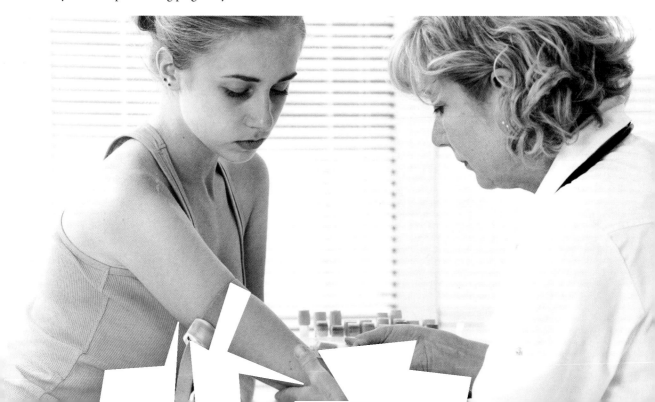

# Complications That Arise in Pregnancy

Some complications that arise in pregnancy are more serious than others and require medical treatment. Other complications resolve with little or no treatment. The following sections discuss the most common complications.

## VAGINAL BLEEDING IN EARLY PREGNANCY

Spotting or light vaginal bleeding in the first trimester occurs in about 20 percent of all pregnancies. In many cases, the bleeding doesn't harm the mother or baby.

What causes bleeding in early pregnancy? Sometimes, the implantation of the fertilized egg into the uterine wall causes slight vaginal bleeding, usually shortly before a menstrual period is expected to begin. Other times, cervical tenderness and an increased blood supply to the pelvis can cause spotting after intercourse. Often, frequent strenuous exercise or a cervical infection causes vaginal bleeding. In rare cases, a condition called molar pregnancy causes brownish vaginal discharge in early pregnancy. In a molar pregnancy, abnormal placental tissue grows into a grape-like cluster; there isn't a baby, even though a pregnancy test is positive.

For about half the women who experience bleeding in early pregnancy, the bleeding stops on its own and many have no further complications. In other cases, the bleeding is serious and sometimes indicates an ectopic pregnancy or possible miscarriage (see below). Expectant parents who have continuous moderate or heavy bleeding are more likely to miscarry than those who experience light bleeding only once.

If you experience any vaginal bleeding during early pregnancy, call your caregiver. If you have spotting or light bleeding for only one day, your caregiver may suggest that you rest and avoid strenuous exercise and sexual intercourse. If you experience heavy bleeding along with cramps or abdominal pain, your caregiver may order an ultrasound scan or blood tests to assess your pregnancy.

## ECTOPIC PREGNANCY

About 1 to 2 percent of pregnancies are *ectopic*. An ectopic pregnancy occurs when the fertilized egg implants itself someplace outside the uterus, usually in the wall of a fallopian tube (called a "tubal pregnancy") but sometimes in the cervix, ovary, or abdomen. This type of pregnancy won't result in a live birth, thus parents feel a similar sense of loss and grief that a miscarriage evokes (see below).

Symptoms of an ectopic pregnancy usually appear in the first six to eight weeks of pregnancy and may include lower abdominal pain or tenderness (or one-sided pelvic pain) and vaginal bleeding. Additional symptoms include nausea, vomiting, dizziness, or a sharp shoulder pain. An untreated tubal pregnancy causes severe abdominal pain and vaginal bleeding that indicates internal bleeding.

To diagnose the problem, the woman has a blood test to check her hormone levels and a high-resolution ultrasound scan to determine the implantation site. Treatment options are laparotomy (traditional surgery) or laparoscopy (minimally invasive surgery) to remove the embryo, or an intravenous (IV) infusion of a medication called methotrexate may be used to end the pregnancy.

If the fallopian tube has ruptured, emergency surgery is needed to stop the bleeding, and sometimes the fallopian tube and ovary are removed.

The likelihood of ectopic pregnancy rises for women whose fallopian tubes are damaged by pelvic infection, disease, or surgery. The majority of women who have an ectopic pregnancy can expect to get pregnant again and carry a healthy baby to term.

## Common Q & A

**Q:** My last pregnancy ended in a miscarriage. What can I do to increase my chances of carrying my next baby to term?

**A:** Before conceiving, try to be in the best possible health. (On our website, http://www .PCNGuide.com, read our article on preconception health.) During preconception and early pregnancy, try to do the following:

- Have a well-balanced diet and take prenatal vitamins.
- Avoid environmental toxins and infections.
- Don't smoke or use recreational drugs. Limit alcohol and caffeine.
- Avoid extremely stressful relationships as much as possible.
- Make arrangements for emotional support and medical monitoring, starting early in pregnancy.

# MISCARRIAGE AND PREGNANCY LOSS

A *miscarriage* (or spontaneous abortion) is the unexpected death and delivery of a baby before the twentieth week of pregnancy. About 15 to 20 percent of known pregnancies end in miscarriage; however, the percentage of early miscarriage (before the thirteenth week of pregnancy) is probably higher because many women might not have realized they were pregnant before the loss occurred.

Although no one knows the specific cause of most miscarriages, the most commonly suspected reason is random chromosomal abnormalities that interfere with the baby's normal development. Other factors that increase the risk include a history of infertility and assisted conception, advanced age of the woman (or man), high body temperature, infection, hormonal imbalance, high intake of alcohol or caffeine, smoking, low body weight along with poor diet, frequent high-impact or strenuous exercise, and extreme emotional stress or physical injury.

Factors that increase the risk of late miscarriages (occurring between the fourteenth and twentieth weeks of pregnancy) include uterine abnormalities, such as an incompetent cervix (see page 130), acute infection (see page 124), placental problems (see page 132), uterine fibroids (see page 124), and certain chronic illnesses (such as autoimmune disorders; uncontrolled diabetes; thyroid conditions; and heart, liver, or kidney disease). Treatment of these possible causes can help prevent a miscarriage.

Signs of a miscarriage include vaginal bleeding and intermittent abdominal pain that often begins in the lower back and develops into abdominal cramping. If you suspect you're having a miscarriage, call your caregiver. You'll be advised to rest, avoid stress, and either wait to see if the bleeding stops or have an ultrasound scan and a blood test to confirm that you're still pregnant.

Once a miscarriage starts, it can't be stopped. If pregnancy tissue is still in the uterus, the miscarriage can be managed in one of three ways:

- *Observation (expectant management).* A woman may choose to let the miscarriage progress without intervention. It may take two weeks or longer for the contents of the uterus to pass. Once the bleeding and cramping has stopped, a follow-up ultrasound scan and pregnancy test are done to verify that the miscarriage is complete. The woman is advised to contact her caregiver immediately if she experiences heavy bleeding, fever, or strong abdominal pains.
- *Medication.* A medication can be given to stimulate the uterus and cause the contents of the uterus to pass more quickly.
- *Surgery.* Dilation and curettage, or D&C, is used to clean out the uterus. D&C is used for women with an infection or heavy bleeding, or those who don't want to wait for the miscarriage to be complete.

If a woman has had a miscarriage and is Rh negative, she may receive a shot of RhoGAM (see page 128).

Sometimes a caregiver discovers that a baby has died before a miscarriage begins. Some women want an immediate end to the pregnancy by having a D&C or receiving medications to expel the baby. Some choose to wait for the miscarriage.

It's normal for a woman to feel shock, grief, and sadness after a miscarriage—especially when the pregnancy was wanted, had been achieved by medical help, or followed a previous miscarriage.

If you experience a miscarriage, you and your partner may need extra rest and support. Even if you hadn't announced your pregnancy to others, seek comfort and help from family and friends as well as from books, online resources, and support groups on pregnancy loss. Talking about your loss with people who have experienced a miscarriage may be a particularly helpful way to ease your pain (see also page 296).

Most women who have one or more miscarriages eventually give birth to healthy babies. As you begin planning your next pregnancy, consider asking your caregiver about medical tests or genetic counseling to determine a possible cause of the miscarriage, to screen for genetic disorders, and to treat a harmful infection or chronic condition. You also may want to seek emotional support to help you manage your fears of another miscarriage, at least until your next pregnancy passes the point at which the miscarriage occurred.

# HIGH BODY TEMPERATURE (FEVER)

Having a high body temperature (an oral temperature over 100.4°F or 38°C) for three to four days may harm your baby, especially in early pregnancy. If you have a prolonged fever, ask your caregiver for advice. Don't take any fever-reducing medication unless your caregiver instructs you to do so. To lower your temperature, drink plenty of cool liquids and take a lukewarm bath or shower or place cool washcloths on your forehead or the back of your neck. If your temperature is higher than 102°F (38.9°C), call your caregiver immediately.

# SEVERE NAUSEA AND VOMITING (HYPEREMESIS GRAVIDARUM)

Hyperemesis gravidarum is persistent, severe nausea and vomiting. While nausea and vomiting is the most common complaint of early pregnancy, the intensity of hyperemesis gravidarum far exceeds that of "morning sickness" (see page 37). This serious condition, which affects about 2 percent of pregnancies, can result in weight loss, dehydration, and changes in blood chemistry.

If you're extremely nauseated and continue to vomit food and fluids for a day or longer, call your caregiver to determine whether the cause is illness or food poisoning. Early management of severe nausea and vomiting may help prevent its progression to hyperemesis gravidarum.

Treatment begins with the same dietary and lifestyle changes recommended for managing morning sickness (see page 113). If this treatment isn't effective, a caregiver may prescribe medications. The American Congress of Obstetricians and Gynecologists (ACOG) recommends beginning with a combination of vitamin $B_6$ and doxylamine, an antihistamine with sedative effects. Other medications can be used if this combination isn't effective.[1] If the vomiting can't be controlled, a woman may need hospitalization to receive IV fluids. Some women feel nauseated throughout pregnancy and continue to take medications at home.

Sometimes, psychological problems can worsen hyperemesis gravidarum; talking with a trained counselor may help resolve the problems and lessen the nausea and vomiting.

Hyperemesis gravidarum can be debilitating, but it's manageable with treatment and only rarely causes lasting effects on you or your pregnancy.

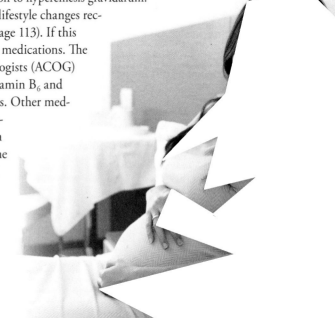

# UTERINE FIBROIDS

Uterine fibroids are benign (noncancerous) tumors of the uterine muscle. Also called "leiomyomas" or "myomas", fibroids are uncommon in women younger than thirty, but they occur in 11 to 18 percent of women ages thirty to forty, and in one-third of women ages forty to sixty. Fibroids typically don't cause problems.[2] Less than 25 percent of childbearing-age women with fibroids experience symptoms such as excessive menstrual bleeding, pelvic pain, or infertility. If symptoms are significant, options include medical treatments (contraceptives such as birth control pills or an IUD or surgery).

Although fibroids typically don't cause problems in pregnancy, possible complications include a slight increased risk of miscarriage, preterm labor, or postpartum hemorrhage. Depending on the number, size, and location, fibroids can sometimes complicate birth. Their presence may slow labor progress or interfere with the baby's movement into a head-down position for birth.

If you've been diagnosed with fibroids, your caregiver will likely watch your pregnancy closely and use ultrasound scans to detect changes in the fibroids' size or number and to determine whether they're affecting your baby's growth. If the fibroids are causing abdominal pain or increased pressure, treatment may include bed rest, applying cold or hot packs, and taking pain medications.

# VENOUS THROMBOSIS

Venous thrombosis is a blood clot that typically occurs in a vein in the leg or pelvis. About 1 in 500 pregnant people experience the condition because pressure from the enlarged uterus slows the flow of blood and because blood changes how it clots to help reduce postpartum bleeding.

A clot that develops in a vein close to the skin is called thrombophlebitis, and it causes warmth, swelling, tenderness, and redness. You may feel or see something that resembles a hard red cord under your skin. Treating thrombophlebitis includes bed rest with the leg elevated, hot packs, special support stockings, and a mild pain reliever.

Deep vein thrombosis (DVT) develops in a big vein that's deeper in the body and is much more serious than thrombophlebitis (but is less common—DVT occurs in about 1 in 2,000 pregnancies). DVT causes leg or pelvic pain and swelling. If a woman has DVT in her calf, she may have increased calf pain when she flexes her toes toward the knee. If you notice symptoms of DVT during pregnancy or after the birth, notify your caregiver immediately.

A person with DVT is at risk for venous thromboembolism (VTE) and possibly a pulmonary embolism, a potentially fatal condition in which a portion of the blood clot breaks loose and travels to a lung. Symptoms of pulmonary embolism include sudden shortness of breath, chest pain, and rapid heart rate. If you have these symptoms, go to an emergency room or call 911.

Your chances of developing VTE increase if you're older than thirty, you or your family has a history of blood clots, or you've recently been on bed rest or been sitting for a very long time.

Treating DVT may require pain medication as well as hospitalization and IV doses of the anticoagulant (blood thinner) Heparin to prevent further clot formation. Heparin doses continue at home.

# INFECTIONS

Although the risk of acquiring a serious infection during pregnancy is low, some infectious diseases can affect your pregnancy or harm your baby. The potential risks depend on the following factors:

- what organism (virus, bacterium, or spore) is causing the infection
- whether you have antibodies to the organism from a prior exposure

- whether the disease is treatable
- when during pregnancy you acquired the infection

Even if you get an infection during pregnancy, your baby might not become infected—and even if your baby gets infected, he might not be harmed.

The following sections provide information on infections that are harmful during pregnancy. For information about other infectious diseases and their effects on pregnancy, visit our website, http://www.PCNGuide.com, or http://www.mothertobaby.org/otis-fact-sheets-s13037.

## Sexually Transmitted Infections (STI)

Some STIs (previously called "sexually transmitted diseases" or "STDs") can cause problems during pregnancy, but if treated early, the risks to the baby are minimal. If you've had multiple sexual partners, you're at greater risk for an STI, such as chlamydia, gonorrhea, genital herpes, hepatitis B, human immunodeficiency virus (HIV), human papillomavirus (HPV), syphilis, and trichomoniasis. If you have or had symptoms of an STI—such as genital sores, abnormal vaginal discharge, or discomfort or difficulty with urination—ask your caregiver if testing and treatment are necessary. Throughout pregnancy, make sure you and your partner practice safer sex to protect against exposure to STIs. An STI contracted in late pregnancy is much riskier for the baby than an STI contracted long before becoming pregnant.

## Group B Streptococcus (GBS)

About 10 to 30 percent of pregnant women are carriers of Group B streptococcus (or are "colonized" with GBS), which means GBS bacteria are present in their bodies, but they don't have signs of infection. Without treatment, about 1 to 2 percent of newborns whose mothers are GBS carriers will develop a GBS infection, which can be life threatening, especially for a premature baby. If these mothers receive antibiotic treatment during labor, their babies' risk of infection drops to 1 in 4,000.

Most caregivers follow the GBS detection and treatment guidelines developed by the CDC in 2010,[3] which recommends screening all pregnant women between the thirty-fifth and thirty-seventh weeks by swabbing the vagina and rectum and having the secretions cultured in a laboratory. If a woman is a GBS carrier, her caregiver treats her with antibiotics during labor and watches her baby closely for signs of infection.

## Ways to Avoid Getting Sick

The best way to prevent complications from an infection is to avoid getting sick. Here are a few guidelines to follow:

- Wash your hands several times each day, especially before eating and after using the toilet. Germs live on doorknobs, handrails, phones, hands, and other surfaces. After touching a germ-covered surface with your hands, you transmit the germs to your food, mouth, nose, and anything else you touch.
- Stay away from sick people as much as possible, especially if your vaccinations aren't up to date.
- Update your vaccinations or have your immune status checked before pregnancy, if possible. Health-care professionals recommend that women avoid certain vaccines—such as chicken pox (varicella zoster) and measles, mumps, and rubella (MMR)—in pregnancy or in the month before conception. During pregnancy, the US Centers for Disease Control and Prevention (CDC) recommends that you get a flu shot and have a Tdap (tetanus, diphtheria, and pertussis) vaccination between twenty-seven and thirty-six weeks. If you'll be traveling internationally during pregnancy, consult with your caregiver about vaccines.
- Eat safe foods. To avoid foodborne diseases, don't eat certain foods during pregnancy (see page 115). Also, wash fruits and vegetables before eating them, adequately cook meats and other foods, and thoroughly clean your food preparation surfaces.

If a woman hasn't been tested or the results aren't known when labor begins, she'll receive antibiotics if she has any of the following conditions:

- preterm labor
- ruptured membranes for more than eighteen hours before labor begins
- fever of 100.4°F (38°C) or higher

GBS is an infection that may come and go during pregnancy. Some women who test negative at thirty-six weeks will test positive at forty-one weeks, so some caregivers recommend a second test if the pregnancy continues past forty-one weeks. Some women who tested positive at thirty-six weeks don't test positive at the birth. Researchers are studying the use of rapid testing during labor to address this situation. However, the treatment protocol recommends that if a woman tested positive at any time during the pregnancy, she should be treated as positive at the birth.

Possible side effects of antibiotics include allergic reactions, but most GBS carriers choose to have the treatment to reduce the risk of infection in their babies. If you receive antibiotics during labor, consider taking probiotic supplements after the birth to minimize side effects such as diarrhea and possible yeast infections. See page 307 to learn more about building a healthy microbiome.[4]

## Bladder and Vaginal Infections

Bladder or vaginal infections increase the risk of preterm labor. Symptoms of a bladder infection (also called "urinary tract infection" or "UTI") include frequent urination, urgency to urinate, blood in the urine, and pain, especially at the end of urination. Symptoms of a vaginal infection include vaginal discomfort or itching and foul-smelling discharge. *Note:* It's normal to have thin, mild-smelling, and whitish vaginal discharge during pregnancy. If you think you have a bladder or vaginal infection, promptly call your caregiver for treatment.

## Listeriosis

Listeriosis is a form of food poisoning that can cause miscarriage, preterm birth, or stillbirth. While rare (1 in 10,000 pregnancies), listeriosis affects pregnant women twenty times more often than it affects other healthy adults. The bacteria live in unpasteurized dairy products, raw or undercooked meats and fish, and in contaminated soil and water. Avoid eating unpasteurized dairy products. Don't eat meat, poultry, eggs, or seafood that isn't cooked thoroughly. Before eating a hot dog or luncheon meat, heat it until it steams. Clean all food preparation surfaces and utensils (see also page 115).

## Toxoplasmosis

Cats are the most common carriers of the *Toxoplasma gondii* parasite, especially outdoor cats that eat rats, mice, and other raw meat. The parasite passes from a cat in its feces, and you can transmit it from your hands to your mouth if you don't wash your hands after handling cats, emptying litter boxes, or working in soil that contains cat feces. You can also ingest the parasite by eating raw or undercooked meat or unwashed root vegetables.

If you've been around cats for many years, you may have become immune to toxoplasmosis, the infection caused by the parasite.

If you contract toxoplasmosis for the first time during pregnancy, you can pass the infection on to your baby. Most infected babies don't have noticeable defects caused by the parasite (such as blindness or mental disability) at birth, but can develop them later on. Although you can treat toxoplasmosis with antibiotics, prevention is the best treatment. Wash your hands after touching a cat, have someone else clean the litter box (and clean it often), and wear gloves when gardening. Also, cook your meat well and wash vegetables thoroughly.

# Diabetes Mellitus and Gestational Diabetes Mellitus

Diabetes mellitus (also called simply "diabetes" or "DM") occurs when someone has trouble making or using insulin, a hormone that helps glucose (sugar) pass from the blood into cells for the body to use as an energy source. There are two types of diabetes: type 1 and type 2. With type 1, the body stops making insulin; with type 2, the body doesn't use insulin effectively. As a result, blood glucose levels rise dramatically and glucose passes into the urine. Without careful management, diabetes can cause serious problems in pregnancy, such as an increased risk of a urinary tract infection (UTI), an overly large baby, preterm birth, stillbirth, and a newborn with hypoglycemia (low blood sugar), jaundice, or breathing difficulties.

When considering getting pregnant, a woman with diabetes needs to balance her medications with her activity level and diet. She may need to adjust her insulin dose or begin taking injections to control her blood glucose levels. She improves her chances of carrying a healthy baby to term if she controls her blood glucose levels before and during pregnancy.

Gestational diabetes mellitus (GDM) is a form of the condition that develops in the second or third trimester. It affects about 4 to 9 percent of women.[5] GDM is related to normal changes in glucose metabolism that promote the baby's growth in the womb. Early detection and appropriate treatment can help prevent the same problems that can arise in pregnancy for a woman with unmanaged type 1 or type 2 diabetes.

Most caregivers use a blood test (glucose challenge test, or GCT) to screen for GDM between the twenty-fourth and twenty-eighth weeks of pregnancy (see page 63). Some caregivers screen for high glucose levels in early pregnancy (often at the first prenatal visit) if a woman has risk factors for diabetes, including a personal or family history of diabetes or GDM, obesity, older than thirty-five, and of African American, Hispanic, Native American, or South or East Asian descent.

To help the test detect the level of glucose accurately, eat a healthy diet and get plenty of rest in the days before your GCT. On the day of your GCT, eat a healthy, nonsugary meal one hour before testing.

If your GCT is positive for high glucose levels, your caregiver will order a glucose tolerance test (GTT) to confirm the diagnosis (see page 141).

If you have GDM, treatment includes a special diet, exercise, and (in some cases) oral medications or insulin injections. The clinic nurse will show you how to check your blood glucose levels. If your caregiver suspects that your baby is overly large or that your placental circulation is affected, your labor may be induced near term. After the birth, your blood glucose will probably return to normal levels; however, about half of the women with GDM develop type 2 diabetes later in life.

# PERINATAL MOOD AND ANXIETY DISORDERS

Perinatal mood and anxiety disorders (PMAD) can arise at any time during pregnancy and the first six months after the birth. Although many people may have heard of postpartum depression, expectant parents should also be aware that they can experience depression, anxiety, or obsessive-compulsive disorder during pregnancy. See page 351 for more information and resources.

# RH (RHESUS) OR RHD BLOOD INCOMPATIBILITY

A characteristic of blood types is the presence or absence of an antigen called the "Rh" or "RhD factor." If your blood type includes a plus sign (such as O+ or A+), the Rh factor is present. If your blood type includes a minus sign (such as O- or A-), the Rh factor is absent. About 15 percent of Caucasians, 3 to 5 percent of people of African descent, and few people of Asian descent are Rh negative.

In early pregnancy, your blood is tested to confirm its type. If you're Rh negative, then your baby's father has his blood tested. If you're Rh positive and your baby's father is Rh negative, or if both of you are Rh positive or Rh negative, all is well. However, if you're Rh negative and your baby's father is Rh positive, then your baby may be Rh positive—and you and your baby are Rh incompatible.

Although you and your baby don't share blood systems, his blood may enter your bloodstream when you give birth or if you experience a miscarriage or have invasive tests. As a result, you may become Rh sensitized and start producing antibodies that may cause mild to severe anemia in your baby. Because your body produces antibodies slowly, the first Rh-incompatible pregnancy is usually unaffected. Without treatment, however, a problem can arise in a future pregnancy if that baby is also Rh positive.

Injecting an Rh-negative mother with Rh-immune globulin (RhoGAM) at the twenty-eighth week of pregnancy can prevent Rh sensitization. If a blood test finds that the baby is Rh positive, the mother receives another dose of RhoGAM within seventy-two hours of the birth. RhoGAM is also given after a miscarriage or abortion, with any invasive procedure such as amniocentesis or chorionic villus sampling (CVS), or if necessary after uterine bleeding or trauma.

Although RhoGAM has made Rh sensitization rare, if you're Rh negative your caregiver will test your blood throughout your pregnancy. If the level of antibodies increases, amniocentesis helps assess how seriously your baby is affected. If the baby is severely anemic, treatment may include early birth and a blood transfusion or, rarely, a blood transfusion in the womb.

# VAGINAL BLEEDING IN LATE PREGNANCY

In late pregnancy, heavy vaginal bleeding may suggest problems with the placenta's attachment to your uterus, such as placenta previa or placental abruption (see pages 132–133). Call your caregiver immediately if you experience fairly heavy bleeding. Slight spotting in late pregnancy may be a normal sign of labor; however, if your pregnancy is less than thirty-seven weeks, the spotting may indicate preterm labor.

# Preterm Labor

A *preterm labor* is one that begins before the thirty-seventh week of pregnancy, and births that result from preterm labor are called "preterm births." About 11 percent of all births are preterm, and most preterm births are near-term (thirty-four to thirty-six weeks). Less than 4 percent of all births occur before thirty-four weeks.

Because preterm babies are immature and underdeveloped, they tend to have more health problems than full-term babies do. Very premature babies have an even greater risk of life-threatening complications (see page 386). Good prenatal care strives to prevent preterm birth by identifying those women most likely to have preterm labor.

## RISK FACTORS FOR PRETERM LABOR

Several factors can increase the risk of preterm labor. However, many women with risk factors carry a baby to term, and some women without any risk factors may have preterm labor.

### Top Risk Factors

- previous preterm labor or birth
- pregnant with multiples
- heavy smoking; abuse of street drugs or prescription medication
- abnormally shaped uterus or previous uterine or cervical surgery

### Other Risk Factors

- maternal medical conditions, including high blood pressure and diabetes
- disease in baby or birth defects
- current infection (see our website, http://www.PCNGuide.com, for more information on infections during pregnancy) or bleeding during pregnancy
- obese or extremely underweight before pregnancy; poor nutrition before or during pregnancy
- use of reproductive technology to become pregnant
- age (younger than sixteen or older than thirty-five), race (African Americans have the highest risk), or low income
- constant emotional stress (domestic violence, extreme poverty, workplace pressures, or other sources of stress)
- high degree of physical stress (heavy lifting, long periods of standing, or very strenuous exercise)

## Decreasing Your Risk of Preterm Labor

Although some of risk factors may be beyond your control (for example, race, age, and medical history), here are steps you can take to reduce your risk of preterm labor:

- Start prenatal care early in pregnancy. Attend all appointments and carefully consider your caregiver's suggestions. Continue treatment for chronic conditions.
- Eat well, stay hydrated, and take any prescribed supplemaents (ask your caregiver about calcium, zinc, and omega-3 fatty acids in particular). Try to reach your suggested weight before becoming pregnant and avoid excessive weight gain during pregnancy.
- Get screened for existing infections and protect against new infections. If you experience symptoms, seek treatment promptly.
- Avoid smoking, secondhand smoke, alcohol, drugs, and hazardous substances.
- Limit strenuous activities and ask others for help when necessary.
- Decrease job or life stresses as much as possible. Seek emotional support from trusted friends and family.

## Signs of Preterm Labor

Because some women without any risk factors deliver their babies early, all pregnant women should know the signs of preterm labor. If you have two or more of these signs, call your caregiver immediately to help you decide whether you're in preterm labor:

- You have uterine contractions that occur every ten minutes, or six contractions in one hour. (See page 131 to learn how to detect contractions.) When checking for contractions, think about your typical uterine activity and remember that contractions of irregular length and frequency are normal in pregnancy. Having persistent, fairly regular contractions (along with other signs) may indicate preterm labor.
- You experience continuous or intermittent menstrual-like cramps, pressure in your lower abdomen and thighs, or a feeling that your baby is pressing down on your vagina.
- There is a dull ache in your lower back that doesn't go away when you change position.
- You have intestinal cramping with or without diarrhea or loose stools.
- You experience a sudden increase or change in vaginal discharge (watery, blood tinged, or with more thin mucus).
- You have a general feeling that something isn't right.

# PREDICTING AND PREVENTING PRETERM LABOR

For years, researchers have tried to find a reliable method to predict preterm labor. More than twenty tests have been developed, but none is accurate enough to justify testing low-risk women who don't have symptoms of preterm labor.

In some high-risk pregnancies, a woman has a transvaginal ultrasound earlier in pregnancy (before twenty-five weeks) to check for cervical changes. If a woman's cervix shortens (begins effacing) months or weeks before term or begins dilating (or "funneling"), the risk of preterm labor increases. She may be diagnosed as having an *incompetent cervix*. A caregiver may recommend *cervical cerclage*, in which the cervix is closed with suture thread. Sutures are removed in late pregnancy.

In some cases, a woman with a shortened cervix receives vaginal progesterone to reduce the risk of preterm labor. A woman with a history of preterm birth may receive progesterone shots. (*Note:* Neither option is effective in parents of multiples or parents at low risk for preterm labor.)

# DIAGNOSING PRETERM LABOR

When you call your caregiver or birthplace to report preterm contractions, you may be asked to drink two large glasses of water and lie on your left side for an hour, then call again if the contractions continue.

Or you may be asked to go to the hospital or clinic, where your contractions will be evaluated with an electronic fetal monitor and you may receive a vaginal exam or ultrasound scan to check your cervix. You may also be tested for infections.

If your cervix isn't changing, you aren't in preterm labor. Instead, you may have an active or irritable uterus. You may be sent home with recommendations to reduce your activity and stress levels or take other steps to reduce uterine activity, including treating any infections.

If an ultrasound scan detects the shortening or opening of the cervix, a caregiver may recommend fetal fibronectin (fFN) testing, blood tests, or saliva tests for certain biochemical markers. If the results of these tests are negative, it's less likely that birth will occur in the next seven to fourteen days than if results are positive.

## TREATMENT TO MANAGE PRETERM LABOR

If your caregiver determines that you're in preterm labor, the following measures may be suggested to try to stop the contractions and prevent a preterm birth:

### Monitor uterine contractions.

You may be hospitalized for electronic monitoring or sent home and asked to continue checking for contractions by hand (see at right) and to watch for other labor signs.

### Reduce activity.

You may be placed on complete bed rest (getting out of bed only when necessary, such as to use the toilet) or asked to decrease activity and increase rest. Although research doesn't show that bed rest reliably stops preterm labor, some caregivers recommend it. Caregivers may also recommend decreasing sexual activity and nipple stimulation, as either can promote preterm labor contractions.

### Treat medical conditions.

Certain infections increase the risk of preterm labor. If you have one, your caregiver may prescribe antibiotics. Your caregiver may also recommend progesterone or cervical cerclage (see page 130).

### Take medication to help stop or postpone labor.

Caregivers sometimes prescribe drugs to relax the uterus (see pages 274–275). These muscle relaxants may delay the birth for up to seven days, providing time to administer other drugs to improve the baby's health.

## WHEN PRETERM BIRTH IS UNAVOIDABLE

If treatment doesn't stop the contractions or cervical dilation, caregivers may suggest measures to help increase a premature baby's chances of a healthy life (see pages 274–275).

If your baby will be born prematurely, your caregiver may want you to give birth in a hospital with a neonatal intensive care unit (NICU). See page 386 to learn more about caring for a premature baby.

## How to Check for Contractions

- Empty your bladder and drink two tall glasses of water.
- Recline with your feet up or lie on your side. Relax.
- Place the tips of all four fingers of one hand on your abdomen at the top of your uterus. When you feel your uterus harden, press on it gently but firmly in several places. If your uterus indents or doesn't feel hard all over, you're not having a contraction. (You're probably feeling your baby's back pressing against your abdomen.)
- Time the contractions for one hour (see page 167). Note their length and frequency.
- If you have six contractions during the hour while you're lying down, call your caregiver.
- Expectant parents at high risk for preterm labor may be asked to check for contractions every day for thirty minutes. Preterm contractions may not be painful or be as obvious as full-term contractions, so pressing fingertips on the uterus may be needed to detect them.

# Complications with the Placenta

A few women develop problems with how and where the placenta attaches to the uterus. The following sections discuss the two most common of these placental complications.

## PLACENTA PREVIA

Less than 1 percent of pregnancies develop placenta previa, a condition in which the placenta lies completely or partially over the cervix. Women with placenta previa can't deliver their babies vaginally; instead, they have planned cesarean births, usually after the thirty-sixth week of pregnancy, but before labor begins.

Normal Placement                Placenta Previa

In early pregnancy, you may learn from an ultrasound scan that your placenta attached to the lower part of your uterus near the cervix (low-lying placenta). In most cases, as your uterus grows, the site where the placenta attached rises away from the cervix. (If the overlap of the placenta onto the cervix is small, it'll probably disappear as the pregnancy progresses. The bigger the overlap, however, the more likely it'll remain.[6])Your caregiver will diagnose you with placenta previa only if a transvaginal ultrasound scan confirms that the placenta continues to cover the cervix later in pregnancy.

Risk factors for placenta previa include a prior cesarean birth, uterine surgery, or abortion; uterine abnormalities; being older than thirty-four; and heavy smoking. The most common symptom of placenta previa is painless vaginal bleeding as cervical changes occur in the last trimester. Bleeding is usually intermittent and ranges from light to heavy. As with any vaginal bleeding during pregnancy, notify your caregiver immediately.

Treatment depends on your symptoms and includes measures to prevent heavy bleeding and decrease the risk of preterm birth. If you haven't had any bleeding, your caregiver will avoid doing vaginal exams and will advise you to avoid sex and heavy exertion. You may be put on bed rest. If you've had vaginal bleeding, you may be hospitalized for close observation and, if blood tests show severe blood loss, have a blood transfusion.

## PLACENTAL ABRUPTION

Another rare condition that occurs in less than 1 percent of pregnancies is placental abruption, in which the placenta partially or almost completely separates from the uterine wall during the third trimester or during labor. The condition can cause significant blood loss in the mother and can deprive the baby of adequate oxygen. Your risk of placental abruption increases if you have any of the following factors:

- extremely high blood pressure or blood clotting disorder
- more than five previous pregnancies
- a history of second trimester bleeding
- a prior abruption
- heavy smoking, drinking, or cocaine use
- severe abdominal trauma

Placental abruption may cause any or all of the following symptoms: vaginal bleeding, continuous severe abdominal pain, lower back pain, tender abdomen, and constant tightening of the uterus. Sometimes, vaginal bleeding is absent if the blood collects high in the uterus.

An ultrasound scan may help determine the degree of separation and its effect on blood flow to the placenta. Assessing the mother's blood pressure and the baby's heart rate helps estimate the severity of the abruption and, along with tests to check how well the mother's blood clots, help determine appropriate treatment. When the abruption is small and the baby remains healthy, bed rest and close observation may be the only treatment. If bleeding is severe and the baby's heart rate shows distress (and if the baby's chances of surviving a preterm birth are high), a woman has an immediate cesarean birth and a blood transfusion if necessary.

# High Blood Pressure and Gestational Hypertension[7]

Your activity level, emotional state, and body position can affect your blood pressure. It's usually lower when you're at rest, lying down, or free of emotional stress. It's usually higher when you're active, upright, or stressed. Short-term changes in your blood pressure are normal; however, blood pressure that stays too high can cause health risks at any age.

Someone with high blood pressure (hypertension) has had at least two consecutive readings that are over 140/90 mmHg. The condition, which affects about 10 percent of pregnant women in the United States, can be chronic or develop during pregnancy. When high blood pressure first appears after the twentieth week of pregnancy and remains high for several readings, it's called *gestational hypertension* (previously called *pregnancy-induced hypertension* or *PIH*).

A pregnant woman with high blood pressure is at risk for serious problems with uterine and placental blood flow and possible damage to other internal organs. Reduced blood flow to the placenta can result in less oxygen and fewer nutrients for the baby and may cause growth problems. Both chronic hypertension (high blood pressure present before pregnancy) and gestational hypertension can cause these problems and can also develop into a more dangerous condition called preeclampsia.

## Treatment for Gestational Hypertension

If you have mild hypertension, your caregiver may advise you to reduce your activity level, avoid stress, count your baby's movements regularly (see page 64), and monitor your blood pressure at home. You'll visit your caregiver more frequently for monitoring (such as weekly blood tests), and your caregiver may recommend that you give birth before your baby reaches full-term, often at thirty-seven weeks. (*Note:* For women with *chronic* hypertension but no other complications, giving birth before thirty-eight weeks isn't recommended.)

## Learning More about Pregnancy Complications

To learn more about a specific disease or condition, ask your caregiver for patient-education handouts that describe your condition or disorder. If handouts aren't available, ask where you can get more information.

You can also search the Internet for websites that provide information about your condition or concern. To ensure the information on a website is accurate and up to date, check several sites to compare data. Also check the expertise of site authors and find out whether the sources they cite are trustworthy or biased. Examples of reliable websites that provide accurate information on a number of pregnancy complications include the following:

- http://www.marchofdimes.org
- http://www.acog.org/Patients
- http://www.childbirthconnection.org
- http://familydoctor.org
- http://www.cochrane.org/reviews/en/subtopics/87.html

# PREECLAMPSIA

*Preeclampsia* is a multiorgan condition with mild to severe symptoms that affects about 5 percent of pregnancies. It typically occurs after the twentieth week of pregnancy.

Mild preeclampsia developed near term may cause fewer health problems than the possibly serious consequences of severe preeclampsia that begins before the thirtieth week of pregnancy.[8] With early diagnosis and aggressive treatment, complications from preeclampsia are generally minimal and both the mother and baby are typically healthy at birth and afterward.

## Signs of Preeclampsia

If you have high blood pressure, you'll be monitored for signs of preeclampsia. A urine test will show proteinuria (protein in the urine), and blood tests may be used to evaluate platelet count and liver and kidney function. You'll be asked to call your caregiver immediately if you experience these signs of preeclampsia:

- sudden puffiness (edema) in your hands or face
- rapid weight gain (more than 2 pounds in one week)
- headache
- visual changes or problems (flashes or spots before the eyes or blurred vision)
- pain in your stomach (epigastric pain) or your right side under your ribs, or possible pain in your shoulder or lower back

Typically, the more systems that are affected or the more symptoms you have, the more severe the condition is. Severe preeclampsia can cause the following complications:

- placental abruption (see page 132)
- HELLP syndrome (hemolysis, elevated liver enzymes, low platelets), which indicates blood and liver complications
- eclampsia, which indicates neurological irritability and imminent convulsions
- seizures, stroke, coma, or even death of mother and baby (in the most severe cases)

## Risk Factors for Preeclampsia

Although the causes of preeclampsia aren't well understood, a combination of factors appears to trigger the condition. The most significant risk factors include the following:

- first pregnancy
- preeclampsia in a previous pregnancy (or a close family member with it)
- personal history of chronic hypertension, diabetes, kidney disease, and certain autoimmune disorders
- obesity
- older than thirty-five or younger than eighteen
- pregnant with multiples
- African descent

## Treating Preeclampsia

If you have preeclampsia, the only cure is the birth of your baby (normal blood pressure usually returns within days or weeks after the birth). However, treatment to avoid further complications is available, based on the severity of the disease and your baby's gestational age and health.

If your symptoms are mild (such as blood pressure over 140/90 mmHG, proteinuria, and fluid retention), treatment is similar to that for gestational hypertension, with additional tests to check your baby's well-being (see page 133).

If you have severe preeclampsia (blood pressure over 160/110 mmHG and proteinuria accompanied by liver, blood, or neurological complications), you'll be hospitalized and given drugs, such as an antihypertensive to lower blood pressure and magnesium sulfate to reduce your risk of seizures. (Visit our website, http://www.PCNGuide .com, for more information on these medications.)

If severe symptoms worsen or don't sufficiently improve with treatment, your caregiver may suggest inducing labor or performing a planned cesarean promptly, rather than allowing the pregnancy to continue to term. If you're less than thirty-four weeks pregnant, your caregiver may recommend transferring you to a hospital with a neonatal intensive care unit to receive corticosteroids to promote your baby's lung development before birth (see page 274).

# REDUCING YOUR RISK OF PREECLAMPSIA

Research suggests that for women at high risk for preeclampsia, taking a low-dose aspirin (50 to 150 milligrams) each day beginning in the second trimester helps reduce the risk. Check with your caregiver before taking aspirin.[9] In addition, studies on folic acid supplementation in the second trimester show a reduced risk of preeclampsia in women who took the supplements in this period.[10]

Strive to eat a healthful diet, exercise in moderation, and gain a moderate amount of weight in pregnancy (see page 111). Attend all prenatal appointments, have the appropriate screening tests, and work with your caregiver to control high blood pressure and treat other early signs of preeclampsia.

# Breech and Other Difficult Presentations

Typically at birth, the baby positions herself so her head is over the cervix; this vertex presentation is the most favorable for a vaginal birth. In about 5 percent of births, however, the baby is in a less favorable presentation.

The rare shoulder presentation (*transverse lie*) occurs in about 1 in 500 births. Because a baby in this position turns to a vertex presentation only occasionally, a cesarean birth is usually necessary. Face and brow presentations occur in less than 1 percent of births, and they usually prolong labor.

The *breech presentation* occurs in 3 to 4 percent of births, although the incidence rises with multiples or premature births. There are three types of breech presentation:

- **Frank:** The baby's buttocks are over the cervix and her legs are straight up toward her face.
- **Complete:** The baby appears to be sitting cross-legged over the cervix.
- **Footling:** One or both of the baby's feet are over the cervix.

In the United States and Canada, breech babies are usually born by cesarean delivery (see page 138). To help avoid a cesarean, many women try to turn their breech babies before the birth by using different self-help techniques or complementary medicine methods. Some women request a medical method called external version or breech version.

The following sections describe these techniques.

## SELF-HELP TECHNIQUES TO TURN A BREECH BABY

If your baby is breech in the thirty-fourth to thirty-sixth week of pregnancy, you may wish to try self-help techniques to encourage him to turn.

The effectiveness of some of these techniques hasn't been formally studied. Others have been studied and found to be mostly ineffective. Nonetheless, these techniques do help some babies turn, and they pose few, if any, risks. (Check with your caregiver before attempting any of them.) Even if their chances of success are low, trying them may decrease your risk of cesarean birth.

*Note:* Please visit http://www.spinningbabies.com for more information on breech and other difficult positions and presentations and what you can try to correct them.

### Breech Tilt Position[11]

In the breech tilt position, your hips are higher than your head. Before trying it, check with your caregiver to make sure you don't have any medical reasons for avoiding it. (If you're in good health and your baby is thriving, your caregiver probably won't object.) Have your partner nearby to help you. Here are three ways to do a breech tilt:

- Lie on your back with knees bent and feet flat on the floor. Raise your pelvis and have your partner place enough firm cushions beneath your buttocks so your hips are 10 to 15 inches higher than your head.
- Lie head down on a wide flat board (such as an ironing board) that's tilted so one end is on a chair and the other is on the floor. If the board is wobbly, have your partner hold it steady and help you get on and off the board.
- Try an exaggerated open knee-chest position (see page 247). From the hands-and-knees position, place a firm cushion or two beneath your knees. Then with your partner's help, carefully lower your chest to the floor or bed so your buttocks are high in the air.

Do the breech tilt position for about ten minutes three times a day, when your baby is active. To ease discomfort, make sure your stomach and bladder are empty. Try to relax your abdominal muscles and visualize your baby somersaulting so her head is in position over your cervix. You may feel your baby squirm as her head presses into the top of your uterus (fundus).

## Use of Sound

Babies can hear well and often respond to sounds. By playing pleasing or familiar sounds so they seem to come from low in your uterus, your baby may move his head down to hear them better.

You can play music by placing headphones or a smartphone or other mobile device on your belly just above your pubic bone. Or your partner can get close to your lower belly and talk or sing to your baby. The sound should be at a comfortable volume. Use this harmless technique for as long as you like.

## Use of Cold on Your Fundus

If your baby's head is near your fundus (the top of your uterus), she may move her head down if the area becomes uncomfortably cold.[12] To do this technique, place an ice pack on your fundus, making sure to have a layer of cloth between the ice pack and your skin. The typical advice is use the ice pack for no longer than twenty minutes at a time, but you may choose to use it for longer periods, if it's comfortable for you. You can also decide how often to use the technique.

# COMPLEMENTARY MEDICINE METHODS

The following methods are used to try to turn a breech baby without the use of medical equipment.

## Acupuncture

Acupuncture is used for numerous health-related purposes, including induction (see page 281). The acupuncture point for turning a breech baby is Urinary Bladder 67, which is located on the outside tip of each little toe. To encourage the baby to change position, a trained acupuncturist places needles on each little toe.

Your acupuncturist may also use moxibustion (see page 281), and you may be taught the technique so you can do it yourself several times each day. Some scientific trials of moxibustion report that its success rate for turning breech babies by the onset of labor is 50 percent.[13]

## Webster Technique

This chiropractic technique involves the analysis of the mother's pelvis, an adjustment of her sacrum, and relief of abdominal muscle tension. The goal is to relieve any *uterine* constraint that may be preventing the baby from moving into a favorable birth position.[14]

Although this technique hasn't been formally studied, its popularity is growing. To find a chiropractor trained in the Webster Technique, visit the website for the International Chiropractic Pediatric Association at http://www.icpa4kids.com.

## Two Views on a Breech Birth

At the thirty-fifth week of pregnancy, when we learned our baby was breech, we went to a chiropractor and an acupuncturist. Fortunately for us, our baby turned head down two weeks later, and we were able to have the birth we'd planned.
—*Megan and Peter*

We'd planned a natural birth, but found out at thirty-five weeks that our baby was breech. We tried acupuncture, moxibustion, lights, talking, and pelvic tilts; nothing worked. We then tried an external version, which also didn't work. So we scheduled a cesarean section for a day after the due date, to allow for our baby's full development. Our caregiver helped us make a cesarean birth plan that would let us have the best possible birth experience.
—*Jamie and Jonathan*

## EXTERNAL VERSION

If self-help techniques or complementary medicine methods aren't successful, you may try an *external version*. This hands-on procedure is done by a physician, who presses on the mother's abdomen to encourage the baby to turn. External version is usually done around the thirty-seventh to thirty-eighth week of pregnancy, but some women consent to the procedure earlier in pregnancy on an experimental basis to evaluate success and safety. Studies of external version indicate that it's a safe procedure with a roughly 65 percent success rate.[15] For 35 percent of women who have the procedure, though, the babies either didn't turn or had turned but resumed a breech presentation and usually were born by cesarean section.

For a detailed description of what to expect during an external version and what you and your partner or doula can do to improve its chances of success, visit http://www.PCNGuide.com.

## BIRTH OPTIONS FOR A BREECH BABY

Although vaginal breech births usually result in healthy babies, they carry greater risks of the following problems than vaginal births with vertex presentations:

- prolapsed cord (see page 289)
- spinal cord injury (rarely), which can occur if the baby's head is tilted back (hyperextended) when it passes through the birth canal
- compressed cord—during a vaginal breech birth, the baby's feet and body are born before her head; as the baby's head comes through the cervix and birth canal, it can compress the cord and reduce the amount of oxygen in the blood
- delayed birth of head—because the baby's feet and buttocks are smaller than her head, they may be born before the cervix dilates enough for her head to pass through; in this event, the birth of her head may be delayed, which may cause the baby distress

Because of these potential complications, cesarean sections have become routine for delivering breech babies in the United States and Canada. The trend toward cesareans began in the 1970s, as improvements in the safety of cesarean surgery led to its increased use. As the number of vaginal breech births declined, fewer caregivers learned the skills to conduct them, which led to a further decline. Then in 2000, a large study found that breech babies born by cesarean had better outcomes than those born vaginally.[16] Consequently, vaginal births of breech babies in many countries plummeted. (Sadly, it was later discovered that the study had many faults that unjustifiably exaggerated the dangers of breech birth, and the reliability of the study's conclusions was brought into question. The authors were criticized for lack of transparency and poor clinical guidelines.)

Newer research has found that for some breech babies, vaginal birth is safer than a cesarean.[17] Those who support these findings urge caregivers to screen for breech babies with high chances of having a safe vaginal birth, then planning vaginal births for those babies, using protocols that allow for an immediate cesarean, if necessary. When caregivers follow this practice guideline, about half of breech babies are born vaginally, the number of complications linked to vaginal breech birth clearly decrease, and both mother and baby do well.

In many major hospitals in Europe and Australia, vaginal breech births are routine. Maternal health-care providers in Canada are striving to make vaginal breech birth a possible option. The Society of Obstetricians and Gynaecologists of Canada has published a practice guideline that supports vaginal breech births under selected circumstances.

In the United States, the number of physicians trained and skilled in vaginal breech birth is very small, so the hospitals where it's possible are few and far between.

For most women, if attempts to turn a breech baby are unsuccessful by the thirty-seventh to thirty-eighth week of pregnancy, it's time to consider a planned cesarean birth. See page 320 to learn how to prepare for the best possible cesarean birth.

# Diagnostic Tests

Caregivers routinely use screening tests in pregnancy to assess the health of the mother and baby. (See page 63 and visit our website, http://www.PCNGuide.com, to learn more about screening tests.) If a screening test shows a potential problem or if you have symptoms of a specific pregnancy complication, your caregiver may suggest a diagnostic test to confirm that you have a problem and to detect its severity. Because the results from one test might not be completely accurate, your caregiver may order several tests to confirm a diagnosis.

Some diagnostic tests have more risks than others. Asking key questions about a test can help you learn its risks and benefits, and knowing this information will help you decide whether to have the test (see page 9).

The following sections describe common diagnostic tests. They're discussed by order of frequency, starting with the ones most commonly used. For more information on these and other diagnostic tests, visit our website.

## TESTS TO DETECT GENETIC DEFECTS AND DISEASES

The following tests can provide helpful information if it's important for you to know in advance whether your baby has a specific genetic problem. These tests are considered invasive, and their potential risks include miscarriage, infection, bleeding, or leaking of amniotic fluid. The general recommendation is to have noninvasive screening tests first (see pages 63 and 66) and have them only if your baby is at high risk for a genetic problem.

### Amniocentesis

Between the fifteenth and twentieth weeks of pregnancy, a needle is inserted into your belly to get a small sample of amniotic fluid. A laboratory then tests the sample to detect Down syndrome, sickle cell anemia, neural tube defects, and other disorders. The results are available in about two weeks. Your caregiver also can use amniocentesis in late pregnancy to assess your baby's lung maturity before a preterm birth.

### Chorionic villus sampling (CVS)

This test examines a small piece from the chorionic villi (the early placenta) to provide information about chromosomal abnormalities in your baby. CVS can be done between the tenth and thirteenth weeks of pregnancy, and results are available after one week.

### Fetal blood sampling

This test (also called cordocentesis or percutaneous umbilical blood sampling) assesses a sample of your baby's blood from the umbilical cord to detect chromosomal defects, blood disorders, and conditions such as infection and anemia. It can be done after the eighteenth week of pregnancy. Results are available in seventy-two hours. Because the test carries more risks than amniocentesis, caregivers use it only when they need confirmation of a diagnosis more quickly than amniocentesis can provide.

# IMAGING TESTS FOR YOUR HEALTH AND YOUR BABY'S WELL-BEING

The following tests allow a noninvasive look at your baby and uterine structures. Except for x-ray, they pose no significant risks to you or your baby.

## Ultrasound scan

An ultrasound scan helps estimate your baby's gestational age and maturity, locates her organs and structures, and detects her presentation and position in the uterus. It also can determine preterm cervical changes and assess amniotic fluid volume when evaluating your baby's well-being. Caregivers often use ultrasound scans in conjunction with other procedures such as external version of a breech baby, CVS, and amniocentesis. (For information about an ultrasound scan as a screening test, see page 65.)

## Magnetic resonance imaging (MRI)

Visual images of the internal structure of your baby can help confirm malformations. MRI also helps assess your internal organs for potential complications. Your caregiver may use MRI when the results of an ultrasound scan are unclear.

## Doppler arterial blood flow studies (velocimetry)

A Doppler ultrasound unit placed on your abdomen provides information about the circulation of blood within and among the uterus, placenta, and your baby. Your caregivers may use this test to identify if your baby is at risk for blood flow complications, such as intrauterine growth restriction (IUGR), anemia, and prematurity from severe preeclampsia.

## X-ray

See page 78.

# TESTS FOR YOUR BABY'S WELL-BEING IN LATE PREGNANCY

The following tests help assess your baby's well-being by monitoring his heart rate.

## Nonstress test (NST)

Your baby's heart rate is monitored for twenty to thirty minutes. (See page 182 for information on monitoring.) This test helps your caregiver predict your baby's well-being. If the results aren't reassuring, your caregiver may recommend other diagnostic tests.

## Biophysical profile (BPP)

The BPP combines information from an NST and an ultrasound scan to assess fetal heart rate, breathing, body movements, muscle tone, and the amount of amniotic fluid. Your caregiver can use BPP to assess if a high-risk or post-date pregnancy can safely continue or if induction should be considered.

## Contraction stress test (CST)

To bring on contractions, you receive Pitocin or are asked to rub your nipples through your clothes to stimulate oxytocin. Your baby's heart rate is monitored to see how he responds. This test can help predict whether he can withstand the stress of labor contractions (if not, a cesarean may be necessary). It's not usually done unless an NST indicates a problem.

Be aware that the results of these are sometimes difficult to interpret and may lead to more testing to further assess your baby's condition.

# TESTS TO DETECT POTENTIAL PREGNANCY PROBLEMS

The following laboratory tests offer information that helps your caregiver make an accurate diagnosis and choose appropriate treatment.

## Glucose tolerance test (GTT)

After fasting for eight hours, you have your blood drawn, then drink a sugary beverage. Your blood is drawn again once every hour for two or three hours. Your caregiver will diagnose GDM if your blood glucose levels are high.

## Vaginal or cervical smear

During a vaginal exam, your caregiver obtains secretions from your vagina or cervical area to detect infectious organisms, premature rupture of membranes, or substances that indicate an increased risk of preterm labor.

## *Key Points to Remember*

- Most pregnancies don't develop complications, and both the mother and baby are healthy at birth and afterward.
- With appropriate prenatal care and self-care during pregnancy, you can decrease your chances of developing serious problems from a chronic condition or from a complication that arises during pregnancy.
- Promptly contact your caregiver if you see any warning signs of pregnancy complications (see page 67). Early treatment helps minimize the severity of any complication.
- Before making decisions about prenatal tests and procedures, be sure you understand how and why they are being done and the benefits, risks, and possible alternatives. Talk to your caregiver and ask questions until you feel that you can make an informed decision. Also, visit our website, http://www.PCNGuide.com, to learn more information about a specific test or procedure.

# CHAPTER 8

# Planning for Birth and Postpartum

Giving birth can be deeply satisfying when you participate fully in the event and your maternity care is respectful, kind, and tailored to your wishes. To help distinguish yourself as an individual with unique preferences and needs, it's important to communicate your priorities and desires to your nurses and caregivers. This chapter shows you ways to discover your options, examine your concerns and priorities, identify your preferences, and discuss them with your caregiver and others involved in your birth and immediate postpartum. With this information, you'll be able to create a written birth plan that effectively communicates your wishes to make your labor, birth, and immediate postpartum safe and rewarding.

You'll also learn how to plan for the postpartum period, so you can arrange for the support, assistance, and sharing of responsibilities that will increase dramatically when you have a baby.

# The Importance of Planning for Birth

A birth plan establishes a line of communication between you and those providing your care, ensuring that they know your priorities and preferences. If everyone understands and respects your wishes, you're more likely to be satisfied with the care you receive than if your wishes are unrecognized.[1]

If you have only one or two caregivers providing all your care—such as a small group of physicians who share on-call duties in one hospital, midwives who belong to a small home birth practice, or a freestanding (unaffiliated with a hospital) birth center—getting to know one another will be easy. The ability to communicate clearly and honestly with one another will strengthen as a personal relationship develops.

If your caregiver belongs to a large group practice—and most maternity caregivers in the United States and Canada do—it's harder to get personalized care, but good communication is still possible. Caregivers who belong to a group practice rotate who's on duty during specific shifts. The caregiver on call attends to all patients from that group practice throughout a shift. Nurses and hospital staff assist the on-call caregiver, but you don't meet them before arriving at the hospital. This system of rotating shifts ensures that everyone involved in your care has had time off for adequate rest. As long as communication among all staff is good, the system is efficient.

During a shift change in a hospital, the nurse whose shift has ended communicates a patient's clinical status directly with the nurse coming on duty. Nurses also communicate directly with the patient's caregiver whenever necessary.

More important than direct spoken communication is the medical chart. If you're planning a hospital birth, your caregiver electronically records information in your chart at each prenatal visit, and frequently during your hospital stay. This chart is read by your on-call caregiver to learn your history and any concerns, medical or otherwise. It becomes a permanent record that's available to you and your caregivers whenever you need medical care in the future.

It's possible that some of your priorities, concerns, and preferences for birth and the postpartum period haven't been recorded clearly in your chart, even if you've discussed them with your caregiver. An excellent way to ensure communication with your nurses is to prepare a birth plan to be placed in your chart. You can also bring copies with you to the hospital.

# Your Birth Plan

A *birth plan* (also called a "birth preference list," "wish list," or "goal sheet") is a one- to two-page letter you write to everyone attending to your care during labor and birth. In it, you describe your concerns and fears for labor and birth, as well as your wishes for the treatment of you, your partner, and your baby. Although a birth plan expresses your priorities and preferences, it's *not* a contract that dictates the actions of everyone involved in your care, nor is it a guarantee that problems won't arise that will require a change in your plan. Instead, a birth plan lets everyone know which safe options are most important to you, which in turn increases your chances of receiving personalized care.[2] The goal of the birth plan is to enhance satisfaction with your birth experience.

## FREQUENTLY ASKED QUESTIONS ABOUT BIRTH PLANS

The following are answers to common questions about birth plans.

### *How does a birth plan help us?*

Preparing a birth plan helps you reflect on how you'll best cope with the unpredictability, stress, and pain of labor and birth. Many safe choices are available to parents, which are discussed on page 149. As you learn about these different care options and treatments, think about what kind of care is important to you. Discuss your birth plan with your caregiver to enhance communication, clarify your expectations, and build trust and understanding.

Perhaps the most important reason to have a birth plan is to provide a way to introduce yourself and your partner to unfamiliar caregivers, nurses, and hospital staff, and to effectively and efficiently communicate your issues, fears, or concerns to all of them. By providing a birth plan for them to read, you free yourself from the need to explain your wishes and expectations each time a new person takes over your care—a clear advantage if you're coping with contractions during a shift change and can't focus on conversation!

### *How does a birth plan help my caregiver?*

A birth plan helps your caregiver understand your goals, preferences, and any special needs. It can also highlight any misunderstandings you may have or unrealistic expectations that aren't possible given your situation. By carefully addressing your priorities and suggesting alternatives where necessary for safety or practical reasons, your caregiver helps you create a birth plan that reflects the flexibility needed if problems arise in labor or birth.

### *How does a birth plan help the nursing staff?*

Because most of the nurses won't have met you before your arrival at the hospital, a birth plan helps them become acquainted with you and individualize your care. Studies show that women often feel disappointment, anger, or depression if their desires and expectations about birth aren't met.[3] A birth plan gives the nurses information about your concerns and preferences, which you expressed before going into labor, when you were calm, comfortable, and able to think clearly. If the nurses know what's important to you, they're better able to meet your needs and help fulfill your wishes.

## In Their Own Words

When my cervix was 9 centimeters dilated, I felt that I couldn't handle the pain anymore and asked for an epidural. Our midwife told me that I could certainly have one, but suggested that a bath might help relieve the pain just as much. This was exactly the sort of help I'd requested in my birth plan, so I knew she was respecting my wishes. I got into the bath and stayed until I was fully dilated.

—Hillary

## Common Q & A

**Q:** What can I do if an intervention is suggested during labor, but it's not in my birth plan?

**A:** If those providing your care recommend treatment that seems to go against your preferences, you or your partner may ask why it's needed. The reason may be that the treatment is the safest way to handle a medical problem that has arisen. Or it's possible that your nurses and unfamiliar caregivers are unaware of your preferences and are following standard protocol. Once they understand your desires and you understand their reasoning for the treatment, you should be able to discuss the matter with them and come to an agreement.

## How do caregivers feel about birth plans?

Reactions to birth plans vary. Some caregivers encourage birth plans and will work with women to follow the plan as much as possible. Others might not be familiar with birth plans. Still others believe that birth plans are unnecessary. These caregivers argue that they wouldn't administer treatment without the woman's consent; therefore, there's no reason for the woman to express her wishes about treatment beforehand. However, these caregivers might not realize how helpful it is for a woman to know in advance whether her desires for care are realistic and acceptable, or how stressful it can be for her to explain her wishes while coping with contractions.

You may need to explain why you're preparing a birth plan. Try to emphasize that you want it to enhance communication and trust among you, your partner, and everyone attending to your care. Let your caregiver know that your plan contains personal information you'd like the staff to be aware of, as well as ways they can best support you.

If you're asked to prepare a birth plan, your caregiver believes that it's an essential part of your care. Your caregiver considers your input and collaboration important for building cooperation and trust. Having a strong relationship with your caregiver increases your satisfaction with the birth experience and can provide reassurance if problems arise during labor or birth that lead to necessary changes in your birth plan.

If your birth plan is received with clear resistance, you'll gain the valuable knowledge that your caregiver doesn't want to know what's important to you and may provide care that goes against your wishes. Beginning on page 18, we discuss your options if you become uncomfortable with your caregiver's approach.

## How do nurses feel about birth plans?

Some nurses believe that birth plans are guides for providing individualized care. If there's not a birth plan in your chart, these nurses will ask you for one.

Other nurses, however, dislike and resist birth plans. Perhaps in the past they were presented with birth plans that seemed unfriendly, bossy, or unrealistic; as a result, they now believe birth plans do more harm than good. Perhaps they worry that a birth plan is the woman's attempt to control the staff or keep them from doing procedures that are essential for safety.

To minimize opposition, follow the advice on page 149 when preparing your birth plan. Be clear that you're not trying to tell the nurses the best way to do their jobs. Instead, you're simply trying to introduce yourself and your preferences so the nurses can take them into account when caring for you.

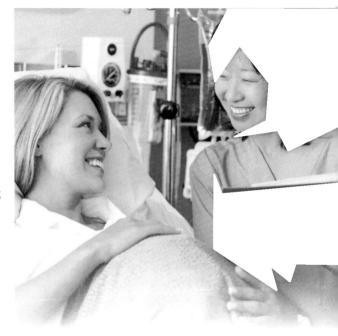

# Preparing Your Birth Plan

In Their Own Words

In these sections, we address the process of writing a birth plan. On our website, at http://www.PCNGuide.com, we offer several sample birth plans to give you ideas for what the final result might look like. Preparing your birth plan is a task that requires plenty of time; ideally, you should begin working on yours a few months before your due date. Follow these four steps.

1. Decide what general approach to maternity care you prefer.
2. Learn about specific options available to you if all is normal and also if unexpected problems arise—minor or major. Select the options you prefer.
3. Make a rough draft of your plan and discuss it with your caregiver.
4. Prepare a brief final birth plan that summarizes your priorities and preferences for both a normal labor and one with medical problems (Plan A and Plan B).

I'd educated myself on what I wanted for labor and birth and knew that the Bradley Method was for me. I had a doctor who was supportive and, after reading my birth plan at the hospital, I was assigned a great nurse who had used the Bradley method herself. My birth plan was followed nearly exactly. I wasn't offered any pain medications, and the nurses were all great.
—*Betsy*

Visit our website, http://www.PCNGuide.com, to see several completed birth plans.

## Step 1: Your Preferred Approach to Maternity Care

To figure out your preferred approach to maternity care, ask yourself this question: Of the following two options, which more closely reflects my thoughts?

### Option A: The Self-Reliant Approach

I want to actively participate in my labor by using nonmedical measures for comfort and labor progress and by taking part in decisions about procedures and other care options. My partner and I are learning about labor and birth, practicing comfort techniques, and attending childbirth classes. We're considering having a doula or another helper with us during labor and birth. I of course will accept medical help if it's truly needed.

### Option B: The Caregiver-Reliant Approach

I want those providing my care to decide how to manage my labor and relieve my pain. I'm more comfortable with appropriate technology and medical resources than with my own knowledge and nonmedical pain-relief techniques. I'll do whatever is asked of me, but I'd like to be kept informed about what's happening to me and my baby and why. I'm not spending much time outside of childbirth classes preparing for labor and birth.

Your preferences may align with one of these approaches, but if they lie somewhere between the two, explain how you'd like to participate and what role you want to play and the role you want your caregiver to play. Choose your caregiver based on these preferences (see chapter 2), or if you already have a caregiver, evaluate the care you're receiving. How does your caregiver respond to your questions? Are you comfortable with the answers? As you learn more about your choices, you may feel happy with your caregiver or you may become uncomfortable with the care you receive. If your caregiver doesn't support your birth plan, you can take one of the following actions:

1. Continue to accept your current care and give up some of your preferences
2. Express your discomfort and try to work out acceptable compromises with your caregiver
3. Change to another caregiver whose care better matches your preferences

## STEP 2: LEARN ABOUT YOUR OPTIONS AND IDENTIFY YOUR PREFERENCES

By reading this book, you can learn about most options and procedures for labor and birth, including key questions to ask about their benefits, tradeoffs, and alternatives (see page 9). Additional resources include other books and websites, maternity caregivers, friends who have given birth, childbirth classes, and hospital tours. Pay attention to whether the resources you use are evidence based (rely on well-designed research, not on opinions or customs). Your childbirth educator or doula should be familiar with the routine practices of maternity care in your area and can be a helpful resource as you prepare and write your birth plan.

As you learn about options, you'll notice those that are natural or low-tech are more compatible with the self-reliant approach, while options that rely on technology and medicine are more compatible with the caregiver-reliant approach. You may discover that you feel strongly about some options; these are good issues to discuss with your caregiver.

On our website, http://www.PCNGuide.com, you can download a birth plan work sheet. It provides a checklist of all the choices you could consider when thinking about your preferences.

## STEP 3: PREPARE A ROUGH DRAFT AND DISCUSS IT WITH YOUR CAREGIVER

Use the following list of topics to prepare a rough draft of your birth plan. (See page 149 for more detailed descriptions of these topics.)

### List of Birth Plan Topics

- basic information
- introducing yourselves
- issues, fears, or concerns
- care preferences for the following situations:
    - managing labor pain
    - normal labor and birth
    - unexpected events, including complications and a cesarean birth
    - postpartum care
    - care of a healthy newborn
    - complications with the newborn

You may need to schedule a longer-than-usual prenatal appointment so you'll have time to discuss your draft with your caregiver and learn whether your plan needs to be revised for clarity, consistency, or safety. This discussion is essential because your caregiver may request modifications to better fit with preferred practices, perceptions of safety, and hospital customs. In most cases, you'll probably be able to reach a compromise that satisfies you both.

# Step 4: Prepare the Final Draft

Revise your rough draft into a final draft. Incorporate any suggestions or modifications from your discussions with your caregiver and others. Use bullet points and keep it brief (ideally one page). A short yet complete birth plan will be easy for your caregiver and nurses to read and understand. It'll also clearly highlight your priorities and preferences.

Don't include lists of procedures that are acceptable and unacceptable to you. If circumstances change during your labor and birth, some "unacceptable" procedures may become necessary and "acceptable." When expressing a preference about a particular procedure, include phrases such as "unless medically necessary" to indicate that you realize that deviations from your birth plan may become necessary.

After completing your birth plan, put yourself in the place of the nurse who will read it. Is your plan friendly, respectful, and flexible (that is, does it indicate your awareness that labor isn't always normal or predictable)? Does the tone promote mutual trust and collaboration? If not, revise the language to help ensure that everyone involved in your care will respond positively to your birth plan.

When you're satisfied with your final draft, make copies for yourself, your partner, your caregiver, the nurses, and your doula. Bring extra copies with you to the hospital.

## Preferences for Managing Labor Pain

Here are examples of preferences for managing labor pain that couples have included in their birth plans:

- I'd prefer to give birth without pain medications. My partner and doula will support me using techniques we learned in childbirth class.
- I'd like to have an epidural as early as possible.
- As long as my labor is progressing normally and I'm coping, I want to avoid pain medications. However, if my labor is prolonged, if complications arise, or if the pain is too great, I may request an epidural.
- I feel strongly about avoiding pain medications. Please don't offer them to me; I'll ask for them if needed.

## Components of Your Birth Plan

Your birth plan should cover the following topics. Limit your discussion of each topic to one short paragraph or a bulleted list that summarizes just the essential points. (Visit our website, http://www.PCNGuide.com, to see several sample birth plans you can use for inspiration.)

### Basic Information

Give your names, due date, and the names of your caregiver, doula, other support people, and your baby's caregiver. You also may include a statement about the limitations of your birth plan, such as, "We realize our birth plan is neither a contract nor a guarantee of an uncomplicated labor. Our highest priority is the health of our baby and me."

### Introducing Yourselves

Tell those providing your care a little about yourselves to help them see the importance of the preferences in your birth plan. For example: "We've been together for six years, and this pregnancy finally happened after three years of trying to conceive. We're hoping for a natural, nonmedicated birth and would value your support."

### Issues, Fears, or Concerns

If you don't have any particular issues, fears, or concerns, you might not need to address this topic. But if you do, here's an opportunity to disclose them. See page 151 for examples.

Your feelings may be influenced by a previous negative experience, such as a miscarriage or a traumatic birth, unpleasant encounters with caregivers or hospitals, or childhood trauma. By disclosing your feelings and the reasons for them, you'll more likely receive treatment that takes your unique needs into account.

## Two Views on Birth Plans

With this pregnancy, I want to create a simple birth plan that includes only what I feel is most important and doesn't bother with what I consider "small stuff."
—Allison

After my first birth, I didn't get to hold my baby right away, and I regretted that. So for this birth, our birth plan is very basic, but there's a whole paragraph about newborn procedures and how I'd like that first hour to go, assuming all is well with me and my baby.
—Maria

## Preferences for Managing Labor Pain

After reading chapters 11, 12, and 13 to learn about self-help and medical measures for pain relief, describe your preferences for managing labor pain as clearly as possible. Use the Pain Medications Preference Scale on page 214 to help describe your needs. It can be hard to predict your choices perfectly, because you don't know how much pain you'll have in labor or how long your labor will last. But describing your prelabor preference can guide the nurse to the types of support to offer.

## Preferences for Normal Labor and Birth

Caregivers always recommend some monitoring of the mother and baby in labor, such as checking the baby's heart rate and the mother's temperature, blood pressure, and contractions.

Some interventions might be routine in hospitals (done for all patients in labor); however, they might not be necessary, especially if there's not an indication of a problem. Examples of such interventions include intravenous (IV) fluids, continuous electronic fetal monitoring, rupturing of the membranes, clamping and cutting the umbilical cord immediately after the birth, and suctioning the baby's nose and mouth. Other routine interventions exist for the convenience of the staff or caregiver, including the supine (lying on back) position for birth and the separation of baby from mother right after the birth for newborn testing and observation. Still other interventions are required by governments, such as administering antibiotics to the baby's eyes and conducting newborn screening.

Find out which routine interventions you're likely to encounter (along with the reasoning behind them). When preparing this section of your birth plan, mention only the preferences that matter to you. You don't have to express an opinion on every intervention, especially those that usually aren't done in your area. For example, you may say, "I prefer to avoid interventions and procedures, including routine ones such as IV fluids and continuous electronic fetal monitoring, and I want to discuss any that are being considered, along with possible alternatives."

## Preferences for Unexpected Events, Including a Cesarean Birth

If a problem arises during labor, birth, or postpartum, you may need undesired medications or interventions to ensure your well-being or your baby's. Under most circumstances, you'll have time to ask key questions (see page 9) such as, "Do we have time to discuss this intervention before I (we) must make a decision?" In rare emergencies, however, the need for immediate action may preclude low-tech measures or even much explanation and discussion.

When creating your birth plan, consider separating it into a Plan A and a Plan B. Plan A covers your preferences when labor and birth go smoothly. Plan B addresses how you'll want possible complications to be handled. For example, you may express preferences for the type of care you'd prefer in the event an unexpected cesarean birth is required. Although it can be disappointing when your Plan A isn't possible, you'll feel better about an intervention if you agree with the need for it, have thought about the possibility, understand your options, and can express your preferences. By being flexible with your birth plan, you'll increase your chances of having a healthy baby and a satisfying birth.

## Preferences for Your Healthy Newborn's Care

If you and your baby are healthy and doing well immediately after the birth, he'll need little more than skin-to-skin contact with you (with a blanket covering you both) and an opportunity to breastfeed; later on, he'll also need a warm environment, diapers, and clothing.

Your caregiver will probably want to do routine observations, tests, and procedures on your newborn to discover any serious congenital disorders or to prevent potentially serious illnesses. When considering the options listed on pages 363–364, balance concerns for your baby's comfort and well-being with the potential benefits and risks of each procedure.

## Preferences for Unexpected Problems with Your Newborn

You may worry about prematurity, illness, birth defects, birth trauma, or even stillbirth. To help manage your concerns, consider in advance how you'd want these misfortunes handled. This way, if a problem does arise, your forethought will prevent having to make such decisions when you're upset and unable to think clearly. Your birth plan can reflect your consideration of these rare possibilities, which increases the likelihood that you'll receive treatment tailored to your preferences (see page 294).

## Preferences for the Postpartum Period in the Hospital

If giving birth in a hospital, your postpartum stay will likely last one to three days. Because the length of your stay is limited, carefully plan how you'll use the time. For example, will you want friends and relatives to visit, or will you prefer to rest and focus on your baby? Will you want help with breastfeeding or formula feeding, diapering, dressing, or bathing your baby? Before leaving the hospital, find out your options for follow-up help with feeding and baby care. See below for more information on creating a postpartum plan.

# A Final Word about Birth Plans

You'll need time for research and thought as you prepare your birth plan. Decisions you make in advance, when you're calm and able to concentrate, will help guide everyone when you need to devote all your energy to coping with labor and birth. When you've finished writing your birth plan, you'll have a fairly complete idea of what you can expect for your care during labor, birth, and the immediate postpartum period. By communicating your priorities and preferences for care both under normal circumstances and if complications arise, you can receive treatment that takes your wishes into account.

## Issues, Fears, and Concerns about Childbirth

Here are examples of issues, fears, and concerns that couples have included in their birth plans:

- We have a history of infertility and miscarriage, so we tend to worry a lot about our baby's well-being and may need to be reassured frequently.
- I'm terrified of needles and will need someone who's understanding, supportive, and very skilled with inserting needles.
- I have trouble trusting strangers. Please introduce yourself and talk with me for a while before you begin my care.
- I'm anxious about labor pain and worry about losing control.
- I'm uncomfortable with the idea of being seen without my clothes on; please help preserve my modesty.
- Vaginal exams are very uncomfortable for me. I may cry when I have them. I need patience and gentleness, and would like as few as possible.

# Your Postpartum Plan

A postpartum plan is quite different from a birth plan in that it's designed for you, your friends, and family to ensure that your needs and your baby's are met in the days or weeks after the birth. You don't need to create as formal a document as your birth plan, but be sure to discuss and write down your needs, plans, and agreements with your partner and friends or relatives who will be helping after the birth.

These first weeks almost surely will be more challenging and stressful than you expected (but also more wondrous). You'll appreciate the help from family, friends, support groups, and professionals such as lactation consultants and doulas. Your postpartum plan will ensure that everyone knows and understands your needs during this time. As you make your plan, think about both parents' needs and how you can work together to meet them and who can help you. Here are some areas to consider:[4]

- rest and sleep
- errands and chores
- helpful advice and companionship from family and friends
- nutritious meals
- sound breastfeeding advice and assistance

## Decisions to Make for Your Postpartum Period

To help ease the transition into parenthood, identify your postpartum needs in advance and plan for how they'll be met. Here are some specific questions to get you thinking:

- What resources are available to help you in the first weeks after the birth, such as classes, support groups, books, and DVDs? Visit our website, http://www.PCNGuide.com, to download a form that helps you keep track of the resources you've found.
- Will your baby be breastfed or formula-fed (see chapter 19)? What help will you need with feeding?
- What help will you need with transportation, housework, meal preparation, shopping, and child care for older children?
- Who will help you? Your partner, relatives, friends, a postpartum doula, or a mother's helper (see page 23)?
- If you're feeling overwhelmed or depressed, whom can you call? Make a list of family, friends, and counselors who can help if necessary (see chapter 17).
- What equipment, supplies, and preparations will you need for your baby? (See page 153 for a list of useful baby items.)
- Will you use cloth or disposable diapers or both? Will you use a diaper service (see page 368)?
- Will you work outside your home after the birth? If so, when will you start? Will you work part-time or full-time? Who will provide child care when you and your partner are at work? Can you and your partner share some or all child-care duties (see page 25)?
- Will you continue to breastfeed while working? Is there a private, comfortable place at work where you can pump your breast milk (see page 430)?
- How will your financial situation change after the birth? Plan and follow a budget, if necessary, to avoid excessive spending and ensure that you can meet expenses.

Develop your postpartum plan from the answers to these questions and from information you've gathered from friends and relatives with experience parenting a newborn.

# Your Postpartum Resource List

After the birth, you'll thank yourself many times over if you take the time now to gather the contact information of people who can help with postpartum care. Visit our website, http://www.PCNGuide.com, to download a template that you can complete. Make several copies of this list for yourself and your partner. Post one on your refrigerator door and program the list into your cell phone. For help preparing your list, consult your caregiver, a postpartum doula, lactation consultant, or your childbirth or parent educator. You can also search the Internet for resources that may help.

# Equipment and Clothing for Your Newborn

If you've ever browsed through a baby boutique or big-box store, you may be overwhelmed by the amount of stuff that's advertised as necessary for proper baby care. However, the number of essentials you really need is modest. Use the following guide to help you acquire the necessary newborn equipment and clothing before your baby's birth. Visit our website, http://www.PCNGuide.com, to download a checklist of this guide. Consider shopping at consignment stores or thrift stores for gently used items. Babies rarely wear out their clothing before they outgrow it, so this option is better for your budget and better for the environment.

### Bed

- A safe sleep space in your bed or your room
- 3–6 lightweight blankets
- Bassinet, co-sleeper, crib, or hammock bed
- 2 sleep sacks or footed pajamas
- 2–4 sheets for the crib or bassinet
- 2–4 waterproof pads for your baby's sleep space, your lap, and diaper-changing areas

### Diapers

- Ask the retailer or diaper service how many diapers to purchase or order for the diaper system you've chosen (see page 368).
- 6–8 washcloths, or a pack of diaper wipes, to clean your baby when diapering
- 6–8 waterproof wraps or pants for use with cloth diapers
- Diaper pail (if using cloth diapers)
- Changing table or foam pad for counter
- Diaper rash ointment (ask your caregiver what to use)

### Bath

- 2–4 hooded towels or soft towels
- Baby bathtub (optional)
- 4–6 baby washcloths
- Cotton swabs for the umbilical cord
- Mild soap and shampoo
- Baby clothing (see page 371)
- 1–2 sweaters or jackets (depending on the season)
- 1–3 pairs of booties or socks
- 4–8 bodysuits or "onesies"
- Hats: 1 knit hat for a newborn and 1 appropriate for the season (sun hat for summer, warm hat for winter)
- 4–8 sleepers ("footies" or one-pieces)—lightweight or heavy, depending on the season

### Travel

- Car seat (see page 367)
- Diaper bag

### Baby equipment (these are optional, but come in handy)

- Thermometer that's safe and accurate for babies (see page 382)
- Birth ball (inflatable exercise ball)
- Dresser
- Blunt-tipped nail scissors or baby nail clippers
- Baby carrier or sling
- Massage oil
- Carriage or stroller
- Baby swing
- Baby monitor (keep at least 10 feet from the crib)

# Preparations for Your Baby's Birth

In addition to writing birth and postpartum plans, you can do many other things to prepare for your baby's birth during the final months of pregnancy. If you're planning to give birth in a hospital or birth center, use the following list to help you get organized. If planning a home birth, many of these tasks are still relevant, but ask your midwife what additional preparations you should make in your home, such as what food and beverages to have available for everyone and what birth supplies to have on hand.

1. Tour your hospital, or backup hospital if you're planning to give birth at a birth center or at home.

2. Preregister at the hospital. (Preregistration may be unnecessary for an out-of-hospital birth.) Sign admission forms, including a general consent form. During labor, you may need to sign additional consent forms for specific procedures. Try to read these forms before you arrive at the hospital in labor, and ask for clarification of information that you don't understand or that makes you uncomfortable.

3. If you have other children, arrange for their care while you're in the hospital or birth center. If you have pets, also arrange for their care while you're away (and for the first few days after you bring your baby home).

4. Pack two bags for the hospital or birth center: one bag for labor and one for the postpartum stay for you and your baby. Visit our website, http://www.PCNGuide.com, to download a checklist of the items listed below. Also make sure items are packed that your partner will need during the labor and after the birth, such as a toothbrush, changes of clothes, pajamas, and a swimsuit (so your partner can accompany you in the shower or bath).

## Items for labor

- this book
- comfort items for labor, such as massage oil, hot water bottle or heating pad, birth ball (if the birthplace doesn't have one), rolling pin, and so on (see chapter 12)
- two nightgowns or long T-shirts (if you don't want to wear a hospital gown) and a pair of warm socks
- hairband, headband, or barrette (to keep your hair off your face)
- toothbrush, toothpaste, and lip balm
- favorite juice, tea, or frozen fruit juice bars
- snacks for you and your partner
- personal comfort items (your own pillow, photos, blanket, and so on)
- phone numbers of people to call after the birth
- camera or video camera (check the birthplace's policies on recording births)
- music (smartphone, iPod or MP3 player, or CDs of relaxing music as well as earbuds or speakers—check the birthplace's available audio equipment and policies on listening to audio devices.)

## Items for your postpartum stay

- nightgowns or pajamas that you can nurse in
- robe and slippers
- cosmetic and grooming aids
- nursing bra
- clothes for the ride home (You won't return to your pre-pregnant size immediately after giving birth, so make sure the clothes are a comfortable size.)
- laptop or tablet, if desired

## Items for your baby to travel home in

- cloth diapers and waterproof diaper cover, or disposable diapers
- undershirt or onesie
- nightgown or stretch suit
- receiving blanket
- warm blanket and cap (if needed)
- car seat (properly installed in your vehicle before labor)

## Key Points to Remember

- Preparing a birth plan will help you and your partner learn about your caregiver, birthplace, and safe care options for normal and complicated labor and birth. Begin preparing your birth plan a few months before your due date.
- By providing a birth plan, you better ensure that everyone can understand your priorities and preferences for care.
- A complete birth plan includes practical information about you; issues, fears, or concerns you may have; and your preferences for managing labor pain, normal labor and birth, unexpected events, postpartum care, and newborn care.
- Think about the assistance and support you'll need during the early weeks and months after the birth. Seek helpful resources for the postpartum period, and use them to prepare your postpartum plan.
- You can use the final months of pregnancy to get organized for your baby's birth.

# CHAPTER 9

# When and How Labor Begins

In the last month or so of pregnancy, babies begin gearing up for life outside the womb. They've grown strong and mature enough to handle body functions independently, such as breathing, eating, and regulating body temperature. Sometime between the thirty-seventh and forty-second week of pregnancy, babies send signals that they're ready to be born. At that point, labor begins. This chapter describes the events and changes that occur in you and your baby during late pregnancy.

# The Last Weeks of Your Pregnancy

As you near the end of pregnancy, you may wish for it to be over. You may feel awkward, tired, fat, hot, and uncomfortable. You and your partner are probably eager to meet your baby and ready to enter the next stage of your lives. If your pregnancy passes your due date, try to remember that labor likely hasn't begun because your baby isn't ready to be born.

No exact time is best for birth. Most normal, healthy births occur after the thirty-seventh week of pregnancy but before the forty-second week. Some healthy babies are ready to be born as early as thirty-seven weeks, but others may need another month before they're ready. It's usually considered safest to let labor start on its own, as long as it falls within this five-week period and mother and baby are doing well.

Some preexisting conditions can override the physiological interaction among the baby, mother, and placenta, leading to births that start earlier or later than ideal. About 11 percent of births in the United States[1] and 8 percent in Canada[2] occur before the thirty-seventh week of pregnancy, and between 5 and 10 percent of births would occur after the forty-second week if labor weren't induced.[3] (See chapter 14 for more information on the effects of labor induction, which bypasses the intricate hormonal processes of normal birth, and on premature and post-mature births.)

## CHANGES IN YOUR BODY TO PREPARE FOR CHILDBIRTH

During the last weeks of pregnancy, your entire body and your baby undergo many changes to prepare for the birth. For example, your breasts start producing more *colostrum* (first breast milk). Your uterus contracts more often and more strongly. You may have contractions when you exercise, sneeze, bump your belly, or for no apparent reason. You may swear that you're in labor only to have the contractions stop. Guided by your changing hormones, these contractions are helping your body prepare for labor.

Your pelvic joints relax, allowing room for your baby to descend into your birth canal. You produce more cervical mucus, and your vaginal wall becomes more elastic. Even though you aren't yet in labor, your body is readying itself to give birth.

Your baby is rapidly storing iron, enough to meet his needs for the next six months (along with the iron he'll consume from your breast milk). He becomes chubby and able to regulate his own temperature. His lungs mature, preparing for breathing without difficulty after the birth.

As your placenta ages, the membrane between your baby's bloodstream and yours becomes more permeable, permitting large molecules such as *antibodies* to reach your baby. Antibodies and other immune properties help protect your baby against diseases to which you're resistant or immune, and the protection lasts for months. If you breastfeed, such protection will continue for as long as you nurse your baby.

Your endocrine (hormone) system controls these changes in your body. When a baby is ready to survive outside the womb, the hormones of both mother and baby cause a chain of events that initiates labor. Other hormones take over once labor is under way, influencing the rest of labor (see chapter 10).

# Key Vocabulary for Late Pregnancy and Labor

During late pregnancy or early labor, your cervix changes so it can dilate, and your baby assumes his birth position (usually head down). To describe and assess these changes and developments, your caregiver may use a special vocabulary. The following sections define terms that you may hear during labor and birth. Being familiar with these words may help you better understand your caregiver's reports on your progress.

## GRAVIDA

*Gravida* refers to a pregnant person. A *primigravida* is pregnant for the first time, and a "gravida 2" or "3" is pregnant for the second or third time.

## PARITY OR PARA

*Parity* describes the condition of having given birth. A *nullipara* (also called a *para 0*) has never given birth, and a *primipara* (also called a *para 1*) has given birth once (this term is often wrongly used to refer to a nullipara). A *multipara* has given birth more than once.

## PRESENTATION

Babies can situate themselves in the uterus in several ways, some more suitable for a straightforward birth than others. *Presentation* or *presenting part* describes the part of your baby that's lying over your cervix and will emerge from your body first. The most favorable and most common presentation (approximately 95 percent of births) is *vertex*, in which the top of your baby's head is down over your cervix. Other presentations are breech (buttocks or feet down—or both) and shoulder, face, brow, or compound (head and hand coming out together) presentations. (See page 136 for further discussion of these rare presentations that may cause labor difficulties.)

## Six Steps to Birth

The following six steps occur before a vaginal birth. The first three steps happen at the same time and usually begin days or weeks before labor starts (prelabor). The last three steps occur in order during labor.

1. Your cervix moves forward.
2. Your cervix ripens.
3. Your cervix effaces.
4. Your cervix dilates.
5. Your baby's head rotates and tucks (chin to chest).
6. Your baby descends through your pelvis, and is born.

## Common Q & A

**Q:** Will a vaginal exam tell me when I can expect labor to begin?

**A:** While a vaginal exam can provide information about the present state of your cervix and how much it has changed, it can't predict when you'll go into labor or how long your labor will last. It's likely—but still uncertain—that a nullipara with a ripe, thin, anterior cervix will soon have a shorter labor. It may be several weeks before labor begins, and labor may last longer than anticipated. It's also possible —but less likely—that a nullipara with a thick, firm cervix might be in labor soon.

## POSITION

*Position* refers to the direction toward which the back of your baby's head (the *occiput*) or other presenting part lies. Here are the most common descriptions of position:

### Occiput anterior (OA)

The back of your baby's head is pointing toward your anterior (front).
*Left (or right) occiput anterior (LOA or ROA)*
The back of your baby's head is toward your left (or right) front.

### Occiput posterior (OP)

The back of your baby's head is directly toward your back.
*Right (or left) occiput posterior (ROP or LOP)*
The back of your baby's head is toward your right (or left) back.
*Right (or left) occiput transverse (ROT or LOT)*
The back of your baby's head is toward your right (or left) side.

Your baby's position may change during labor between OA, OT, and OP, although by birth most babies move to the OA position and are born vaginally. These variations in presentation and position may mean that your baby doesn't fit as well as possible, which can slow labor or cause back pain. During labor, the goal is to help your baby find her way through your pelvis more easily or quickly by using positions, movements, and hands-on techniques. See page 238 for more information.

## STATION AND DESCENT

The downward movement of your baby into your pelvis is called *descent*. The location of the top of your baby's head (or other presenting part) within your pelvis is called *station*. It's measured in centimeters, in relation to the middle of your pelvis (the ischial spines), which is referred to as 0 station (see illustration). During late pregnancy, if your baby's head is still "floating" above the level of your pubic bone, it may be as high as a −4 (minus four) station (4 centimeters above the middle of your pelvis).

For primigravidas, some descent—either gradual or sudden—usually takes place several weeks before the onset of labor. This process is called *lightening* or *dropping*. These terms refer to the decreased pressure in your chest and upper abdomen, and the increased pressure on your bladder. Primigravidas may begin labor at a -1 or 0 station. *Engagement* describes when your baby is at 0 station and fixed in your pelvis. It can be determined by your caregiver by palpating your abdomen or by a vaginal exam. For multiparas, it's common for labor to begin with their babies still "floating."

For all babies, however, most descent takes place during pushing in late labor. If your baby's head is at a +1 (plus one) or +2 (plus two) station, it's 1 or 2 centimeters below the middle of your pelvis. When her head is at your vaginal opening and on its way out, it's at a +4 station.

# CERVICAL CHANGES

Changing levels and interactions of hormones cause your cervix to change gradually, beginning before labor and ending just before your baby's birth. Your caregiver can assess these changes during a vaginal exam and evaluate your body's readiness for labor as well as the progress of your labor.

Because these cervical assessments are subjective, they may vary if more than one person examines you. You may become confused or discouraged if examined within a short time by two people whose assessments differ. If the same caregiver checks your cervix each time, you can rely on that person's assessment of your progress.

The following paragraphs describe the changes your cervix undergoes during the labor process.

### Your cervix moves forward

Usually weeks before labor begins, your cervix is high and posterior (pointing toward your back); as labor approaches, your cervix gradually moves forward to an anterior position (pointing toward your front). See illustration at right.

Anterior Cervix    Posterior Cervix

### Your cervix *ripens* (softens)

During pregnancy and prelabor, when your cervix is still firm, it doesn't change during Braxton-Hicks (practice) contractions. Before ripening, your cervix is like a muscle that contracts when the uterus does, so it remains closed. When your cervix begins to ripen and its consistency changes, it no longer contracts when your uterus does. Contractions begin to efface and eventually dilate your cervix. Ripening may begin weeks before labor starts or just a few days before. This window of time helps explain why some women's cervixes dilate in late pregnancy, while others don't dilate until after a period of strong, frequent contractions.

### Your cervix *effaces* (thins or shortens)

The cervix of a primigravida usually effaces a lot before it dilates. The cervix of a multigravida typically effaces and dilates at the same time.

*Effacement* is measured either as a percentage or as a length in centimeters. Zero percent effacement means that your cervix is 3 to 4 centimeters long and hasn't begun to thin. Fifty percent effacement, or 2 centimeters long, means that your cervix has thinned about halfway; 100 percent effacement, or "paper-thin," means that your cervix has thinned completely. Make sure you don't confuse the centimeters of effacement with centimeters of dilation!

### The cervix *dilates* (opens)

Although your cervix usually dilates before labor begins (1 to 2 centimeters in primigravidas and up to 4 centimeters in multigravidas), most dilation occurs during labor. Dilation is measured in centimeters. When your cervix has opened the width of a fingertip, it's 1 centimeter dilated; when fully dilated, it's about 10 centimeters.

| | | | | |
|---|---|---|---|---|
| Effacement | none | 50% | 90% | 100% |
| Dialation | none | 2–3 cm | 5 cm | 9 cm |
| Position | Left Occiput Anterior (LOA) | | | Occiput Anterior (OA) |

# How to Distinguish between Prelabor and Early Labor

As you near the end of pregnancy, your uterus becomes more active, and you'll be aware of contractions. One of your biggest challenges is to figure out whether these contractions signal labor or prelabor. For most women, the shift is subtle and gradual from prelabor contractions (Braxton-Hicks contractions, which tighten your uterus but don't cause dilation—see page 39) to labor contractions (ones that dilate your cervix). For a few women, this shift is obvious if their membranes rupture (bag of waters breaks) with a gush before contractions begin, or if their contractions begin suddenly and intensely.

## PRELABOR

During *prelabor*, contractions can last thirty to forty seconds each and occur ten to twenty minutes apart, or they may last up to two minutes each and occur five minutes apart. Some women barely notice prelabor contractions, while others need to use distraction, slow breathing, tension release, and other comfort techniques to get through them (see chapter 12).

## Events of Late Pregnancy That Are Guided by Hormones

During approximately the last six weeks of pregnancy, the mother's body prepares to give birth and the baby prepares to thrive outside the womb. Once the baby's lungs reach maturity, the baby is ready to breathe air. The lungs begin to secrete a substance called 'surfactant' into the amniotic fluid, which begins the following chain of events that are guided by the baby's and mother's hormones:

1. The baby's brain secretes corticotrophin-releasing hormone (CRH), which goes to the baby's pituitary gland and stimulates it to secrete adrenocorticotropic hormone (ACTH). ACTH makes the adrenal glands secrete androgen, a steroid hormone, into the mother's bloodstream and onto the placenta.
2. The androgen is converted into estrogen, which causes the uterus, membranes, and placenta to produce prostaglandins, leading to cervical ripening and opening.
3. These hormones cause changes in the uterine muscles, increasing the number of oxytocin receptors by 100 to 200 percent and making the uterus more sensitive to oxytocin, which increases the frequency of contractions.
4. As the uterus contracts, it tightens around the baby and causes the ripe, thin cervix to open or dilate. Nerve fibers carry impulses from the cervix to the mother's pituitary gland, causing it to produce more oxytocin (as well as other labor hormones—see chapter 12) and build the momentum of labor.

This process ensures that, usually, birth takes place under the following circumstances:
• The baby is ready for life outside the womb.
• The placenta is no longer able to meet the increasing requirements of the growing baby.
• The placenta shifts its role to hastening the end of pregnancy (the birth of the baby).
• The uterus is ready to push out the baby.
• The mother is ready to nourish and nurture the baby.

In short, labor is initiated when the baby is ready to be born. When you understand how important a baby's maturity is to starting labor, you may wonder why anyone would want to interfere in this elegant process by inducing labor without a clear medical reason. (For more on labor induction, see chapter 13.)

The distinguishing feature of prelabor contractions is that they're nonprogressing; that is, they change very little in length, frequency, and intensity over time. They may even subside for a while and resume later. See page 171 for more tips on distinguishing between prelabor and labor contractions. Prelabor may last for a few hours to a day; if it lasts longer than a day, it's considered a *prolonged prelabor*, which can be tiring and discouraging (see page 175).

As puzzling and frustrating as prelabor contractions may be, try to recognize that they're doing the essential work of preparing your cervix to dilate by moving it forward and causing ripening and effacement.

You may wonder why it matters whether you're in prelabor or labor. You have to deal with these contractions, whatever they're called! From a clinical standpoint, the status of your contractions and your cervix usually determines when you can be admitted to the hospital or birth center. For a normal pregnancy, maternity care providers consider prelabor and early dilation no different than the events of late pregnancy. If you arrive at your birthplace with prelabor contractions and a cervix that hasn't yet dilated to 3 or 4 centimeters, you'll likely be sent home with instructions on when to return. For a home birth, your midwife probably won't stay with you if you're in prelabor, although the birth assistant may. See Signs of Labor on page 165 for more advice on when to call your hospital or caregiver and when to go to your birthplace.

If you're not admitted to the hospital or birth center because you're still in prelabor, you may feel embarrassed, disappointed, or upset. To overcome these negative feelings, try to focus on helpful ways to get through prelabor. See page 172 for practical suggestions on restful, distracting, and pleasant activities to make both prelabor and early labor positive experiences.

**Events of Late Pregnancy: 34-40 weeks**

**Fetus**
- Stores iron
- Gains weight, fat, strength
- Temperature regulation
- Gains mother's immunities
- Brain cortex doubles in size
- Lungs mature
- Secretes adrenal hormones, cortisol

**Pre-Labor Events**
- Assumes birth position
- Engagement

**Labor Events**
- Head flexion, rotation
- Molding, rotation descent

**Mother & Uterus**
- ↑ Colostrum
- Pelvic joints relax
- Interrupted sleep
- Frequent urination
- ↑ Braxton-Hicks contractions
- ↑ Vaginal mucus
- ↑ sensitivity to oxytocin
- Restless backache
- "Nesting urge"
- Soft BMs
- Nonprogressing contractions
- Cervix ripens, effaces
- Bloody show
- Labor pain
- Progressing contractions
- Dilation
- Rupture of membranes
- Expulsive contractions
- Pushing
- Placental separation

**B I R T H !**

**Placenta & Membranes**
- Large molecules cross to fetus (immunities)
- Converts adrenal hormones to estrogen
- ↑ Estrogen
- ↓ Progesterone
- ↑ Prostaglandin
- ↓ Amniotic fluid

**~ 34 Weeks**

Penny Simkin
© Penny Simkin, 2011-2013

# A NOTE TO FATHERS AND PARTNERS

The events of prelabor can be difficult to understand, making this time challenging for everyone. However, prelabor can be a pleasant experience with support, guidance, and the right attitude. Join your pregnant partner in distracting activities and try to remain patient, cheerful, and attentive. If you become confused or frustrated, contact your doula or a friend who has been through labor. This person can offer support, reassurance, and companionship.

# SIGNS OF LABOR

Recognizing the signs of labor is the best way to ensure that you don't mistake prelabor contractions for labor contractions. The signs of labor are divided into three categories: *possible signs, prelabor signs,* and *positive signs.* You might or might not experience all categories of signs.

*Caution:* If you're at least thirty-seven weeks pregnant, these are all normal healthy signs of labor. However, if you're less than thirty-seven weeks pregnant and have two or more possible signs along with six contractions in an hour, whether or not the contractions are progressing, call your caregiver. You may be in preterm labor. Your caregiver may ask you to try resting, taking a bath, or drinking water to stop your contractions. If they don't stop, you'll probably be asked to go to the hospital for further assessment (see page 179).

## *Possible Signs*

Possible signs of labor occur in late pregnancy and may indicate that the hormonal changes described on page 162 are underway (but cervical changes aren't yet occurring). These signs occur intermittently for days or weeks, but they don't indicate labor.

### Restless back pain that comes and goes

This vague, nagging back pain is often accompanied by a feeling of uneasiness or restlessness. You're unable to be comfortable in any position for long. This pain differs from the postural back pain that you may feel after standing or sitting for a while. It may resemble the back pain you feel before a menstrual period and may occur off and on for days. If restless back pain is the only symptom you have, don't get too excited. By itself it doesn't indicate labor or even prelabor.

### Mild to moderate abdominal cramping

These cramps may be similar to menstrual cramps and may be accompanied by discomfort in your thighs. With time, they may progress into distinct contractions, or they may stop.

### Frequent, soft bowel movements

This sign may be accompanied by intestinal cramps or an upset stomach. It's probably due to increased levels of prostaglandins, which cause your lower digestive tract to clear itself in order to make room for your baby as she descends.

### Nesting urge

In this sudden burst of energy, you focus on getting your "nest" ready. Whether you scrub every floor in your home, shop extensively, tie up all loose ends at work, or spruce up your baby's room, you do it with a sense of urgency. Your behavior may seem reasonable to you at the time, but it may surprise others. In fact, you might not recognize it as a nesting urge until after the birth.

Think of the extra energy as a sign that you'll have strength to handle labor, but try to avoid doing exhausting activities.

## *Prelabor Signs*

Prelabor signs indicate that your cervix is probably moving forward, ripening, or effacing. These signs may progress into positive labor signs the same day they begin, or they may simply alert you that labor will begin in a few days or weeks.

### Nonprogressing contractions

These contractions occur regularly and may last for a short time or may continue for hours without changing in length, strength, or frequency. They don't dilate your cervix, but probably prepare it for dilation. (See page 162 for more information on prelabor contractions.) Although nonprogressing contractions can be strong, long, and frequent, they're most likely to be mild and occur eight to twenty minutes apart. Try to be patient and maintain normal activity—eat, drink, and alternate between resting and doing distracting activities.

### Bloody show (vaginal discharge)

Throughout pregnancy, your cervix contains thick mucus, which may be loosened and released when your cervix begins effacing and dilating. Sometimes this loosened mucus appears as a sticky plug. More often, the mucus becomes thin and liquid (*leukorrhea*). It may be tinged with blood from small blood vessels in your cervix that broke as your cervix thinned and opened. Bloody show can appear before any other labor sign or it might not appear until hours after contractions have begun. You continue to pass bloody show throughout labor.

In late pregnancy, you may pass brownish, bloody discharge within twenty-four hours after a vaginal exam or sexual intercourse, both of which can cause harmless cervical bleeding. It's easy to mistake this discharge for bloody show. If you're unsure, note the appearance of the blood. After an exam or intercourse, it's usually brownish, like dried blood. If it's mostly mucus mixed with pink or bright red blood, it's bloody show. However, if it's more blood than mucus or your vagina is dripping blood, you may have a larger broken blood vessel or a more serious problem. In that case, call your caregiver immediately.

### Leaking of amniotic fluid

Your membranes (bag of waters or amniotic sac) may begin to leak before labor. Loss of amniotic fluid may occur as leaking or a gush from the vagina. It occurs in about 10 percent of pregnancies. Leaking may mean that you've developed a small hole in the bag high in your uterus and amniotic fluid is seeping out. If your underwear feels damp and you notice leaking when walking or changing position, let your caregiver know. Your caregiver may ask to examine you, to confirm that you're leaking amniotic fluid. (It may be urine or liquid mucus.) If you have Group B streptococcus (GBS—see page 125), your caregiver may want to give you antibiotics after your membranes have ruptured or begin to leak.

## *Positive Signs*

Positive signs of labor include contractions that become longer, stronger, and more frequent (*progressing contractions),* and that might or might not be accompanied by *rupture of the membranes* in a gush of fluid. These are the *only* reliable signs that labor has begun and that (with few exceptions) your cervix is dilating.

## Signs of Labor

**Possible signs**
- Restless back pain
- Diarrhea or soft bowel movements
- Cramps
- Nesting urge

**Prelabor signs**
- Nonprogressing contractions
- Leaking or trickle of amniotic fluid
- Bloody show

**Positive signs**
- Progressing contractions*
- Rupture of membranes in a gush of amniotic fluid
- Cervix dilated more than 4 centimeters

\* See the Early Labor Record on page 167 for instructions on determining whether your contractions are progressing.

## Progressing contractions

The purpose of progressing contractions is to dilate your cervix and push your baby down and out of your uterus. Unlike nonprogressing contractions, over time these become longer, stronger, and more frequent (or at least two of these three changes)—regardless of whether your prelabor contractions were twenty minutes apart and lasted thirty seconds each, or they were five minutes apart and lasted a minute each. The point is, these contractions become stronger and harder to manage than your earlier contractions.

In early labor, your contractions probably feel like abdominal tightening with some back pain. As labor advances, your contractions likely become painful. (See page 171 for further description of contractions.) If you've given birth before, you may have contractions that come and go for several hours until their pattern becomes continual and progressive. These intermittent contractions can make it difficult to determine whether your contractions are progressing. To help you decide, time your contractions and save the record to determine if they're progressing over time (see page 167).

## Rupture of membranes (ROM) with a gush of amniotic fluid

Also known as "when your bag of waters breaks," ROM doesn't occur in most pregnancies until the active phase of labor or later. However, about 6 percent of labors begin when ROM occurs with a gush of ½ to 1 cup of amniotic fluid. If ROM occurs this way, you may think you've lost control of your bladder. You may even hear a popping sound before feeling the wetness. Contractions usually start within hours of ROM. If your membranes rupture before you have contractions, follow these guidelines:

1.  Describe the amount of fluid (a trickle or a gush). Note the time and the color and odor of the fluid. Amniotic fluid is normally clear and practically odorless. A strong foul odor may mean infection. Brownish or greenish fluid is a sign that your baby has experienced stress (see page 183).

2.  Notify your caregiver or call the hospital immediately. Your caregiver may recommend one of two actions: inducing labor or waiting for labor to begin on its own. Labor may be induced soon after ROM if it occurs at term and especially if you tested positive for GBS (in which case, your caregiver will also recommend antibiotic treatment—see page 125). See page 9 for the key questions to ask about induction. Also see page 277 for more information on induction.

    Instead of induction, your caregiver may recommend waiting several hours to see if you go into labor spontaneously or if you can get labor to start. (For suggestions, see page 280.) If ROM occurs before term, your caregiver may take steps to try to prevent labor.

3.  After ROM, don't put anything into your vagina (such as tampons or fingers) and don't have sexual intercourse; doing so increases the risk of infection. Vaginal exams also increase the risk of infection, so try to limit the number of exams you have after ROM. It's fine to take a bath for comfort or pain relief after ROM. Research hasn't found that vaginal exposure to bath water causes infection.[4]

    *Caution:* On rare occasions (between 1.7 and 6.4 per 1,000 births[5]), the baby's umbilical cord prolapses (slips through the mother's cervix into the vagina) when the membranes rupture with a gush. This event requires immediate medical intervention because the baby may press against the cord and cut off his own oxygen supply. (See page 289 for further information on prolapsed cord.)

## Changes in your cervix confirmed by vaginal exam

Before admitting you to the hospital, your caregiver or nurse will check you for changes in cervical position, ripening, effacement, or dilation (3 to 4 centimeters with progressing contractions is a common indicator for admission). After ROM, your caregiver should postpone this exam until there are clear, positive signs of active labor (see page 165) to reduce the chance of infection.

# Early Labor Record

To help you decide whether you're in labor, keep an Early Labor Record. See the sample on the right. Keeping track of your contractions helps you decide when to call your caregiver or go to the hospital or birth center. (See page 177 to learn about the 4-1-1 or 5-1-1 rule.) Many women begin timing contractions when they can't walk or talk through them or when they need to use slow or light breathing (see pages 243 and 244).

Either you or your partner can time your contractions. To time them manually, you need a watch or clock with a second hand and a pencil and paper. When a contraction begins, write down the time (hour, minutes, and seconds). When the contraction ends, write down how long it

## Written Sample of an Early Labor Record

Contractions on **May 8th**

| Starting time | Duration (in seconds) | Interval or frequency (minutes since beginning of last contraction) | Comments |
|---|---|---|---|
| 1:54:10 a.m. | 40 seconds | — | Bloody show noted at 6 p.m. |
| 2:03:00 a.m. | 45 seconds | 9 minutes | Can't sleep |
| 2:10:15 a.m. | 45 seconds | 7 minutes | Loose BM, back pain |
| 2:17:30 a.m. | 50 seconds | 7 minutes | Stronger! |

lasted in seconds (duration). Note the length of time from the beginning of one contraction to the beginning of the next (interval or frequency). This information tells you how often your contractions are occurring. You can also include comments about the intensity of contractions, your appetite and the foods you've eaten, breathing rhythms used, bloody show, status of your membranes (have they ruptured?), and so on.

Instead of using paper and pencil, you may prefer to search the Internet for online tools to record your contractions or download one of the many apps to your smartphone. Most apps allow you to press a button when the contraction begins and ends, and it does the math for you to figure out the pattern. Practice using the app before labor. You can also enter information about activities and how you're feeling. You can send the information to others, if you wish.

Time five to six contractions in a row. Then stop timing them until their pattern seems to have changed (this change may take many hours or just a few), at which time you can resume timing. If your contractions are progressing, you're probably in labor. If they're not progressing, you're probably still in prelabor.

## *Key Points to Remember*

- Your baby and your body play key roles in the complex interaction of factors that trigger labor.
- It can be difficult to determine whether you're in labor. Recognizing the signs helps you figure out if you're in labor or still in prelabor.
- The most reliable signs of labor to look for are progressing contractions (ones that become longer, stronger, and more frequent over time) and the rupture of your membranes in a gush of amniotic fluid. To confirm that you're in labor, your caregiver may also check for cervical dilation.

# CHAPTER 10

# What Childbirth Is Really Like

When labor begins, all the information you've gathered and the plans you've made will suddenly merge with the reality of childbirth—a physical and emotional experience that's often unpredictable and uncontrollable. You'll be glad you took the time during pregnancy to learn how to work with your labor and birth and to figure out your preferences and needs. This chapter describes the sequence of events that occurs in a normal, healthy labor and birth. It also discusses how you'll respond to each stage of labor and how your partner can best support you as you welcome your baby into the world.

# Stages and Phases of Labor

Labor marks your baby's transition to an independent existence and your transition to parenthood. Even before labor begins, changes occur that prepare your body for it. During prelabor, which may last for days or weeks, your cervix moves forward, ripens (softens), and effaces (thins or shortens). (See page 161.) Over the course of labor, your uterus contracts; your cervix continues to ripen and efface, and it begins to dilate; your baby rotates and moves down your birth canal; and you give birth to your baby and placenta.

Labor is divided into four stages. The *first stage* (dilation) begins with contractions that are becoming longer, stronger, and more frequent (progressing) and ends when your cervix is completely dilated. It has three phases: early labor, active labor, and transition. The *second stage* (birth) begins when your cervix is fully dilated and ends when your baby is born. The *third stage* is the delivery of the placenta. The *fourth stage* (recovery) lasts for a few hours after birth, until your condition has stabilized. The entire process (excluding prelabor) can take anywhere from a few hours to a day or longer.

*Note:* On page 444 is the Road Map of Labor, a visual summary of the stages of labor with reminders of comfort techniques appropriate to each stage. It's accompanied by a chart that summarizes key information from chapters 9–14 into a "cheat sheet" you can use in labor for quick reference.

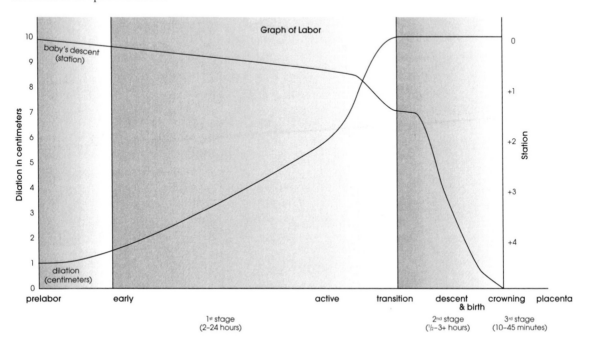

# First Stage of Labor: Dilation

When your contractions are progressing and your ripening, effacing cervix begins to dilate, you're in the first stage of labor. In early labor, your cervix dilates to about 6 centimeters. In active labor, it dilates to 8 centimeters. In transition, it completely dilates to 10 centimeters. Each successive phase becomes shorter and more intense than the previous phase. Each phase has recognizable characteristics that present unique physical and emotional challenges.

The first stage typically lasts between two and twenty-four hours. For a first-time mother, the average length is twelve and a half hours but can safely last for twice as long. For a woman who has given birth before, the first stage usually lasts half that amount of time (if labor wasn't induced). For some women, the first stage may be much slower or quicker than average. See pages 175 and 177 to learn more about handling these challenges.

## LABOR CONTRACTIONS

Throughout the first stage, your contractions become increasingly intense. But what exactly is a labor *contraction*? By the end of your pregnancy, your uterus has become the largest and strongest muscle in your body. When it contracts, it hardens and bulges as any other muscle does, and the muscle fibers shorten and pull your ripe, effaced cervix open. The sensation you feel during this process may be mild and uncomfortable or it may be intense and painful.

Contractions are involuntary; you can't control them. Each contraction builds to a peak, remains at peak for about half the contraction length, then gradually disappears, allowing your uterus (and you) to rest until the next contraction begins. A series of contractions follows a wavelike pattern: building, cresting, fading away, then building again. The frequency of contractions increases until your cervix is completely dilated.

In early labor, contractions usually feel like dull lower back pain or abdominal cramps. Very early contractions are usually short and mild, lasting thirty to forty seconds. The resting time between them may be as long as fifteen or twenty minutes. These contractions may make it difficult to tell whether you're in labor or in prelabor (see chapter 9).

As labor progresses, contractions become markedly stronger and longer. By the end of the first stage, contractions usually are very intense and last as long as ninety seconds to two minutes. When trying to cope with the intensity of labor, remind yourself that every contraction ends.

## What Is Normal Labor Progress?

The American Congress of Obstetricians and Gynecologists (ACOG) and the Society of Maternal-Fetal Medicine (SMFM) recently released a statement on ways to safely prevent cesareans for first-time mothers. Recommendations were based on compelling new research on labor progress and other related topics.[5] One recommendation was redefining active labor as beginning at 6 centimeters dilation instead of 4 centimeters. Another was waiting to recommend a cesarean because of prolonged labor until after several hours have passed since 6 centimeters dilation and other means to augment labor have been tried. These recommendations assume, of course, that mother and baby are tolerating labor well (see chapter 15). This concept of "6 is the new 4" will clearly reduce the number of cesareans, to the benefit of mothers and their babies.

## Two Views on Getting through Early Labor

The first contraction woke me at 3:25 AM. For most of that day, I had a contraction every ten minutes or so. The pain was mild, so my husband and I thought it was best just to go about our business as though it were any other day. We ran some errands, ate a nice meal, and napped. It was a relaxing time.
—Joy

My first contractions weren't very strong or frequent. To take my mind off the contractions, I took a shower, walked my dog, watched a movie, and just tried to relax. That night, after an entire day with little change in my labor, I tried to slow down the contractions with a bath so I could sleep. The bath helped, and I slept off and on for several hours.
—Katie

# First Phase: Early Labor

*Early labor* or the *latent phase* is usually the longest phase in the first stage, often because contractions are further apart, shorter, and less intense than they'll be later in labor. During early labor, your cervix becomes fully effaced and dilates to 6 centimeters.[2] You'll probably spend most of this phase at or near home. Because this is the "waiting and wondering" phase, review chapter 9 and use the Early Labor Record on page 167 to help you decide whether you're in early labor or still in prelabor.

The best way to cope with early labor is to ignore the phase until your mind or body no longer lets you do so. At that point, use coping techniques to help you enter a confident, optimistic state of mind. This mind-set can influence the interactions of hormones in a way that optimizes labor progress (see page 174).[3]

## GETTING THROUGH EARLY LABOR

When you begin early labor, you may feel excited and a bit nervous. You'll probably want your partner nearby to provide support, now that labor feels real to you. The key to coping with this phase is to avoid assuming your labor is progressing much faster than it really is. Try not to focus too much on each contraction. In fact, if you can ignore these early contractions, do so! Becoming preoccupied with early contractions often has the unwelcome effect of making your entire labor seem longer than you were anticipating.

Rest if you're tired or if it's nighttime. Otherwise, try to keep busy doing activities that are fun, calming, or distracting (but not exhausting). Here are some activities that may appeal to you:

- Pack your bag to take to the hospital or birth center (see page 155) or prepare your home if you're planning a home birth.
- Meditate or use guided visualization.
- Have a massage. During contractions, it's natural to tense up your body. Tension increases your perception of pain. Releasing tension with early contractions gets you into the habit of relaxing your muscles for later phases, when contractions will be more intense (see page 232).
- Take a long shower (but not a bath because a bath might stop your contractions when they are just beginning to progress).[4]
- Consume easy-to-digest foods and drinks that appeal to you, such as soup, broth, and herbal tea, as well as high-carbohydrate foods, such as fruit, pasta, toast, rice, and waffles.
- Go for a walk, visit with friends, listen to music, write in your journal, e-mail relatives, watch a movie, dance, or play cards or other games.
- Do a preplanned "early labor project," such as working on a hobby, gardening, laundering and sorting your baby's clothes, preparing one-dish meals to freeze and enjoy after the birth, or baking a birthday cake to welcome your new arrival. Be sure to have all the necessary equipment and ingredients on hand.

# THE THREE Rs: RELAXATION, RHYTHM, AND RITUAL

After several hours (or even a day or longer) of prelabor and early labor, you'll at last reach a point when you're unable to ignore your contractions. You can't walk or talk through a contraction without having to pause at its peak. Activities are no longer distracting or fun. This point marks a shift in your coping strategy. Instead of using distracting activities to cope with contractions, you instead begin using your planned ritual—relax, breathe, and focus. (See page 224 to learn about the Three Rs: relaxation, rhythm, and ritual.)

## Common Q & A

**Q:** My mother said labor went by pretty quickly when she gave birth to me. Will my labor progress as fast as hers did?

**A:** It might—or it might not. The answer depends on many variables, including whose body build and other characteristics you inherited, your overall health, and characteristics that your baby inherited from his father.

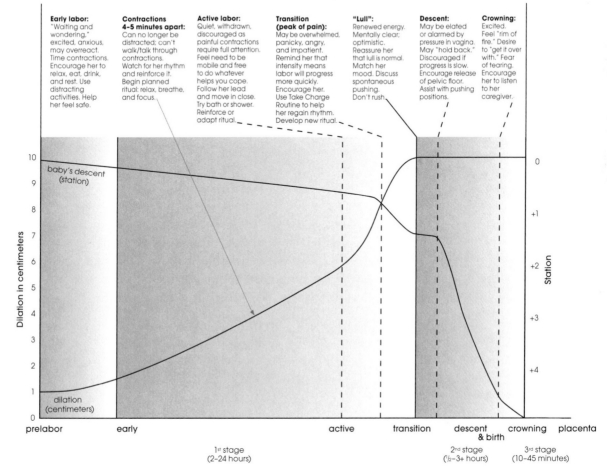

**Your emotions during labor**
How your partner can help

**Early labor:**
"Waiting and wondering," excited, anxious, may overreact. Time contractions. Encourage her to relax, eat, drink, and rest. Use distracting activities. Help her feel safe.

**Contractions 4–5 minutes apart:**
Can no longer be distracted; can't walk/talk through contractions. Watch for her rhythm and reinforce it. Begin planned ritual: relax, breathe, and focus.

**Active labor:**
Quiet, withdrawn, discouraged as painful contractions require full attention. Feel need to be mobile and free to do whatever helps you cope. Follow her lead and move in close. Try bath or shower. Reinforce or adapt ritual.

**Transition (peak of pain):**
May be overwhelmed, panicky, angry, and impatient. Remind her that intensity means labor will progress more quickly. Encourage her. Use Take Charge Routine to help her regain rhythm. Develop new ritual.

**"Lull":**
Renewed energy. Mentally clear; optimistic. Reassure her that lull is normal. Match her mood. Discuss spontaneous pushing. Don't rush.

**Descent:**
May be elated or alarmed by pressure in vagina. May "hold back." Discouraged if progress is slow. Encourage release of pelvic floor. Assist with pushing positions.

**Crowning:**
Excited. Feel "rim of fire." Desire to "get it over with." Fear of tearing. Encourage her to listen to her caregiver.

Dilation in centimeters — 10, 9, 8, 7, 6, 5, 4, 3, 2, 1, 0

baby's descent (station)

dilation (centimeters)

Station — 0, +1, +2, +3, +4

prelabor   early   active   transition   descent & birth   crowning   placenta

1st stage (2–24 hours)   2nd stage (½–3+ hours)   3rd stage (10–45 minutes)

## Hormones in Labor

Before, during, and after labor, your body produces several hormones:

- *Oxytocin,* the "love hormone," which plays a major role in orgasm, breast-feeding, and childbirth. In labor, it causes contractions and helps with progress.
- *Beta-endorphins,* your body's pain-killers, which are secreted when you experience pain, stress, and physical exertion. They help you transcend pain and enter a trance state that's sometimes called the "birth zone."
- Stress hormones (*catecholamines*), which counteract oxytocin and can slow contractions, leading to a prolonged labor.
- *Prolactin,* which is produced after the birth. It's necessary for milk production, and it calms and elevates your mood.

To decrease stress hormones and increase oxytocin and beta-endorphins during labor, the following are essential: confidence, a sense of safety, privacy, quietness, familiar places and faces, supportive interactions with others, and feeling loved (and reciprocating that feeling) through touch, massage, kissing, and caressing. Conversely, the following increase stress hormones and decrease oxytocin and beta-endorphins: anxiety, fear, anger, decision making, frequent disturbances, and feeling watched or judged.[1] Partners play a huge role in this process. If they remain present, attentive, and loving—even if they're not always sure exactly what to do—it makes a positive difference to the laboring woman. For more information about hormones and optimal hormonal interactions, read the booklet *Pathway to a Healthy Birth* by Sarah Buckley, available at http://www.childbirthconnection.org.

## A NOTE TO FATHERS AND PARTNERS

Early labor is an exciting time for you as well. If the birth will occur in a hospital or birth center, make sure her bags (and yours) are packed and stowed in your vehicle, and check that there's enough fuel in the tank. If you're planning a home birth, make sure you have the birth supplies that the midwife requested, as well as enough food and beverages for everyone. Have comfort items ready and accessible. Tidy your home so your partner and the midwife can move about during labor without having to navigate around clutter. Make sure your vehicle has enough fuel, in case a transfer to the hospital is necessary.

Help your partner through early labor contractions by following her lead. If she becomes quiet and uncommunicative during contractions, you should also become quiet. Don't ask her questions during contractions, and try not to act more excited than she is. However, if she becomes chatty, active, and excited between contractions, respond in kind.

Be aware of how she's coping during contractions, but don't hover or stare at her—this may have the unintended but annoying effect of making her feel watched. If you notice that she's tensing any area of her body during a contraction, help her recognize the tension by firmly touching the area, or by telling her about it between contractions in a gentle, nonjudgmental way. For example, "I noticed you seemed to tense up in your shoulders with that contraction. With the next one, try to breathe away any tension in your shoulders with each exhalation."

Look for rhythm in her breathing and movements during contractions, and try to match her rhythm with your touch, movements, and voice. Offer her water after every contraction or two. She might not want to drink it, but be sure to make it available. See appendix B for suggestions on ways you can help throughout labor, and see chapter 12 for information on comfort measures. Working with your partner during early labor contractions will pay off later, when her contractions become more challenging.

# Prolonged Prelabor or Early Labor

Sometimes, labor is *prolonged* (takes a long time to get started). If early labor seems slow, you might not truly be in labor yet. It can be difficult to distinguish between a long prelabor (in which your contractions aren't progressing and your cervix isn't dilating) and a slow early labor (in which contractions and cervical dilation are happening, but progression is slower than usual). The best way to know for sure is to time your contractions (see page 167). You're not considered to be in labor until your contractions have changed over the past few hours in at least two of the following ways:

- becoming longer
- getting stronger
- occurring closer together than before

How much time must pass before early labor is considered prolonged? Historically, caregivers were taught that early labor is prolonged if contractions continue for longer than twenty hours.[6] Today's caregivers recognize that a long early labor isn't itself a clinical risk.[7] However, if early labor is taking a physical or psychological toll on the woman, then it's prolonged—regardless of the amount of time that has passed—and the focus must be on supporting her with reassurance, comfort, companionship, rest, and nourishment.

If your early labor is prolonged, you may become tired and discouraged, but don't assume that your entire labor will be slow or that no progress is being made. These contractions may be allowing your cervix to ripen, efface, and move forward—changes that are necessary before significant dilation can take place (see page 161). Prolonged early labor is *not* a labor complication. In most cases, labor progresses normally as soon as it reaches the active phase.

Here are some possible causes for short, weak, or widely spaced contractions:

- Your cervix is still moving forward, ripening, or effacing.
- Your cervix is scarred from a previous surgery, cone biopsy, or another cervical procedure. For your cervix to dilate, it may require many frequent and intense contractions to overcome the resistance caused by the scar tissue.
- Your baby is malpositioned, such as occiput posterior (see page 286) or with a raised chin. If this is the case, you may also have back pain. Your contractions may seem irregular or they may couple (occur in pairs, with a short break between the first and second contractions).
- You're tense, anxious, exhausted, or distressed, all of which increase the levels of stress hormones that can hinder labor progress (see page 174). Several factors can cause stress, including a previous unresolved emotional or physical trauma, a previous difficult birth experience, grief from a miscarriage or abortion, a stressful relationship (with your partner, caregiver, or relatives), and fears about your own or your baby's well-being.

## In Their Own Words

After ten hours of mild contractions that were six minutes apart, I called the hospital to see if I could come in for medication to help me sleep. An examination showed that my cervix was 3 centimeters dilated and 100 percent effaced. My midwife gave me three options: get a morphine shot and go home to sleep, get the shot and sleep in an unused room upstairs, or be admitted and get an epidural. I chose to get the shot and go home, where I was able to sleep for a couple hours. When I woke up, contractions were strong, so I headed to the hospital. My cervix was 6 centimeters dilated, so I was admitted.

—Carrie

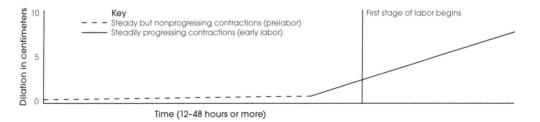

## What You Can Do

If early labor is prolonged, here are some suggestions to help you cope mentally and physically as you wait for your labor to progress:

- Try not to become discouraged or depressed by your slow progress. Try to accept it as temporary and appropriate for your body at this time.
- Nurture yourself with food, drink, and loving support.
- Alternate labor-stimulating activities with restful, distracting activities (see page 172).
- Don't time every contraction. Instead, time six contractions in a row, then wait until the pattern of your contractions seems to have changed before timing another series.
- If you have irregular or coupling contractions or back pain, assume that your baby isn't in an ideal position for birth. Use the techniques described on pages 247–248 to relieve back pain and move your baby. Once your baby is in a better position, your pattern of contractions should improve, and labor progress should speed up.
- If you're worried or tense, talk with your partner, caregiver, or other supportive person. Talking with someone may help you put your concerns into perspective. If all else fails, having a good cry—in private or with a compassionate companion—can help release any overwhelming sadness or anxiety.
- If you have a vaginal exam, ask your caregiver whether your cervix has moved forward, is ripe, and how much it has effaced. If your cervix hasn't changed much, you need patience and stamina to allow early contractions to complete these changes before they can dilate your cervix.

*Note:* If you know or suspect that you'll be very worried or tense in labor, talk with your caregiver, doula, counselor, or childbirth educator during pregnancy to help you identify and address potential sources of stress. Together, you can plan ways to cope with the stress during labor, such as using relaxation techniques, visualizations, massage, and slow breathing to calm yourself (see chapter 12). Also, talk about your feelings with a trusted friend or family member or a counselor.

## Medical Care for a Prolonged Early Labor

Despite your best efforts to cope with a prolonged early labor, if you become exhausted or have made little or no progress for more than twenty-four hours, you and your caregiver may need to decide whether to turn to medical interventions. There are two major approaches:

- Using medications to stop contractions or to help you rest. Your caregiver may recommend drugs such as tranquilizers, sedatives, uterine relaxants, morphine, or alcohol.
- Using medications or procedures to stimulate more effective contractions. Your caregiver may suggest stripping your membranes, mechanically ripening or dilating your cervix, breaking your bag of waters, ripening your cervix with prostaglandins, or inducing labor with Pitocin (see pages 281–283).

These medications and procedures can affect your baby and have undesired side effects for you, so they shouldn't be used without good reason. To help you make an informed decision, ask your caregiver the key questions about the risks and benefits (see page 9).

If scar tissue on your cervix is causing a prolonged and very painful early labor, you likely need medical help. Your caregiver may quickly massage your cervix open a few centimeters. If this procedure is successful, your cervix begins dilating, and your labor progress may then continue normally. The procedure is painful, and you may need to follow the Take Charge Routine (see page 186).

# Rapid Labor

Some women—especially those who've given birth before—have rapid labors. These labors begin with contractions that are only three or four minutes apart, and quickly become stronger, longer, and more frequent. If your labor progresses this quickly, see page 276 for more information on what to do.

## When to Go to Your Birthplace or Call Your Midwife

During your last month of pregnancy your caregiver will tell you when and whom to call if you think you're in labor. Depending on your caregiver and birthplace, you may call the hospital maternity unit, an answering service, or your caregiver's direct line.

Your caregiver probably will recommend the following:

- If this is your first baby, call when your membranes rupture (or may have ruptured), or follow the *4-1-1 or 5-1-1* rule. This rule means that your contractions are intense enough to require you to focus and breathe rhythmically, and are four or five minutes apart, each lasting at least *one minute* for a period of *one hour*. Whether you follow 4-1-1 or 5-1-1 depends on your caregiver's advice and how long it takes you to get to your birthplace or for your midwife to come to your home.
- If you've given birth before, ask your caregiver for recommendations based on your previous experience. Typically, you'll call your caregiver or hospital maternity unit when your membranes rupture or when you're having progressing contractions and other signs of labor (for example, bloody show or soft bowel movements with contractions). Because you've given birth before, you're likely to quickly shift from early labor to active labor. Consequently, you don't necessarily need to wait for 5-1-1: You may be advised to go to the hospital or birth center as soon as your contractions are five minutes apart.
- If you have a condition that requires hospital observation during early labor, call whenever you suspect labor. Examples include positive Group B streptococcus (GBS), a herpes sore, and any high-risk condition. See chapter 14 for information on these potential complications.
- Regardless of the status of your labor, you may always call your caregiver or the hospital maternity unit if you're anxious, have questions, or live far from the birthplace (or your home birth midwife lives far from you).

When you do call, be ready to report the following information that you've noted in your Early Labor Record (see page 167):

- how long your contractions last (duration)
- how many minutes apart they are (interval or frequency)
- how strong the contractions seem (intensity)—can you talk through them or do you need to use your planned ritual
- how long your contractions have been like this
- status of your membranes (bag of waters)—have they ruptured and was there a color or strong odor to the fluid
- presence of bloody show
- other information that will help your caregiver know about you and your pregnancy

The nurse or caregiver who takes your call uses this information to determine whether to tell you come to the hospital or birth center, or recommend that you stay home until further changes have occurred. If you're having a home birth, your midwife uses this information to decide whether to come to your home immediately or later, when your labor has further progressed.

## In Their Own Words

After a nurse examined me, she said I was still in early labor and told my partner and me to go home and rest. When we got home, he went to bed, but I couldn't sleep and found many tasks to complete around the house. Having some privacy and quiet time plus keeping active did allow my labor to progress, and I was admitted to the hospital just four hours later.
—Jennifer

# Second Phase: Active Labor

## GETTING INTO ACTIVE LABOR

By the time your contractions have reached the 4-1-1 or 5-1-1 (or even closer) pattern, (see page 177), you're probably shifting from early labor to *active labor*. During this shift, contractions typically become more painful (requiring your active coping skills), but cervical dilation may still be rather gradual. Your uterus seems to know that it's time for labor to progress, but your cervix hasn't yet "gotten the message." Strong contractions are required for a while before the cervix opens from about 4 centimeters to about 6 centimeters. Once it does, you're in active labor, and dilation typically speeds up.

## GETTING THROUGH THE ACTIVE PHASE

Active labor may be emotionally challenging for you. Your contractions have intensified and require your full attention to manage. You may feel discouraged when you think about how long it's taken your cervix to dilate just over halfway, and you may assume labor will continue as slowly until your cervix dilates to 10 centimeters. (It won't!) You may feel trapped, as you realize that your contractions are beyond your control and will continue to intensify until your cervix is fully dilated. You may weep because you feel overwhelmed. These reactions to this demanding phase are normal.

Although active labor can be challenging, you're *not* doomed to suffer through it. You can manage this phase (and cope better afterward) if the following are true:

- You recognize that 6 centimeters is a landmark, after which progress typically speeds up.
- You're allowed to labor in an environment that fosters privacy, preserves your modesty, and minimizes disturbances. When you're undisturbed, you can focus inward and find your spontaneous rituals (see page 225) to help you get through contractions.
- You have support people who unconditionally accept your coping style and assist you whenever needed. In this phase, you become serious, quiet, and preoccupied. During contractions, your partner and others should focus on you—they shouldn't talk among themselves or to you, unless you request a response. Remember that keeping a rhythm is essential to your coping. If everyone in your care team keeps your rhythm, you'll feel their support. (If you feel that someone isn't acting in a way that contributes to your emotional well-being, ask that person to leave the room.)
- You have the freedom to move about and seek comfort in whatever ways you find helpful.

## A Note to Fathers and Partners

Figure out how to help your laboring partner by following her lead. Just as in early labor, be attentive to her, but don't disturb her. If she wants silence during contractions (or all the time), keep quiet. Match her mood. Observe and support her ritual during contractions (see page 225). She may want you to help her cope by slow dancing or walking with her, stroking her, moaning with her, matching her rhythm by swaying or by moving your head, keeping eye contact with her, or counting her breaths. Or she may be so inwardly focused that she wants only your calm presence, perhaps allowing you to hold her hand or offer her a beverage between contractions. See appendix B for suggestions on ways you can help your partner.

If she seems disappointed with her progress, encourage her to be patient and trust that she's doing well. If you're discouraged with her progress, take her caregiver or doula aside (so you're out of her earshot) and ask about her well-being. Once labor progress speeds up, you'll both feel encouraged.

## Arriving at the Hospital or Birth Center

After you've called to report the information in your Early Labor Record (see page 167) and are told to go to the hospital or birth center, make sure you have your bag and several copies of your birth plan (see chapter 8), and head to the birthplace. Do *not* drive yourself; have your partner drive. If you know beforehand that your partner might not be able to drive you, recruit someone else.

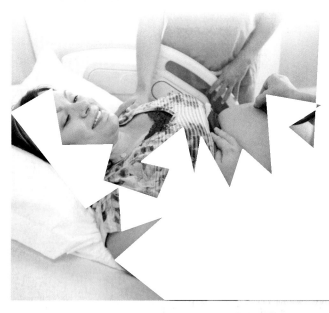

The ride to the birthplace may be challenging and uncomfortable. You'll probably be more aware of every bump and pothole than ever before! Your partner should drive carefully and not speed. Try to think of the trip as a way to confirm whether you need to be at the birthplace. Focus your breathing on something in the vehicle to give you a rhythm to follow. For example, your partner can nod in rhythm with your breathing or count your breaths.

If giving birth in a hospital, find out ahead of time which entrance to use. If you arrive in the middle of the night, the emergency room may be the only open entrance. Once you're in the hospital, walk to the maternity unit or use a wheelchair if necessary.

When you arrive at the birth center or the hospital's maternity unit, an admitting nurse should greet you, then take you either to a birthing room or the *triage* (observation) area, where your condition, your pattern of contractions, your dilation (with a vaginal exam), and your baby's well-being will be assessed. This information helps the nurse decide whether to admit you. If you think your bag of waters has broken, the nurse should avoid doing a vaginal exam because of the increased chance of infection; instead, you may be given a sterile speculum exam to obtain a sample of your amniotic fluid for diagnosis. (See page 165 for information on amniotic fluid.)

If the nurse decides that you're still in very early labor, you may be advised to leave the hospital or birth center until your labor pattern changes. You should follow this advice. If you stay at the birthplace, your labor progress is likely to dominate your thoughts, which can make your entire labor seem extremely long. You or your caregiver may begin to consider interventions simply to "do something," not for medical indications. If you leave

# IV Fluids in Normal Labor

Many women require an IV (intravenous catheter) at some point during their labor—for example, if they need medications such as Pitocin or antibiotics, if they choose to take pain medications, or if they become dehydrated. At some hospitals, it's routine to insert an IV in all laboring women shortly after they're admitted. In other hospitals, an IV is inserted only when needed. During a prenatal appointment, ask your caregiver what to expect and what options you may have.

IV catheters carry a few risks such as overhydration (too much fluid), which can slow labor and cause tissue swelling that can last for days after birth. In addition an IV catheter can limit (but not prohibit) your mobility in labor because you're connected to a wheeled pole that holds the bag of fluids. Ask whether the catheter can be "capped" (called a *Heparin Lock* or saline flush) and hooked to an IV bag and pole only when needed.

the birthplace, you can keep busy at home until your labor pattern changes. Also, your labor is likely to progress more readily when you're in an environment that feels safe, secure, and familiar.

It's natural to become discouraged when learning that you can't be admitted, especially if you're tired and are finding your contractions difficult to cope with. You may feel concerned, angry, ignored, or frustrated. You may worry that you won't return to the birthplace in time. Talk with the admitting nurse for reassurance, help with coping strategies, medication options to help you rest, or other suggestions if you don't want to return home (such as taking a walk near the birthplace or going to the cafeteria). As you wait for your labor pattern to change, focus on resting between contractions and on ways to relax or distract yourself during contractions. (See pages 175–176 for a discussion on prolonged prelabor.)

When you meet the criteria for admission, you're taken to your birthing room. Your labor nurse may assess you, take your medical history, get urine and blood samples, and check your baby's heart rate and position. You change into a hospital gown (or your own) and get an identification bracelet. You may have an *intravenous (IV) catheter* inserted. The nurse begins monitoring your contractions and your baby's heart rate (see page 182) for twenty to thirty minutes.

In some ways, admission to a freestanding birth center (unaffiliated with a hospital) is similar to admission to a hospital maternity unit. You're assessed in the same way; however, your midwife makes the assessments, not a nurse. You wear your own clothing and don't receive an identification bracelet.

Traveling to your birthplace and checking in during active labor create a major disturbance in your coping strategy. A good way to prepare for this disruption is to practice comfort techniques (see chapter 12) in noisy, busy environments *before* labor. That way, you may be able to continue coping during the ride and the admitting procedures as best you can, then return to your ideal focused state once you're settled in your room.

## INITIAL PROCEDURES FOR A HOME BIRTH

After receiving your call and deciding it's time to come to your home, your midwife assesses your progress in a way that's similar to how an admitting nurse makes assessments (see above). Your midwife brings needed supplies for the birth as well as safety supplies, such as medical implements, medications, an oxygen tank, and other essential equipment. Depending on your labor progress, your midwife may remain with you or may leave your home for a while (but stay within a reasonably close distance). Your midwife may work with an assistant, who remains with you if your midwife leaves for a time during early labor.

## Working with Your Labor

After your midwife or labor nurse finishes assessing you, make yourself as comfortable as possible. Continue your planned coping ritual or you may discover a spontaneous one (see page 225). Use comfort measures as appropriate (see page 226). Empty your bladder every hour or so; a full bladder increases discomfort and can slow labor. Make sure to keep yourself hydrated by sipping water every few contractions or by sucking on a frozen fruit juice bar or ice chips.

Try not to lie in bed throughout your labor. Lying in bed may increase the pain of your contractions and slow labor progress.[8] Unless you need to rest or your contractions are coming so fast that you can't move, try to periodically move about in bed or take advantage of gravity by standing and walking in your room and in the hall. (See pages 238–239 for a discussion of positions.) *Note:* If you choose to receive pain medications, your mobility may be limited (see chapter 13).

Continue slow breathing (see page 243) for as long as it helps you relax. Switch to light breathing or one of the adaptations (see pages 244–246) if your breathing begins to feel labored, if you can't keep your breathing rate slow, or if you can't maintain your rhythm, even after renewed efforts and active encouragement from your partner. Light breathing may be better suited for demanding contractions than slow breathing, just as short, quick breaths are better suited for demanding physical exercise than long, deep breaths are. By tuning in to your contractions, you can adapt your breathing rhythms as needed.

## Monitoring You and Your Baby during Normal Labor

Whether you labor in a hospital, birth center, or at home, expect your caregivers to monitor you and your baby closely, watching for signs that all is well or that signal potential problems that may require medical attention. As long as your labor is normal and your baby is doing well, you don't need medical procedures. Visit our website, http://www.PCNGuide.com, to learn more about monitoring and other hospital procedures.

### Monitoring You

Throughout labor, your nurse or caregiver regularly checks and records your blood pressure, temperature, pulse, urine output, fluid intake, activity, and emotional state. You may also receive vaginal exams periodically to determine the effacement and dilation of your cervix and the station, presentation, and position of your baby. These results are recorded on an electronic or paper chart that shows your labor progress. Your nurse or caregiver observes the frequency and intensity of your contractions either by hand or by an electronic monitor (see below).

## *Monitoring Your Baby with Fetal Heart Rate Monitoring*

During labor, many things influence your baby's heart rate: your contractions, fetal activity and movements, location of the umbilical cord, medications, your body temperature, your position, and other factors. The normal fetal heart rate (FHR) range is between 120 and 160 beats per minute. FHR varies within this range in response to changes in the amount of oxygen that's available. If your baby is handling labor well, he has a "reactive" heart rate, which means the heart rate either is unchanged, or it naturally slows down to compensate for the temporary reductions in oxygen during a contraction and speeds up between contractions. This response shows that he's handling labor well.

Your baby's heart rate can be monitored either by *auscultation* (listening) or by *electronic fetal monitoring (EFM)*. With auscultation, your nurse or caregiver listens to your baby's heartbeat during and between contractions with a Doppler, a handheld ultrasound stethoscope. (Some caregivers may use a fetal stethoscope.) At the same time, this person may place a hand on your abdomen to feel your contractions, noting whether your baby's heart rate speeds up or slows down and recording the findings.

There are two types of EFM. The commonly used external EFM uses belts to place two sensors on your abdomen. One uses ultrasound to detect the baby's heartbeat. The other is a pressure-sensitive device called a tocodynamometer, which senses the length of your contractions. Internal EFM is used only if external EFM isn't picking up accurate signals. During a vaginal exam, an electrode is placed on the baby's scalp to monitor the heartbeat electronically, and a fluid-filled tube called an intrauterine pressure catheter is placed in your uterus to detect the length and strength of your contractions. With both types of sensors, data from the monitors is displayed on video screens in your room or at the nurses' station (or both), is stored electronically, and can be printed out (see illustration).

In all birth centers and home births, auscultation is used. Many hospital midwives also use it. Most caregivers at hospitals prefer EFM because it lets nurses monitor many women at the same time from the nurses' station (an advantage when the nursing staff is overextended) and frees them from having to record a baby's heart rate by hand. Plus, the record is stored electronically. EFM may limit your contact with your nurse and may keep you in bed. By comparison, auscultation may feel more personal because your nurse focuses on you—not a screen—to monitor you and your baby, and it may work better with your coping strategy because you're not restrained from moving about by the EFM device.

Obstetrical associations in the United States and Canada endorse the protocol of intermittent auscultation for low-risk women, typically for one minute during and after a contraction every fifteen to thirty minutes in the first stage and every five to fifteen minutes during the second stage.[9] However, many hospitals follow a protocol of twenty minutes of EFM when you're first admitted to the hospital, followed by fifteen minutes of EFM each hour, as long as your baby's heart rate remains normal. If you're considered high risk—or if you have pain medications, Pitocin, or other interventions that may affect your baby's heart rate—you'll typically be placed on continuous EFM.

Studies show that for healthy low-risk pregnant women who have no medical interventions, their babies do just as well when checked by auscultation as when monitored by EFM (continuous or intermittent), even

Baby's heart rate

Mother's contractions

though auscultation doesn't give as much data. Having twenty minutes of EFM when admitted, continuous EFM, internal monitoring, or a combination of these factors lead to more forceps deliveries, vacuum extractions, and cesareans—without improving the health of babies at birth. For example, cesareans are often done for "indeterminate heart rate," but it may turn out the baby is actually doing well.[10]

During pregnancy, check whether your caregiver or hospital uses continuous EFM and under what circumstances. If continuous EFM is routine, check whether the hospital offers wireless (or telemetry) EFM, which allows staff to monitor you continuously while you're out of bed, walking around, or even in the tub.

For more information on the different types and techniques of monitoring, visit our website http://www.PCNGuide.com.

Depending on the maturity and health of your baby, his ability to handle labor varies. Some babies show signs of possible stress, known as *indeterminate fetal heart rate*, or if more extreme, *abnormal heart rate* (formerly known as *fetal intolerance of labor*). When FHR is indeterminate or abnormal, close observation, measures to increase oxygen (for example, having you breathe oxygen and rolling to your side to achieve the best flow of oxygen-rich blood to your placenta), and further testing help caregivers identify those few babies who aren't tolerating labor well and may need immediate medical intervention or delivery (see page 288).

## Evaluating Your Amniotic Fluid

When your membranes rupture, the appearance of your amniotic fluid can provide some clues on your baby's condition. Normal fluid is clear and has a slightly fleshy odor. If your fluid has the strong odor of old fish, you may have an infection. If your fluid is green or dark, your baby has expelled meconium (fetal bowel movement), which *may* indicate that she has experienced (or is experiencing) a lack of oxygen. The presence of meconium in amniotic fluid isn't uncommon; it occurs in 20 percent of all labors. If your fluid shows signs of meconium, your caregiver will observe your baby's heart rate frequently to assess her well-being and may ask a pediatrician to attend the birth as a precaution. It does *not* necessarily mean that your baby is in trouble.

If your baby has expelled meconium, the protocol may be to suction his nose and mouth at birth, although this practice isn't supported by research (see page 195).

# Third Phase: Transition

As its name suggests, you *transition* from the first to the second stage of labor during this phase. Your cervix is reaching complete dilation, and your baby is beginning to descend into your birth canal. At this time, your contractions are longer (ninety seconds to two minutes), much stronger, and closer together (two to three minutes apart). Although your labor is still technically in the first stage, your body shows some signs of the second stage. Your emotions and physical sensations are intense. You feel tired, restless, irritable, and totally consumed by your efforts to cope. You may lose your ritual (see page 225). Your body begins secreting high levels of adrenaline, which may lead to a "fight or flight" response (temporary fear, nausea, vomiting, agitation, hot flashes, chills, and trembling), but this hormone is beneficial because you become more alert and have renewed strength and energy just when you need to push out your baby.[11]

Involuntary spasms (precursors of bearing down) may stimulate your diaphragm, causing you to hiccup, grunt, or belch. You may find yourself holding your breath and straining or grunting during each contraction; this reaction is called the "urge to push." (See page 188 for more information.) Your back or thighs may ache. Increased pressure may cause your legs or even your whole body to tremble, and it may also cause heavy vaginal discharge of bloody mucus. Despite the intensity and pain of contractions during transition, you may doze between contractions, as though your body is conserving all energy for managing them.

Transition often lasts less than an hour (usually between five and twenty contractions).

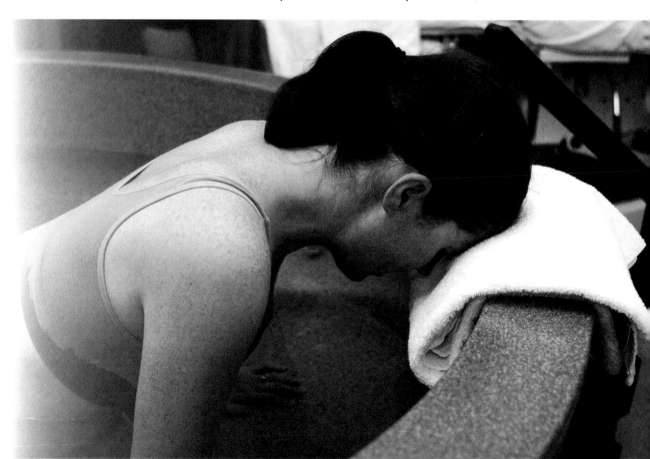

# Getting through Transition

During transition, you become focused only on your labor; nothing else matters. The intensity of your labor may frighten you. You may feel that transition will last forever and you can't cope much longer. In this phase, the encouragement and support from your partner, doula, and caregivers are essential.

Your responses to transition (such as fear, nausea, despair, or crying) are natural and unique to your labor. Your goal at this time isn't necessarily to remain calm, still, and relaxed during contractions. Instead, your aim is to maintain a coping ritual, with the help of your partner or doula if necessary (see page 186). You may rhythmically sway from side to side, tap your fingers or feet, stroke your belly, or rock back and forth. Or you may want your partner to stroke you or murmur rhythmically in your ear. You may find that moaning during contractions helps release tension. Or you may remain still and quiet during your contractions. Between contractions, try to relax and rest, if only for a few seconds.

You might like your partner to hold you close, or you might not want to be touched. You may want your partner to provide only eye contact and verbal encouragement. You may find hot, damp towels on your lower abdomen soothing. If you're sweating, your partner can fan you or wipe your face, neck, and chest with a cool, damp cloth. If you're able to doze between contractions, your partner can help you focus and begin breathing rhythmically as soon as the next contraction begins so the intensity doesn't overwhelm you.

If you recognize that you're in transition, you can cope better with this phase. If you think your cervix is only 5 or 6 centimeters dilated, you may become discouraged and worry that you have hours of demanding contractions to go. However, when you and your partner recognize the signs of transition described on page 184, your progress can encourage you. You can see that the challenges of transition lead to the second stage of labor, when your mental state will improve as the birth of your baby draws closer.

## *Pain Medications during Transition*

You can get through transition without pain medications, especially if you have the following: a desire for a nonmedicated labor; knowledge of what to expect and how to cope; recognition that you're close to pushing (and will soon be able to actually *do* something in response to your contractions); good support; and a labor that's progressing normally. Some women, however, find that transition is too much for them to handle; the pain is too great, they're exhausted, or they lose control or panic. If you have this response, or if you have no interest in avoiding pain medications, drugs are usually an option (see chapter 13). Contractions during transition are about as painful as they're going to be—if you can cope with them, you'll probably be able to cope with the rest of labor, if you wish.

While there's no shame in wanting medical help during this phase, don't take pain medications just because you fear that the intensity of your labor is abnormal. Remember that these strong emotional responses and intense contractions are completely normal in transition. Before deciding on pain medications, first find out how far your labor has progressed. Because transition typically lasts less than an hour (ten to twenty contractions), you may decide that pain medications are unnecessary.

## In Their Own Words

It's hard to watch your girlfriend be in pain and know there's nothing you can do. I just stayed strong for her and let her know I wouldn't leave her side. Observing the confidence in the staff and seeing my girlfriend smile when our son was born let me know that everything was fine.
—*Tom*

## Take Charge Routine for Partners

Use this routine when the birthing woman is in despair, weeping, crying out for help, or ready to give up. Also use this technique when she's overwhelmed with pain, can't relax, and can't regain her coping rhythm or ritual.

- Keep your composure. Your touch should be firm and confident. Your voice should be calm and reassuring. Give simple, concise directions. Don't ask her questions.
- Stay close to her. Remain by her side with your face near hers.
- Anchor her. Hold her hand or cradle her in your arms.
- Immediately when the contraction begins, make eye contact with her. To help her focus, tell her to open her eyes and look at your face or your hand.
- Immediately, give her a rhythm to follow with her breathing or moaning; move your hand or head to set a pace for her to follow (about one breath per each second or two). If she loses the rhythm, say, "Breathe with me; follow my hand. That's the way, just like that." Nod in time with her breathing to reinforce the rhythm.
- Between contractions, encourage her. Acknowledge that labor is difficult, but not impossible. Tell her to look at you the moment she feels the next contraction so you can help her.
- Repeat yourself. She might not be able to do what you tell her for more than a few seconds, but repeating your instructions will help her continue.

## *Premature Urge to Push in Transition*

In this phase you may develop an urge to push (see page 188), which may feel as though you need to have a bowel movement (because your baby's head is pressing against your rectum). You may also start catching your breath and grunting (making "pushing sounds"). When you first feel an urge to push, let your nurse or caregiver know. Try not to push until you've been assessed. If your cervix isn't completely dilated or is almost dilated except for one thickened area (a "lip" of cervix), you may be asked not to push.

While it's usually okay to bear down a little, doing so isn't worthwhile before your cervix is fully dilated. In fact, pushing too hard too early may cause your cervix to swell and slow your labor progress. You may find it difficult and uncomfortable to keep from pushing when the urge is strong. Try blowing or panting to keep from holding your breath (see page 246). Also try changing positions, such as to the hands-and-knees, side-lying, or other positions that neutralize the effects of gravity. Sometimes this urge is uncontrollable, no matter what you do. Often, a less-than-ideal-position of the baby's head, or even a hand up by her head, is the cause for the urge. Sometimes, an epidural is the only way to relieve it.

## A NOTE TO FATHERS AND PARTNERS

Transition is probably the most difficult challenge that you'll ever see your laboring partner experience. Her pain and discouragement may trouble you, but remember that her intense sensations and emotions are normal and unlikely to last for long. She and the baby are all right. Ask for reassurance and encouragement from your doula, nurse, or caregiver.

Your job during this phase is simple but vital: Help her keep a rhythm (see page 224). Listen closely for whatever rhythm she may have and help her maintain it. She may need you to give her a rhythm to follow. (See the Take Charge Routine at left.) Don't mistake rhythmic moans, groans, or other intense sounds for cries of agony. If they're rhythmic, she's coping. See appendix B for other ways to help your partner throughout labor.

If she begins catching her breath and grunting (making pushing sounds), she may have an urge to push. Call her nurse or caregiver. She may be in the second stage of labor and ready to push!

# Short, Fast Labor

Occasionally, a woman's entire labor lasts only six hours or less. Contractions may have started at three or four minutes apart, lasted a minute each, and were already so intense that the woman couldn't cope with them.

A labor this fast is rare among first-time mothers, but a few may have labors that are as short as three hours. Short, fast labors are much more common for women who have given birth before. If your labor progresses quickly and a *precipitate birth* is imminent, forget the 4-1-1 or 5-1-1 rule (see page 177)—call your caregiver!

Although a quick labor may sound appealing, it presents its own challenges. Early labor may pass unnoticed or so quickly that you suddenly find yourself in active labor without time to prepare psychologically. Your first noticeable contractions may be long and painful. You may feel confused, unprepared, and even panicky, especially if you think what you're experiencing is early labor. You may quickly lose faith in your ability to handle the rest of labor.

If you've planned a hospital birth, you may hurry to the hospital while trying to cope with strong, almost continuous contractions. At the hospital, you're probably met by unfamiliar caregivers, who spark a flurry of activity. You may feel anxious and alone if your partner can't accompany you. Even if your partner is with you, you may want to give up and take any medication available to make the pain disappear or at least become manageable. Your partner is probably caught off guard and shocked by the sudden intensity of your labor, especially if assuming you're experiencing early labor.

## WHAT YOU CAN DO IF YOUR LABOR IS RAPID

If it's clear that your baby will be born quickly, don't give up on your ability to cope. Try not to tense up during contractions and use slow breathing (see page 243). If slow breathing doesn't help you, use light breathing (see page 244) or moan or bellow rhythmically. Consent to a vaginal exam before making any decision about pain medication; your cervix may have already dilated to 8 or 10 centimeters. If your labor has progressed this rapidly, anesthesia may be unnecessary or may take effect too late to provide relief before your baby's birth. Rely on your partner, doula, and staff to help you cope with contractions and to reassure you that you and your baby are doing well.

In a rapid labor, contractions are intense and effective, and you may have the urge to push before the staff is ready. It may feel chaotic as they run around to get ready for the birth! Lie on your side and pant, trying not to push, if possible. Doing so gives your birth canal and perineum more time to stretch, decreasing the likelihood of tearing your vagina.

After the birth, you'll probably be relieved that you and your baby are safe, but stunned that the entire event passed so quickly. You may also feel disappointment because you weren't able to fully appreciate the experience, to use all the breathing and relaxation techniques you learned, or to share the birth with your partner as you planned. You may need to discuss the sequence of events with your caregiver and partner so you can process the birth and come to terms with it.

Although very few babies are born on the way to the hospital or birth center, in the unlikely event that you start to give birth before you leave home or on the way to the birthplace, or before your home birth midwife arrives, you and your partner should know how to safely catch your baby. See page 275 for more information.

# Second Stage of Labor: Birth of Your Baby

As soon as your cervix has dilated completely, you're in the second stage of labor. A new sequence of events begins: Your baby gradually leaves your uterus, rotates within your pelvis, descends through your vagina, and is born.

The second stage typically lasts between fifteen minutes to more than three hours. For a first-time mother, the average time is ninety minutes to two hours. For a mother who has given birth before, the second stage is usually faster than it was for her first birth. If you have an epidural, it's likely to take an hour or so longer.

## SIGNS OF THE SECOND STAGE

During the second stage, the pain of your contractions lessens and the interval between them increases. You calm down and can think clearly again. You experience renewed energy and become optimistic and aware of those around you. Now you can collect yourself for pushing your baby out.

### Urge to Push

The *urge to push* is the most significant sign of the second stage. It's a combination of forceful sensations and reflex (involuntary) actions caused by the pressure of your baby in your vagina during contractions. The urge to push occurs several times with each contraction and indicates that your uterine muscles are pushing your baby downward. When you have the urge, you experience a compelling need to grunt or hold your breath and bear down. At first, it may feel like a strong urge to have a bowel movement, but the sensation will change as your baby moves deeper into the birth canal.

You may have an urge to push immediately when your cervix is fully dilated or you may get a brief rest. It depends on various factors, including the degree and speed of your baby's descent, her station and position within your pelvis, and your body position. If your cervix is fully dilated, you generally can begin pushing when you feel the urge. If it's not fully dilated but is very ripe and effaced, you may be asked not to push, but to bear down only enough to satisfy the urge (see page 246).

For many women, responding to the urge to push is one of the most satisfying aspects of the birth experience; some women even have an orgasm when giving birth. Others find pushing painful and exhausting, while many are simply relieved to be able to start pushing.

*Note:* Some women don't feel a strong (or any) urge to push in this stage. Usually, time or changing to an upright position can strengthen the urge. Also, if you receive pain medication, especially epidural anesthesia, you might not feel the urge to push or it might be a vague sensation.

# THREE KEY CONCEPTS FOR THE SECOND STAGE

During the second stage, the following three key concepts should guide you and your caregiver: *Don't rush. Push when you have an urge. Use different positions.*

## Don't Rush

Although you and your caregiver are anxious to have your baby born, don't use prolonged pushing (see below). By holding your breath and bearing down only when you can't resist the urge, you're working with your uterus and not wasting effort. You're also allowing time for your vagina to stretch open gradually, which decreases the likelihood of vaginal bruising or tearing.[12]

## Push When You Have the Urge

The following are descriptions of different ways to push.

### Expulsion breathing and spontaneous bearing down

Use when you have an urge to push. With *spontaneous bearing down,* you naturally bear down or strain for five to six seconds at a time and take several breaths between efforts. This type of pushing makes more oxygen available to your baby than if you hold your breath and bear down for as long as possible.

### Delayed pushing (passive descent or laboring down)

Use when you have an epidural. Your uterus will be pushing your baby down and into a good position, but you won't feel the need to push. With *delayed pushing*, you try to rest and refrain from pushing until your baby's head can be seen at your vaginal opening (crowning) or until you feel the urge to push. (Many women with epidurals feel the urge near the time of birth.) This way, if your baby is occiput posterior (see page 286) or his head is tilted (either is a likely occurrence if you have an epidural), you avoid forcing him too deeply into your pelvis before he can reposition himself. *Delayed pushing* usually means a longer second stage, but as long as your baby is doing well, research shows that waiting an hour or two before pushing with an epidural gives your baby time to gradually reposition until his head is visible.[13] Delayed pushing is also much less tiring for you, and greatly improves your chances of a spontaneous vaginal birth (without vacuum extraction, forceps delivery, or a cesarean).

When it's time to push, your nurse or caregiver will tell you when and how long to push during each contraction.

### Directed pushing

Use if you can't feel your contractions, if delayed pushing isn't an option because of concerns for your baby, or if spontaneous pushing isn't effective. With *directed pushing*, your caregiver will tell you when, how long, and how hard to push. (See page 251 for more information on directed pushing.)

### Prolonged pushing

Prolonged pushing differs from directed pushing in the length of time you're expected to hold your breath and bear down (ten seconds or more, instead of five to seven seconds).

Not long ago, standard maternity care required that women push for as long and as hard as they could in order to push out the baby as quickly as possible. Many maternity caregivers are still more comfortable advocating prolonged pushing than spontaneous bearing down. Research shows, however, that prolonged, forceful pushing usually isn't necessary and may cause problems including exhaustion of the mother, overstretching of pelvic ligaments and muscles, possible perineal tears, later urinary incontinence (leaking of urine), concerns with the baby's heart rate, and failure of the baby to rotate or descend.[14]

Prolonged pushing, especially in the supine position (on your back), can also decrease the oxygen available to your baby and may cause your blood pressure to drop, both of which can increase the need for a faster delivery with an episiotomy. The second stage may last slightly longer with spontaneous or directed pushing than with prolonged pushing, but babies usually remain in good condition throughout the process, because you spend much less time actually pushing.[15]

Prolonged pushing is best reserved for women with inadequate progress in the second stage, even after trying different positions, or for women whose babies are already in distress and may require interventions (such as a forceps delivery, vacuum extraction, or cesarean) unless they're pushed out quickly. Well before your due date, discuss prolonged pushing with your caregiver. Include your preferences regarding routine prolonged pushing in your birth plan and discuss them with the staff when you arrive at the hospital or birth center. See pages 250–252 for more discussion on pushing techniques.

## Use Different Positions

As long as your labor is progressing well in the second stage and your baby is fine, use whatever positions seem most comfortable to you. If your caregiver is concerned about your progress or your baby's well-being, you may be encouraged to try a different position. Even if it's uncomfortable, this new position may correct the problem and avoid the need for further interventions.

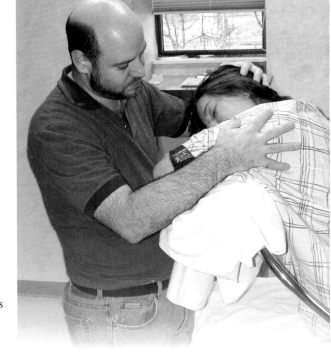

If your second stage is rapid, help slow down labor by trying a position that neutralizes the effects of gravity, such as side-lying, hands-and-knees, or kneeling over the birth ball. If progress is prolonged, try positions that take advantage of gravity. Be prepared and willing to change positions every twenty to thirty minutes. (See pages 239–240 for descriptions of positions.)

Some caregivers are comfortable with women giving birth in any position they desire. However, most caregivers prefer a position that they're used to (usually semi-sitting or on the back),[16] which might not be the best position for comfort or progress. During pregnancy, discuss your options with your caregiver. If only one position is allowed, plan to use several other positions throughout early second stage to aid labor progress. During second stage, if pushing is prolonged, ask whether a change in position might help resolve the situation.

*Note:* If you've received pain medications, your mobility and choice of positions may be limited (see chapter 13).

# Phases of the Second Stage

The second stage has three phases: resting, descent, and crowning and birth. These three phases share characteristics with the three phases of the first stage. High spirits, little pain, and slow progress characterize the first phases of both stages. Intense contractions, total mental absorption, and steady progress characterize the second phases. Lastly, intense sensations and confusion characterize the third phases.

| Resting | Descent | Crowning and birth |
|:---:|:---:|:---:|
| (latent) | (active) | (transition) |

## *Resting Phase*

After the intensity of transition, your uterus may stop contracting for ten to twenty minutes, allowing you to rest, clear your head, recoup your energy, and grow excited for your baby's imminent arrival. This resting phase is normal and may occur because your baby's head has slipped into your birth canal, causing your uterus, which had been stretched tightly around your baby, to slacken. Your uterus needs a few minutes to adjust to the change, but once it begins to tighten around the rest of your baby's body, strong contractions resume and your urge to push becomes powerful.

The resting phase doesn't occur in all labors. If your baby is low in your pelvis when the second stage begins, or if she's descending rapidly, your body may skip this resting phase or make it brief. Even if this phase doesn't offer you much rest, you probably still become clearheaded and emotionally recharged as you move into the second stage.

If the resting phase lasts longer than fifteen to twenty minutes, try using a position that enhances the effects of gravity to bring on an urge to push. Or your caregiver may direct your pushing, asking you to hold your breath and bear down even if you don't have an urge. Directed pushing may frustrate both you and your caregiver, as labor progress rarely occurs without the urge to push. However, directed pushing may be worth trying before using a medical intervention such as Pitocin (see page 282). If you and your baby are doing well, you may also ask if it's appropriate to wait longer for the urge to push.

## *Descent Phase*

During this phase, your baby descends into your birth canal and likely completes rotation to the occiput anterior position (see page 286). At this time, powerful contractions make your urge to push irresistible. You may find bearing down thrilling and rewarding because you can feel progress. Or you may feel alarmed by the full, bulging, stretching feeling in your perineum. If so, you may unintentionally tense your pelvic floor and "hold back" (see page 194), afraid to let your baby descend. When pushing, it's important to relax your pelvic floor and bulge your perineum (see page 91). Prenatal perineal massage (see page 252) is excellent preparation for the second stage because it teaches you to relax your perineum while it's being stretched. Your partner can help you during this

## Two Views on Crowning and the Birth

When our baby, Grace, finally crowned, I knew my wife could push her out, even though she was feeling exhausted. Sure enough, she tapped into a source of strength that probably surprised her as much as it did me, and pushed our daughter out. Grace was so slimy! But she was so gorgeous, I cried when I saw her.
—Ryan

When I began pushing, Jacob was holding my left hand and the nurse was murmuring instructions in my right ear. I didn't feel that my contractions were coming close enough together. I could feel a burning sensation as my baby's head slowly moved down. Everything seemed in slow motion. Finally, with a rush of pain and a huge relief, my daughter came out.
—Paige

phase by reminding you to relax, open up, bulge your bottom, or ease your baby out. This type of encouragement is usually more helpful than being told to push, push, push!

In this phase, you may need several contractions before you can push effectively. If you have trouble figuring out where to focus your efforts when pushing, ask your caregiver to use a warm compress to help direct you. Once the baby's head is visible, using a mirror to watch what happens when you push may also help you figure out how to push more effectively. (*Note:* To avoid being disappointed, don't use the mirror before there's any sign of the baby.)

Clenching your jaw and clamping your lips together are signs that you're also tensing the muscles in your vagina. By relaxing your face and mouth, you may be able to relax your vagina. If you let yourself release tension and push despite the pain, you'll find that pushing feels better than holding back.

As this phase progresses, the joy and anticipation you feel give you renewed strength. Your perineum begins to bulge, your labia part, and your vagina opens as your baby's head descends each time you bear down. Between pushes, your vagina partially closes and your baby's head retreats. With another contraction, your baby moves farther down, his head becomes clearly visible, and you may be able to see it in a mirror. You may want to reach down and touch his soft, wrinkled head. The normal squeezing of your baby's head by your vagina causes the scalp to wrinkle until his head moves farther down your birth canal.

### Crowning and Birth Phase

The third phase of the second stage is the crowning of your baby's head and her birth. It begins when your baby's head no longer retreats from your vaginal opening between pushes, and it ends when her body completely exits yours. During this phase, your vaginal opening stretches to its maximum, which likely causes a stinging, burning sensation called the "rim of fire." To reduce the risk of a vaginal tear or a rapid birth, you may need to stop pushing to let your vagina and perineum gradually stretch around your baby's head as it emerges. Depending on the speed of the birth, your caregiver may direct you to push only moderately or to push only between contractions. You may be asked not to push at all (see page 246). Your caregiver may support your perineum with warm compresses to prevent your baby's head from coming too rapidly and to help your perineum stretch gradually.

Although research finds clear problems with routine episiotomy, some caregivers still commonly perform them to enlarge the vaginal opening. See page 292 for more information.

## Protecting Your Perineum from a Large Tear or an Episiotomy

Many women worry that pushing will damage their vaginal tissues, or they fear that an episiotomy will be needed. Here are research-based actions you can take to protect your perineum:

- Choose a caregiver who prefers to avoid episiotomies and has a low rate of doing the procedure (less than 15 percent).
- Good nutrition promotes healthy tissues, so eat well during pregnancy.
- Perform perineal massage regularly for a few weeks before the birth (see page 252).
- When you push, use spontaneous bearing down for only five to seven seconds each time.
- Use pushing positions that put minimal strain on your perineum, such as side-lying, kneeling, or hands-and-knees (see pages 239–240).
- Listen to your caregiver's directions to pant and avoid pushing while your baby's head and shoulders are born.

## Holding Back during the Descent Phase

During the second stage, you may tense your pelvic floor (at least briefly) in response to the stretching sensations you feel when your baby's head is in your birth canal. Holding back is normal and usually passes quickly once you feel your baby descending. You may have trouble letting go for one or more of the following reasons:

**The pressure of your baby's head within your vagina alarms you, and you find it difficult to give in to it.**
Remind yourself that holding back tends to increase pain and slow progress. You'll feel so much better after letting go! Listen to your partner, doula, and caregiver when they encourage you to let go and let your baby out.

Try sitting on the toilet for a few contractions. This position may help your perineal muscles release naturally because it's associated with "letting go" of urine or a bowel movement.

Warm compresses on your perineum can help because the moist heat promotes relaxation and relieves the stretching sensation. This simple, inexpensive comfort measure also alleviates perineal pain and reduces the risks of tearing and urinary incontinence (see page 346).[17] In addition, having a warm cloth pressed on your perineum reassures you that your caregiver will help guide your baby out. Before your due date, discuss using warm compresses during labor with your caregiver and include the option in your birth plan (see chapter 8).

*Note:* During this phase, some caregivers use their fingers to stretch a woman's perineum. While this practice may help her push more effectively, research finds that it's often very painful and is no more effective for enlarging the vaginal outlet and preventing a tear than the use of warm compresses or even no treatment.[18]

**You're uncomfortable with having people stare at your perineum.**
Try to recognize that they're watching the progress of your baby, but ask to be covered as much as possible. For example, warm compresses can conceal your perineum as they help relax and stretch it.

**You fear you'll have a bowel movement while pushing.**
Because your baby presses on your rectum while descending, it's not unusual to pass a small amount of stool when you push. When this happens, your nurse or caregiver interprets it as labor progress. You might not even be aware of it, because your caregiver wipes away and removes the stool discreetly. Sitting on the toilet for a few contractions may help you dismiss this fear and relax. Try not to prevent passing stool. Holding back eventually will fail, and it may be more painful than letting the stool pass.

**If you've been sexually abused, the sensations of your baby in your vagina may remind you of your abuse.**
With a history of abuse, it's normal to make that association. However, the birth of your baby and previous sexual abuse are vastly different. Abuse may have caused pain and injury in your vagina, but it may help to remind yourself that you can push your pain out of your body as you push your baby out. Your baby becomes your ally in healing. Because it's important to separate your abuse from the birth of your child, see page 56 for more information on sexual abuse and childbearing.

# Your Baby's Birth

The second stage of labor ends with your baby's birth. If your baby's position is head down, first the crown of his head emerges, followed by his brow and face. After his head is out, it rotates to the side to allow his shoulders to slip more easily through your pelvis. One shoulder emerges, followed by the rest of his body, perhaps rather quickly. You or your partner may want to help catch your baby.

Your baby's body may appear bluish at first and may be streaked with blood, mucus, and *vernix caseosa* (a white, creamy substance that protected your baby's skin in your womb). With your baby's first breath, his skin color quickly becomes normal. All babies, regardless of skin color, experience this change in the first minutes of life, as respiration and circulation become stable. See chapter 18 for more information on your newborn's appearance.

Your caregiver's or birthplace's policy may require suctioning the nose and mouth of all babies immediately after birth. If the baby expelled meconium during labor, many caregivers suction the baby's nose, mouth, and trachea (windpipe) when the head is born and before the first breath. The belief is that suctioning prevents the baby from inhaling meconium and developing breathing problems or meconium aspiration syndrome. However, studies find that healthy vigorous newborns don't benefit from these procedures, and aggressive suctioning can cause abrasions in the baby's nose and mouth.[19] During pregnancy, discuss your caregiver's or birthplace's policy on suctioning and include your preferences in your birth plan (see chapter 8).

While you await the delivery of the placenta, your baby may be dried and immediately placed on your abdomen or in your arms. The umbilical cord is typically clamped and cut around this time; however, there are long-term advantages for your baby if cord clamping is delayed (see page 197).[20] The custom in some hospitals is to assess a newborn's well-being while he's in a baby warmer in the birthing room. Research shows, though, that

newborns are warmer and begin breastfeeding earlier when kept skin-to-skin with their mothers; in addition, most women report greater satisfaction when they have their babies with them immediately after the birth than if they're separated from them.[21] Before the birth, find out your hospital's custom on the use of baby warmers; in your birth plan, express your preference to hold your baby immediately after the birth (if he's doing well). Your nurse or caregiver can assess your baby while he's in your arms or at a later time, after he's had at least an hour of skin-to-skin contact with you.

## YOUR REACTIONS AFTER THE BIRTH

After your baby is born, your first response may be, "It's over! No more contractions!" and you may feel grateful and relieved that your baby is finally out of your body. These feelings may initially overtake your interest in your baby, especially if you had a long, tiring labor.

Conversely, you may temporarily forget about your labor and birth the moment you see or hear your newborn. You may be surprised or awed by your baby's appearance. You may hold your breath in suspense until you hear her begin to cry and breathe, then smile with relief and joy. If your caregiver needs to inspect your perineum and check for separation of the placenta, you may find the procedures uncomfortable and distracting, and you

## In Their Own Words

After my baby was placed on my chest, my body began shaking uncontrollably. The lights were turned back on, and I opened my eyes to stare at this slimy, squirmy thing that had been living inside of me. I always thought I'd need medication, but everything went so fast that I had a natural birth. It was an amazing, scary, and wonderful experience—something I will never forget.
—*Mary Ann*

may be unable to focus completely on your baby. Use light breathing to manage the discomfort. After your caregiver has finished these tasks, you can return your total attention to your baby.

## A NOTE TO FATHERS AND PARTNERS

The birth of your baby requires great physical effort by your laboring partner, even if she has an epidural. Here are ways you can assist her during this stage:

- Help her change positions and physically support her as needed.
- Encourage her to relax her pelvic floor as she pushes.
- Cheer her on as she pushes, but be sure you don't make it impossible for her to hear her caregiver's directions!

When your baby is born, you may experience happiness, exhaustion, relief, wonder, joy, and love for your partner and your baby—all at the same time. Your baby becomes the focus of your attention.

If your baby has to be taken away immediately after the birth (probably because of concerns for his well-being or because the staff want to check him carefully in a baby warmer in the room), stay with him so you can report what you see being done to him to your partner. Talk to your baby; he knows your voice and hearing it calms him. You might want to take photos to show your partner.

# Third Stage of Labor: Delivery of the Placenta

Typically lasting between ten and thirty minutes, the third stage is much shorter and less painful than the earlier stages. It begins with the birth of your baby and ends when the placenta is delivered. The following sections describe what you can expect, and discuss the care your newborn will receive immediately after the birth.

## WHAT YOU CAN EXPECT

After your baby is born, contractions stop briefly, then resume and cause your placenta to separate from your uterine wall. Although these contractions are typically much less intense than those before your baby's birth, you still may need to use relaxation techniques and rhythmic breathing. Or you may be so engrossed in your baby that you hardly notice these contractions. Your caregiver will probably direct you to give a few small pushes to deliver the placenta. You may appreciate seeing the placenta after it's delivered; after all, it's an amazing organ that allowed your baby to thrive in your womb.

## NEWBORN ASSESSMENT WITH THE APGAR SCORE

Within one minute after the birth and again at five minutes, your caregiver evaluates your baby's well-being with a routine assessment called the *Apgar score*, which can be done while you hold your baby. As soon as your baby is breathing and dried off, your caregiver considers five factors and gives a score of zero to two points for each one (see page 197). A score of seven to ten indicates that your baby is in good condition. Babies seldom receive a ten on the first score (most babies' hands and feet are bluish for a while after the birth). If your baby's first score is six or less, your caregiver may have her taken to the baby warmer in the birthing room for stimulation or possibly oxygen. The five-minute score is usually higher than the first score, indicating improvement with time or medical assistance.

While Apgar scores help detect babies who need immediate medical attention, they can't predict a baby's overall health or long-term well-being. Your nurse or caregiver performs a thorough newborn exam (within twenty-four hours after birth) to more accurately assess your baby's condition.

## Apgar Score

| Sign | 0 points | 1 point | 2 points |
|---|---|---|---|
| Heart rate | Absent | Fewer than 100 beats per minute | More than 100 beats per minute |
| Respiratory effort | Absent | Slow, irregular | Good, crying |
| Muscle tone | Limp | Arms and legs flexed | Active movement |
| Reflexes, irritability (your baby's reaction when made uncomfortable, as with a mild pinch | No response | Grimace | Sneezing, coughing, pulling away |
| Skin color | Bluish-gray, pale all over | Normal skin color, except bluish hands and feet | Normal skin color all over |

## CLAMPING AND CUTTING THE UMBILICAL CORD[22]

Soon after birth, your baby's umbilical cord is clamped, then cut with scissors. The cord has no nerve endings, so cutting it is painless for your baby. Your partner may cut the cord.

The timing of cord clamping and cutting affects your baby's blood volume. Before birth, your baby's blood circulates via the cord to and from the placenta, allowing the exchange of oxygen, nutrients, and other substances. At birth, approximately one-third of your baby's blood is in the placenta.[23] Over the first few minutes after birth, this blood is transferred to your baby (placental transfusion). The blood vessels in the cord are gradually compressed by a substance called Wharton's jelly, which expands when the cord is exposed to air. Delaying clamping until the cord stops pulsating allows your baby to receive as much blood as possible. Some blood remains in the placenta after pulsation stops. If the cord is clamped immediately, which is still a common practice, your baby doesn't receive a large portion of his blood from the placenta.

For years, obstetricians and others had been taught that placental blood was "extra" and that if it got to the baby, it could lead to jaundice (see page 383). Recent research has shown that, after delayed cord clamping, red blood cells are increased in the baby and bilirubin levels are somewhat higher. These levels, however, were still within the normal range and didn't result in more jaundice diagnoses. In fact, delayed clamping benefits the baby by helping increase iron levels in the blood and reducing anemia and related problems for the first six months. Additional advantages include improvement of the baby's early breathing and more rapid separation and delivery of the placenta by decreasing its size.[24]

To achieve the optimal blood volume, the baby is placed on the mother's abdomen (level with the placenta) until the cord stops pulsating. Then it's clamped and cut. Holding the baby high above or low below the mother may change the speed of placental transfusion and the amount of blood that reaches the baby.[25]

In challenging situations, the baby may benefit even more from delayed cord clamping. Some hospitals are waiting a few minutes to clamp and cut the cord after a cesarean.[26] For a premature baby, or a baby who needs

## Does Cord Blood Banking Interfere with Delayed Cord Clamping?

Cord blood is usually extracted immediately after birth, which could prevent the baby from getting the full blood supply. However, according to several prominent cord blood banks and the American Academy of Pediatrics, delayed cord clamping is possible. Caregivers can wait until the cord stops pulsating, which indicates that blood flow to the baby has stopped. Then, direct extraction of blood from the placenta—not the cord—will provide sufficient blood in most cases.

If you're interested in learning more about cord blood collection, donation, or storage, ask your caregiver, contact your local blood bank, or search the Internet for unbiased sources of information. Do this research well before your due date.

medical attention or resuscitation, delaying cord clamping may be especially beneficial.[27] If needed, procedures can be carried out with the cord intact, and the baby continues to benefit from oxygenated blood transferring to him while remaining next to his mother. Sometimes, in serious cases, the cord must be cut early to move the baby to emergency equipment.

During pregnancy, discuss delayed cord clamping and cutting with your caregiver and include your preferences in your birth plan.

## COLLECTION AND STORAGE OF UMBILICAL CORD BLOOD

Blood in the umbilical cord is a rich source of stem cells, which generate and continually renew supplies of red cells, platelets, and white cells. Stem cells make it possible for a person to use oxygen, clot blood, and fight infection. Umbilical cord stem cells are easier to match to another person's tissue than the mature stem cells found in bone marrow. As a result, cord blood stem cells can be used to successfully treat people with such diseases as immune deficiencies, severe inherited anemia, childhood leukemia, and other cancers. Stem cells are also used in the search for cures of these diseases.

Cord blood can be collected after the baby's cord is cut. After collection, the stem cells are separated from the blood in a laboratory and stored according to the parents' choice. The American Academy of Pediatrics (AAP) encourages parents to donate cord blood to public blood banks and cautions against using private cord blood banks.[28] The reason is because most conditions that cord blood stem cells may help treat (such as precancerous changes and genetic abnormalities) already exist in the baby's cord  blood, which means the baby's stored cord blood stem cells won't help treat the condition if it develops later. (The AAP also points out that private cord blood storage is expensive, and marketers sometimes play on the "emotional vulnerability of pregnant women and their families and friends" in recruiting efforts.[29]) Publicly donated cord blood is tested for disease and genetic abnormalities before being approved for use.

# Fourth Stage of Labor: Recovery and Family Bonding

The fourth stage of labor begins just after the birth of the placenta and lasts until your condition is stable, typically an hour or two after the birth. (This stage may take longer if you had anesthesia, if your labor was difficult or prolonged, or if you had a cesarean.)

When this stage proceeds normally, you and your baby belong together, skin to skin, for the first hour or longer. During this time, you help each other with the dramatic physiological and psychological transition from pregnant woman to mother and fetus to infant. This interaction is called mutual regulation and is crucial for your newborn's adjustment and for establishing breastfeeding. Your partner's role is to facilitate mutual regulation by helping you with comfortable positions to hold your baby, kissing and caressing both of you, and encouraging family members and friends to respect the need for leaving you undisturbed.

## Your Hormones[30]

A cocktail of hormones—oxytocin, endorphins, prolactin—flow through your body, protecting you from excessive bleeding, giving you loving feelings toward your partner and your baby, making you feel protective and unselfish toward your baby. Your partner's hormones are also altered by being with your baby in these early minutes of life.

## Your Baby's Hormones[31]

After birth, catecholamines (stress hormones) stimulate your baby's adaptation to life outside your uterus. These hormones cause fluid in her lungs to be absorbed so she can breathe easily. They also jump-start her ability to regulate her temperature, make her alert, and heighten her reflexes for the first few hours. During that time, she begins feeding, exploring her world, and seeing you for the first time.

During labor, your baby produced beta-endorphins; after the birth, she produces prolactin. She also begins producing oxytocin (the "love hormone") in synchrony with you. These three hormones help strengthen the bond between you, increase her interest in breastfeeding, and stimulate you to care for her. Other people also can produce oxytocin—although to lesser degrees than what you produce—by holding your baby skin-to-skin, keeping eye contact with her, and caring for her.

By snuggling with your baby after the birth, the skin-to-skin contact allows for mutual regulation of hormones as you adjust to your new lives together.

## Your Physical Adjustment

After you deliver the placenta, your caregiver checks your perineum and birth canal for bleeding. If you had a vaginal tear or an episiotomy during the birth, your tissues are stitched to speed healing, a procedure that typically lasts less than thirty minutes. Unless you were already given anesthesia in labor, you receive a local anesthetic by injection before your perineum is stitched. Although the stitching should be painless, the injection may sting and you may need to use rhythmic breathing to manage the discomfort. (See page 326 for information on caring for your perineum.)

After the birth, your uterus continues to contract, beginning the process of *involution* (returning to its nonpregnant size). You begin passing *lochia*, the heavy red discharge consisting of the extra blood and fluid that supported your pregnancy and the uterine lining that sustained your baby. A maternity pad is necessary to absorb the flow. (See page 325 for more information on involution and lochia.)

## How to Massage Your Uterus

1. Empty your bladder. Lie on your back and check your uterus by pressing on the area below your navel. If your uterus feels as firm as a grapefruit, you don't need to massage it. If you can't feel your uterus, it has relaxed and softened. Proceed to the next step.

- With one hand slightly cupped, massage your lower abdomen firmly with small circular movements until you feel your uterus contract and become firm. This action may be painful (but probably less so than if someone else does it). If you can't make your uterus contract, tell your nurse or caregiver. Your uterus will be massaged to make it contract. See page 348 to learn what's done if your uterus doesn't contract or you have excessive bleeding.

Because your uterus can bleed excessively if it's not firm, do this massage every few hours for the first couple of days after the birth. Afterward, you may periodically check to see if your uterus needs massage to keep it contracted.

Your nurse or caregiver checks your uterus frequently and massages your uterus firmly to make sure it remains firm and contracted. (If your uterus is relaxed, some of the uterine blood vessels may open and bleed.) Uterine (fundal) massage can be painful, and you may want to do it yourself to control the amount of pressure used and reduce pain. See page 199 or ask your nurse for instructions.

Your contractions during involution may be painful, especially if you've given birth before. Although these *afterpains* are common and aren't nearly as intense as labor contractions, you may need to use slow breathing to help manage them.

After your baby's birth, your legs may tremble for a while, which is normal. A warm blanket may reduce the trembling. You may also realize that you missed some meals during the hard work of labor. Be sure to eat and drink to satisfy your hunger and quench your thirst.

## YOUR BABY'S PHYSICAL ADJUSTMENT

Immediately after birth, your baby begins breathing on her own; her circulation is rerouted to supply much more blood and oxygen to her lungs; her body temperature is regulated by your warm skin and her own hormones. She squirms and coughs to clear mucus and fluid from her airway. She sees, smells, hears, feels, and tastes her mother. She becomes calm and alert, staring intently at your face. Sing the song that you sang to her while pregnant; see if she responds by turning toward you.

After a few minutes, she begins to wriggle, bob her head, and move her legs and arms as if crawling. If undisturbed, she'll eventually find her way to your breast, lick and nuzzle it, and begin to suckle. (Most babies are ready to suckle within twenty to sixty minutes after the birth.) See page 400 to learn more about your baby's first feeding. This stimulation to your breast prevents excessive bleeding by encouraging your uterus to contract.

## ENTERING PARENTHOOD

A main characteristic of the fourth stage is that you and your partner are no longer *expectant* parents—you're *parents*! After the birth of your baby, you don't get a chance to regroup before you begin parenting your child. This new role starts immediately and, along with other postpartum changes to your life, may overwhelm or bewilder you. In chapters 16, 18, and 19, you'll learn about feeding and caring for your baby as well as your emotional and physical adjustment after his birth.

Enjoy your baby's first hours of awake time. He's likely alert, calm, and bright-eyed. If the light isn't too bright, he'll stare, particularly at your face. (If the light is too bright, ask someone to dim them or use your hand to shield your baby's eyes.) As your baby cuddles with you, gazes into your face, or suckles at your breast, your curiosity will give way to fascination. These moments are a time for falling in love with each other. Your partner also will want to hold your baby close, perhaps skin-to-skin, and bond with him. Family-centered and baby-friendly hospitals (see page 12) encourage parents and babies to stay together as much as possible after the birth, unless problems develop that require separation. The caregiver performs routine observations or procedures on a healthy, normal baby while the newborn is in his parent's arms. Before your due date, check your hospital's policy on newborn procedures. If caregivers routinely send healthy newborns to the nursery, ask your caregiver to issue an order to delay or bypass your baby's admission to the nursery.

A few hours after the birth, your baby will probably fall deeply asleep. You and your partner may do the same, as exhilaration gives way to fatigue. At that time, someone who's alert should periodically observe your baby's vital signs and yours, including skin color, pulse, respiration, blood pressure, and temperature. Your partner may be as exhausted as you and unable to take on this responsibility until after getting some rest. In the hospital, a nurse does this job. After a home birth, the midwife or a birth assistant makes initial observations before passing the job on to an informed and rested friend or relative.

## Processing Your Birth Experience

Your birth experience isn't really over until you've had a chance to think about and understand it. Giving birth to your child will become one of the most vivid and poignant memories you'll ever have. In order to create a complete story of the experience, you need to compare and contrast your feelings, thoughts, and impressions with those of others who attended the birth, getting answers to any questions, and looking at photos taken during labor and birth. At some point, you may want to tell your story to people who didn't attend the birth but are eager to hear about it. You may even want to write the story or draw or paint a picture of it—each option is a great way to preserve this special memory for you and your child.

Depending on your birth experience, processing it may take weeks, months, or even years. If your birth experience was particularly difficult or disappointing, processing it may take longer than processing a straightforward and satisfying experience. Dealing with a difficult birth may also bring up strong, disturbing feelings. If this is the case for you, talk about your experience with your caregiver, doula, childbirth educator, or a counselor knowledgeable about childbirth. This person can help you gain perspective and come to terms with your birth experience. See page 350 for further discussion on disappointing birth experiences.

# Key Points to Remember

- By understanding what happens in each stage of labor, you can anticipate and appreciate the physical accomplishments of each stage, respond well to the accompanying emotional hurdles, and cope with increasingly intense contractions.
- Expect the unexpected in labor. Know that you can take steps to respond to any variation in labor.
- Your labor partner's presence and support are vital to your ability to cope with labor.
- A doula can guide you and your partner through labor and assist you with measures for comfort and progress.
- Your baby also labors. The two of you labor together, accomplish the birth together, and adjust together to your new roles afterward. Throughout, your partner offers support and assistance.
- See page 444 for the Road Map of Labor and a quick reference chart that summarizes the stages of labor and briefly explains what you can do during each stage to help labor progress and increase your comfort.

# CHAPTER 11

# Labor Pain and Options for Pain Relief

When new parents were asked to describe the sensations of childbirth, some used words that depicted a positive experience, such as *exhilarating, empowering,* and even *orgasmic;* others used words that portrayed a negative experience, such as *painful, exhausting,* and *traumatic.* For still others, childbirth wasn't a particularly transformative event, and they used words such as *tedious, uncomfortable,* and *manageable* to describe the experience.

The preparations you make during pregnancy can influence the kind of birth experience you'll have. You're more likely to have a positive birth experience if you learn about your pain relief options, practice a variety of coping techniques, and arrange for continuous labor support from people who respect your preferences for pain relief. This chapter describes labor pain and provides an overview of your options for coping with it so you can have the best possible birth experience. See chapter 12 to learn specific nondrug coping techniques you can practice in pregnancy and use in labor. See chapter 13 for more details on pain medications.

# Why Labor Is Painful

In almost all pregnancies, labor begins with mild contractions that come and go. As labor progresses, the contractions occur more frequently and their intensity increases. Although a few women have reported experiencing little to no pain during labor, the process is painful for most people. The following physical changes contribute to labor pain:

- reduced oxygen supply to the uterine muscle during contractions, which creates a buildup of waste products, such as lactic acid, that in turn causes pain (the pain disappears as soon as the contraction stops)
- stretching of the cervix as it dilates; pressure of the baby on the cervix
- tension and stretching of the ligaments of the uterus and pelvic joints
- pressure of the baby on the urethra, bladder, and rectum
- stretching of the pelvic floor muscles and vaginal tissues during the birth

Although these changes can hurt, the pain isn't a sign of injury. Instead, it's an expected side effect of the normal labor process that lets women efficiently and effectively push their babies out into the world. For this reason, labor pain is often called "pain with a purpose."[1]

# Your Perception of Pain

Simply understanding the physical reasons for labor pain and acknowledging that labor pain is normal and temporary can allow women to work with their bodies and prevent the pain from overwhelming them. The following sections describe theories about pain perception.

## THE GATE CONTROL THEORY OF PAIN

The Gate Control Theory helps explain how distractions help reduce pain. You've probably had some of the following experiences:

- a headache that goes away when you're watching an exciting movie, but returns when the movie ends
- the pain from dental work that's eased when listening to music through headphones
- the pain of physical exertion that's eased when you focus on a rhythm (counting or singing out loud or in your head)
- a bumped elbow that hurts less when you rub it

Although the pain stimulus never goes away in these examples, your awareness of it decreases when your brain receives other stimuli (*pain modifiers*). Your brain is so busy processing those other messages that it can't pay as much attention to painful sensations.

During labor, you can use this approach to make pain more manageable by increasing pleasant stimuli—such as massage, music, aromatherapy, or a heating pad —and focusing on these distractions. (You can also use an uncomfortable sensation to distract you from pain—see page 229.)

# THE NEUROMATRIX THEORY OF PAIN

The Neuromatrix Theory is an expansion of the Gate Control Theory and takes into account all possible factors that can influence how pain is felt and interpreted.[2] It helps explain why women differ in their reactions to labor pain and why some women find comfort measures more helpful than other women do. The theory acknowledges that painful and nonpainful stimuli aren't the only factors that affect perception of the pain. Other factors include past experiences of pain or trauma, chronic pain or painful medical conditions, anxiety, personality, and cultural or familial attitudes toward pain.

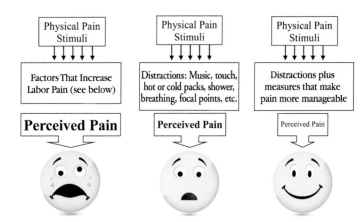

## *Factors That Increase Labor Pain*

**Physical factors**

- hunger or thirst
- fatigue
- muscle tension
- full bladder
- discomfort from staying in the same position for too long
- hospital policies or procedures that limit mobility or ability to use coping techniques

**Emotional or mental factors**

- fear, anxiety, loneliness, or feeling watched or judged (all of these emotions can cause the release of excessive stress hormones and make labor longer or more painful than usual—see page 232)
- lack of confidence and preparation
- ignorance or misinformation about labor and birth
- unsupportive staff, friends, or family members
- feeling powerless to make decisions or feeling that your decisions aren't being respected
- expectations for labor and birth that don't match the actual experience

**Variations during labor**

- rapid intense labor, with little break between contractions
- prolonged, tiring labor; exhaustion
- coupling contractions (occur in pairs with little break between the first and second contractions) or a baby that's malpositioned (see page 286)
- medical interventions such as IV placement or Pitocin

## Different Views on Labor Pain

When asked to describe the pain experienced in labor, new mothers had many different responses. Here are a few examples:

*I'd first feel cramping in my back, then it'd move around to my front and my whole belly would tighten. Later in labor, I could feel the cramping even in my thighs.*

*The contractions were just really intense. My body demanded my complete attention, like it does when I sneeze, orgasm, or vomit. The contractions were all my body would let me think about right then.*

*The best way to describe labor pain is that it's like the kind of aching pain you get when you do something that requires a lot of effort such as doing a chin-up or holding an advanced yoga pose for a long time. Your muscles burn as they get tired. That's what my uterus felt like.*

## Measures That Make Labor Pain More Manageable

To counteract the following factors that increase labor pain, be aware of them in advance, make plans to manage them (see examples below), and ensure that your support people are aware of them and work to minimize their impact on you.

### Physical Factors

- Eat and drink enough to stave off hunger and thirst.
- Rest, if possible, and change positions frequently.

### Emotional Factors

- Dim the lights and arrange for minimal interruptions to increase your sense of privacy.
- Take childbirth classes to learn about birth and choose caregivers and support people you trust and who will respect your decisions. If past trauma has made you fearful, get counseling before the birth to help you learn skills to manage the fear. Visit our website, http://www.PCNGuide.com, to download a work sheet to help with this process. *Variation:* Use comfort measures and positions that enhance labor progress (see page 247).

A number of specialized comfort measures are particularly helpful in labor, such as massage, relaxation techniques, breathing techniques, positions, and movement. See chapter 12 for details. However, the comfort measures that are most effective for you may be similar to coping measures you've used throughout your life. To help you prepare for coping with labor pain, ask yourself these questions and brainstorm as many answers as you can:

- What comforts you when you're sick?
- When you were a child, what did your parents do when you were sick that made you feel better? (Or what do you wish they had done?)
- What do you do during heavy physical exertion to help you keep going?
- What soothes the pain of a headache or sore muscles?
- What helps you feel safe in an unfamiliar situation?
- What calms you when you're stressed?
- What kind of support from others best helps you? Your answers to these questions will give you clues about what you'll find most helpful in labor. Visit our website to download a work sheet to help track your observations.

# Pain versus Suffering in Labor

While pain is a natural part of the labor process, suffering certainly isn't. *Pain* is a mildly to severely unpleasant physical sensation that might or might not be associated with physical damage. *Suffering* is a debilitating emotional state that might be associated with pain or with another cause such as grief, humiliation, or defeat.

You can have pain without suffering. For example, during a strenuous workout, you may experience the pain that accompanies exertion. You know why your body hurts, but you also associate the pain with improved physical conditioning, which makes the pain manageable. ("No pain, no gain.")

In the same way, many women experience intense pain during labor but don't feel as though they're suffering. They associate the pain with normal labor progress, and they have the support needed to cope. Although labor is very challenging, they can "work with labor pain" because it feels manageable to them.[3] If they make it through labor and birth without pain medication, they may feel the same exhilaration a mountain climber experiences upon reaching the summit.

Not everyone in labor, however, has this positive experience. Some women do suffer in labor. Suffering includes any of the following experiences:

- a perceived threat to your body or psyche
- helplessness and loss of control
- the inability to cope with a distressing situation
- fear of dying or of the death of the baby[4]

## *Rating Your Intensity of Pain and Your Ability to Cope*

In many hospitals, the staff use a very helpful tool called a pain intensity scale to assess how much pain a patient is experiencing during a medical procedure or postoperative recovery. By rating the intensity of pain, the patient can alert staff of potential problems that are then treated with pain medications. During labor, however, pain is a normal and expected part of the process, and women have a range of preferences for how they want to manage the pain, which don't always include pain medications.

**Pain Intensity Scale**

| No Pain | | | | | Moderate Pain | | | | | Worst Possible Pain |
|---|---|---|---|---|---|---|---|---|---|---|
| 0 | 1 | 2 | 3 | 4 | 5 | 6 | 7 | 8 | 9 | 10 |

Another way to assess labor pain is by using a pain coping scale. A low score means the pain isn't that unpleasant and you're coping fine. A high score indicates the pain is very unpleasant and you're not coping. After you rate your pain on the pain intensity scale, then rate how well you're coping.

**Pain Coping Scale**

| No need to cope | | Easy to cope | | | Able to do Three Rs (see page 206) | | Need lots of help | | | Can't do it |
|---|---|---|---|---|---|---|---|---|---|---|
| 10 | 9 | 8 | 7 | 6 | 5 | 4 | 3 | 2 | 1 | 0 |

Pain does *not* equal suffering. Suffering equals inability to cope with pain.

## CONTROL IN LABOR

For many pregnant women, the possibility of losing control of themselves during labor is the most upsetting part of childbirth. They worry that the pain will be so intense they'll do or say things they'll regret later. They've seen movies or heard stories in which a laboring woman panics, screams, or says hurtful things to those around her. Some expectant mothers plan to dull labor pain with anesthesia to prevent themselves from behaving in a way that's socially unacceptable.

Childbirth is emotionally transformative and physically demanding. Just as someone who's completing a marathon might not be able to engage in polite social conversation, you may find that coping with labor and maintaining the Three Rs (see page 224) takes your complete attention. You may cry or yell, but women typically don't behave in ways that are completely uncharacteristic for them. When your needs are respected and you're allowed to express yourself freely, you can cope well with labor.

### Releasing Control versus Losing Control

Just as you can't control how your body digests food, you can't consciously control your contractions. You can, however, control how you respond to them. For example, during pregnancy you may prepare for labor by practicing a certain breathing technique and making sure you'll have access to a bathtub. When labor begins, though, you may find yourself breathing in a different, unplanned rhythm and wanting to walk rather than soak in the tub.

Instead of forcing yourself to follow your plans, you *choose* to give them up—that is, you release control and allow yourself to discover new ways of coping that help you work in harmony with the labor process. Releasing control is a matter of responding to your labor in the moment, as it unfolds.

Conversely, losing control in labor comes from feeling overwhelmed and helpless when labor doesn't go as expected, or from feeling that you're being excluded from the decision-making process. To help avoid feeling powerless in your care, learn about your options for childbirth well before labor begins (see chapter 2), ask your caregiver the key questions on page 9 for any interventions, and make sure your decisions are reflected in your birth plan (see chapter 8).

# Options for Pain Relief

While some women want a drug-free birth, others can't imagine giving birth without pain medications. Most women's opinions fall in between these two extremes: They want to minimize the amount of strong pain medications they receive during labor, yet they don't want the pain to overwhelm them. The information in this section will help you clarify your own opinions.

## STOCKING YOUR TOOLBOX

To effectively manage labor pain, it's essential to have a "toolbox" of coping options. During pregnancy, you can read books on childbirth and take childbirth classes to help you stock your toolbox with options such as the following:

- coping skills you've used throughout your life to comfort yourself when you're sick, tired, worried, in pain, or physically exerting yourself (see page 206)
- self-help skills that you can practice during pregnancy to lessen labor pain or help you cope with it, such as breathing techniques, relaxation techniques, and visualization and attention focusing (see chapter 12), as well as positions that enhance comfort and labor progress (see pages 238–240).
- comfort items that you can use at the birthplace, such as your own pillow or clothes, snacks and beverages, heating pads and cold packs, birth ball, and shower or bathtub (see page 230)
- hands-on support from your partner or doula, such as massage, gentle stroking, and acupressure (see page 231)
- changes to the environment to make it more comfortable, such as dimming the lights, playing music, using pleasing scents or aromatherapy, and asking for minimal disruptions
- pain medications, including intravenous (IV) narcotics (see page 261) and epidural or spinal analgesia (see chapter 13).

Before labor, you may think you know which coping techniques will work best for you. During labor, however, you may discover that those options don't work as well as expected. This is why it's important to learn a variety of coping techniques: the technique you never imagined you'd use may be the one that helps you the most!

## AVAILABILITY OF PAIN-RELIEF OPTIONS

Your options for pain relief depend on where you plan to give birth. If you'll give birth at home or in a freestanding (unaffiliated with a hospital) birth center, you can use most nondrug coping techniques, but you won't have access to pain medications such as epidural analgesia. If you'll give birth in a hospital, medications will be available. Hospital policies and available equipment might or might not support comfort techniques, such as eating in labor, mobility, baths, and showers.

To learn what pain-relief options are available at your birthplace, visit our website, http://www.PCNGuide .com, to find lists of questions to ask during your prenatal care appointments, hospital tour, and childbirth classes. If you're considering using pain medications, ask your caregiver which ones are typically available. Lastly, make sure to discuss the risks and benefits of pain medications with your caregiver (see page 259) so you can better make an informed decision.

# EFFECTIVENESS OF VARIOUS PAIN-RELIEF OPTIONS

Expectant parents may wonder how effective pain medications and various nondrug techniques are. Subjective experiences of new mothers and objective research can answer that question.

## What New Mothers Say

The following table summarizes the effectiveness of various pain-relief options. The ratings are based on reports given by women who were surveyed in the first year after giving birth.[5]

|  | Percent who used the option | Percent who said the option was very helpful | Percent who said the option was somewhat helpful |
|---|---|---|---|
| Epidural or spinal analgesia | 76% | 81% | 10% |
| Immersion in tub or pool | 6% | 48% | 43% |
| Hands-on techniques (such as massage) | 20% | 40% | 51% |
| IV narcotics | 22% | 40% | 35% |
| Birth ball | 7% | 34% | 33% |
| Shower | 4% | 33% | 45% |
| Application of heat or cold | 6% | 31% | 50% |
| Mental strategies (such as relaxation) | 25% | 28% | 49% |
| Position changes | 42% | 23% | 54% |
| Changes to environment (such as dimming lights) | 4% | 21% | 57% |
| Breathing techniques | 49% | 21% | 56% |

This table shows that the majority of women received epidural or spinal analgesia, and most found the medications very helpful. However, this option wasn't the only effective one. All the options proved somewhat to very helpful for the majority of women who used them. For example, the total percentage of women who found pain relief from immersion in a tub or from hands-on techniques equaled the total percentage of women who found pain relief from epidural or spinal analgesia (91 percent).

Unfortunately, nondrug measures weren't used as often as medications, perhaps because the women surveyed either didn't know about them or hadn't learned to use them, or their caregivers didn't encourage their use during labor.

## What the Research Shows

Pain has two components: how intense it is and how unpleasant it is.[6] Intensity is about the quality of the pain (where it's located and how much it hurts), and unpleasantness is about how well you're managing pain versus how desperately you want to escape from it.

A 2014 review of the research on nondrug pain-coping techniques divided them into three categories and found these results.[7]

- **Gate Control Theory** (see page 204): Applying pain-free stimuli on the painful area (such as massage, bath, positions, or warm packs) blocks some of the pain intensity. Those who used these techniques were less likely to use epidurals and Pitocin and had lower pain scores.

- **Counter-irritation** (see page 229): Creating pain or discomfort anywhere on the body (such as applying ice, acupressure, or sterile water injections) causes the release of endorphins, which reduce the perceived intensity of the pain. Those who used these techniques were much less likely to use epidurals, had lower pain scores, and were more satisfied with birth.
- **Central Nervous System Control**: Techniques such as focusing attention elsewhere, prenatal education, relaxation, hypnosis, and continuous labor support help reduce the unpleasantness of pain. Those who used these techniques were less likely to use epidurals and Pitocin, less likely to need instrumental or cesarean delivery, and have a higher satisfaction with birth.

Visit our website, http://www.PCNGuide.com, to see a chart that summarizes other research reviews that examined individual comfort techniques.

## Nonmedicated Labor versus Medicated Labor

The following chart compares a labor that's managed by using nondrug coping techniques with one that's managed with medications. This comparison helps you see how your labor may differ based on the choices you make.

| | Nonmedicated labor | Medicated labor | |
|---|---|---|---|
| Pain-relief option used | Nondrug coping techniques* | IV narcotics | Epidural analgesia |
| | | | |
| How it affects your experience of pain | Increases pain-relieving endorphins, enhances oxytocin production, decreases muscle tension, eases anxiety or fear, distracts your attention from the pain, and enhances your mood. Helps you feel that you can "work with your labor pain." | Blocks pain receptors in the brain so pain messages aren't recognized or interpreted as pain. Pain intensity at the peak of the contraction might not be reduced by narcotics and might be hard to manage. Reduces pain. | Blocks nerve endings so they don't send pain messages to the brain. Light doses eliminate contraction pain (but not all the pain of pushing) and dull other sensations. Heavy doses also cause numbness and inability to move your legs. Relieves pain. |
| Feedback from women who used it | "It was really challenging to handle the contractions. I finally discovered that if I got on my hands and knees and rocked and roared, I could do it. It was as though I'd found my inner tiger!" | "I felt fuzzy-headed and slept between contractions. During the peak of a contraction, I'd wake up, cry out, and rock back and forth while my husband rubbed my back. Then I'd doze off again." | "After I got the epidural, it was great. No more pain! But then it seemed as though labor took forever, and we were sitting around watching TV—it wasn't quite what I thought birth would be." |
| How it affects your mental state | You're fully focused on coping with the contractions and are less aware of surroundings. | You're relaxed, drowsy, foggy, or disoriented. You may hallucinate. | You return to your normal, everyday mental state. You may be chatty or may sleep through much of labor, if tired. |

|  | Nonmedicated labor | Medicated labor | |
|---|---|---|---|
| Pain-relief option used | Nondrug coping techniques* | IV narcotics | Epidural analgesia |
| How it affects your mobility | You're fully mobile to find comfort: You can walk, rock, sway, sit, and so on. You may need to keep moving in order to cope with pain. | Mobility may be limited by policy, by equipment, or if you're unsafe standing because you're dizzy or groggy. | You're rarely allowed out of bed. Movement in bed is limited by equipment and lack of sensation. You may need assistance to move at all. |
| What you'll need from your support people | You'll need their continuous presence; active, hands-on assistance with massage, movement, and positions; encouraging words; and more. | You'll need some assistance with movement and mental reorientation (if you're foggy) and help coping at the peak of contractions. | You'll need companionship to help pass the time, manage anxieties, identify contractions, and guide pushing. |
| Equipment and precautions required | None (However, you may choose to use the tub, shower, birth ball, rocking chair, cold packs, or heating pads. In addition, you'll have periodic monitoring of your baby, contractions, blood pressure, and vital signs.) | Intravenous (IV) fluids, electronic fetal monitors (EFM) to continuously check your baby's heart rate; equipment to frequently monitor your blood pressure, respiration, and vital signs; oxygen supply and mask. | Epidural catheter and pump; IV fluids; EFM to continuously monitor your baby's heart rate; equipment to frequently monitor your blood pressure, respiration, and vital signs; oxygen supply and mask; pulse oximeter; bladder catheter. |
| Impact on labor progress | Usually promotes labor progress. | May slow normal labor.** | Likely to slow normal labor progress (may require Pitocin).** |
| Timing | Can be used at any time during labor and birth. | Best used in active labor. Effects last 45 to 90 minutes. Can be repeated once. Not used if birth is expected to occur within 2 hours. | Can be used at any time except if birth is anticipated soon—for example, within 30 minutes. Once started, the medications usually stay in effect until after your baby is born. |
| Availability | Anytime, anyplace | All hospitals, anytime | Some hospitals, anytime; other hospitals, limited hours and an anesthesiologist must be called in at night. Not available in some US hospitals. |
| Possible risks to you | None (But you'll still have labor pain.) | Some (see page 261) | Some (see page 262) |
| Possible risks to your baby | None | Some (see page 261) | Some (see page 262) |
| Cost | Free or inexpensive | Moderate | Expensive |
| Best option for you if... | You're committed to a nonmedicated labor or want to delay use of medication, have a supportive staff, have made necessary preparations, and have recruited a support team. | You want only an hour or two of moderate pain relief, or feel that you're coping well at the peak of contractions but want to feel that you have a longer rest between contractions. | You want to experience the least amount of pain and are willing to have more medical interventions to minimize the adverse side effects of the epidural; or if you require painful interventions for safety or progress. |

* It's assumed that you'll use a variety of techniques from among those listed on page 209 and described in chapter 12.

** Occasionally, epidural analgesia may speed up a prolonged labor if the labor was slow because of extreme muscle tension, fear, or pain-related anxiety.

# COMBINING TECHNIQUES

You can increase the overall effectiveness of these techniques by using several compatible ones at the same time and shifting to others whenever you desire. The 2014 review cited previously found that the most effective pain relief came from combining continuous labor support (such as a doula) with other techniques.[8]

When planning your coping ritual, consider trying various nondrug methods first. Nondrug methods are free, easy to use, have few side effects, can be easily discontinued or replaced by other measures, and let you work with your body and take an active role in childbirth. Pain medications—especially epidural analgesia—can effectively minimize or eliminate labor pain, but they're also expensive and have possible side effects and risks that may complicate labor and birth. If nondrug techniques aren't enough to help you cope as labor progresses, you can always request pain medication. (If planning an out-of-hospital birth, know that you'll need to transfer to a hospital to receive pain medication.)

# Determining Your Preferences for Pain Relief

The following are factors that help determine whether you'll use or avoid pain medications in labor.

## Preference

Do you prefer to give birth without drugs, or do you prefer to use medications? How strongly do you feel about this preference? Your views may be influenced by past experiences with pain, your expectations about how challenging labor will be, your confidence in your ability to cope, and whether you want to rely on your own resources or prefer to turn over management of your labor to others. (See the Pain Medication Preference Scale on page 214.)

## Preparation

You're better able to cope with labor pain if you have complete information on all available options for pain relief, and have had opportunities to learn, practice, and adapt nonmedicated comfort measures. Without such preparation, you're more likely to need pain medications.

## Support

You're more likely to avoid, postpone, or minimize your use of pain medications if you have the following:
- a partner or doula (see page 220) who encourages you and helps with self-help comfort measures
- support staff who are skilled in comfort measures
- a caregiver who's patient and encouraging

## Luck

The nature of labor affects the use of medications. The more uncomplicated your labor is, the better your chances are for a nonmedicated birth. If your labor is prolonged, complicated, or includes the use of potentially painful interventions (such as Pitocin or cesarean section), you're likely to need medications.

## Two Views on Managing Labor Pain

I wanted to be able to use pain medications. But Ben was worried about the side effects. We talked with our caregiver about how to minimize the possible side effects and risks and created a plan that we were both comfortable with.
—Ann

Ashley really wanted to have a "natural" labor. But I knew it'd be hard for me to see her in pain. I worried that I'd talk her into getting drugs. Luckily, we have a friend who had given birth without pain medications. She came with us to the hospital and helped us both cope with natural labor.
—Nick

# DEFINING YOUR PREFERENCES WITH THE PAIN MEDICATION PREFERENCE SCALE (PMPS)

Even though it's impossible to know how painful labor will be for you, the PMPS lets you determine how strongly you feel about medications and under what circumstances you'll use them. Whatever your preferences, address them in your birth plan (see chapter 8) and remind your caregiver and hospital staff of them during labor.

## Pain Medication Preference Scale (PMPS)

| Rating | Your preference | How your partner, doula, and others can help you |
|---|---|---|
| +10 | I don't want to feel any pain. I prefer to be numb and to get anesthesia before labor even begins (typically not possible). | Discuss your wishes and fears with you. <br><br> Explain that you'll have some pain, even with anesthesia, and plan how you can cope. <br><br> Promise to help you get medications as soon as possible. |
| +9 | I want as much medication as I can have. I fear labor pain and don't want to experience any pain and stress. | Same as for +10 rating, plus: <br><br> Help you write a birth plan that expresses your fears and preferences. <br><br> Review circumstances when an epidural may be delayed and how to cope while waiting. <br><br> Ensure that someone will always be there to help you. |
| +7 | I want pain medications as early in labor as my caregiver will allow, and definitely before labor becomes painful. | Same as for +9 rating, plus: <br><br> Help you learn the policies on timing of doses. <br><br> Help you use relaxation techniques and comfort measures to cope in early labor and while waiting for the anesthesiologist. |
| +5 | I want epidural analgesia in active labor (cervix dilated 5 to 6 centimeters). I'll try to cope until then, perhaps with narcotic medications. | Same as for +7 rating, plus: <br><br> Help you with relaxation techniques and comfort measures in early labor. <br><br> Suggest medications when you're in active labor. |
| +3 | I want to use some pain medications, but I also plan to use self-help comfort measures for as much of labor as I can. | Same as for +5 rating, plus: <br><br> Help you with self-help measures. <br><br> Help you get medications if you decide you want them. |
| 0 | I have no opinion on pain medications or preference for or against them (a rare attitude among pregnant women, although not rare among partners). | Help you become informed about labor pain, comfort measures, and medications. |

## Pain Medication Preference Scale (PMPS)

| Rating | Your preference | How your partner, doula, and others can help you |
|---|---|---|
| -3 | I'd like to avoid pain medications if I can. If I find labor too painful, I'd like to use as little medication as possible, but won't feel guilty for taking it. | Emphasize coping techniques.<br><br>Avoid suggesting pain medications.<br><br>Avoid trying to talk you out of medications if you request them.<br><br>Suggest half doses of narcotics or a light epidural. |
| -5 | I really don't want to use pain medications so I can avoid their side effects on my baby, my labor, and myself. I'll accept them only if labor is complicated or long. | Same as for -3 rating, plus:<br><br>Prepare to play a very active role in your labor support.<br><br>Practice comfort measures with you.<br><br>Avoid suggesting drugs, even if you appear to be having trouble coping. Suggest other nondrug options instead.<br><br>Be aware of your code word (see page 217), which alerts your partner to stop suggesting other options.<br><br>Help you accept pain medications if you're exhausted, can't keep a rhythm during contractions (see page 224), or if none of the comfort measures help. |
| -7 | I strongly desire a nonmedicated childbirth because of its benefits to my baby and my labor, and the gratification of meeting the personal challenge. I'll be disappointed if I use drugs. | Same as for -5 rating, plus:<br><br>Help you enlist the support of your caregiver and request a nurse who will help with natural birth.<br><br>Plan and rehearse ways to get through discouraging times. |
| -9 | I definitely don't want pain medications. If I ask for them, I want my support team and the staff to refuse and insist I continue without drugs. | Same as for -7 rating, plus:<br><br>Explore with you the reasons for your feelings.<br><br>Explain that if you change your mind, staff can't deny your requests for medications.<br><br>Reinforce that it's your decision to use or avoid pain medications. |
| -10 | I want no medication, even for a cesarean section (an impossible extreme). | Same as for -9 rating, plus:<br><br>Help you gain a realistic understanding of the risks and benefits of pain medications.<br><br>Explain that there are situations in which pain medications are required, and plan how you can cope if such a situation arises. |

## Using the PMPS with Your Labor Support Partner

During pregnancy, review the PMPS with your partner. First, read the statements under "Your Preference" and find the one that best describes how you feel. Keep your selection to yourself. Next, have your partner read these statements and mentally choose the one that's closest to what your partner *wishes* you'd choose. Then, reveal your selections to each other and discuss them to clarify how you'll work together to achieve your goal. Also discuss the tips in the third column to plan how your partner can help you cope with labor and support your preferences. If your partner is uncertain about supporting you, consider having an additional support person.

# BEING FLEXIBLE WITH YOUR PLAN FOR PAIN RELIEF

While it's helpful to plan for pain relief, it's also important to be flexible with your plan in case labor doesn't go as expected and your preferences are no longer possible or necessary. For example, if you planned to use medications, you may find that labor is easier than anticipated and you don't need drugs. Or your labor may progress faster than expected, leaving no time for medications—or you may be one of the unlucky few for whom medications don't provide adequate pain relief, in which case you'll need to try nondrug comfort techniques instead. If you planned for a nonmedicated birth, you may find labor to be more challenging than expected, or you may have unexpected interventions that make it difficult to give birth without pain medications.

Most women have particular times in labor when they doubt their ability to cope (see page 218). If you begin to doubt yourself, your partner can remind you of these predictable challenges to help you regain confidence. If your doubt turns into dismay and you ask for pain medications, your partner should remember your pain medication preferences. If you'd said you wanted pain medications, your partner should help you get them. If you'd planned to delay receiving medications, your partner should suggest trying another coping technique for four or five contractions before helping you get drugs. If you'd planned a nonmedicated birth, your partner should continue to encourage you to cope unless you say your code word (see page 217).

# Preparing to Labor without Pain Medications

If having a drug-free labor is your goal, the following suggestions can help you avoid pain medications or minimize your need for them:

- During pregnancy, confirm that your partner understands your preferences and feels capable of helping you achieve your goals. If your partner doesn't, ask someone who does to accompany you both in labor to provide support.

- Choose a birthplace that supports nonmedicated birth and has non-medical tools available to provide pain relief and comfort (such as birth balls and large bathtubs). Choose a caregiver with experience supporting women who labor without pain medications. Ask both the birthplace and the caregiver what percentage of their clients use pain medications. If most women do, the staff may have little skill or experience supporting women who don't.

- Learn the comfort techniques in chapter 12. Practice the relaxation and self-help comfort techniques with your partner or support person.

- Take childbirth classes that focus on learning and practicing comfort techniques.

- Consider hiring a birth doula to guide and reassure you and your partner (see page 220). Studies show that a doula's presence and guidance reduce a laboring woman's need for pain medications.[9]

- State your wishes in your birth plan (see chapter 8). Ask hospital staff to avoid offering you pain medications and instead provide you with encouragement, advice for labor progress, and ideas for comfort measures. (You can, of course, receive medications if you ask for them.)

- Avoid or minimize interventions that can increase labor pain (such as induction and augmentation) or that limit your mobility (such as continuous electronic fetal monitoring and IV fluids).

- Consider having a *code word* to communicate that you've changed your mind and you no longer want to labor without medications. Women with a strong desire for a nonmedicated birth (rating a –5 to –7 on the Pain Medication Preference Scale—see page 214) often use a code word so they're free to complain, vocalize, cry, or curse without others misunderstanding their actions as a plea for pain medications. For example, one woman told her support team that if she said "I can't" or "This is too hard," she was really saying "I need more support." But if she said her code word *uncle*, her partner knew to help her get pain medications.

- If you want to use a code word, make sure it isn't one that's commonly said in a childbirth setting or associated with pain or pain relief, such as *I need drugs*. That way, you'll avoid having others mistakenly believe you want pain medications if you happen to say those words during labor. Instead, choose a code word that's unrelated to childbirth, such as *pumpernickel*. Let everyone attending to your labor know what your code word is as well as its purpose.

## Epidural Birth versus Nonmedicated Birth

Here's one woman's account of her birth experiences:

*For my first birth, I'd planned to labor without drugs, but in transition I panicked and accepted an epidural. Soon we were cracking jokes and watching for my next contraction on the monitor. I didn't feel any pain, but I also felt a little detached from the experience. Almost immediately after Hannah was born, I just wanted to sleep.*

*For my next birth, when contractions got intense and I felt that I couldn't possibly do it, my support people encouraged me that I could—and I did, even though it was hard. I felt so alive afterward. Some friends still think I was crazy for not having an epidural. My only response is that I've given birth with drugs and without, and nothing compares to the euphoria I experienced with a drug-free birth.*

- Know the predictable challenges of labor and prepare for ways to manage them without medications:
  - As you move from early labor to active labor (when your cervix dilates from about 4 to 6 centimeters), your contractions will become painful, but you'll realize you still have a long way to go before your baby is born. You may feel that labor is beyond your control. Try to adapt your breathing, movements, or activities in whatever way will help you cope. (See chapter 12 for ideas.) You may find that if you can release control, you'll spontaneously discover new ways of coping.
  - When your cervix has dilated to 6 to 7 centimeters, your contractions may become very intense. Don't expect to feel peaceful and relaxed during contractions. If you can relax *between* contractions and can maintain a rhythm in your breathing, movements, or activities during contractions, you'll be coping well. Remember that as labor intensifies, progress speeds up. (See the graph on page 284.)
  - As you move from active labor to transition, when your cervix dilates to 7 or 8 centimeters, you may need to rely heavily on your support team to help you keep your rhythm. Your partner can remind you that your contractions are about as painful as they'll become (although they may become more frequent). If you can cope at this time, you can probably manage the rest of your labor without pain medications—as long as you want to do so and your labor continues to progress normally.

If you begin to struggle with the pain at any point in labor, you and your support team should have a contingency plan for coping. See page 219 for more information.

# A Note to Fathers and Partners

It's easy to neglect your own needs when caring for a woman in labor, especially one who's laboring without pain medications. By taking care of yourself, you can help your partner meet the demands of labor. Stay hydrated and keep up your energy by eating nutritious snacks. Conserve your strength when physically supporting your partner (for example, sit or lean against something whenever possible, rather than standing), use good body mechanics (for example, lift with your legs, not your back), and work within your body's limitations (visit our website, http://www.PCNGuide.com, for more information). Let others provide support, especially if you need the rest. Maintaining your stamina will help you provide the invaluable contribution that only you can make during the birth of your baby.[10]

# Contingency Plan

What if you plan to give birth without pain medications, but begin to have second thoughts during labor? If you truly don't want to labor any longer without drugs, you can say your code word (see page 217) and your support people should help you ask for pain medications. However, if you're struggling to cope but still don't want to receive drugs, here are ideas to try:

- Change your environment. Take a walk or a shower, dim the lights, or put on some relaxing music.
- Change your ritual or your breathing techniques (see pages 224 and 241).
- Consider contacting another supportive friend or relative to be with you.
- Eat something or drink a sugary beverage. Sometimes all you need for pain relief is a quick energy boost.
- Find out how far your cervix has dilated. Labor may be difficult because you're making rapid progress!
- Don't base your decision to use pain medications on your experience with just one hard contraction. First try a new comfort technique (see chapter 12 for ideas) *for four or five contractions in a row.* During this time, your endorphins may kick in and labor may feel manageable again. (See page 174 for more information on endorphins.)

If your labor is still too intense after trying all these suggestions, you may choose to receive pain medications. If you do, try not to feel disappointed in yourself or feel that you've failed in some way because you didn't reach your goal. Take comfort in the fact that many women in this situation have reported feeling better about their decision because they'd first tried everything possible to manage without drugs, but were wise enough to change their minds when the pain led to suffering.

## The Invaluable Birth Doula

When considering options for pain relief, don't overlook the important services that a birth doula can provide. Unlike the nursing staff, who must concentrate on completing clinical tasks while providing care, a doula can focus solely on you and your partner, making sure you're both coping well.

This person (usually a woman) knows all the comfort measures and when to use them. From her meetings with you before the birth, she'll know your birth plan (see chapter 8), your pain medication preferences, your likes and dislikes, and your hopes for birth. She'll know what to say and do to comfort and encourage you—and what not to say and do. For example, one woman told her doula, "Don't tell me 'you're doing great' when I'm clearly not. Please acknowledge what I'm feeling by saying, 'I can see that it hurts, and I know it's hard, but we can do this together.'"

Women hire doulas for many reasons. One woman without a partner hired a doula to be her primary support person. Another woman hired a doula because her own mother couldn't attend the birth and she wanted a mother figure with her during labor—someone who had given birth and had supported many women through labor. Another wanted someone to help her and her partner with comfort measures so she was less likely to use pain medications. One had a lot of fear and anxiety, partially because of a history of sexual abuse, and knew she needed more emotional support than the nursing staff could provide.

Some couples hire a doula just as much for the partner as for the laboring woman, especially if the partner isn't completely comfortable with the demands of labor support and needs a guide or helper, or wants someone else to take over the role of primary support person. A doula can provide backup support if the partner has a medical condition, becomes queasy at the sight of blood, has physical limitations, or simply wants to avoid the pressure of having to learn and remember all the comfort measures. One woman said, "We want our doula to be the brain, so my partner can stop thinking and problem-solving and focus on emotional support."

A doula can also do any necessary tasks, allowing the partner to focus on providing primary support. For example, the doula can run errands and fetch food, beverages, and comfort items such as ice packs. She can take photos. She can report progress and developments to the couple's friends and family. She can massage the woman's back while her partner helps her maintain a rhythm. She can continue support so the partner can eat, get some air, or take a much-needed nap. For more information on doulas, see page 20.

*Note:* Doulas might not be available in every area, and not all birthplaces welcome doulas. If a doula isn't available or allowed (or you don't want one), trusted relatives or friends can do many of the things a doula can do, especially if they attend childbirth classes with you and your partner.

# Preparing to Labor with Pain Medications

It's wise to learn about pain medications during pregnancy, whether or not you plan to use them during labor. That way, if the need for medications arises in labor, you'll already have some knowledge about them and can make an informed decision about their use.

Because both you and your baby are affected if you take pain medications, you and your caregiver should evaluate all possible risks and benefits of a drug. You should also be informed of "trade-offs"—extra precautions or interventions that may accompany pain medications to ensure their safety. (See chapter 13 to learn more about medications.)

## THE IMPORTANCE OF LEARNING COMFORT TECHNIQUES WHEN PLANNING FOR AN EPIDURAL

If your Pain Medication Preference Scale rating is +5 or higher (see page 214) and you're planning for an early epidural, you may think you don't need to learn self-help techniques to relieve pain. Keep in mind, however, that it's likely you'll have at least a few painful contractions before the epidural takes effect. It's also possible to have a failed epidural (see page 269) or that even if your epidural is effective, you'll still feel strong, painful sensations deep in your pelvis when pushing. For these reasons, it's wise to have other pain-coping tools in your "toolbox."

## *Key Points to Remember*

- Labor pain is a physical sensation that many women can manage by using coping techniques and receiving continued respectful support. Suffering is an emotional response that includes feelings of helplessness, fear, and panic. No one should suffer in labor.
- Well before the birth, learn about your pain relief options and discuss your preferences with your caregiver to help you and your support team plan how to meet your needs in labor.
- Even if you're planning to use pain medications, it's still wise to learn the comfort techniques in chapter 12, because you'll need ways to cope with contractions before heading to the hospital or while waiting to receive pain medications, or if the drugs turn out to be ineffective for you. Some comfort techniques—such as relaxation, breathing patterns, massage, and some movements—are more effective if you practice and adapt them well before labor begins.

# CHAPTER 12

# Comfort Techniques for Pain Relief and Labor Progress

As your due date approaches, you may wonder how you'll cope when your contractions become intense, or what you can do if your labor becomes slow or extra challenging. Comfort techniques, such as rhythmic breathing, body positions, and relaxation exercises, can help you cope with labor pain and maintain progress with less need for intervention.

This chapter describes how you and your partner can practice and adapt comfort techniques during pregnancy so they can help you effectively manage the pain and stress of labor. Instead of using pain medications, you may use just these techniques to keep your pain at a manageable level. Or you may use them along with pain medications to enhance your comfort and reduce the amount of medication you need. In either case, comfort techniques can help make the birth of your child a rewarding, fulfilling, and joyful experience by allowing you to participate in the event more fully.

# Finding Your Own Way to Cope with Labor Pain: The Three Rs

Every woman responds to labor pain in her own way. Your response will depend on the nature of your labor, your coping style, your goals and expectations, and how prepared you feel for labor.[1] Although you can learn about labor from other people, such as your caregiver or childbirth classes, only you can develop your own approach to handling labor pain. You have your own learning style, values, and ways of dealing with change, stress, and pain. With the help of your support team, you can adapt the following comfort techniques to suit your labor and modify them to match your personality and preferences.

## THE THREE RS: RELAXATION, RHYTHM, AND RITUAL

Although every woman responds to labor differently, those who cope well have three behaviors in common: relaxation, rhythm, and ritual. These Three Rs describe the instinctual coping behaviors observed in hundreds of women who were managing labor well.

### Relaxation

Women use relaxation in various ways. They may move about between contractions and let their muscles relax during contractions. They may become active during contractions (for example, swaying, rocking, and stroking their bellies) and relax only between contractions. Or they may remain quiet and unresponsive to their surroundings during and between contractions for all or part of labor. (For information on relaxation techniques, see pages 234–237.)

### Rhythm

Women who cope well in labor rely on *rhythm* in various forms. Rhythmic activity calms the mind and lets a woman work well with her body. For example, she may rhythmically breathe, moan, or chant during contractions. She may rhythmically repeat some words in her head or sing silently to herself. She may rhythmically tap or stroke something or someone. She may rock, sway, or dance in rhythm.

A partner's (or doula's) role is to enhance your rhythm and reinforce it through contractions. For example, if you're breathing and swaying in rhythm, your partner can follow the same rhythm when rubbing your back. If you start to lose the rhythm during a contraction, your partner can help you reconnect to it. If you aren't coping well, your partner can help you find rhythm by dancing with you or directing you to breathe rhythmically.

### Rituals—Planned and Spontaneous

In labor, *ritual* is the repetition of a meaningful rhythmic activity during contractions. Relaxation, breathing (see page 241), and attention-focusing (see page 226) are common rituals that childbirth educators teach expectant parents. These planned rituals help establish an effective coping style in early labor.

A partner's behavior and actions can influence the effectiveness of a ritual. If your partner is part of your ritual, nothing should be done to change it as long as it has a rhythm. Given the anxiety and uncertainty of labor, having someone act in the same way during each contraction will be enormously reassuring to you. Your partner's job may include maintaining eye contact with you; holding, touching, or stroking you; swaying with you; repeating the same words or phrases; or counting your breaths through each contraction. If your coping style is to focus inward, your partner's job simply may be to remain close by and do little but protect you from interruption.

It's difficult to know beforehand exactly what rituals you'll need in labor. Most women spontaneously adapt their planned rituals as labor progresses and intensifies. If they feel uninhibited and are free to move (change positions, walk, rock, and so on), they'll adjust a ritual or find a new one to help them cope.

If you begin to feel overwhelmed and can't carry on with a ritual, look to your support team for help. Your partner, doula, or caregiver may be able to help you reestablish a ritual or create a new one.

If you plan to give birth in a hospital, be aware that it may be difficult to find your own ritual if hospital policies or routine medical procedures limit your options or interrupt your rhythm. Make sure to practice a rhythmic activity that you can maintain during disturbances, such as self-talk (silent or vocal), tapping, or stroking. Your partner or doula can help you focus by maintaining the rhythm you established before the interruption or by using the Take Charge Routine (see page 186).

## Unplanned Rituals

The following are examples of unplanned rituals discovered by women in labor:

- rocking in a rocking chair in rhythm with her breathing
- silently repeating, "Be still like the mountain; flow like the river"
- having her partner stroke her lower leg in rhythm with her breathing
- having her partner softly count her breaths and point out when she has passed the halfway point of the contraction
- having her partner continuously repeat a word or phrase with her (One couple said, "Ruuusssh!" together through many hours of labor.)
- having her partner move with her in a way that she finds comforting (One couple walked everywhere during labor—in the park, grocery store, and hospital. With every contraction, they'd stop, embrace, and sway.)

# Comfort Techniques for Labor

Most pain is associated with injury, illness, or stress. Labor pain, however, is associated with a normal, healthy body function. Recognizing that labor pain is a productive part of the birthing process is key to keeping the pain manageable.

As you prepare for labor, remember the Three Rs (see page 224) and plan to use them to relax or feel secure. Think about what helps you relax, such as listening to music, having a massage, hearing soothing voices, taking a warm bath or shower, meditating, praying, humming, recalling pleasant places, or visualizing empowering images. Tell your support team what activities you're most likely to find helpful. Then think about the people and objects that help you feel safe and comfortable, such as your partner, mother, sister, friend, or doula, as well as your pillow, nightgown, pajamas, or favorite photo. Consider asking those trusted people for support and packing those items to take with you.

When rehearsing, try the following comfort techniques. Visit our website, http://www.PCNGuide.com, to download a checklist of comfort techniques; use it to record all the ones you prefer, as your preferences may change in labor. During labor, use the Road Map of Labor (see page 444) as a quick, visual reminder of options for comfort techniques.

## TUNING IN AND TUNING OUT

To cope with labor, you may find it most helpful to tune in to the pain by focusing on it, accepting it, and tailoring your response to it. Or you may prefer to tune out the pain by using distraction techniques, concentrating on outside stimuli, or performing mental activities.

## ATTENTION FOCUSING

During contractions, focus your attention to calm yourself and help keep your mind from wandering to pain or anxiety. (See page 204 to learn why distraction can help.) The following sections describe attention-focusing techniques that laboring women have used. Some were planned before labor began, but many were unplanned.

### Visualization

Closing your eyes and visualizing an encouraging or empowering image can help you cope with labor pain. Here are suggestions:
- Picture your uterine muscles contracting and pulling your cervix open. Visualize your baby pressing your cervix open.
- Imagine calm, pleasant places or recall happy, peaceful events.
- Picture yourself as lightly breathing above your contractions, as if you're a gull soaring above choppy waves.
- Visualize each contraction as a hurdle to clear, a steep hill to climb, a race to run, or a wave to ride.

### Cognitive Attention Focusing

By focusing on a mental activity, such as thinking or saying the words of a song, poem, verse, or prayer, you can direct your attention to the activity and away from the labor pain. You may plan this activity in advance. One woman imagined herself as the "Little Engine That Could" and planned to say as each contraction built to a peak, "I think I can, I think I can."[2] As each contraction subsided, she planned to repeat, "I thought I could, I thought I could."

Conversely, you might not think of doing this activity until you're in labor and find yourself choosing a word or phrase on the spot. One woman began rhythmically stroking her belly and chanting, "Keep stirring and you won't boil over." The day before she went into labor, she had become distracted while making fudge and had allowed the ingredients to boil over, so repeating this phrase helped her not become overwhelmed by contractions.

Some women combine cognitive attention focusing with physical activity. For example, they'll rhythmically count along with swaying, walking, dancing, or tapping.

## *Visual Focus*

Instead of closing your eyes to visualize, you may prefer to focus on a positive image within your sight. Here are some suggestions:

- Look at your partner's face, a picture, a reminder of your baby (a toy or a bootie), a flower, or the view from your window. One woman chose to stare at a hole in her pillowcase—not an inspiring image, but it worked for her!
- Focus on a line, such as the edge of a window casing, and visually follow that line around the object during each contraction.

## *Sounds*

Many laboring women use sounds as a way to focus their attention. To use this technique, try listening to your favorite music, your partner's soothing voice, repeated rhythms, recorded visualizations, or a recording of rhythmic environmental sounds such as a pounding surf, rainfall, or babbling brook. Or you can make your own rhythmic sounds by moaning, sighing, counting your breaths, singing, reciting poems or prayers, or chanting. See page 245 for more information on vocalizing.

## BATHS AND SHOWERS

A long soaking bath, whirlpool bath, or shower can be a marvelous comfort measure during labor. The warmth and buoyancy of the bathwater or the gentle massage provided by the showerhead or whirlpool jets can help your body relax.

If you take a bath during labor, you may get instant relief or it may take up to twenty minutes before you feel relaxed. (Try to stay in the water for at least this long before giving up and trying another pain relief option.) When in the water, you can lean back against a bath pillow or folded towels. If the tub is large enough and you're uncomfortable sitting up or lying on your back, try kneeling and leaning over the side of the tub (especially helpful for back pain) or lying on your side with your head elevated on a bath pillow.

### Advice from the Authors

If you're planning a home birth, be aware that long showers or soaks in a large tub may use up your regular hot water supply before you're ready to get out of the water. To ensure you'll have enough hot water, turn up the temperature on your water heater in advance. As a precaution against burns, leave a note that warns of the hot water temperature by each faucet in your home, and make sure to keep small children away from faucets.

## Water Births

The idea of giving birth in the water appeals to some expectant parents as a relaxing and gentle way to bring a baby into the world, and they seek out a birthplace and caregiver that support this option. Sometimes a woman who hadn't planned ahead for a water birth discovers during labor that the bath is so relaxing and helpful for relieving pain, she doesn't want to leave the water when she's ready to push. If she's giving birth in a hospital, she might not have the choice to stay in the bath. Many US and Canadian hospitals allow women to labor in the water, but few have policies supporting birth in the water. Conversely, caregivers who attend births at homes or at freestanding birth centers are often comfortable with water birth.

Although the leadership among caregivers in hospitals agree with out-of-hospital caregivers that laboring in water is a reasonable option, the groups disagree on the safety of water birth.[7] (Many hospital administrators (and caregivers) have the following objections to water births:

- the caregiver's need to master new techniques to facilitate birth positions and to protect the woman's perineum
- the physical agility needed by the caregiver to deliver the baby
- extra difficulty managing complications that arise during the birth[8]
- concerns about the baby's safety and other practical concerns, such as extra precautions for infection control (for example, shoulder-length gloves for caregivers) and insufficient room around the tub for access to the woman

Although these concerns can be addressed, few US and Canadian hospitals do so. If you're interested in learning more about water birth, visit http://www.waterbirth.org.

In addition to relieving pain, taking a bath may lower blood pressure if it's elevated and can affect labor progress. For example, taking a warm bath in early labor may slow down your contractions,[3] which is helpful if you need to rest. As a result, however, you may need a medical intervention such as the medication Pitocin to speed up labor later on.

In active labor, taking a bath often reduces stress hormones such as adrenalin, which may speed up labor progress.[4] Be sure the water temperature stays around your normal body temperature: 98°F to 99°F (36.7°C to 37.2°C).[5] This temperature is warm enough that you can comfortably stay in the water for an extended period, but not so warm that you become overheated. You and your baby will benefit from this precaution. If you become overheated, your baby will as well. His heart rate may increase, which signals the need to leave the bath and lower the water temperature before returning. Stay in the bath for no longer than ninety minutes at a time. Get out of the bath, walk around or sit for a while, then return to the bath if you wish.

You may choose to talk a shower instead of a bath. Showers don't slow labor and don't tend to raise body temperature. If you take a shower, lean against the shower wall or sit on a towel-covered stool or birth ball so you can rest. Direct the spray where it best relieves tension. (Directing it against your lower back helps relieve back pain.) If you like (and if there's room), your partner can accompany you in the shower or tub to provide additional comfort measures such as massage. (If you'll be birthing in a hospital or birth center, make sure your partner packs a swimsuit.)

In the past, maternity care experts believed that letting a woman bathe after her membranes had ruptured would lead to infection; however, the results of several studies show that this belief is false.[6]

## FOODS AND FLUIDS

To keep up your energy in early labor, eat high-carbohydrate foods that appeal to you, such as fruit, pasta, toast, rice, and waffles. Also eat and drink easy-to-digest foods and beverages, such as soup, broth, and herbal tea. In active labor, you may be less interested in food; however, hunger and low blood sugar levels decrease the tolerance for pain.

Find out your caregiver's advice on eating during labor. At home births, freestanding birth centers, and some hospitals, you'll be encouraged to eat. Other hospitals restrict eating but permit patients to drink clear fluids. If your hospital has this policy, try clear broths, frozen fruit juice bars, tea, juice, sports drinks, and plenty of water to quench your thirst and provide you some calories. Because a full bladder may slow labor and increase pain, be sure to empty your bladder often.

A few hospitals don't permit even healthy, low-risk women to eat *or* drink in labor, in case they require general anesthesia; however, a recent review of the research found no clear disadvantages of eating or drinking in labor for low-risk women. It concluded that women should be free to eat and drink as they wish.[9]

If your caregiver won't permit you to drink fluids or you're vomiting, you'll probably receive fluids intravenously (IV) to prevent dehydration. You may develop a very dry mouth; sucking on ice chips, a frozen fruit juice bar, or a sour lollipop will help moisten it. You may also try brushing your teeth or rinsing your mouth with cold water or mouthwash.

## HEAT AND COLD

An electric heating pad or hot-water bottle on your lower abdomen or back relieves labor pain. Another soothing heat source is a cloth bag or sock filled with uncooked rice or other grain and heated in a microwave. To relieve perineal pain or tension while pushing, your partner or caregiver can soak washcloths in hot water, wring them out, and apply them wherever you need relief. If you'll be birthing in a hospital, check for any restrictions on heating devices brought from home. (If so, only warm wet washcloths or hospital-supplied items such as gel packs will be allowed.)

A cold pack on your lower back can relieve back pain, too. Examples include a bag of ice cubes or frozen peas, frozen wet washcloths, cold cans of soda, or—best of all—frozen gel packs used to treat athletic injuries (preferably those with straps so you can move around while wearing one). When using a cold pack, wear a warm robe or use a blanket to avoid feeling chilled.

During labor, your tolerance for heat and cold might be affected, and you might not notice that a compress is too hot or cold for your skin. To check that the temperature is safe, have your partner hold the compress for several seconds. Have one or more layers of cloth between your skin and the heat source or cold pack to protect your skin and to let you adapt to the temperature change gradually. If you're given pain medication that causes loss of sensation (such as epidural anesthesia), avoid using heat or cold on numbed areas.

## COUNTER-IRRITATION

When in pain, you might unconsciously start biting your lip, digging your nails into your palms, or pounding your fist on your thigh. These examples of counter-irritation cause an uncomfortable sensation that *you control* to distract your attention from the pain that you can't. They also cause the body to produce more endorphins (pain-relieving hormones).

In some cultures, "birth combs" are used in labor. These are wide-tooth wooden combs or hairbrushes that a laboring woman squeezes in her hands during contractions. The goal is that the pressure of the comb on the palm will draw the woman's attention away from labor pain and help make it feel more manageable. Other examples of counter-irritation include a transcutaneous electrical nerve stimulation, or TENS, unit (see page 249) and acupressure (see page 231).

If a laboring woman uses counter-irritation in a way that might be harmful, her partner can try placing a comb or hairbrush in her hand or finding some other item she can use to produce a little discomfort without causing injury.

## COMFORT ITEMS

The following is a list of items that can provide comfort during labor. You may already have some; most others are easy to find.

- rolling pin or rolling massage devices, plus other massage aids (for back pain—see page 249)
- gardening foam knee pad (for kneeling on the bed, floor, or in the tub)
- shawl or rebozo (for abdominal lift—see page 247)
- warm fleece wrap and socks (hospitals typically provide only light cotton blankets)
- fan (labor is often hard, sweaty work)
- audio player (listening to favorite music or motivating dialogue can provide encouragement and comfort)
- TENS unit (see page 249)
- two wide-toothed combs (one to hold in each hand for counter-irritation)
- birth ball (see below)
- other personal items that comfort you

### Birth Ball

A *birth ball* is a large inflatable plastic ball that pro-vides a soft yet firm place to sit or lean comfortably. Usually known as a physical therapy or fitness ball, it requires you to have proper posture when you sit on it.

To help relax your torso and perineum in labor, sit on the ball and sway your hips from side to side during and between contractions. To help relieve back pain or reposition your baby if necessary, place the ball on your bed, then either kneel on the bed or stand next to it and lean over the ball. Sway your hips from side to side or from front to back. The ball allows such movement to be comforting and almost effortless—a definite advantage when you're tired from the hard work of labor.

Many hospitals and birth centers provide birth balls, but you may wish to have your own so you can use it during pregnancy for exercise, comfort, and backache relief as well as to get familiar with using it before labor. Also, gently bouncing on the ball while holding your newborn will be a wonderful way to soothe him (see page 373).

Birth balls are available at many chain discount retailers, physical therapy clinics, sporting goods stores, and birth supply companies. They usually come with a hand pump, but they can be inflated to the desired firmness with a party balloon pump or air compressor. A ball with a 65-centimeter diameter is best for a woman of average height (63 to 70 inches). A much shorter woman may require a 55-centimeter ball, and a much taller woman may require a 75-centimeter ball. Make sure the strength of the ball can hold at least 300 pounds.

Practice using a birth ball before labor begins. Put one hand on the ball as you carefully lower yourself onto it. Use your other hand to hold on to someone or a stable object. With practice, you'll be able to use the ball without support. Because the ball may get sticky or pick up germs from being on the floor, cover it with a towel before sitting or leaning on it.

Peanut-shaped balls are also used in labor in some of the same ways as the round birth ball. They come in various sizes) and are particularly useful to a woman in bed with an epidural. The peanut shape helps keep her legs spread, which gives the baby more room to move down the birth canal and out.[10]

# Massage and Touch

Massage and touch are effective ways to direct your attention away from labor pain and can convey encouragement, reassurance, and love. Having someone firmly stroke, rub, or knead your neck, shoulders, feet, or hands can be soothing. Having someone lightly stroke your back or thighs can also help with relaxation and pain relief. You may find relief if someone presses firmly on tense areas such as your hips, thighs, shoulders, hands, or lower back. Other tactile ways to focus your attention away from pain include tightly embracing your partner or directing the spray from a handheld showerhead onto tense areas.

To relax and relieve pain by yourself, try lightly and rhythmically stroking your belly in circles. When following the lower curve of your uterus, imagine that you're stroking your baby's head. To make your hands slide more easily on your skin, dust your palms with cornstarch or use unscented massage oil.

## Warning about Acupressure

Maternity care experts advise against pressing on the Hoku and Spleen 6 points before the due date, because doing so can cause preterm contractions. During pregnancy, partners should find these points on their own bodies but not press them on the woman's body until after the thirty-eighth week of pregnancy.

## Crisscross Massage

The crisscross massage can ease back pain and relax your lower back muscles during or between contractions. Practice this technique in pregnancy so it's most helpful during labor.

Kneel forward on your hands and knees or lean over a birth ball or onto a counter or chair. Flex your hips so your thighs are about 90 degrees from your spine. Your partner stands or kneels next to you, facing your side, then places a hand on each side of your body, below your ribs (not on the ribs—that hurts!), at the narrowest part of your waist, with the fingers on the far hand pointing down and the fingers on the near hand pointing up. (See illustration.)

Next, your partner firmly presses into your sides, then moves each hand up and over your back, following your waistline with each hand passing the other as it continues to the other hand's starting place. Your partner then uses the same firm pressure to return the hands to their original starting positions. Repeat this motion for as long as you like, trying to match the movements with the rhythm of your breathing. Most women favor pressure on their sides, which relieves the ligaments that support the uterus.

## Acupressure for Comfort and Progress in Labor

*Acupressure* may help reduce labor pain, increase contractions, and increase your satisfaction with pain relief in labor.[11] Hoku and Spleen 6 are the two most popular points. The Hoku point is on the back of your hand, in the V formed where the bones extending below your thumb and index finger come together. The Spleen 6 point is on the inner side of your leg, about the width of four fingers above your inner anklebone. See the illustration at right.

Press your thumb steadily into the point for ten to sixty seconds, then rest for the same length of time before pressing again. Repeat this pattern three to six times whenever you want during labor. Be aware that these spots are sensitive and may hurt a bit when pressed.

## A NOTE TO FATHERS AND PARTNERS

Practicing comfort measures and relaxation techniques during pregnancy not only allows you and your pregnant partner to adapt them to your own style, but it also increases the likelihood that you'll remember how to do them when under the stress of labor.

Here are suggestions for how you can practice together. Many of these tips will also be useful in labor.

- To signal the beginning of a practice contraction, your pregnant partner tells you, "Here it comes," or begins to breathe rhythmically. You both practice coping techniques for the next thirty to sixty seconds, until she says, "It's over." Take turns starting the contractions so you both get used to beginning a coping technique whether you're ready or not.

- To understand the effectiveness of a comfort measure, try this experiment: Each of you holds an ice cube in one hand for a minute. Note how it feels. Then hold the ice cube in the other hand for another minute while breathing rhythmically and counting your breaths, or using another comfort measure. Was there a difference in the discomfort you felt? Many people clearly note less awareness of discomfort when using coping techniques.

- If the above experiment helps your partner realize the effectiveness of a comfort measure, suggest that she hold ice cubes to simulate contractions as you practice other comfort measures together. It may help her determine which techniques are most effective.

- While practicing, try to detect any tension your partner is holding. Help her relax by touching or massaging her, talking to her, reminding her to move around, or breathing with her.

- Be aware of your facial expressions, tone of voice, and way of touching your partner. You'll convey anxiety if you look troubled or distressed, if you speak loudly in a worried voice, or if you rub her brusquely or distractedly. You'll convey reassurance by having a confident expression, speaking soothingly, and massaging smoothly and slowly.

# Relaxation and Tension Release

Relaxation is the art of recognizing and releasing muscle tension; it's the key to finding comfort during labor. Remaining relaxed is especially important during early labor, when contractions are usually manageable. If you consciously release muscle tension during early contractions, you'll establish a habit of keeping relaxed during the intense contractions of active labor and transition. Conversely, if you tense up during early contractions, you'll have trouble relaxing in later labor.

Here are just some of the benefits of relaxation during labor:

### Conserves energy and reduces fatigue

If you don't consciously relax your muscles during contractions, you'll probably unconsciously tense them. Tension wastes energy and increases pain and fatigue.

### Calms your mind and reduces stress

A relaxed body leads to a relaxed state of mind, which in turn reduces stress. Anxiety, anger, or fear causes stress in labor, which produces excessive *catecholamines* (stress hormones such as adrenaline). High levels of these hormones can prolong your labor and can harm your baby by decreasing the blood flow to your uterus (see page 174).[12]

**Reduces pain**

Contracted muscles become painful when deprived of oxygen. Relaxing tense muscles frees more oxygen to reach your uterus, which may decrease labor pain. In addition, consciously releasing tension focuses your attention away from the contractions and reduces your awareness of pain.

## Recognizing Muscle Tension

To release muscle tension, you first need to be able to recognize it.
Try this exercise:

1.  Sit on a chair or the floor.
2.  Make a tight fist with your right hand. Pay attention to how hard the muscles in your forearm feel. Touch them with your left hand.
3.  Relax your right hand, letting it droop. Notice how soft the forearm muscles feel.
4.  Raise your shoulders toward your ears and tense up. Notice how tight you feel when your shoulders are tense.
5.  Lower your shoulders and relax. Then relax even further. Do you notice an additional release? You can often release residual muscle tension when you become aware of it.

## Two Views on Comfort Measures

By the time we reached the hospital, my contractions were quite stunning! I was 3 centimeters dilated. I used the birth ball, but it seemed to increase the pain. The whirlpool tub saved me! I spent an hour in there, which helped me relax. When I got out of the tub, I'd dilated to 10 centimeters, so I could push.
—*Clarissa*

Once labor began, it felt natural and empowering to use the tub, birth ball, and breathing and vocal rhythms to process the pain. Thanks to those comfort measures and my doula's and my husband's gentle coaching, I was very aware throughout labor.
—*Susan*

## Practicing Tension Release with Your Partner

Your partner also can learn how to recognize when you're tense and when you're relaxed by using the following methods:

*   Observation (How do you look when you're anxious, uncomfortable, calm, content, or asleep?)
*   Touch (How do your muscles feel? Hard or soft?)
*   "Floating a limb" (Your partner lifts one of your arms or legs while you let it be heavy and loose. Once supporting its full weight, your partner moves it slowly, bending and straightening the joints, feeling for the looseness and heaviness that signal relaxation. Don't "help" your partner with lifting your arm or leg.)

Help your partner practice spotting muscle tension by deliberately tightening your muscles and having your partner locate the tense spot. If your body is assessed calmly and gently, you'll develop confidence in your partner's ability to help you relax in labor.

Once your partner has located the tension, find out what releases it. Your partner may touch or massage the area, place a warm compress on it, or simply remind you to let those muscles relax. As you practice together, you'll learn which muscles you tense most often (and thus may be the most difficult to relax). You may discover that you frequently tense your shoulders, forehead, mouth, jaw, or fists. These areas, or *tension spots*, should receive special attention as you practice relaxation and especially during labor.

# Relaxation Techniques

Once you can recognize muscle tension, the next step is to learn how to release it. By focusing on different parts of your body and consciously releasing the tension, you can relax both your body and mind.

Some women are able to relax more easily than others, but almost anyone can learn to relax with practice. The following sections describe several techniques. Try them all at least once, then practice those that appeal to you and seem to best relax you.

When you first begin practicing, lie on your side with plenty of pillows supporting you, or sit in a comfortable chair with your head and arms supported. After you've mastered the relaxation technique in this position, practice it while sitting up, lying down, standing, and walking. You'll use various positions during labor, so you'll need to be able to relax in any position.

Begin practicing a relaxation technique in a quiet, calm area. As you master the technique, progress to practicing it in louder, more active surroundings. Especially if laboring in a hospital, you'll need to be able to relax in a noisy, busy environment.

When you're done practicing a technique, stretch your arms and legs and rise slowly (if seated or lying down) to avoid becoming lightheaded or dizzy.

## PASSIVE RELAXATION

This exercise calls for your partner to guide you through steps to relax your entire body, while you rest in a comfortable position. (If your partner is unavailable, use a relaxation recording or app to guide you.) Consider playing pleasant, relaxing music each time you practice. Playing the same music in labor will help create a familiar and relaxed environment that you'll find comforting.

Before beginning, try this simple relaxation awareness exercise: Take in a long breath and hold it for a few seconds. Notice the tension in your chest and abdomen while you hold your breath. Now release your breath as if you're sighing, and notice the release of tension as you release your breath. Every exhalation is a relaxing breath.

### Practicing Passive Relaxation

As you practice this exercise, breathe as you do when falling asleep—slowly, easily, and fully. Your body and mind release tension and thought, your breathing slows, and you pause slightly at the end of each inhalation and exhalation. (To see this process in action, observe the way someone else's breathing gradually slows when falling asleep.)

Lie on your side or sit in a semireclined position with the floor or bed supporting your head and limbs. Take your time getting comfortable. You may want to put pillows under or between your knees, beneath your head, or under your belly to increase comfort and support.

Next, ask your partner read the following script in a calm, relaxed voice, letting you spend two or three breaths releasing the tension in each area of focus to allow time for your tension to slip away.

# Script for Passive Relaxation

- Yawn or exhale completely.
- Focus on your toes and feet. Imagine that you're breathing away any tension there. Feel how warm and relaxed they are.
- Now think about your ankles. Notice how floppy and loose they are. They're relaxed and comfortable.
- Now focus on your lower legs. Let those muscles become loose and soft. Good.
- And now, your knees. They're supported and relaxed—you're not holding your legs in any position. Wiggle them to see how relaxed they are.
- Think about your thighs. Those strong muscles are soft and relaxed because they have no work to do right now, and they're fully supported. Good.
- And now think about your buttocks and perineum. This area needs to be especially relaxed during labor and birth, so just let it become soft and yielding. When the time is right, your baby will travel down the birth canal, and the tissues of your perineum will spread to let your baby make her way out. You'll release, letting your perineum relax and open for your baby.
- Focus on your lower back. Imagine that someone with strong, warm hands is giving you a lovely backrub. It feels so good. Your muscles are relaxing, and your lower back is comfortable. Notice the tension leaving your back.
- Let your thoughts turn to your belly. Let those muscles relax. Let your belly rise and fall as you breathe in and out. Good. Now let's move your focus deeper to your baby within your uterus. She's floating or wiggling and squirming in the warm water of your womb—a safe place where you're meeting all your baby's needs for nourishment, oxygen, warmth, movement, and stimulation. Your baby hears your heartbeat, your voice, my voice, music, and other interesting sounds. What excellent care you're giving your baby. You're the perfect mother—meeting all your baby's needs!
- Now focus on your chest. As you inhale, your chest swells easily, making room for the air. As you exhale, your chest relaxes to help the air flow out. Breathe easily and slowly, letting the air flow in and flow out, almost as though you're asleep. Good.
- Take a moment to focus on your breathing again—inhaling through your nose and exhaling through your mouth—slowly and easily, letting the air flow in and out. At the top of an inhalation, notice that little tension in your chest, which you can release with an exhalation. Listen as you exhale. Your breath sounds relaxed and calm, almost as if you were asleep. Every exhalation is relaxing. Use your exhalations to breathe away any tension. Good.
- And now focus on your shoulders and upper back. Imagine you've just had them massaged. Breathe any tension away and feel the warmth and softness as the tension slips away.
- Now focus on your arms. As you exhale, let your arms go limp—from your shoulders, all the way down your arms, to your wrists, hands, and fingers. Let them become heavy, loose, and relaxed.
- And now your neck. All the muscles in your neck are soft because they don't have to hold your head in any position. Your head is either comfortably balanced or completely supported, so just let your neck relax. Good.
- Focus on your lips and jaw. They're slack and relaxed. You're not holding your mouth closed or open. It's comfortable; no tension there.
- And now your eyes and eyelids. You're not keeping your eyes open or closed. They're the way they want to be. Your eyes are unfocused and still. Your eyelids are relaxed and heavy.
- Focus on your brow and scalp. No worries there! Think about how warm and relaxed they are. You have a calm, peaceful expression on your face, reflecting a calm, peaceful feeling inside.
- We've gone all the way from your toes to the top of your head. Take a few moments to enjoy these feelings of calmness and well-being. You can relax this way anytime—before bedtime, during an afternoon rest, or during a quiet break. This is how you'll want to feel in labor. Of course, during labor, you won't lie down all the time. You'll walk, sit up, shower, and change positions. But whenever a contraction comes, you'll let yourself relax all the muscles you don't need to hold yourself in a particular position, and you can let your mind relax, giving you a confident, peaceful feeling. This feeling will help you yield to contractions, letting you focus on breathing and finding comfort through each one.
- And now it's time to end the exercise. Gradually open your eyes, stretch, and tune in to your surroundings. Take your time. There's no need to rush.

# Relaxation Countdown

Once you've learned to recognize muscle tension and have mastered passive relaxation, use the following technique to release tension quickly. This exercise uses your breathing to create a wave of relaxation that passes from your head to your toes. It's particularly helpful when you want to fall back to sleep, when you're stressed, or when you're trying to relax after a contraction.

## *Practicing the Relaxation Countdown*

Inhale through your nose. As you exhale through your mouth, release muscle tension in the following order. By the time you count down to one, you'll be fully relaxed.

5.  Head, neck, and shoulders
4.  Arms, hands, and fingers
3.  Chest and abdomen
2.  Back, buttocks, and perineum
1.  Legs, feet, and toes

At first, use five slow breaths (one for each of the five areas) to count down to total body relaxation. Then try to relax all five areas while slowly exhaling one deep breath (rapid relaxation countdown).

During labor, you can use the first or last breath of each contraction as a rapid relaxation countdown to maximize tension release and reduce discomfort or pain.

# Touch Relaxation

For this technique, you release tension in response to your partner's comforting touch. During pregnancy, this exercise is a pleasurable way to practice relaxation. During labor, you'll use your partner's touching, stroking, or massaging as a cue to relax.

Lie on your side or sit in a comfortable position. Next, contract a set of muscles (for example, stiffen one arm or leg) and have your partner touch the tense area. Release the tension and relax into your partner's hand. Imagine the tension leaving that part of your body.

Have your partner try the following types of touch. Tell your partner which types you prefer, but be sure to practice all of them. Your preference may change during labor.

**Still touch**

Your partner places a relaxed hand on the tense area, molding it around the muscles, while you release the muscle tension until you're relaxed.

**Firm pressure**

Your partner firmly presses on the tense area, gradually increasing the pressure as you inhale, then gradually relaxes the pressure as you release the tension while exhaling. The pressure should feel good.

### Stroking

Your partner lightly strokes the tense area as you let the tension flow out. If stroking your arms or legs, your partner strokes toward your fingers or toes. When stroking your belly, your partner may make circles.

### Massage

Your partner firmly rubs or kneads your tense muscles.

While doing each technique, give your partner feedback on the amount of pressure that feels best to you. Your partner should always keep one hand in contact with your body whenever using a touch relaxation technique. When your eyes are closed, it'll be hard for you to relax if your partner's touch disappears, leaving you to wonder where and when it'll reappear.

## *Practicing Touch Relaxation*

Practice contracting the following muscle groups, then releasing them in response to your partner's touch.

- brow and eyes
- jaw
- neck
- shoulders
- arms and hands
- abdomen
- buttocks
- legs and feet

# ROVING BODY CHECK

Sometimes you may think you're entirely relaxed, but you're still retaining tension in one or more areas of your body. This exercise helps you systematically release tension throughout your entire body, allowing for deeper relaxation. It's similar to the Passive Relaxation exercise on page 235, except that you do it by yourself.

## *Practicing the Roving Body Check*

Get into a comfortable position and begin breathing slowly, rhythmically, and easily. Focus on one area of your body with each breath. As you inhale through your nose, notice any tension in that area. As you exhale through your mouth, deliberately release that tension. Then focus on another area. Repeat, moving your attention from one area to another in the following order or in the opposite order, whichever you prefer:

1. Brow, eyes, and eyelids
2. Jaw and lips
3. Neck and shoulders
4. Right arm and hand
5. Left arm and hand
6. Upper back
7. Lower back
8. Buttocks and perineum
9. Right leg and foot
10. Left leg and foot

Use the roving body check during or between labor contractions to make sure you're releasing tension throughout your body. Your partner can help by telling you which area to relax with each exhalation, or by touching or stroking a different area with each exhalation. You may prefer to have your partner focus only on those areas you know are tense.

# RELAXING IN DIFFERENT POSITIONS AND WHILE ACTIVE

During labor, you'll use various positions and frequently move around to find comfort and to help your labor progress. For this reason, it's important to practice relaxation techniques when you're not lying down and inactive. Different positions require different muscle groups to support you, and your aim is to completely relax the muscles you don't need to use while in a position. For example, you can't relax your legs while standing, but you can relax your shoulders, arms, and face.

# Movement and Positions for Labor

Moving around and changing positions allow you to discover ways to be comfortable during labor. The use of different positions may speed up a slow labor by changing the shape of your pelvis and by using gravity, both of which help your baby rotate and descend into your birth canal. Changing positions can also affect your mind-set during labor. For example, being in an upright position may give you a greater sense of control and active involvement in your labor than when you're lying down.

The following chart describes positions and movements for labor. Plan to change positions at least every thirty minutes, especially if your labor progress is slow.

| Position or movement | | What this position or movement does |
|---|---|---|
| **Positions and Movements for the First Stage of Labor** | | |
| Standing | | Takes advantage of gravity. |
| | | Makes contractions less painful and more productive. |
| | | Helps your baby descend by lining him up with the angle of your pelvis. |
| | | May speed up labor if you've been lying down. |
| | | May increase your urge to push during the second stage of labor. |
| Walking | | Same as standing, plus: |
| | | Causes rhythmic shifts in the shape of your pelvis, nudging your baby to find her way through it. |
| | | Can be tiring if you walk for too long. |
| Standing and leaning forward on your partner, bed, or birth ball | | Same as standing, plus: |
| | | Relieves back pain. |
| | | Is a good position for a back rub. |
| | | May be more restful than standing. |
| | | Encourages repositioning if your baby is occiput posterior (OP—see page 286). |
| Slow dancing | | Same as walking, plus: |
| | | Enhances your sense of well-being, because a loved one is embracing you. |
| | | Increases comfort through rhythm and music. |
| | | Is a good position for your partner to give back pressure. |
| Lunge (see page 248) | | Widens one side of your pelvis (the side toward which you lunge). |
| | | Encourages an OP baby to rotate. |
| | | Can be done while standing or kneeling. Try lunging for one contraction to the left and one to the right. Continue for 5 or 6 contractions in the direction that feels better. |
| Sitting upright* | | Is a good resting position. |
| | | Uses gravity (to a degree). |

| Position or movement | | What this position or movement does |
|---|---|---|
| Sitting and swaying on birth ball | | Same as sitting upright, plus: |
| | | Relaxes torso and pelvic floor. |
| | | Encourages rhythmic movement. |
| | | Movement may improve labor progress. |
| Sitting or rocking in chair | | Same as sitting upright, plus: |
| | | May speed up your labor because of the rhythmic rocking movement. |
| | | May increase your comfort. |
| Sitting, leaning forward with support | | Same as sitting upright, plus: |
| | | Relieves back pain. |
| Open knee-chest position (see page 247) | | If your baby is OP and you use the position in early labor, gravity will encourage your baby to back his head out of your pelvis and rotate. |
| | | Helps in early labor to relieve back pain. |
| | | In later labor, reduces pressure on your cervix if it's swollen. |

### Positions and Movements for Either First or Second Stage of Labor

| | | |
|---|---|---|
| Sitting on toilet or commode | | Same as sitting upright, plus: |
| | | Encourages pelvic floor relaxation. |
| | | Helps with effective pushing and prevents holding back (because of the position's association with bearing down to have a bowel movement). |
| Semi-sitting* | | Same as sitting upright, plus: |
| | | Is an easy position to get into (on the bed or delivery table). |
| | | Is a common birthing position. |
| | | Disadvantages: May increase pre-existing back pain and slows down expansion of the pelvis. |
| Hands-and-knees* | | Helps relieve back pain. |
| | | Helps your baby rotate if she's OP. |
| | | Allows for pelvic tilts (see page 247). |
| | | May reduce premature urge to push. |
| | | May slow a rapid second stage of labor because the position neutralizes the effects of gravity. |
| Hands-and-knees* with forward/back movement | | Same as hands and knees, plus: |
| | | May aid descent of baby. |
| | | Enlarge front-to-back dimensions of pelvis. |

| Position or movement | | What this position or movement does |
|---|---|---|
| Side-lying* | | Is an excellent resting position. |
| | | Helps lower your blood pressure. |
| | | Is a safe position if you've received pain medications. |
| | | Neutralizes the effects of gravity, making the position useful for slowing a rapid labor. |
| | | In the second stage, allows your sacrum to shift to create a wider opening for your baby's descent. |
| Side-lying lunge or "semiprone" (lower leg extended, upper leg raised and flexed ) | | Same as side-lying, plus: |
| | | Widens upper side of pelvis. |
| | | Shifts gravity from side-lying position. |
| | | Encourages baby to rotate. |
| | | Extra room in pelvis may aid descent. |

Positions and Movements for the Second Stage of Labor

| | | |
|---|---|---|
| Squatting | | Takes advantage of gravity. |
| | | Widens your pelvic outlet (but may diminish your pelvic inlet, which is why this position is best to do in the second stage and not the first). |
| | | May enable your baby to rotate and descend in a difficult birth. |
| | | Is helpful if you don't feel an urge to push. |
| | | Allows you the freedom to shift your weight for comfort. |
| Lap squatting | | Same as squatting, plus: |
| | | Reduces strain on knees and ankles (compared to squatting). |
| | | Allows more support and requires less effort. |
| | | Enhances your sense of well-being, because your loved one is embracing you. |
| | | Disadvantage: If you're much heavier than your partner, this position might not be possible. |
| Supported squat | | Allows greater mobility of pelvic joints than any other position, and eliminates external pressure (from the bed, chair, and so on). |
| | | Takes advantage of gravity. |
| | | Lengthens your trunk, allowing more room for your baby to maneuver into position. |
| | | Allows your baby's head to change the shape of your pelvis. |
| | | Disadvantage: Requires your partner to have strength enough to support you for long periods. |
| Dangle | | Same as the supported squat, except your partner sits with legs braced and well supported, making this position easier to sustain. |

For more information on labor positions, see pages 247–248.

* Can be used if you receive epidural anesthesia (although you may need support).

# Breathing Techniques as Comfort Measures

When you swim, run, practice yoga, sing, or play a musical instrument, you need to regulate your breathing to perform effectively and efficiently. In this way, labor is no different from any other activity that requires physical coordination and mental discipline. Each childbirth preparation method focuses on some form of breath awareness because of the following benefits:

- Enhances relaxation.
- Helps reduce pain by supplying your muscles with oxygen.
- Provides a focus to calm you and distract you from pain. Breathing won't make labor pain completely disappear, but it'll help make pain more manageable.

Most people who have taken childbirth classes use slow and light breathing rhythms (or a variation on them) in labor. The rhythm you'll use to breathe during labor depends on your preferences and on the nature and intensity of your contractions. In early labor, you'll likely use slow breathing for as long as it relaxes you. You may continue to breathe slowly for your entire labor, or you may switch to light breathing or some variation in late labor.

During pregnancy, experiment with all of these breathing techniques. You can't be sure that your favorite techniques *before* labor will be the same *during* labor. Practice rhythmic breathing in the positions shown on pages 238–240.

Each breathing technique includes an illustration next to the description. The curved line at the bottom of each illustration shows the contraction, which begins subtly and builds in intensity, then fades away. The typical length of a contraction in labor is shown in seconds, listed below the curved line. The top line shows the pattern of inhalations and exhalations.

You can combine rhythmic breathing with other comfort measures, such as moaning, movement, massage, tension release, hot or cold packs, bath, shower, and so on. Through practice, experimentation, and adaptation, you'll discover how best to use and adapt the techniques to help you relax in labor.

## Advice from the Authors

### Tips for Partners When Using Breathing Techniques

During a one-minute practice contraction, interject encouraging words or phrases as you count your pregnant partner's breaths. For example, say, "One, okay. Two, good. Three, let go. Four, just like that. Five, great...." Repeat the same encouraging words as the contraction continues.

During labor, the number of breaths she'll take to get through a contraction won't vary significantly from one contraction to the next. Counting her breaths can help you know how much longer a contraction will last. Point out when she has passed the halfway point—information she'll be encouraged to receive. You'll also be able to tell when the contraction is subsiding, because her breathing will ease after passing the peak. As one woman recalled, "Having my partner tell me when a contraction was half over seemed to shorten it and cut its intensity in half. I knew that when I had passed the peak, I could make it the rest of the way."

# AVOIDING HYPERVENTILATION

A common problem that may bother you temporarily when you begin exploring new ways to breathe is *hyperventilation* or overbreathing. While rarely serious, hyperventilation makes you feel lightheaded or dizzy, or it can make your fingers, feet, or the area around your mouth tingle. You may feel panicky, as if you can't get enough air.

What causes hyperventilation? Breathing too deeply or too quickly (or both) makes you feel as if you need more oxygen. In response, you may gulp air. Paradoxically, you wind up with too little carbon dioxide, which changes the balance of oxygen and carbon dioxide in your blood and may cause hyperventilation.

To prevent hyperventilation, breathe more lightly or more slowly. If you've mastered rhythmic breathing before labor begins, you're very unlikely to hyperventilate during labor. Without even thinking about it, you'll adapt the pace and depth of your breathing to your changing needs in labor. Here are some general principles that will keep you from hyperventilating when practicing breathing techniques:

- Try to relax your shoulders, face, and lips (and as much of your body as possible).
- Try not to rush your breathing.
- Try to keep your inhalations silent. If they're noisy, you're likely moving too much air.
- Your exhalations should be slightly audible, but not forced. They should *sound* relaxed.
- Always pause at the end of an inhalation and at the end of the exhalation, before inhaling again. It's almost as if you're waiting for the air to "turn around" before you inhale or exhale.
- As you adjust the rate of your breathing, also adjust the depth of your breaths. The slower you breathe, the deeper your breaths should be. The quicker you breathe, the shallower your breaths should be to prevent hyperventilation.

If you (or your partner) experience hyperventilation, try these suggestions to correct it:

- If you're feeling dizzy, hold your breath for ten to twenty seconds to allow the amount of carbon dioxide in your blood to return to normal levels.
- Breathe into your cupped hands, a paper bag, or a surgical mask (available if you're in a hospital). Breathing your own carbon dioxide helps restore levels to normal quickly.
- Talk to yourself. "I'm feeling panicky. I *feel* I can't get enough air, but I actually can. Even if I think I'm in danger, I'm not. No one dies of a panic attack. I know what to do. I need to hold my breath or make myself breathe slowly, and I will feel better soon."
- Your partner can help you pace your breathing with a visual cue (such as by moving a hand as though conducting an orchestra to keep a rhythm), by talking to you in time with your breathing, by using rhythmic stroking, or by breathing with you.

# Slow Breathing

In labor, slow breathing can help calm you. The keys to the technique are keeping an even rhythm and trying to release tension during exhalations. Begin using slow breathing when your contractions become so intense that you can't walk or talk through them or can't be distracted from them. Use slow breathing for as long as it comforts you—probably until you're well into the first stage of labor and possibly throughout your entire labor. Shift to light breathing or a variation if slow breathing no longer seems to work or you have trouble keeping your breathing slow.

## *Using Slow Breathing in Labor*

1. As soon as a contraction begins, signal your partner with a nod or by saying, "Here it comes." Inhale fully and easily and sigh as you exhale, releasing all tension. You may think of this first breath as your "organizing" breath—you block everything out and focus only on your planned ritual (see page 224) of slow breathing combined with tension release and positive mental activity. Your partner will note the time if timing contractions (see page 167).
2. Focus your attention (see page 226).
3. Inhale slowly through your nose and exhale completely through your mouth. Pause for a moment before you inhale again. Take about five to twelve breaths per minute (about half the normal resting breathing rate for most people).
4. Inhale quietly, but keep your mouth slightly open and relaxed when exhaling so someone nearby can hear your breath. In labor, you may also vocalize or moan as you exhale.
5. Keep your shoulders down and relaxed. Relax your chest and belly so they can swell as you inhale. Your partner should touch or stroke you, talk to you in the rhythm of your breathing, or just sit quietly nearby, following your lead as to what feels good.
6. Signal to your partner as the contraction ends or take a final deep breath.
7. Completely relax, change positions, chat, sip liquids, and do whatever you need to feel comfortable.

## *Rehearsing Slow Breathing for Labor*

Rehearse slow breathing until you're confident in your ability to use the technique for sixty to ninety seconds at a time (the typical length of a contraction). Practice in different positions. Combine with the Roving Body Check (see page 237).

You may find it uncomfortable to inhale through your nose and exhale through your mouth. If so, breathe only through your nose or mouth. You may find that you prefer letting your belly expand first, then your chest, as you inhale deeply (belly breathing). Or you may prefer letting only your chest expand as you inhale (deep chest breathing). However you practice slow breathing, make sure it's rhythmic, calming, and relaxing.

# LIGHT BREATHING

Light breathing helps you manage labor pain when you can no longer relax during contractions, when the contractions are too painful with slow breathing, or when you instinctively speed up your breathing. In active labor, let your responses to contractions help you decide when to begin using light breathing. Your partner may suggest switching to light breathing if you're losing your rhythm, tensing, grimacing, clenching your fists, or crying out at the peak of a contraction.

## *Using Light Breathing in Labor*

1.  As soon as you feel a contraction begin, take a quick, shallow inhalation and signal to your partner that the contraction has begun. Exhale quickly to release all tension—go completely limp.
2.  Focus your attention (see pages 226–227).
3.  Take short, light, and shallow breaths, inhaling and exhaling through your mouth—one breath every second or two (about five to ten breaths in ten seconds). Keep your inhalations quiet and exhale audibly by releasing short "puffs" of air or by making light sounds. Continue light breathing in a steady rhythm, pausing after each exhalation (but not pausing at the end of each inhalation, as you do with slow breathing). Let the contraction guide the rate and depth of your breathing. Keep your mouth and shoulders relaxed. Continue breathing in this way until the contraction ends.
4.  When the contraction ends, use your last exhalation to "sigh" the contraction away. Then signal your partner that the contraction is over.
5.  Completely relax and do whatever you need to feel comfortable, such as change positions, sip liquids, and so on.

## *Rehearsing Light Breathing for Labor*

When you first begin to practice light breathing, you may feel that the technique isn't right for you. It may make you tense or feel as though you're not getting enough air. In our experience, however, expectant parents who practice and master light breathing *before* labor typically don't hyperventilate *during* labor and can adapt their breathing to meet the demands of the contraction.

Keep in mind that light breathing will come more naturally as your labor becomes more intense. Just as running makes you breathe faster to meet your oxygen needs, the rising intensity and frequency of contractions will increase your need for oxygen, which will naturally guide your breathing rate during labor.

Begin practicing light breathing by taking one breath every second or two. Continue at this rate for thirty seconds to two minutes. When you can do light breathing effortlessly for two minutes, try the adaptations described in the following sections.

## *Note:*

-   If you become lightheaded or dizzy while rehearsing, try to focus on your exhalations, perhaps by making small sounds while exhaling, such as "hee-hee-hee" or "puh-puh-puh." Keep your inhalations silent. By doing so, your body will naturally inhale as much air as it needs.
-   Breathing lightly through an open mouth may cause dryness. To help moisten the air that you breathe, try touching the tip of your tongue to the roof of your mouth a bit behind your teeth, or hold a moist washcloth near your mouth. During labor, you may also try sipping water or other fluids between contractions, or sucking on ice or a frozen fruit juice bar. Brushing your teeth or rinsing your mouth occasionally may also help relieve a dry mouth.
-   It takes a little practice to become comfortable with light breathing, but many women say it was very helpful during labor.

# Adaptations of the Breathing Techniques

The following are ways to adapt rhythmic breathing by combining slow and light breathing patterns. During labor, try switching to one of these techniques to help you cope if you become overwhelmed or exhausted, can't relax, or begin to despair. You may even discover a spontaneous rhythmic pattern of your own in labor.

## Vocal Breathing

This technique combines slow or light breathing with vocalization. As you exhale with each rhythmic breath, you moan, sigh, count, sing, or recite poems, affirming phrases, chants, or other words. For example, one woman found that repeating, "One, two, three, *Max!*" (her baby's name) let her maintain a rhythm and keep a sense of control during contractions. Another woman chanted, "Epidural, epidural" during contractions because she felt that as long as she could say the word, she didn't need the epidural.

Making low-pitched rhythmic sounds such as moaning is an effective technique for maintaining a sense of control while releasing tension. High-pitched, nonrhythmic sounds *could* indicate fear and stress. However, if your sounds are rhythmic—whether high- or low-pitched—and you find them helpful, you're coping well. If you're feeling scared or frantic, your support team can help you lower the pitch by moaning with you and help you keep your rhythm with the Take Charge Routine (see page 186). If your vocalizations are loud, your support team should keep the doors to your room closed so you can continue "shouting down the pain" (as one woman called it) without worrying about disturbing others.

## Contraction-Tailored Breathing

For this technique, use the intensity of the contraction to guide the rate and depth of your breathing. Breathe slowly when each contraction begins. As the contraction intensifies, quicken and lighten your breathing past the peak. As the contraction subsides, gradually slow and deepen your breathing. Think of each exhalation as a way to relax completely.

If your contractions peak quickly, this technique won't help you cope. Instead, use light breathing throughout each contraction.

## Slide Breathing

Some women, especially those with a respiratory condition such as asthma, find that the quicker pace of light breathing makes them uncomfortable and tense, regardless of how often they practice. If you can't master light breathing after several attempts (see page 244), slide breathing is a good alternative. To do this technique, inhale deeply and slowly, then exhale with three or four light puffs of air. Pause, then repeat this process. To help guide your breathing, say "in" to yourself as you inhale, drawing out the word to match the length of your inhalation, then say "out" with each puff of air you exhale. Although the deep inhalations make slide breathing similar to slow breathing, the change in rhythm provides a different focus.

## Variable Breathing

Because variable breathing combines light, shallow breathing with a longer or more pronounced exhalation, it's sometimes called "pant-pant-BLOW" or "hee-hee-HOO" breathing. Variable breathing is an option for women who still feel uncomfortable or short of breath with light breathing even after practice. It's also helpful for women who prefer structured breathing patterns.

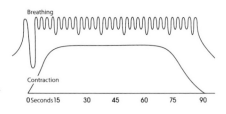

With variable breathing, use light breathing for two to four breaths, then take another light inhalation followed by a long, slow, emphasized exhalation (the "blow"). This last exhalation helps you steady your rhythm and release tension. Some women emphasize it by making a drawn-out "hoo" or "puh" sound.

Find a comfortable pattern and then repeat it throughout the contraction. To help keep your rhythm, your partner can count your breaths: "One, two, three, BLOW!" Or you can count your breaths to yourself as a way to focus your attention.

## Rehearsing Breathing Adaptations for Labor

When practicing breathing techniques, include your favorite adaptations and practice them in various positions. Relax for only thirty seconds or so between practice contractions to prepare for the brief rest you'll experience between contractions during late labor, when contractions may last two minutes or they may occur in pairs with little break between the first and second contractions (coupling). Be prepared to use light breathing or its adaptations for up to three minutes.

# BREATHING TECHNIQUES FOR A PREMATURE URGE TO PUSH

During labor, you may have an early urge to push at the peak of a contraction. This urge is considered premature if it occurs before your cervix is completely dilated. Whenever you have an urge to push, alert your nurse or caregiver so dilation can be confirmed by observing your behavior or by vaginal exam. If dilation isn't complete, you'll probably be asked not to push to prevent the cervix from swelling and slowing progress. (Some caregivers tell clients to push gently, just enough to satisfy the strong urge.)

To avoid pushing, lift your chin and either pant or blow lightly until the urge subsides. You may find it helpful to say "puh, puh, puh" or "hoo, hoo, hoo" with each exhalation. When the urge to push passes, resume rhythmic breathing. Also, changing positions can help reduce the premature urge to push (Try hands-and-knees, side-lying, and open knee-chest positions. See page 247.)

Being asked to stop pushing can be upsetting when the urge to push is strong and seems uncontrollable. As one woman cried out, "I'm not pushing, but my body is. I'm trying but can't stop it!" These breathing techniques won't take away your body's urge to push. Instead, they'll help you keep from holding your breath and bearing down with the urge, which could increase swelling.

*Note:* The other time during labor when you might be asked to stop pushing is when your baby's head is crowning. See page 193.

## Rehearsing Breathing Techniques to Avoid Pushing

When rehearsing breathing techniques, occasionally practice a premature urge to push. Hold your breath or grunt as you breathe to signal to your partner that you have an urge to push. Your partner can remind you how to resist the urge until it passes. Rehearsing this technique can be silly and fun, but it's also good preparation.

# Comfort Techniques for Back Pain, Slow Labor, or an Extra-challenging Labor

Certain circumstances may make it challenging to cope. You may experience back labor and feel contractions more in your back than in your uterus. Your contractions may begin to couple (occur in pairs with little break between the first and second contractions) or become irregular. Your may have a prolonged labor and feel discouraged and fatigued. Your baby's position in your pelvis may cause back pain and may slow labor progress (see page 286). On the Road Map of Labor (see page 444), this kind of labor is depicted as the rough, rocky detour.

The following sections describe measures that can help you cope with an extra-challenging labor.

## POSITIONS AND MOVEMENT

To reduce back pain or help speed up a slow labor, use positions and movements to ease back pain and to encourage your baby to change to a position that's a better fit in your pelvis.

### Open Knee-Chest Position

Get onto your hands and knees, then lower your head and chest to the floor or bed. Move your knees back enough so your hips are high in the air. Try to remain in this position for thirty minutes—very difficult to do without help. Your partner can help support you as shown. This position is best used during prelabor or very early labor to help eliminate back pain and possibly reposition an OP baby.

### Leaning Forward

Positions that allow you to lean forward may help your baby find a better-fitting position and keep him there. Examples include leaning over a birth ball, the labor bed, or a counter (while kneeling, standing, or sitting). The hands-and-knees position is also effective. These positions also relieve back pain by easing the pressure of your baby's head against your sacrum.

### Pelvic Tilts on Hands and Knees

While kneeling and leaning forward over a birth ball or a chair seat, rock your pelvis forward and back or move your hips in a circle (also see page 92). The motion helps change your baby's position in relation to your pelvis, and the position encourages her to rotate to a favorable OA position.

### Abdominal Lift

While standing, interlace your fingers and place your hands palms up, beneath your belly and against your pubic bone. During contractions, bend your knees (to tilt your pelvis slightly) and use your hands to lift your abdomen up and slightly in. This movement often relieves back pain while improving the position of your baby.

Because the abdominal lift can be hard work for you, your partner can do it using a woven shawl or rebozo. Fold the shawl so it's about 5 inches wide, then position it around your waist and below your belly (the same place that you'd put your hands). Have your partner stand behind you and cross the ends of the shawl behind your back. During the contraction, your partner will pull on each end of the shawl to lift your belly. Adjust both the shawl and the strength of your partner's pulling so the lift feels good.

*Caution:* If your baby wiggles a lot during the abdominal lift, he may be experiencing uncomfortable pressure. Discontinue the lift and use another comfort technique.

## Standing, Walking, Slow Dancing, and Stair Climbing

These movements take advantage of gravity and help align your baby with the upper part of your pelvis (pelvic inlet) and encourage her descent into the birth canal. Moving also allows your pelvis to change shape slightly, which encourages your baby to rotate.

## Asymmetrical Positions: Lunge, Side-Lying, and Semiprone

The lunge, side-lying, and semiprone are *asymmetrical* because one side of your body is doing something different from the other side. Try them on both sides. If you're more comfortable on one side than on the other, use that side. If you have no clear preference, alternate sides.

### Lunge

The lunge is usually done during contractions. Find a sturdy chair that won't move when you lean against it. Stand in front of the chair, facing to the side. Lift the foot that's closest to the chair and set it on the seat, with your toes pointing toward the back of the chair (so they're at a 90 degree angle from the direction your body is facing). Remaining upright, slowly and rhythmically lunge sideways toward the chair (by further flexing your knee) and return to the starting position. You should feel a stretch in your inner thighs. Lunge sideways and back throughout the contraction, then rest. Repeat for five to seven contractions.

### Side-lying

Lie on your side with your hips flexed and your knees bent. Place a pillow between your knees. Try switching sides about every thirty minutes whenever you're awake, as long as your baby's heart rate is normal.

### Semiprone

Lie on your side with your lower arm behind you and your lower leg out straight. Flex the hip of your upper leg and bend the knee, resting it on a doubled-up pillow. Roll slightly toward your front. Alternate this position with side-lying when you must remain in bed.

## A NOTE TO FATHERS AND PARTNERS ABOUT RELIEVING BACK PAIN

The following measures can help reduce the laboring woman's back pain and make her more comfortable. If any measure causes her more pain or doesn't help, stop and try another comfort measure.

## Counterpressure

Throughout each contraction, use your fist or the heel of your hand to steadily press on the woman's lower back. Hold the front of one of her hips with one hand (to help keep her balance) and press steadily and firmly in one spot on her lower back 4 to 6 inches below her waist, slightly away from her spine. The exact spot will vary over the course of the labor; she'll let you know where to press to give her the best relief. Use as much pressure as she wants. Between contractions, rest or massage the area you pressed.

## Double Hip Squeeze

Have the laboring woman kneel and lean forward on a birth ball or chair, or get on her hands and knees. During a contraction, stand close behind her, then press on the roundest part of each buttock with your palms. To relieve pelvic pressure and ease back pain, apply steady pressure (instead of pressing and releasing repeatedly) as you try to press her hips together. Try other places on her hips to press and apply as much pressure as she needs.

If another person is available to help, the two-person double hip squeeze is easier to do. Instead of standing behind the laboring woman, you and the other support person stand on opposite sides of her, facing each other. You each place one hand on the roundest part of the closer buttock, then together press on her buttocks. Be sure to coordinate timing and amount of pressure. Ask your partner if the pressure feels even, and adjust accordingly.

## Knee Press

Have the laboring woman sit upright in a chair that won't slide when you press your weight against it. If necessary, elevate her feet so her thighs are parallel to the floor. Kneel in front of her and cup a hand over each knee. Lean toward her so your hands press straight back toward her hip joints. Keep the pressure steady throughout the contraction.

# OTHER COMFORT MEASURES TO REDUCE BACK PAIN

Heat and cold (see page 229) are excellent comfort measures to relieve back pain, as are baths and showers (see page 227). The following sections describe additional measures that you may want to try.

## Rolling Pressure

Have your partner move a rolling pin over your lower back. This is a soothing way to relieve back pain and muscle tension during and between contractions. You may find additional relief if your partner uses a can of frozen juice, a cold can of soda, or a hollow rolling pin filled with ice, because the cold helps numb the area. If the rolling object is cold, make sure there's a layer of cloth on your back so the object isn't in direct contact with your skin.

## Transcutaneous Electrical Nerve Stimulation (TENS)

TENS relieves back pain during contractions by creating tingling, buzzing, or prickly sensations on your skin. According to the Gate Control Theory of Pain (see page 204), TENS reduces your awareness of pain by increasing your awareness of other distracting sensations. TENS is a type of counter-irritant that takes the focus off labor pain (see page 229). Another theory to explain the effectiveness of TENS is that it gradually increases endorphin production in the area where it's applied. Endorphins are your body's natural pain relievers that block transmission of pain signals. If TENS begins in early labor, the level of endorphins in the lower back will increase by the time labor intensifies. Many women find TENS helpful for relieving back pain, but some don't.

TENS devices are simple to use. Four stimulating pads are placed on the back and then connected to a small handheld battery-operated generator that produces tingling, buzzing, or prickly sensations. Models vary but all have controls to regulate the intensity of the sensation and to switch the pattern of the stimulation between a continuous mode to use during contractions, and an intermittent burst mode for between contractions.

Either you or your partner can hold and control the device. Between contractions, set the intensity to the level that feels comfortable and set the stimulation to burst mode. When the contraction begins, change the stimulation to continuous mode. When the contraction ends, switch it back to burst mode. As your back pain increases, increase the intensity.

Specially designed maternity TENS devices are widely available in Canada and the United Kingdom, but are hard to find in stores in the United States. You may be able to learn more about TENS from a physical therapist who uses it to treat numerous pain conditions. If you plan to hire a birth doula (see page 20), she may be trained to use TENS and have a device to loan you. Or you can purchase a maternity TENS device online. Use the term "maternity TENS" to search for retailers and to find videos and other information.

Although there are no known harmful side effects of TENS, be sure to check with your caregiver before using it.

# Comfort Techniques for the Second Stage of Labor (Pushing)

Many of the comfort techniques used during the first stage of labor are also helpful during the second stage. Here are some ideas specific for helping you find comfort when pushing out your baby. Each pushing technique includes an illustration. The line at the bottom shows a uterine contraction, as seen on a monitor when a mother is pushing. You'll see how the intensity peaks as she is actively pushing, and drops when she stops pushing to take a quick breath. The top line shows the pattern of inhalations and exhalations. In the spontaneous pushing diagram, she's taking small breaths while she pushes. In the directed pushing diagram, she's holding her breath while pushing.

## WORKING WITH THE URGE TO PUSH IN LABOR

Around the time your cervix becomes completely dilated, your breathing rhythm will change and you'll feel pressure on your pelvic floor as your baby moves deep into your pelvis. These developments will cause you to have an irresistible urge to push. At first, you may mistake this urge for the need to have a bowel movement (see page 188).

*Note:* If you have an epidural, you'll feel the urge to push much less clearly or you might not feel it at all. See pages 251–252 and page 189 for more information on directed or delayed pushing with an epidural.

## SPONTANEOUS BEARING DOWN

Your responses to contractions during the second stage will depend on the sensations you feel. You'll probably feel several strong surges (irresistible and involuntary urges to push) during each contraction. Each surge will last five to seven seconds. During a surge, you'll use *expulsion breathing*. Simply breathe using whatever technique suits you, until you have an urge to push and your body begins bearing down (a spontaneous reaction to the urge). Bear down for as long as you feel the urge. Then breathe lightly until either you feel another urge or the contraction ends. Expect to bear down three to five times per contraction, with each effort lasting about five to seven seconds. Between contractions, rest and relax.

How hard you bear down in response to an urge is similar to how hard you sneeze in response to an irritant in your nose. Both sneezing and spontaneous bearing down are involuntary reflexes. Sometimes you need one tiny sneeze to clear an irritant; other times, you need several explosive sneezes. Sometimes you need to gently bear down; other times, you'll feel compelled to push with all your strength.

Spontaneous bearing down is recommended if labor is progressing normally and you haven't had an epidural. If you have an epidural, you'll use delayed pushing (see page 189) or directed pushing (see page 251). Epidurals diminish the pushing sensations and the effectiveness of your ability to spontaneously bear down.

## Using Spontaneous Bearing Down in Labor

Here are steps that explain how to use spontaneous bearing down in labor.

1. As the contraction begins, start slow or light breathing (see pages 243 and 244).

2. Focus on a positive image, such as your baby moving down and out of your uterus.

3. Breathe rhythmically as the contraction intensifies. When you can no longer resist the urge to push, bear down or strain while holding your breath or while slowly releasing air by grunting or vocalizing, whichever feels best. *Relax your pelvic floor* (see page 91)! Your partner may need to remind you to relax your perineum.

4.  Exhale when the urge passes (usually after five to seven seconds) and breathe rhythmically for several seconds until you feel another urge to push. Then, bear down again. The urge to push will come in waves during the contraction, giving you time to "breathe for your baby" (that is, to oxygenate your blood to provide enough oxygen for your baby between urges).

5.  When the contraction ends, slowly lie or sit back (or stand up if squatting) and take one or two relaxing breaths.

## *Rehearsing Spontaneous Bearing Down for Labor*

When practicing comfort techniques for the second stage of labor, bear down just enough to feel your pelvic floor bulge (see page 91). Don't bear down forcefully. To practice more effectively, use different positions and imagine what will be happening when you're pushing in labor. Visualize your baby descending and rotating into your birth canal. Remind yourself that contractions are proof that your baby is working to be born, and it's important to relax and bulge your pelvic floor.

# DIRECTED PUSHING

Unlike with spontaneous bearing down, when you push in response to an urge, directed pushing is bearing down when someone tells you to do so. You'll use this type of pushing in the following circumstances:

•   You've had an epidural and don't feel contractions.

•   You don't have an urge to push, or you're not pushing effectively when spontaneously bearing down, even after trying gravity-enhancing positions, such as squatting, sitting, dangling, lap squatting, or standing upright (see pages 238–240).

•   Directed pushing is routine for your hospital or for your caregiver.

Directed pushing is typically more forceful than spontaneous bearing down, which means it may be more stressful for both you and your baby. For this reason, many caregivers reserve this type of pushing for births that may require forceps delivery or vacuum extraction. Before the birth, check whether directed pushing is routine for your caregiver or birthplace. If it is, find out when and under what circumstances it's used.

## *Using Directed Pushing in Labor*

Here are the steps that explain how to use directed pushing in labor. Your caregiver, nurse, or partner will tell you when, how long, and how hard to push. You can use various positions to do directed pushing.

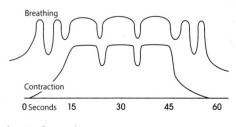

•   At the beginning of a contraction, take two or three breaths. When you're told to push, inhale and hold your breath. Curl forward, tucking your chin on your chest, and bear down, tightening your abdominal muscles.

•   Relax your pelvic floor muscles. Bear down for five to seven seconds. Quickly exhale as directed, then take another few breaths.

•   Repeat steps 1 and 2 until the contraction subsides.

•   When the contraction ends, slowly lie or sit back (or stand up if squatting), rest, and breathe normally.

*Note:* Directed pushing will continue for each contraction until your baby's head is almost out. At that point, your caregiver may tell you to stop pushing to allow your baby's head to pass slowly through your vaginal opening. Relax and stop pushing, using the techniques described on page 246. To decrease your risk of developing a vaginal tear, breathe lightly and quickly to keep from bearing down.

## *Rehearsing Directed Pushing for Labor*

With directed pushing, you'll be told when and how hard to push, so you need to practice this technique only enough to coordinate holding your breath with bearing down gently and bulging your pelvis (see page 91), as your partner coaches you through the contractions as described above. You may find it helpful to occasionally hold your breath and bulge your perineum during perineal massage (see below).

## PROLONGED DIRECTED PUSHING

In labor, prolonged directed pushing requires you to hold your breath and push hard for ten seconds, take a quick breath, and do it again throughout the contraction. Babies don't tolerate prolonged bearing down as well as they do shorter efforts with longer breaks in between for you to catch your breath. Caregivers generally don't recommend the technique, but sometimes circumstances (such as weaker contractions or a malpositioned baby) may require it as a way to possibly avoid forceps delivery or vacuum extraction (see page 292). Because you'd use prolonged directed pushing only under your caregiver's guidance, there's no need to practice it before labor.

## POSITIONS FOR THE SECOND STAGE OF LABOR

Just as moving around and changing positions can help with labor progress and pain relief during the first stage of labor, these comfort measures can help you during the second stage. Until you're in labor and ready to push your baby out, you won't know which positions will feel right. Try to practice spontaneous bearing down (see page 250) in all the positions shown on pages 238–240 so you're prepared to effectively bear down while in any of them.

If your baby descends rapidly, you might not have the time or desire to change positions; however, if your second stage progresses slowly, you'll have a chance to try many positions.

Other factors may influence the positions you can try during the second stage, such as your caregiver's preferences or your willingness and freedom to change positions. Some procedures and equipment may impair your mobility, including electronic fetal monitors, catheters, anesthetics, IV equipment, and narrow beds. But with help and encouragement, you can safely work around these obstacles.

Discuss birthing positions when preparing your birth plan (see chapter 8). Although some caregivers are comfortable with any birthing position a woman chooses to use,[13] most are confident only with the supine (woman lying on her back) or semi-sitting position for delivery. To help with labor progress until your baby is close to being born, discuss a plan to use various positions that enlarge the pelvic outlet and make room for your baby.

## PERINEAL MASSAGE

Prenatal *perineal massage* stretches the inner tissue of your lower vagina. It teaches you to respond to pressure in your vagina by relaxing your pelvic floor muscles. In this way, it's a rehearsal for responding to the sensations of vaginal stretching during birth.

Perineal massage is also thought to enhance the hormonal changes that soften connective tissue during late pregnancy, which can reduce your chances of needing an episiotomy or developing a serious tear during birth.[14] Massaging your perineum a few times each week during the last five to six weeks of pregnancy may help you avoid an episiotomy or serious tear.

Some caregivers aren't familiar with the benefits of perineal massage and don't recommend it. Even if their caregivers recommend perineal massage, some women find it distasteful and don't want to do it. Others, however, feel the massage is worthwhile if it can reduce the chances of an episiotomy or a serious tear. Some even find it enjoyable, especially after they've learned to relax while it's done.

*Note:* If you have vaginitis, a genital herpes sore, or another vaginal problem, perineal massage may worsen the condition. Wait until the problem is completely gone before beginning perineal massage.

## How to Do Perineal Massage

You or your partner can do this massage with clean hands and short fingernails. If either of you has rough skin, consider using disposable vinyl or latex gloves. If doing the massage yourself, you may want to use a mirror at first to help you see your perineum.

1. Get into a semi-sitting position (if your partner is doing the massage—see page 239 for a description of the position) or stand with one foot on the side of the tub or a chair (if doing the massage yourself).

2. Use a squeeze bottle to squirt vegetable oil on your thumb or partner's index finger(s). (Dipping your fingers into the oil can contaminate it.) Wheat germ oil has a high vitamin E content, which may be soothing on your skin. You can also use another vegetable oil or a water-based lubricant such as K-Y Jelly. Don't use baby oil, mineral oil, petroleum jelly, or hand lotion—many women who used these products reported that their skin didn't tolerate them well.

3. Place your thumb well inside your vagina, or have your partner place an index finger (one at first, then both as you become comfortable), well inside your vagina (up to the second knuckle). Do a few Kegel exercises (see page 90) so you can feel your pelvic floor muscles tense. Relax the muscles. Curl your thumb (or the finger, if your partner is doing it), and gently pull it outward and downward toward your anus, then rhythmically move it within your vagina in a U motion. Focus on relaxing your pelvic floor muscles. If the pressure is too great and you can't relax, reduce the pressure. Do this massage for about three minutes. At first, your vaginal wall will feel tight. After a few days of practice, you'll find that you can tolerate the sensation and can increase the stretching.

4. Concentrate on relaxing your muscles as you feel the pressure and stretching. As you become comfortable with the massage, increase the pressure just enough to make the tissue begin to sting or burn slightly. (The same sensation will occur as your baby's head is being born.)

5. Know that this massage isn't meant to be painful. If it is, reduce the pressure and stretching until you can relax during the massage. If you have questions after trying the massage, ask your caregiver, childbirth educator, or someone who's familiar with this technique for advice.

# Practice Time as a Rehearsal for Labor

When taking the time to practice these comfort techniques with your partner, try to think of it as a rehearsal for labor. Discuss when you may use the techniques and why. Review what you've learned about the emotional and physical events of labor (see appendix B). Most importantly, learn how to work together to use the techniques effectively and adapt them to fit your needs.

## AMOUNT OF PRACTICE TIME

You don't have to practice every day to master comfort techniques, especially if you and your partner attend childbirth classes together. Practice enough so you're completely comfortable with each technique and have time to figure out any adaptations you may want to use. Then, review them periodically so they become familiar and easy.

## SUGGESTED PRACTICE SEQUENCE

The following sequence will help you master the techniques discussed in this and other chapters. (Visit our website, http://www.PCNGuide.com, for an additional practice guide.) You may choose to take a few months to complete the sequence, or you may decide to begin closer to your due date and finish it in a few weeks. Either way, practicing these exercises, breathing rhythms, and relaxation techniques will increase your confidence in your ability to handle labor and birth.

1. Conditioning exercises (see pages 89): continue practicing these exercises until the birth
2. Comfort measures for discomforts (see page 98): use as needed
3. Body awareness exercises (see page 233)
4. Passive relaxation (see page 235)
5. Relaxation countdown (see page 236): at first, use several breaths to relax, then work toward relaxing with one breath
6. Perineal massage (see page 253): during the last five to six weeks of pregnancy, do five to six times a week
7. Slow breathing (see page 243)
8. Touch relaxation (see page 236)
9. Roving body check (see page 237): practice this exercise by yourself and with your partner's direction
10. Slow breathing with roving body check (see pages 243 and 237)

11. Attention focusing (see page 226)
12. Crisscross back massage (see page 231)
13. Possible positions for the first stage of labor (see pages 238–239): practice slow breathing in each position
14. Light breathing (see page 244): experiment with the depth and rate of your breathing to find what works for you
15. Adaptations of slow and light breathing—contraction-tailored, vocal, slide, and variable breathing (see pages 245–246)
16. Variety of positions for the first stage of labor (see pages 238–239) while practicing breathing adaptations
17. Ways to decrease back pain in labor (see pages 247–249): practice the double hip squeeze, counterpressure, abdominal lift, open knee-chest position, knee press, and lunge; combine these techniques with breathing patterns
18. Ways to avoid pushing (see page 246)
19. Spontaneous bearing down and directed pushing (see pages 250–252): practice gently bearing down and incorporate the bulging exercise (see page 91); occasionally, practice panting to avoid pushing in the middle of a practice contraction
20. Positions for the second stage of labor (see pages 239–240): try the positions while practicing spontaneous bearing down (expulsion breathing)
21. Labor rehearsal: practice all the coping techniques during a series of pretend contractions; your partner can help by observing you and helping you fully relax in all positions.

## *Key Points to Remember*

- Women respond to labor differently, but those who cope well use the Three Rs in some way: they relax during or between contractions; they move, breathe, and vocalize in rhythm; and they have a ritual during which they repeat the same rhythmic activities through many contractions.
- Figure out which comfort techniques may be most effective in labor by practicing them with your partner during pregnancy. Have pretend contractions while practicing techniques to make each practice session a rehearsal for labor.
- Mastering several comfort techniques and adapting them to suit your needs will increase your confidence and ability to cope with labor pain.
- When you're in labor, be prepared to discover and use unplanned coping techniques and rituals.

# CHAPTER 13

# Medications for Pain Relief during Labor

Many expectant parents plan to use pain medications in labor. Some begin labor uncertain of their pain medication preferences (see page 214). Still others hope to avoid pain medications, but decide to use them during labor.

The goal of using medications is to relieve pain without compromising labor progress or the well-being of the baby. Some medications can also allow the laboring parent to think clearly. For many families, these benefits lead to a positive and satisfying labor. Medications, however, make labor a much more medicalized experience, with more routine interventions and a risk of side effects to the drugs. For some families, these tradeoffs lead to a less satisfying labor.

The effects of pain medications on a mother and baby are influenced by the drugs used, how much is given, how they're administered, the mother's response to them, and the baby's condition during labor. This chapter discusses the options for medications, their benefits and risks, and how best to support labor progress when using them.

# Weighing the Risks and Benefits of Pain Medications

The benefits of pain medications include an increased ability to relax and sleep, and the reduction or elimination of pain. If pain medications are used judiciously and with current methods, the side effects are often mild, manageable, and familiar to hospital staff.

However, as with all interventions, pain medications have potential risks. Examples include itching, nausea, prolonged labor, fever in the mother and baby, and variations in fetal heart rate. While these risks are typically moderate, they may require additional interventions that have their own potential side effects. If you use pain medications in labor, your caregiver will be aware of all potential risks and take measures to either prevent or manage them. (Visit our website, http://www.PCNGuide.com, for more information.)

As you consider the risks and benefits of laboring with pain medications, keep the following factors in mind:

• While medications can minimize pain or even eliminate it for some portion of your labor, they generally can't prevent you from feeling *any* pain throughout your entire labor.

• Any medication you receive affects your baby. Because his liver and kidneys are immature, the effects of some drugs last longer for him than for you. A medication's effects depend on the drug, the amount received, how and when it's given, and other factors.

• Pain medications affect your labor progress. On one hand, they often slow contractions and may increase your need for other medical interventions. On the other hand, if labor progress is abnormally slow, drugs may speed up progress by letting you relax.

• Special precautions are required with pain medications to prevent, minimize, or treat side effects. For example, the following interventions are necessary more often when pain medications are used: restriction to bed, restriction of eating and drinking, IV fluids, Pitocin augmentation, administration of oxygen, frequent monitoring of blood pressure and blood oxygen levels, bladder catheterization, and continuous electronic fetal monitoring (EFM).

• Several factors influence which medication is right for you, including the nature of your pain, stage of labor, allergies or medical conditions, other medications you use regularly, unusual anatomical conditions of your spine or lower back, and availability of anesthesia services at your birthplace. Tell your caregiver if you've ever had an allergy or reaction to medication.

# Key Vocabulary of Pain Medications

Each drug has specific characteristics that make it safe and effective for pain relief in particular phases of labor. The following describe key terms for medications that can relieve labor pain:

## ROUTE OF ADMINISTRATION

How you receive a medication is its route of administration. *Oral medication* is a pill or liquid you swallow; *inhalation medication* is a gas you breathe. *Intramuscular (IM) medication* is a shot given into muscle, while *intravenous (IV) medication* is an injection into a vein, often through an IV catheter (see page 180). Lastly, *neuraxial medications* are drugs that are injected into the space surrounding the spinal cord (neuraxis), such as epidurals and spinals. How quickly a medication takes effect depends on the route of administration.

## AREA OF EFFECT

Medications may be *systemic* (affecting your entire body), *regional* (affecting a large area of your body), or *local* (affecting a specific, relatively small part of your body). In general, you need more medication to get the desired results with a systemic medication than with a regional or local medication.

## TYPE OF EFFECT

*Analgesia* is any effect that reduces your perception of pain. In this chapter, this term refers specifically to medications that act on the brain so you don't interpret stimuli as pain. *Anesthesia* indicates a loss of sensation, including pain sensation. Anesthetics block nerve endings from sending pain impulses to your brain.

## Questions to Ask Your Caregiver about Pain Medications

During a prenatal visit, ask these questions about pain medications:

- What medications are most commonly used for pain relief? How is each medication given?
- How does each medication relieve pain? How effective is it?
- What are the potential risks or undesirable side effects of the drug on me, my baby, or labor progress? What precautions do you take to prevent, control, or treat side effects?
- What are my alternatives to pain medications?

Be aware that the answers you receive may vary depending on whom you ask. For example, an anesthesiologist, who is trained in the best pharmaceutical solutions to relieving pain, will likely believe that the side effects of pain medications are manageable and their benefits outweigh any potential risks. A home birth midwife who's familiar with non-drug coping techniques may recommend using them first because they're low-cost, low-risk, and can be done anywhere.

Supplement the information you learn from your caregiver with additional research-based sources of information (such as this book and our website, http://www.PCNGuide.com) to help you make an informed decision about pain medications.

# Systemic Medications

Systemic medications come in many forms, including pills, injections, and gases. All are absorbed into your bloodstream and affect your entire body. The desired effect is to reduce your pain, but there may be side effects.

Systemic medications may affect your baby as well, because the placenta can't screen them out. The extent of the effects depends on the type and amount of medication used, the time between the last dose and the birth, and your baby's health. If a healthy, full-term baby and a premature, ill, or distressed baby were each exposed to the same amount of medication during labor, the healthy baby would show fewer side effects.

The medication or its byproducts might not disappear from your baby's bloodstream for hours or days, and neurobehavioral changes may be present during the first few days after birth. These changes may be obvious, or they may be noticeable only to professionals who use highly sensitive tests to examine your baby.

*General anesthesia* is a systemic medication that causes a total loss of sensation and consciousness. It's used for only a small percentage of cesarean births. (Visit our website to learn more about this and other systemic medications, such as sedatives, tranquilizers, and nitrous oxide.) Intravenous (IV) narcotics are the systemic medications used most commonly in labor.

# IV or IM Narcotics or Narcotic-Like Medications[1]

*Narcotics and narcotic-like drugs* (such as morphine, fentanyl, or Stadol) reduce the transmission of pain messages to the pain receptors in your brain.

## Benefits

The *analgesic* effect is often described as "taking the edge off the pain." It may take you longer to notice that a contraction has started, and it may seem to fade away sooner. The peak of a contraction, however, may still be intense enough that you feel the pain despite the narcotics.

Narcotics may work well for you if you're handling the pain at the peak of a contraction but want to feel as if you have a longer break between contractions so you can rest. You may even be able to doze between contractions and wake up to manage the peak.

*Note:* Narcotics might not work well for you if you *can't* handle the pain at the peak of a contraction, or if you can handle the pain only when you can feel the start of the contraction and can begin using a coping ritual before the peak occurs. If you do use narcotics and doze between contractions, your partner or doula can help you prepare for the pain by noting the start of the contraction (as indicated by a monitor or by your wincing or moaning), awakening or alerting you, and guiding you to use rhythmic breathing (see page 241) before the peak.

## Tradeoffs

IV fluids, continuous electronic fetal monitoring (EFM), and restriction to bed may be necessary when narcotics are used. Narcotics may cause sleepiness or lethargy, and they may cause a hazy feeling, disorientation, or euphoria. Some people find the sensation relaxing or pleasant, while others feel mentally out of control, which may make it difficult to use self-help techniques.

## Possible side effects

Common side effects include itching, nausea, vomiting, and lowered blood pressure. Narcotics may slow labor and cause variations in your baby's heart rate. You can receive a drug called a narcotic antagonist to reduce these side effects, but it'll reduce pain relief. After the birth, the narcotics in your baby's bloodstream may cause her to breathe slowly and have poor muscle tone. She can receive a narcotic antagonist if needed. Visit our website, http://www.PCNGuide.com, for more information on possible side effects.

## Timing

The effects of narcotics last for sixty to ninety minutes. Narcotics are used in early to active labor, when it's believed that the birth is at least two hours away. This timing allows the narcotic effects on your baby to fade before the birth.

## Comparing options[2]

Compared to regional analgesia (such as an epidural), IV and IM narcotics provide less effective pain relief for a shorter time. They may also cause more side effects in general, because more medication is given. (Epidurals, however, may have a higher risk of forceps delivery or vacuum extraction.)

## Two Views on Narcotics

Initially, fentanyl made me feel drunk. I was a little dizzy, and I don't think I was mentally all there. The contractions were still very painful, but more manageable, especially in the hot tub. About an hour later, my cervix was dilated to 6 centimeters, and I got another dose of fentanyl. The pain continued getting stronger, and I got a third dose, which unfortunately wasn't effective at all.
—Sami

Within two hours of being admitted, I asked for drugs because the pain was making me very anxious. The Nubain helped me relax and focus on my breathing for the next wave of contractions. I completely lost track of time as I found myself instinctively using rhythm to cope. My cervix was checked ninety minutes later, and it had dilated to 7 centimeters. I was assured that an epidural was still an option, and the anesthesiologist was called.
—Jennifer

# Local and Regional Anesthetics

Local or regional anesthetics (often called "blocks") cause reduced feeling or numbness in a particular area of your body. When an anesthetic drug is injected near specific nerves, it blocks the transmission of sensations along them. It also affects muscle control, blood flow, and temperature in the affected area to a degree. Lower doses of an anesthetic eliminate or dull pain while allowing some muscle control. Higher doses remove both sensation and the ability to use your muscles. Local and regional anesthetics don't affect your mental state. Most anesthetic drug names end with the suffix "-caine," such as lidocaine and bupivacaine.

## LOCAL ANESTHETICS (PERINEAL BLOCK)

Local anesthetics block sensation in a small area near nerve endings. They're injected into the skin, mucous membranes, or muscles. During the pushing stage, they're typically injected in the perineum (perineal block). They can be injected in the cervix (paracervical block) or the vagina (pudendal block), but these blocks are rarely used.

### Benefits

Perineal blocks numb the perineum for an episiotomy or forceps delivery (see page 292) or for stitches after an episiotomy or laceration.

### Tradeoff

The injections may be painful.

epidural
and spinal
blocks

local block

### Possible side effects

If a perineal block is given during the repair of an episiotomy or lacerations, the side effects are minimal (barring an allergic reaction). If it's given early in the second stage (which is rare), the medication could affect the baby's heart rate during labor or his reflexes at birth.

### Timing

Local anesthetics are given during the late second stage or in the third stage

# Regional (Neuraxial) Analgesia: Epidurals and Spinals[3]

*Neuraxial medications* are injected in your lower back near nerve roots in the spinal column. The medications affect the region of your body to which these nerves and their branches go. The region can be as small as your abdomen and lower back, or as large as the area from your chest to your toes. The medications are often a combination of an anesthetic medication (see page 269) and a narcotic-like analgesic such as fentanyl, which enhances the overall numbing effect. *Spinal analgesia* is an injection that takes effect quickly and lasts for an hour or two. An *epidural catheter* is a tube placed in the lower back through which medication is given for as long as it's needed.

## Benefits

The American Congress of Obstetricians and Gynecologists (ACOG) and the American Academy of Pediatrics (AAP) have stated that among all options for medicated pain relief, the epidural is the most effective for reducing pain while allowing the woman to stay alert and actively participate in her labor.[4] Among women who receive an epidurals, almost all (over 90 percent) have significant pain relief for at least some of their labor. (See page 269 for information about the possibility of a failed epidural.) Once the epidural takes effect, the medications typically continue to provide relief for the rest of labor.

Because of the locations of the injection sites, much smaller amounts of medication can be used than are needed for systemic analgesia. With neuraxial medications, people typically have fewer side effects and have a higher level of satisfaction. At birth, their babies are more alert, breathe better, and have better muscle tone than babies born with high doses of systemic narcotic-like medications.[5]

## Tradeoffs

To minimize the side effects of neuraxial medications, various additional precautions and interventions must be used to maintain safety. For example, an epidural is accompanied by IV fluids, a bladder catheter, and continuous monitoring of blood pressure, contractions, and fetal heart rate. Eating and drinking are restricted and you're typically confined to bed. Along with the effects of the medications, the accompanying medical equipment significantly reduces mobility (you might not be able to change positions in bed without assistance) and contributes to the feeling that the birth has become a medical event.

## Common Q & A

**Q:** Is it ever too late for an epidural?

**A:** You may have heard that it's best to receive an epidural in early labor because you won't be able to receive one in late labor. It's true that if your labor is progressing quickly and birth is anticipated within thirty to sixty minutes, your caregiver may recommend against an epidural. However, if labor progress is slow, it's possible to receive an epidural even during transition or the second stage.

If comfort techniques are helping you cope, don't feel that you have to get an epidural in early labor because you fear it'll be your only chance to get one. Keep using comfort techniques for as long as they help you manage contractions. If you decide later that you want an epidural, it's very likely that you'll be able to get one.

## Possible side effects[6]

The most common side effects during labor and birth include decreased blood pressure, itching, nausea, a longer labor, a longer pushing stage, and fever. These effects may lead to further interventions (such as oxygen, Pitocin augmentation, vacuum extraction, or forceps delivery) and secondary side effects on both you and your baby (such as uterine hyperstimulation or variations in fetal heart rate).

Some people worry that an injection near the spinal cord may carry the risk of paralysis or even death; however, these outcomes are so rare, they're nearly nonexistent. After the birth, about 1 percent of mothers have a severe headache. Most research shows that regional analgesia has little long-term effect on the baby.[7] If the mother had a fever during labor, the baby may have a fever after birth and may be tested for infection (see below).

When observing initial breastfeeding sessions, some lactation consultants report subtle changes in the alertness and muscle tone of babies who were exposed to neuraxial medications. (Compared to babies who weren't exposed to these drugs, their sucks were marginally weaker and they initiated feeding behavior slightly less often.) Some research indicates that women who had an epidural may be more likely to give up breastfeeding earlier than women who had a nonmedicated birth.[8] These problems can be overcome by early and frequent skin-to-skin contact between the mother and baby, and by starting breastfeeding within the first hour after the birth. Current methods of epidural analgesia focus on finding a balance between maximizing pain relief and minimizing side effects. Caregivers and nurses are trained to recognize and treat side effects when they occur. With an "ideal" epidural, your pain is significantly reduced, you and your baby experience few side effects, you have at least a slight urge to push, and you can move your legs and change positions with assistance.

Whether you'll have few or many side effects can't be predicted or controlled. Many factors will influence your experience, including the skills of the anesthesiologist who administers the epidural, your and your baby's physical state and well-being, and how your body reacts to medications. Visit our website, http://www.PCNGuide.com, for more information on side effects.

## Timing

Many caregivers recommend that clients wait to receive an epidural until they're in active labor with strong, regular contractions and good labor progress. These caregivers believe waiting until that point to administer an epidural reduces the chance it'll slow labor progress. Most anesthesiologists, however, believe an epidural can be given at any point in labor because, even if it may slow labor, the mother will be more comfortable.[9] Some caregivers use a *combined spinal-epidural* or *CSE* (see page 265).

## PROCEDURE FOR EPIDURALS AND SPINALS

If you decide to receive an epidural or a spinal, here's the procedure you can expect:

1.  The anesthesiologist might or might not be immediately available. The contractions you experience while waiting for the requested relief may seem especially intense, and you may need extra support to manage them.

2.  You may receive IV fluids to help reduce the risk of a drop in blood pressure and to allow for administration of additional medications, if needed. This procedure can take ten to twenty minutes. If you have an IV in already, your nurse can increase the flow.

3.  When the anesthesiologist arrives, you're asked to either lie curled on your side or sit up and lean forward to curve your back. The anesthesiologist then cleans your lower back with an antiseptic and numbs your skin with a shot of local anesthetic. This preparation, along with the delicate placement of the epidural catheter or spinal needle, can take ten minutes or longer. You may need extra support to help you sit or lie still during contractions. If you can't stay still during the peak of a contraction, the anesthesiologist can pause until the pain subsides.

4.  Where and how the anesthesiologist places the needle or catheter in your back depends on the type of block.

    - **Spinal analgesia**
    A single injection of an anesthetic or narcotic is given with a needle that's inserted through the dura (the tough membrane that surrounds your spinal cord) into the *intrathecal space*, which is filled with cerebrospinal fluid. (See the illustration at right.) A *spinal block* takes effect within minutes and lasts a few hours.

    - **Epidural catheter**
    A needle is inserted into the epidural space, just outside the dura. A thin plastic tube (catheter) is threaded through the needle, the needle is removed, the catheter is taped to your back, and a test dose of medications is given through the catheter to ensure you don't react poorly to the drugs. The catheter is attached to a pump device that steadily releases small amounts of anesthetic or analgesic. Within a few

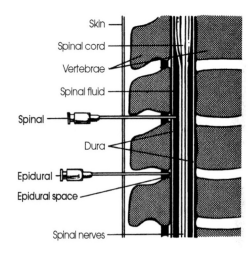

    minutes, tingling and numbness are noticeable; within fifteen minutes, you're likely to be completely numb from the top of your uterus to your pelvis or even from your chest to your toes. (The effects sometimes take longer to be felt, and the catheter may need to be repositioned to yield the best effects.) The catheter remains in place and pain relief continues throughout the rest of your labor.

    - **Combined spinal-epidural (CSE)**
    The epidural needle is inserted, then the smaller spinal needle is inserted through it and into the intrathecal space. A spinal narcotic is given. The spinal needle is then removed and the epidural catheter is inserted for later use. The spinal narcotic takes effect in about five minutes and lasts a few hours. When you need more relief, medication is given through the epidural catheter.

5.  Your temperature, blood pressure, pulse, and blood oxygen levels are checked frequently, and your contractions and fetal heart rate are closely monitored. You may also have an electrocardiogram (EKG) to monitor your heart function.

6.    Many people receive excellent pain relief with epidural analgesia and don't experience any side effects beyond the tradeoffs described on page 263. However, if monitoring indicates that you or your baby are reacting poorly to neuraxial medications, then more interventions may be necessary.

For example, if your blood pressure drops significantly, your baby's heart rate will also decrease. To improve your oxygen levels and increase your baby's heart rate, your nurse or caregiver will turn you onto your side, place an oxygen mask on your face, and ask you to breathe deeply. While the oxygen mask may concern you and your partner, it almost always corrects the problem quickly. If not, you may also be given medications or additional IV fluids to raise your blood pressure.

Managing side effects often causes a "cascade of interventions," in which the use of one intervention leads to additional side effects that necessitate even more interventions. For example, if epidural medications cause your contractions to slow down, you may receive Pitocin to stimulate them—which may overstimulate your uterus, which can lead to variations in your baby's heart rate, which may increase your need of a cesarean section. (The research, however, doesn't indicate that, by themselves, epidurals increase the risk of cesarean.) To be able to make an informed decision about any pain relief option, you need to acknowledge the possibility of these unintended side effects.

As another example, your chances of fever increase when you have epidural anesthesia, because the medications alter your ability to regulate your temperature. The longer the epidural is in place, the higher your risk of fever is. When you have a fever, the fetal heart rate may increase to a worrisome level, a problem that may require an intervention. If you have a fever during labor, your baby may have one at birth. If she does, her fever can't be assumed to be a result of the epidural, because fever can also be associated with infection. Your baby will be checked for infection with blood tests and possibly a spinal tap. She may be kept in the special care nursery and given antibiotics for two days, until her test results are known. Although the testing and preventive treatment will separate you from your baby and can be worrisome, test results will likely show that your baby is fine.

See the chart on our website, http://www.PCNGuide.com, for more information about the effects and side effects of regional medications.

# OPTIONS FOR EPIDURALS

The types of epidurals offered vary among hospitals. Typically, you aren't allowed to choose which type you'll get. Ask your caregiver what the hospital's standard protocol for epidurals is so you'll know what to expect.

### Anesthetic-only or narcotic-only epidurals

These types of epidurals aren't typically done, because combining medications provides better benefits with fewer side effects. Anesthetic-only epidurals can reduce the mother's mobility and reduce her urge to push, leading to slower labors and more forceps deliveries or vacuum extraction. Narcotic-only epidurals don't provide as much pain relief without an anesthetic.

### Epidural with combination of anesthetic and narcotic

This is the most common type of epidural. You may receive medications by continuous drip, from a series of doses called intermittent boluses (a method that's becoming uncommon), or by patient-controlled epidural analgesia (see below).

## Patient-controlled epidural analgesia (PCEA)

PCEA allows you to press a button attached to your epidural pump to give yourself more medication when you need it. When patients are allowed to control their dosage, they tend to use less medication and are more satisfied with the epidural experience than when the dosage is controlled for them. Although you have some control over the flow of medication with PCEA, the device has a timer that limits the number of doses, which are carefully measured so you can't overdose. (*Note:* Patient-controlled analgesia, or PCA, may also be available for IV narcotics.) PCEA is available in most large hospitals.[10]

## Combined spinal-epidural (CSE)

CSE uses a spinal narcotic in early labor (which may allow for more mobility), then an epidural later in labor, when you need more pain relief. Advantages of CSE over epidural by continuous drip include quicker pain relief,[11] much less medication, generally fewer side effects (mild itching is likely), and more mobility. While often available at university-based teaching hospitals, CSE is uncommon at community hospitals.

## Light or late epidural

You can reduce some side effects by delaying an epidural until you're in active labor (late epidural) and requesting a low concentration of the medications (light epidural).

Policies for managing labor with an epidural also vary among hospitals. Ask your caregiver about the following measures:

### Movement
Ask whether you'll be able to move with an epidural and whether movement in bed is encouraged.

### Food and drink
Many hospitals allow people with epidurals to consume only ice chips; however, the American Society of Anesthesiologists recommends allowing clear fluids. Sometimes policies depend on whether you're considered high risk or low risk. Ask your caregiver what you'll be allowed to consume.

### Delayed pushing (also called passive descent or laboring down)
Rather than pushing as soon as your cervix is fully dilated, you may wait to push until your baby's head is visible at the vaginal outlet. Delayed pushing has been proven to reduce vaginal tears, forceps delivery, vacuum extraction, and the need for a cesarean section. It also won't harm your baby. Ask whether delayed pushing is common practice.

### Lowering the dosage or discontinuing the epidural
By slowing or stopping the flow of epidural medications at the beginning of the second stage of labor, you may be able to bear down more effectively. (However, labor pain may be intolerable when it returns.)

---

## Different Views on Epidurals

When asked about epidurals, new mothers had many different responses. Here are a few examples:

*For me, comfort techniques weren't enough and the fentanyl wasn't much help, so I just rested on my side in bed for a while and did my breathing exercises. Sometime later the epidural came—relief at last! I even slept. I think the epidural slowed things down, but I was grateful that the pain was so much less.*

*I had twenty hours of labor with a great support team and without drugs. I was coping with the pain okay, but I was exhausted. So I got an epidural and slept. My son was born ten hours later, after four hours of pushing. I was glad to get the epidural, but the birth was definitely a much more medical experience than I'd expected.*

*I'd hoped the epidural would take away all my pain, but it didn't. I was pretty numb overall, but this one spot on my belly hurt a LOT. It was almost harder to cope with that window of pain than it'd been to cope with regular contractions. Luckily, James remembered all the comfort techniques we learned, and helped coach me through the contractions.*

# A Note to Fathers and Partners

When your laboring partner has an epidural, her shift from intense effort and pain to complete physical relaxation may be sudden. At that point, you may think that she no longer needs your support. You may begin thinking about taking a nap or going for a walk; however, your job isn't done. Even though your partner may be more comfortable physically, she still needs your emotional support. If you shift your attention away once the epidural has taken effect, she may feel as though you're abandoning her.

To reassure your partner, stay with her and relax together. Do things that soothe her such as holding her hand or brushing her hair. An epidural may leave your partner feeling disconnected from the birth experience; talk with her about the labor and your baby to help her reconnect with events. (Resist the temptation to turn on the TV, post status updates online, or text everyone you know!) If she's anxious, listen to her fears, acknowledge them, and reassure her. If she falls asleep, she'll probably be restless. She'll be reassured by your staying awake or at least staying in the room so she can wake you if she needs anything.

Help her change positions as much as possible to assist with labor progress and baby's position. If she has a light epidural, she may be able to get on her hands and knees on the bed with assistance and if you remain by her side to help keep her steady. If she has CSE, she may be allowed to stand.

Your partner may also experience discomforts that are caused by the medications, such as itching, nausea, and feeling overheated or chilled. Make her more comfortable by giving her a massage, helping her change positions, covering her with a warm blanket, placing a cool cloth on her forehead, or giving her ice chips or sips of water (if allowed). Do *not*, however, place heating pads or ice packs on any part of her body that's affected by the epidural. The medications will affect her sense of temperature, and she might not be able to tell if a heating pad or cold pack is damaging her skin.

Be aware that some side effects of epidurals may lead to other interventions or may require a decision from your partner on how to manage the problem. Try to stay calm and supportive so you can help her make decisions that are best for her.

Even with pain relief, your partner may experience intense pressure or burning during the pushing stage. Reassure her that these sensations are normal and signal that your baby will be born soon. If you're holding up one of her legs as she pushes, be careful not to pull it back too far. Think about her hips' normal range of motion, and don't force her leg beyond that point so you avoid straining her hips, thighs, or lower back. (Your partner will be unable to tell you when her muscles are straining because the medications will have numbed all sensation.)

After the birth, help your partner get lots of early skin-to-skin contact with your baby so breastfeeding can begin in the first hour.

Occasionally, epidurals don't provide effective pain relief (see page 269). Be sure to alert the staff if this situation occurs. They may be able to fix the problem. If your partner is among the few women for whom an epidural doesn't relieve pain, even after multiple attempts to correct the problem, she'll need your support to help cope with the pain and to deal with the disappointment that the epidural failed her.

# Failed Epidurals

Although epidurals are very effective for most people who use them, they can pose challenges for some. As many as 13 percent of epidurals don't provide complete pain relief when first inserted, while 7 percent may provide good pain relief initially but fade over time. Some epidurals provide only minimal pain relief; others allow for "windows" of pain, in which most of the area is numbed but one spot still has sensation and the person can fully feel the pain in that area. Given how the catheter is placed, CSE is less likely to fail than an epidural, but it still fails up to 9 percent of the time.[12]

If you have a problem with your epidural, the staff may be able to fix it by changing your position, increasing the medication, or repositioning the epidural catheter. These measures have resulted in good pain relief for nearly all women with epidurals (98.8 percent).[13] However, while the staff works to correct the problem, comfort measures can help you cope.

When you're unprepared to manage labor pain, your inability to cope can make you feel that you're suffering, which in turn can create a very unhappy memory of what should be one of the best days of your life. Learn self-help techniques in chapter 12 so you can manage these challenges and have a more satisfying birth. As a bonus, these techniques can help you deal with other challenging or painful situations at other times in your life.

## *Key Points to Remember*

- To minimize possible side effects of pain medications, try using coping techniques first (see chapter 12). Use them for as long as they're effective, before starting medications.
- IV or IM narcotics reduce pain for a short time, but they may cause itching, nausea, and disorientation.
- Epidural analgesia provides effective and satisfying pain relief for most people, but it requires more monitoring and routine interventions. Common side effects include reduced blood pressure, fever, slower labor, and a longer pushing stage.
- Although an epidural can help relieve labor pain substantially, labor support is still needed and appreciated.

# CHAPTER 14

# When Childbirth Becomes Complicated

Most healthy pregnant women will have normal childbirth experiences: Labor progresses without significant delay, and the baby is healthy, tolerates contractions well, and is in a position that's favorable for birth. For some women or babies, however, complications can arise during labor or birth. In these cases, the well-being of the mother and baby may improve with interventions such as medications, technology, or surgery. While it's never easy to think about the possibility of problems, knowing how to address them can reduce anxiety and help you work with your caregiver should they arise.

This chapter describes conditions and events that can complicate labor or birth, as well as procedures that may resolve them. If your pregnancy is considered to be high risk, you're likely to need some of these interventions. If your pregnancy is low risk, it's still wise to learn about possible complications and available interventions, because problems can develop unexpectedly during your labor or birth.

It's important to understand your caregiver's concerns and recommendations, as well as the reasons for them. With this knowledge, you can best help decide a safe plan of action (if there's more than one) and prepare for how you'll work with your caregiver to have the best possible birth experience.

# Labor Complications and Interventions

Compared to a normal labor, a *complicated labor* is longer, more painful, or more difficult, and may require medical help to ensure the well-being of the mother and baby.

Few labor complications pose serious problems that require immediate medical attention. If a potential problem arises in labor, such as slow cervical dilation, it may be resolved easily with time, patience, and simple techniques used by the mother or the staff. The problem becomes a complication only if simple approaches don't resolve it. To identify, prevent, or treat a complication, caregivers may use *interventions* such as induction, continuous electronic fetal monitoring, episiotomy, cesarean, or instrumental delivery.

For every complication, multiple possible interventions are available that may resolve it. When deciding which interventions to use, caregivers consider many factors:

- the circumstances of the woman's pregnancy and labor
- the woman's preferences or concerns regarding interventions
- current scientific evidence on the effectiveness of interventions, as well as their benefits and risks
- hospital policies and customs on interventions
- legal liability issues
- the caregiver's training and experience
- professional standards on interventions
- professional peer pressure to use interventions
- cost of interventions as well as staff availability to do them

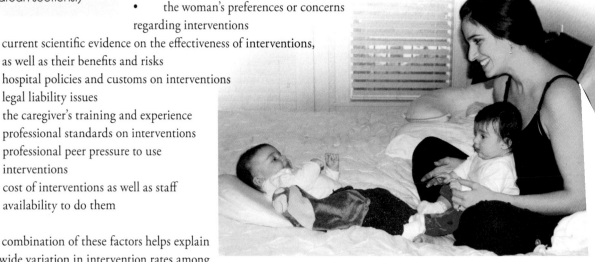

The combination of these factors helps explain the wide variation in intervention rates among different caregivers and hospitals across the United States and Canada. Childbirth classes can provide general information about these topics. However, during your prenatal visits, discuss any problems that come up and ask the key questions on page 9 to help you make informed decisions about interventions. That way, you'll know what to expect if a complication arises in your labor.

The following sections cover complications in roughly the order they appear in pregnancy, labor, and birth.

# Pregnancy Complications That Affect Labor

The following sections discuss issues in pregnancy that can cause problems during labor. These include gestational hypertension, preeclampsia, and a pregnancy with multiples.

## MULTIPLES (TWINS, TRIPLETS, OR MORE)

When compared to a singleton pregnancy (only one baby), a multiple pregnancy is at higher risk for complications, such as preterm rupture of the membranes, preterm labor, preeclampsia, prolonged labor, prolapsed cord, postpartum hemorrhage, and babies who are premature or small for their gestational age. Although labor with multiples often progresses normally, the birth is usually more complicated than the birth of a single baby.

The risk of these difficulties increases as the number of babies increases. If you're pregnant with multiples, expect more medical supervision and more interventions than a woman pregnant with a single baby.

Timing the birth of multiples is a controversial topic. Some caregivers believe that waiting for labor to begin on its own can harm the babies' well-being; they argue that multiples are born healthier if labor is induced or a cesarean section is scheduled between the thirty-seventh and thirty-ninth weeks of pregnancy. Studies of these claims, however, have found inconsistent results. Other caregivers believe that the process of labor and birth best benefits mother and babies; they wait for labor to begin spontaneously while monitoring the pregnancy and the babies' well-being closely.[1]

With vaginal births of multiples, caregivers may recommend routinely placing an epidural catheter in the mother, in case a possibly painful intervention is needed to deliver one or more of the babies (such as forceps delivery). Although twins are often born vaginally at term, the rate of cesarean birth for twins is higher than for single babies. It's rare for triplets or more to be born vaginally at term. See chapter 15 for more information on cesarean birth.

### Vaginal Birth of Twins

If you're pregnant with twins, expect to receive an ultrasound scan during labor to identify your babies' presentations (the parts of their bodies that will emerge first from the birth canal). The results help your caregiver determine whether a vaginal birth or cesarean birth is best for your babies' well-being and your own. Vaginal births usually occur in an operating room in case a cesarean becomes necessary.

For a vaginal birth, the most favorable presentation is vertex (head down), and in most cases both babies are vertex at the time of the birth. However, if both babies are breech (buttocks, legs, or feet over the cervix), a cesarean is usually performed. If the first baby is vertex and the second baby is breech, your caregiver may attempt to turn the second baby after the vaginal birth of the first, or the second baby may be born in the breech presentation. The birth of the second baby usually occurs within five to thirty minutes after the first, and the delivery of the placenta (or placentas) occurs after both babies are born.

## GESTATIONAL HYPERTENSION AND PREECLAMPSIA

If you have gestational hypertension, expect your caregiver to monitor your blood pressure and your baby's well-being closely throughout your pregnancy. (To learn more about hypertension and preeclampsia, see page 133.) If the condition is mild and stable, your pregnancy is typically allowed to continue. However, hypertension rarely improves and often worsens as pregnancy continues. In severe cases of preeclampsia, or when blood tests indicate HELLP syndrome (see page 135), care during labor usually focuses on keeping blood pressure down and preventing seizures from eclampsia.

Caregivers commonly recommend inducing labor in women with preeclampsia, because ending the pregnancy is the first step to fixing the problem. Some caregivers also recommend an epidural because of its suspected side effect of lowering blood pressure; however, studies haven't shown this practice to be effective.

# Problems during Transition from Pregnancy to Labor

The following sections describe issues that can arise as a pregnancy transitions into labor. They include preterm labor and preterm birth, rapid unattended birth, and the need or wish to start labor before it begins on its own.

## PRETERM LABOR AND PREMATURE BIRTH

A labor is preterm if it begins before the thirty-seventh week of pregnancy. If a preterm labor isn't stopped, a premature birth occurs. The younger a premature baby's gestational age, the more problems she's likely to have. If you experience signs of preterm labor (see page 130), *call your caregiver immediately!* Methods used to prevent a premature birth are more likely to succeed if preterm labor is detected before your cervix has dilated to 2 centimeters.

Some women are at higher risk for preterm labor, but it can happen to anyone. For a full discussion of risk factors and ways to reduce your risk, see page 129.

If you think you're experiencing preterm labor but aren't sure, contact your caregiver. You'll be assessed to confirm whether you're in preterm labor (see chapter 7 for more information).

### What to Expect If You Have Preterm Labor

If you're more than thirty-four weeks pregnant and birth is unavoidable, your labor may be allowed to progress with extra monitoring. Because preterm labor is a high-risk condition, it usually involves the specialized skills of an obstetrician. If your caregiver isn't an obstetrician and you develop preterm labor, an obstetrician may work closely with your caregiver to manage the problem. If a premature birth is unavoidable, a pediatrician or neonatologist (a pediatrician specialized in the medical care of newborns) will likely be present at the birth for immediate evaluation and treatment of your baby.

If you're less than thirty-four weeks and if your cervix is changing, expect the following:

- Your caregiver will withdraw a small amount of amniotic fluid from your uterus (*amniocentesis*) and analyze the surfactant levels to check whether your baby's lungs are mature enough to allow him to breathe on his own after the birth.

- If your baby's lungs aren't mature and birth seems unavoidable, the focus of care shifts to prevention of *respiratory distress syndrome (RDS)*—the most common complication of premature birth. Your caregiver may try to delay the birth for a day or two to allow time for *corticosteroids* to speed up the maturing of your baby's lungs.[2] The administration of these medications has reduced the incidence of RDS by 40 to 60 percent. Corticosteroids also help decrease intracranial bleeding (brain hemorrhage) in a newborn.

- The drugs given to the mother to stop or slow preterm labor are powerful and have strong side effects. Although the highest doses are usually used only for a day or two, lower doses, combined with bed rest, may be used for a longer period to keep preterm contractions from increasing in frequency and intensity. The following drugs are used to prevent preterm labor:
  - beta-mimetic agents (terbutaline and ritodrine)[3]
  - calcium channel blockers (nifedipine)[4]
  - prostaglandin inhibitors (naproxen and indomethacin)
  - oxytocin receptor antagonists (atosiban)[5]
- Once a preterm labor is established, giving the mother systemic pain medications (such as narcotics or narcotic-like drugs) usually isn't recommended because these drugs can affect the baby's heart rate and sometimes his breathing after the birth. Therefore, in early labor, plan to use relaxation and breathing patterns for pain relief. In active labor or during the birth, you can continue these techniques or you can request regional anesthesia (epidural), which has less effect on newborns than systemic pain medications have.

### In Their Own Words

I went into labor with my second child two weeks early. My husband and I headed to the hospital, but I was ready to push before we arrived. We'd called 911, then called my doula, who told my husband what to do and coached me to breathe and tell my two-year-old that I was okay. The ambulance arrived just as the baby was born. We were all fine, but continued on to the hospital for observation and rest. Labor and birth took just an hour from beginning to end. What an adventure!

—*Kirsti*

If your baby is born prematurely, he may need special care. See page 294.

## Rapid Unattended Birth

Some women's labors are much faster than usual. They *begin* with intense contractions that are less than four minutes apart and progress rapidly. If your labor is this fast, head for your birthplace immediately (do *not* drive yourself—have someone else drive), or if planning a home birth, call your midwife.

If your labor progresses so quickly that you push and strain involuntarily and can see your baby's head at your vaginal opening or feel him coming down the birth canal, stay at home—don't travel. It's better to have shelter and essential supplies to help with an unattended birth than it is to rush to your birthplace and risk having an unattended birth in the car on the way. If, however, you decide to travel to your birthplace and you begin to give birth on the way, the driver should pull over to the side of the road, help you deliver your baby (see page 276), and then drive you both to the hospital.

### Possible Problems after a Rapid Unattended Birth

Usually after a rapid birth, both the mother and baby are fine; however, complications may develop and medical professionals should assess the mother and baby as soon as possible after the birth. If you have a rapid birth, medical help is likely only minutes away. In the meantime, you may be able to help fix the following potential problems or prevent them from worsening:

#### If your baby doesn't breathe spontaneously

First, have someone call 911, if possible. Place your baby on his stomach with his head lower than his body, then rub his back briskly but gently. If he doesn't respond within thirty seconds, hold his ankles together and smack the soles of his feet. If your baby still doesn't breathe, check for mucus in his mouth with your finger. If you know how to give infant CPR, do so while waiting for medical assistance.

## Quick Checklist for a Rapid Unattended Birth

Do as many of the following tasks as possible if you expect a rapid birth without the attendance of a medical professional. A rapid birth can be hectic, but try to remember to use what you've learned about the birth process, as well as relaxation and breathing techniques.

1. Get help, if possible. Call your partner, your caregiver, the hospital, or 911. If your partner can't be with you in person, try to get someone else—a neighbor or even a child—to assist you.
2. Gather clean sheets, towels or paper towels, tissues, and extra clothing to be used during the birth and for your baby.
3. Wash your hands.
4. Remove all clothing from your bottom and vaginal area.
5. Lie on your side or sit leaning back. Make sure you're in a clean place with enough room for your baby to rest as she slips out of your body.
6. Put a sheet, towel, or some clothing under your bottom.
7. Try not to hold your breath if your body is pushing. Keep panting through each contraction until your baby is born.
8. After your baby is born:
   - Wipe away any mucus from her nose and mouth. Remove any membranes covering her face.
   - Wipe her head and body to dry her.
   - Place her on your bare abdomen or chest to keep her warm.
   - Cover your baby and yourself using cloths, towels, or clothing.
9. Don't clamp or cut the cord.
10. Put your baby to your breast, and let her breastfeed, if possible.
11. If you're at home, await the birth of the placenta. (If the placenta isn't expelled in fifteen to twenty minutes, try kneeling to see if gravity can help it come out. If it doesn't, go to the hospital.) If you're in a car, have your partner or another person drive you and your baby to the hospital.
12. Place the placenta nearby in a bowl, newspaper, or cloth. (It'll still be attached to the cord and your baby.)
13. Place towels or a pad between your legs to absorb the blood flow.
14. Go to the hospital or get medical help as soon as possible to check both you and your baby. A medical professional will also cut the umbilical cord and check your placenta.

*Note:* The medical emergency team may arrive in time to help you with some of these tasks.

### If you have excessive bleeding from your vagina

Some bleeding normally occurs after labor and birth, both before and after the placenta is expelled. However, excessive bleeding (more than 500 milliliters or 2 cups) may mean a postpartum hemorrhage, especially if you begin to have symptoms of shock such as rapid pulse, pale skin, trembling, faintness, feeling cold, and sweating. Don't try to measure the amount of blood; your symptoms are a better sign of shock. If you or your partner suspect that you have a postpartum hemorrhage, call 911. You or your partner should firmly massage your fundus (the top of your uterus) in a circle until the uterus contracts, and encourage your baby to nurse (or you or your partner can stroke your nipples) to stimulate the release of oxytocin, a hormone that causes contractions. To avoid shock, lie down and elevate your hips so they're higher than your head. Get to the hospital or call for an ambulance if you haven't already done so.

# The Need or Wish to Start Labor

The need or wish to start labor sometimes makes it impossible to let labor start on its own. If so, women consent to or request *induction*, or the initiation of labor. (If a woman is already in labor, but it's progressing too slowly, her caregiver may recommend *augmentation*, or speeding up a labor. See page 285.)

## *Common Medical Reasons for Induction*

If your caregiver knows or suspects that the well-being of you or your baby is at risk, you'll both be closely monitored and may undergo tests to assess your health and your baby's maturity and well-being (see page 141). If monitoring or test results suggest that the risks of continuing the pregnancy outweigh the risks of induction, your caregiver will likely recommend induction. Not all caregivers see the degree of risk in the same way. Here are common medical reasons for recommending induction:[6]

### Post-date pregnancy

A *post-date*, or prolonged, pregnancy is one that has lasted to at least forty-two weeks. (Many caregivers shorten it to forty-one weeks.) After forty-two weeks gestation, the risk of *postmaturity* increases and the risk of stillbirth gradually rises. Tests that assess babies' well-being can help identify some of those at risk (see page 141).

### Ruptured membranes

After a woman's bag of waters breaks, her risk of infection increases. Induction may be recommended if her labor doesn't start on its own within twenty-four hours (or sooner if she has tested positive for Group B strep—see page 125).

### Lack of growth in the baby

If a caregiver observes signs that the baby is no longer thriving in the uterus, induction is recommended.

### Genital herpes

If a woman is having frequent outbreaks of genital herpes in late pregnancy, her caregiver may plan to induce labor between outbreaks to avoid a cesarean birth.

### Illness in the mother

Some illnesses, such as gestational hypertension or diabetes, can affect the health of the mother or the pregnancy, especially if the illness worsens over time (see chapter 7).

### Fear of macrosomia (big baby)

In some pregnancies, ultrasound scans suggest that the baby is large for his mother's size and build, or is growing rapidly. Some of these women and their caregivers worry that the baby may grow too big to fit through the pelvis or will experience *shoulder dystocia*, a rare and serious situation in which the baby's head is born but the shoulders become stuck within the pelvis. To avoid either complication, these women consent to induction.

Studies on the accuracy of ultrasound estimates of fetal weight, however, have found a margin of error of at least 10 percent. Ultrasound scans often overestimate the baby's size. In addition, even if a baby is large, his size won't necessarily cause problems with the birth. Of all cases of shoulder dystocia, 70 percent occur in babies of average or small size. Furthermore, when compared to letting labor begin on its own, inducing labor because of a suspected large baby more often causes labor to stop (*arrest of labor*), increasing the need for a cesarean delivery. For these reasons, professional obstetrical and midwifery organizations don't include macrosomia on their lists of medical reasons to induce labor.[7] They conclude that using ultrasound to estimate fetal weight should be minimized.[8]

## Elective Induction

Sometimes, women request induction—or their caregivers recommend it—for nonmedical reasons. This type of induction is called a social or *elective induction*.[9] Common reasons for elective induction are discussed below:

### Convenience for the caregiver's call schedule

If a woman has been seeing a caregiver in a group practice, she may want labor to begin when her caregiver is on call and avoid having an unknown caregiver attend the birth. Many caregivers prefer inducing their clients' labors so they can attend the births. In some group practices, the caregiver who attends the birth receives the largest share of the maternity care fee.

### Convenience for the family's schedule, support needs, or circumstances

Many women choose induction so the birth will fit into their family's schedule or into the schedules of those who can help after the birth. Induction may especially appeal to women who live far from a hospital, those who need to arrange for the care of other children during the birth, or those who have had a previous rapid birth and want to better control the timing of this birth.

### Discomfort in late pregnancy

Induction often appeals to women who are uncomfortable in the late trimester and are impatient for pregnancy to end.

### Pregnancy reaches thirty-nine weeks

A pregnancy reaches term at thirty-seven weeks, but inductions at that time are too early for babies whose development may still be premature (have problems with breathing, temperature control, suckling ability, and more). Recently, a consensus was reached stating that induction at thirty-seven weeks is too early for the baby without a medical reason. Thirty-nine weeks is the minimum gestation that's acceptable for elective induction,[10] and the American Congress of Obstetricians and Gynecologists (ACOG) advocates waiting until forty-one weeks to induce without medical reason.[11]

## *Reasons to Think Carefully before Requesting or Consenting to Induction*

About 23 percent of labors in the United States are induced.[12] In a recent study of more than 130,000 low-risk labors, 10 percent were *electively* induced.[13] Although induction may sound tempting when you're anxious to get labor started, consider the following facts:

Induction bypasses the baby's ability to start labor at the best time. Labor should begin when your baby's lungs have matured enough that she can breathe safely on her own after birth, and when other hormonal changes are triggered that prepare your cervix to open and your uterus to push your baby out so the two of you thrive (see page 162). Weigh these considerations against any reasons you or your caregiver has for ending pregnancy:

- Induction leads to a more medicalized birth, with more interventions such as intravenous (IV) fluids and continuous electronic fetal monitoring (EFM), and fewer options for natural coping techniques such as the freedom to move around and using the tub for pain relief.
- Induction may make contractions more painful than normal, which may increase the need for pain medications.
- Induction can cause a premature birth if done too early, especially for a pregnancy without a clear due date (see pages 386–387). Elective inductions have contributed significantly to the high rate of prematurity in the United States; however, the rate is gradually dropping as more caregivers discourage elective induction.
- All methods of induction carry possible risks, especially uterine hyperstimulation (contractions that are too strong or too frequent) and the higher likelihood that the baby won't tolerate labor (as shown by EFM).
- Induction doesn't guarantee labor will start. If induction fails, a cesarean section typically is performed. When compared to first-time mothers whose labors began on their own, those who had elective induction (or whose cervixes weren't ripe before induction) were two to four times more likely to have had a cesarean.[14]

If you're considering an elective induction, or if your caregiver recommends induction, ask the key questions on page 9. Ask whether there's a desired time frame for an induction to work and under what circumstances an induction is considered a failure. Ask if waiting for labor to begin is possible after a failed induction or if an immediate cesarean is required. If you're uncomfortable with your caregiver's advice, see page 18 for suggestions. Good communication can usually resolve disagreements.

Once you're thoroughly informed about the procedure, you may decide to wait for labor to begin on its own or postpone induction until later in pregnancy. Or you may consent to induction after concluding its benefits outweigh the potential risks. Whatever you decide, you'll have made an informed decision that's best for you.

### Medical Conditions That Rule Out Induction

In some cases, induction isn't possible because a medical condition compromises the procedure's safety. Examples of such conditions include a genital herpes outbreak, placenta previa (see page 132), previous surgery to remove uterine fibroids, or a baby with a transverse presentation (lying sideways). If you have any of these conditions, your caregiver won't induce your labor.

## Two Views on Medical Induction

The most frustrating thing after receiving Pitocin was how it affected my ability to move around. First I got an IV for the Pitocin and fluids. Then I got an epidural, which meant I was hooked up to monitors and stuck in bed. Next I had a blood pressure cuff put on, and then I got a bladder catheter. All those wires and tubes made it really hard to move.
—Mary

During labor, my contractions repeatedly slowed down whenever I rested, so I walked around to get them going again. Ultimately, my doctor convinced me to use a very low dose of Pitocin so my contractions would become regular. They did, and my baby was at last born after twenty-one hours of labor.
—Melissa

## Nonmedical Methods for Induction

If your caregiver recommends induction, you may have a few days to try nonmedical methods to start labor on your own. Although most of these methods have had little scientific evaluation and are less likely to start labor than medical methods, they're generally simpler and easier to do than medical induction. They also pose milder risks, although some have unpleasant side effects.[15] Even if only partially effective, they may cause enough cervical changes to allow for a successful medical induction.

The following sections briefly describe self-help techniques and complementary medicine methods for inducing labor. (Visit our website, http://www.PCNGuide.com, to learn more.) Before trying these methods, discuss them with your caregiver. Some of the techniques may be inappropriate under some circumstances, and your caregiver may have advice regarding their use. If you think your caregiver might not support your decision, phrase your question carefully. For example, instead of asking, "Do you think I should try castor oil or acupuncture?" try asking, "Is there any medical reason why I shouldn't try castor oil or acupuncture?" That way, you can get specific reasons if your caregiver disapproves of a technique.

*Note:* If you don't have time to try nonmedical induction methods, if you don't wish to try them, or if they don't work, your next step is medical induction. See page 281.

### Self-Help Techniques

The following are actions you can take to try to start labor on your own.

#### Walking

Long walks may sometimes help start labor, but don't exhaust yourself. Walking is more effective for speeding up a slow labor than it is at starting it.

#### Intercourse or orgasm

Sexual intercourse and clitoral stimulation (manual or oral) may help start labor. Sexual excitement, particularly orgasm, causes the release of oxytocin and prostaglandins, two hormones that cause uterine contractions and may start labor. Semen also contains prostaglandins. If using this method, frequent sexual activity is more effective than a single act. Try to forget your goal of starting labor and just enjoy the sexual experiences.

*Note:* If your bag of waters has broken, don't have vaginal intercourse or put anything into your vagina, to minimize the risk of infection.

#### Nipple stimulation

Nipple stimulation causes the release of oxytocin, which causes contractions that may start labor.[16] To stimulate your nipples, lightly stroke them, have your partner gently caress or suck on them, or use a breast pump. You may feel contractions within minutes, or you may have to stimulate your nipples for hours (off and on, but perhaps continuously) before experiencing steady contractions.

*Caution:* Occasionally, nipple stimulation causes contractions that last too long (longer than sixty seconds), occur too frequently (more than two in ten minutes), or are too painful. If you have this reaction, stop stimulating your nipples.

#### Castor oil

Labor may start if the bowels are stimulated to empty. *Castor oil* is a strong laxative that causes powerful bowel cramps and contractions. It's thought to increase prostaglandin production, which may start uterine contractions.[17] Visit our website for directions on using castor oil. Other mixtures containing ingredients such as verbena oil are sometimes used, but little scientific study of their usefulness or side effects has been done.

#### Acupressure

Firm finger or thumb pressure on particular acupressure points may start or speed up contractions (see page 231).

## Complementary Medicine Methods

The following methods are often used along with conventional medicine methods.

### Herbal tea and tinctures

Various herbal teas and tinctures can induce labor; however, these ingredients may also cause undesired side effects. (Visit our website for more information.) Use this method only with the guidance of a knowledgeable professional and your caregiver.

### Homeopathic remedies

*Homeopathy* uses diluted derivatives of certain natural substances to stimulate the body to respond in a way that heals or corrects a specific problem such as a labor that won't start. Although side effects are unlikely, these remedies are best administered by a trained homeopathic practitioner.

### Acupuncture

*Acupuncture* is an ancient Chinese medicine technique that uses needles placed at strategic points along meridians, or energy flow lines, in the body. It has no known risks. Little scientific research has been done on the effectiveness of acupuncture to ripen the cervix or start labor, and the few studies have mixed results.[18] (Visit our website for more information.) An acupuncturist may also use *moxibustion*, which doesn't use needles but instead uses burning herbs placed close to the acupuncture point.

## Medical Methods of Induction

Induction is more likely to succeed if the cervix is favorable— ripe, anterior, and partially effaced and dilated. The cervix is unfavorable for induction if it's firm, posterior, and not effaced (see page 161). Some caregivers use a scale called the Bishop score to describe the condition of the cervix. The choice of induction method depends on the condition of the cervix and on the philosophy and preferences of the caregiver and hospital. Ask your caregiver which method will be used so you'll know what to expect and ask the key questions on page 9).

### Medical Nondrug Methods

The following are brief descriptions of methods for ripening the cervix or inducing labor without the use of medications. Visit our website to learn more.

### Balloon dilators

These devices have been found to help start labor by ripening and thinning the cervix and causing some dilation.[19] A balloon catheter called the Foley (originally designed to empty the bladder) is placed within the cervix, or a double balloon *cervical ripening device* is placed with one balloon in the uterus and a second one in the vagina. Water is injected into the balloon(s) to put pressure on the cervix, causing it to thin and begin dilating. The device remains in place until it either slips out as the cervix begins to open or it's removed after twelve hours. Although effective, the balloons may cause discomfort.

## Two Options If Induction Doesn't Work

Occasionally, labor can take a long time to start with induction. If your membranes haven't been ruptured, two options are possible.

**Option One: Serial Induction**

Pitocin is discontinued at night to allow you to eat and sleep. The advantage of *serial induction* is that it may improve your chances of a vaginal birth. The disadvantage, however, is that it may take several days for labor to start, which can be emotionally and physically draining for you and your partner. Extra support and patience are essential. Today, caregivers rely on serial induction less often than in the past, mainly because having one family occupy a birthing room for days is costly to both the family and the hospital.

**Option Two: Artificial Ruptures of Membranes (AROM)**

Your membranes are ruptured and your dose of Pitocin may be increased quickly. This more aggressive approach may start labor, but it must do so within a certain time frame (twelve to twenty-four hours). If you don't have steady dilation within this period, the induction is considered a failure and a cesarean section becomes necessary.

# Risks and Benefits of Artificial Rupture of Membranes (AROM)

## AROM for Induction

When the cervix is ripe, AROM increases the chance of starting labor, especially when used with Pitocin. However, the risk of infection increases after AROM, so if labor doesn't progress after the procedure, a cesarean section is performed.

For elective induction, consider trying Pitocin without AROM. If Pitocin doesn't start labor, it can be discontinued and tried again in a day or two.

## AROM to Augment Active Labor

During contractions in active labor, your bag of waters may bulge through your cervix. Performing AROM is intended to cause your baby's head to press more firmly on your cervix, can make contractions suddenly more painful and augment (speed up) labor progress. Recent studies found that routine AROM doesn't shorten labor and may result in a greater chance of a cesarean.[21] Without AROM, the membranes often remain intact until late first stage or the second stage of labor, and then break spontaneously.

If your caregiver suggests AROM to augment labor, ask the key questions on page 9. If labor is progressing well, you might not need AROM. If labor is progressing slowly and your baby is in a favorable position, then AROM may help speed up progress. If labor is progressing slowly because your baby is an unfavorable position (see page 286), AROM is unlikely to improve progress and may prevent your baby from moving into a favorable position and potentially causing a longer or more painful labor.[22] Try other options first. Your bag of waters provides your baby some cushioning, room, and time to move into a more favorable position.

## Stripping (or sweeping) the membranes

The caregiver inserts a finger into the cervix to loosen the bag of waters from the uterine wall to prompt the release of hormones that start contractions. Your caregiver may suggest this intervention if you're near or past your due date and your cervix is very ripe and dilated at least the width of a finger. Although the procedure is painful (it feels like a vigorous vaginal exam) and may cause slight bleeding, cramping, and (rarely) unintended rupture of the membranes, studies have found that it reduces the time until labor begins.[20]

## Artificial rupture of membranes (AROM)

Also called *amniotomy*, AROM is a procedure in which the caregiver breaks the bag of waters with an amnio-hook, a long plastic device that resembles a crochet needle. It's done either alone or with Pitocin to start labor or to speed up progress in active labor. AROM is rarely successful if the cervix is unfavorable (see page 281), in which case the caregiver uses cervical ripening techniques (see below) before trying AROM. See sidebar at left for more information.

## Medications to Induce or Augment Labor

*Pitocin* (also called Syntocinon and commonly referred to as "Pit") is a synthetic version of oxytocin, the hormone that your body releases to start labor. Pitocin is used for medical induction, and it's sometimes used to help augment a slow labor by increasing the frequency and intensity of contractions. It's administered intravenously, allowing the dosage to be increased, reduced, or stopped, if necessary.

Although Pitocin causes your uterus to contract, it doesn't ripen your cervix. If your cervix is unfavorable for induction, cervical ripening methods are necessary before receiving Pitocin. Visit our website, http://www.PCNGuide.com, for more information.

## Medications to Ripen the Cervix

*Synthetic prostaglandins* are medications that mimic prostaglandin, which is a hormone normally released by the body to ripen the cervix. They're used when the cervix is unfavorable for induction (see page 281).

One type of synthetic prostaglandin is prostaglandin E2, which releases the medication over a period of hours in a tampon-like device (Cervidil). The device can be removed if it causes problems.

Another type of synthetic prostaglandin is prostaglandin E1 or *misoprostol (Cytotec)*. It comes either in a pill that's taken orally or in a gelatin capsule that's placed next to the cervix. See page 283 for more information.

Misoprostol and other synthetic prostaglandins have potential undesirable side effects. (Visit our website for more information.) Prostaglandins shouldn't be placed in the vagina after membranes have ruptured. (Misoprostol can be given orally to minimize the risk of infection.[23]) Guidelines from the ACOG state that women with a prior cesarean birth shouldn't use prostaglandins, because of the increased risk of uterine rupture.[24]

## Procedure for Medical Induction

If you've consented to a medical induction, here's what you may expect:

- You may be asked to call the hospital before leaving home for your scheduled appointment. The hospital staff can't predict the number of women who will be in labor. If the maternity unit is especially busy, you may be told to call back in a few hours to confirm that they have room for you. Be prepared for this possibility so you aren't overly frustrated and disappointed if your appointment is postponed at the last minute.
- Be prepared to wait. It may take a few hours to ripen your cervix. Depending on the techniques used, the reasons for the induction, and policies in your hospital, you may be able to leave the hospital and return periodically for assessment. Once your cervix is ripe, Pitocin (and possibly AROM) is used to stimulate contractions; it sometimes takes several hours to a day to bring on effective labor contractions. Make sure you bring magazines, books, puzzles, needlework, or other projects with you to pass the time.
- While you're in the hospital, expect to have intravenous fluids containing Pitocin and continuous electronic fetal monitoring (EFM) to keep track of your contractions and record how well your baby tolerates them. Continuous EFM restricts your ability to use self-help comfort measures. Ask to use *wireless (or telemetry) monitoring*, which allows you to walk and use the shower or bath. If wireless EFM isn't available, try to move around as best you can. Also, ask to have the IV fluids hung from a pole on wheels to allow you to walk.
- Expect to become hungry if hospital policy restricts eating while receiving Pitocin. The drug increases the risk of a cesarean section, and many hospitals restrict any food, to reduce your risks if you need general anesthesia. (See page 228 for more on eating during labor.) If your induction takes more than a day, you'll probably get a chance to eat.[26]
- Be prepared for contractions that become intense soon after they begin, especially if Pitocin doses are increased quickly. You may ask if you can receive lower doses that are increased gradually, in hopes of simulating early labor and better coping with the contractions. However, this method prolongs labor. Weigh these complex choices with your caregiver.

## The Strange Story of Misoprostol (Cytotec)[25]

In the mid-1990s, misoprostol was introduced as a quick, inexpensive way to ripen the cervix and induce labor. A drug company had introduced the medication for the treatment of stomach ulcers. Its use for labor induction was never approved by the FDA, and it continues to be considered "off-label."

Misoprostol seemed to be a success, because it helped induce labor quickly; however, along with fast labors came severe contractions (uterine hyperstimulation) and distressed babies. Many mothers and babies suffered physical harm, and some died. Many women found misoprostol-induced labor to be traumatic.

After several years of controversy, extensive research determined that overly high doses had caused the dangerous side effects of misoprostol. If it's given in low doses (typically 25 micrograms for vaginal use and 50 micrograms for oral use) and no more frequently than every four to six hours, misoprostol is about as safe (and much less expensive) than other ripening methods. Sometimes, low doses are all that's needed to ripen the cervix and start labor; however, misoprostol is usually used along with Pitocin and AROM. If labor hasn't progressed with repeated doses, or if the baby becomes distressed, the drug is discontinued.

If your caregiver recommends misoprostol, ask the key questions on page 9 so you can make an informed decision about whether it's right for you.

# Challenges That Arise in Labor

The following sections describe issues that can challenge labor progress, including possible causes of prolonged active labor and self-help measures and medical approaches for resolving them. Concerns about the baby's well-being in labor are also addressed.

## PROLONGED ACTIVE LABOR

In the first stage of labor, the early phase is prolonged if it takes longer than usual for the cervix to dilate to 5 or 6 centimeters and enter the active phase. Prolonged early labor generally doesn't cause problems for the mother or baby, and usually resolves with time, self-care, and changes to the environment that reduce stress and increase the body's release of oxytocin, the hormone that causes contractions. (See page 175 for information on prolonged early labor.)

Typically in active labor, cervical dilation speeds up, contractions become more painful, and labor progresses with each contraction. If labor slows or stops in this phase, it may indicate problems with the mother or baby. By using the self-help measures described in the next section (and the measures for prolonged early labor described on page 175), a woman may speed up prolonged active labor. However, if these measures don't work, medical interventions may be required.

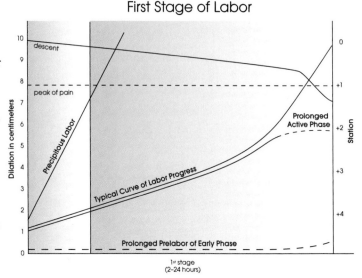

First Stage of Labor

## *Causes of Slow Labor and Self-Help Measures to Speed Up Active Labor*

In many cases, you may be able to solve the problem on your own, depending on how rested you are, the amount of pain you have, your state of mind, and whether you have emotional support and encouragement. The way to speed up active labor depends on which of the following factors is causing the delay:

### Full bladder

Empty your bladder every hour or so. A full bladder can delay labor progress, increase pain, and possibly cause problems with urination after the birth. If for some reason, you can't empty your bladder, a catheter (a tube that's run through your urethra to your bladder), may be necessary.

### Medications

If you've received pain medications or other drugs that may have slowed your labor, allow time for them to wear off, if it's safe to do so.

### Immobility

If you've been lying in one position for a long time, walk or stand to let gravity help your baby descend. Or shift from lying on one side to sitting or to the hands-and-knees position. Use these positions even if you're attached to an IV line and an electronic fetal monitor.

## Ineffective contractions

To enhance the effectiveness of contractions, try acupressure, nipple stimulation, walking, and standing.

## Unfavorable presentation or position of baby

To improve the presentation or position of your baby within your pelvis (see page 136), try the techniques described on page 287.

## Dehydration and lack of nourishment

To keep hydrated and provide fuel for the hard work of labor, drink enough fluids to prevent thirst and eat foods that give you energy (if allowed). If you're vomiting frequently IV fluids may help prevent dehydration and get labor moving again.

## Exhaustion or stress

If you're discouraged, anxious, fearful, or exhausted, you need reassurance, encouragement, a safe and nurturing environment, and help with comfort measures and relaxation techniques (see chapter 12). A doula can relieve your emotional stress and uncertainty, and can reassure and guide both you and your partner (see page 20). You can also reduce stress and build confidence by referring to the information you've learned in this book and in other resources, or in your childbirth classes. Lastly, don't forget your nurses and hospital staff—their help can keep you going.

## Advice from the Authors

Remember that "6 is the new 4"—active labor isn't prolonged until the cervix has dilated to 6 centimeters and labor hasn't progressed further for several hours. As authors of this book, our goal is to improve your chances of having a healthy vaginal birth. This new approach to normal active labor may mean longer labors for some women, but it also means that most women will have a better chance for a vaginal birth, which is safer for both mother and baby under these circumstances and leads to a quicker, easier recovery.

## *Medical Care for Prolonged Active Labor*

Until recently, a normal active labor was believed to begin when the cervix had dilated to 4 centimeters, after which time dilation would speed up significantly. Active labor was considered prolonged if dilation continued at a rate of less than 1.2 centimeters per hour (for a first-time mother) or 1.5 centimeters per hour (for a woman who's given birth before). In that case, actions were taken to speed up labor (for example, AROM and Pitocin). If those interventions didn't work in a reasonable amount of time, the labor was labeled "failure to progress" and a cesarean delivery was performed.

This definition of prolonged active labor, however, has become outdated. It was based on studies of labor progress that took place in the 1950s, when childbearing women were generally younger and weighed less than women today.[27] Maternity care was also different. Medications for pain relief differed from those available today. Fewer inductions and cesareans were performed, and instrumental deliveries were more common.

Numerous studies of healthy normal labor patterns in today's women with modern labor management have found that dilation can take five to seven hours to progress from 4 to 6 centimeters—three times longer than the rate found in the studies done over half a century ago.[28] Labor typically speeds up around 6 (not 4) centimeters in both first-time mothers and those who've given birth before. These studies show that diagnosing slow labor progress and performing a cesarean before the cervix has dilated 6 centimeters is premature, unnecessary, and harmful, unless other medical problems arise that make a cesarean necessary. In 2014 the ACOG recommended that a cesarean for failure to progress shouldn't be considered until labor hasn't progressed in the four to six hours *after* the cervix has dilated to at least 6 centimeters, even with AROM and Pitocin.[29]

Unfortunately, cesareans for failure to progress are still done in many hospitals if labor progress stops or remains slow at 4 or 5 centimeters. When this out-of-date practice is completely abandoned, the cesarean rate will go down significantly.

What happens if labor progress from 4 to 6 centimeters is slow? Your caregiver's goal is to maintain the well-being of you and your baby. You may receive vaginal exams to check dilation and your baby's descent or rotation. Some caregivers may assess the position of your baby with an ultrasound scan, which is more accurate than a vaginal exam. Your baby's heart rate is monitored closely, possibly with continuous electronic fetal monitoring. If you and your baby are tolerating labor, you can use self-help techniques (see page 284) to determine the cause of the delay and help resolve the problem. If your or your baby's ability to tolerate a long labor is a concern, medical treatment may include IV fluids to prevent or treat dehydration, medications for relaxation and pain relief, rupture of your membranes (see page 282), or Pitocin to speed up labor.

In a planned home birth or birth at a birth center, a transfer to the hospital will be necessary if you need Pitocin or if your baby isn't tolerating a long labor well. Prolonged active labor is the most common reason for transfer to the hospital during labor in a first-time mother who has planned for an out-of-hospital birth.

If your baby's heart rate shows that he isn't tolerating labor well, or if your labor doesn't speed up after several hours of receiving Pitocin, you and your caregiver may decide a cesarean delivery is necessary.

## Slow Active Labor Caused by Your Baby's Position

One of the most common reasons for prolonged labor is that the baby is in an unfavorable position (*malposition*) and doesn't fit into the pelvis well. The most favorable position for birth is the baby's head down (vertex presentation) and facing the mother's back (occiput anterior, or OA, position). See page 160 for more information.

While about 70 percent of babies begin labor in an OA position, about 25 percent are in the OP position (the baby faces the mother's front). When the baby is OP, cervical dilation and the baby's descent might not progress efficiently, and labor may take longer for the baby to rotate into position for birth. Sometimes, the baby's head is tilted to the side with one ear close to a shoulder (*asynclitism*), or he may have a hand by his cheek or under his chin. Both of these subtle malpositions can slow dilation and descent, because the head doesn't press evenly against the cervix. The baby also doesn't fit through the pelvis as well, because the side of the head or the head and the hand are larger than the crown of the head.

By the transition phase of labor, most babies in a malposition have moved to OA. At birth, only 3 to 5 percent of babies are OP. When low in the birth canal, some OP or asynclitic babies can be repositioned by the caregiver, who reaches inside the vagina and manually rotates the baby's head to the OA position. This procedure has a significant success rate.[30] Other babies are born in the "persistent OP" position (sometimes called "sunny side up") or in the "persistent asynclitic" position. Still others are born vaginally by vacuum extraction or forceps delivery, or are born by cesarean delivery.

Less common and more serious problems arise if the baby's brow, face, shoulder, buttocks, or feet are coming out the birth canal first (*malpresentation*). See page 136 for more information.

### Identifying a Malposition

It isn't easy to diagnose problems with the baby's position, especially by vaginal exam or by feeling the baby through the mother's belly. Even seasoned caregivers and nurses often misidentify position.[31] Ultrasound is a more accurate way to identify a baby's position. Some hospitals have portable ultrasound devices on the maternity floor and can identify position in less than a minute.

Clues that suggest problems with position include delayed dilation or uneven dilation, in which most of the cervix dilates completely but the rest of it doesn't, creating a "cervical lip." Another clue is a swollen cervix that

seems to have closed a few centimeters. You can also assume your baby
is malpositioned if you experience any of the following:

- Your labor slows after a period of good progress.
- You have irregular or coupling contractions (occur in pairs with
  a short break between the first and second contractions).
- You have back pain that occurs during and sometimes between
  contractions (back labor).

Although back pain sometimes occurs when the baby is well-positioned,
it's more likely if he's malpositioned. If you have pain in your lower back,
it's probably caused by your baby's head pressing unevenly on your sacrum,
straining your sacroiliac joints. Sometimes, back pain is caused by variations
in the anatomy of your pelvis or spine. Be aware that a prolonged labor with
back pain is exhausting and discouraging. Support from your partner and
others is key to coping with back labor.

### What You Can Do If Your Baby Is Malpositioned

At any point in labor, try the positions and comfort measures described on pages 247–249 to help your baby find
her way into and through your pelvis and to manage any back pain. On the Road Map of Labor (see page 444),
reminders of these techniques on the rocky "detour for back pain" are given. If you continue using these positions
and comfort measures for an hour or two at a time, you may be able to keep the pain tolerable and guide your
baby into a favorable position. Once your baby's head fits into your pelvis, back pain often decreases and labor
progress improves.

## Medical Approaches to Relieve Back Pain

If you continue to have intense back pain even while using the positions and comfort measures described on
pages 247–249, here are a few medical approaches that may help relieve the pain.

### Sterile Water Block

If you have severe back pain but want to minimize use of pain medications, the *sterile water
block* is a simple and promising option. Your caregiver or nurse injects tiny amounts of sterile
water into four places on your lower back. The procedure provides almost immediate pain
relief by rapidly increasing endorphin production in the area around the injection sites. The
effects last for an hour or two, and the procedure can be repeated. Be aware that the first
injections may feel like bee stings for up to thirty seconds, but additional injections may be
less noticeable. While the sterile water block can relieve back pain, it doesn't relieve abdominal pain.[32]

    If you're interested in the sterile water block, discuss it with your caregiver. Despite its benefits, the procedure
isn't widely used in North America, even though any nurse, physician, or midwife has the skills to do it.

### Medications for Pain Relief

If you have severe back pain during a prolonged active labor, you can request an epidural block, spinal narcotics,
or other medications (see chapter 13). In particular, an epidural can offer you almost total pain relief until very
late in labor, which may give you an opportunity to sleep. It can also reduce your body's production of stress
hormones, which may be slowing your labor. Under these circumstances, an epidural may make a vaginal birth
possible and help you avoid a cesarean for failure to progress.

## In Their Own Words

According to several ultrasound
scans, my baby had turned a
couple times during labor, from
face-up (OP) to face-down (OA)
and back again. At the time of
the birth, she was face-up, which
gave me a lot of back pain.
Luckily, we had a friend present
who was training to be a doula.
She did a wonderful job massaging my back during contractions,
which made the pain tolerable.
—Linda

## CONCERNS ABOUT THE BABY'S WELL-BEING

Going through labor is good for babies and helps most healthy full-term babies get a better start in life. Contractions jump-start many processes that improve a baby's transition to life outside the womb, such as breathing, temperature regulation, alertness, and suckling. See page 182 to learn how a baby's response to labor is monitored.

During a contraction, the baby's heart rate changes in response to how much oxygen is available. Most babies handle the variations well. However, a few babies don't tolerate labor well, and their heart rate patterns show that they might not be getting the ideal amount of oxygen during contractions. If the baby's heart rate patterns are categorized as indeterminate or abnormal, she may require closer monitoring, further testing, or immediate intervention such as a cesarean. See page 182 for more information.

The presence of *meconium* (a baby's first bowel movement) in the amniotic fluid may also indicate that a baby's heart rate has adjusted—or is adjusting— to the varying amount of available oxygen during contractions. When a baby's oxygen supply is low, her intestines contract to send oxygen-rich blood to other areas of her body that need oxygen the most (such as her brain). This contracting expels meconium from the intestines into the amniotic fluid, giving the fluid's normally clear color a brownish or greenish tint. (If a lot of meconium is present, the fluid becomes dark brown or black and thick.) When a woman's bag of waters breaks, the caregiver notes the presence of meconium and assesses the baby's health. See page 183 for more information.

EFM and the presence of meconium don't always mean that a baby is oxygen-deprived. However, caregivers won't hesitate to take measures to improve the baby's well-being if either assessment shows distress.

### Medical Care for Babies Who Show Signs of Distress

If a baby's heart rate pattern is considered indeterminate, he might or might not be adjusting well to the varying amounts of oxygen during contractions. Sometimes the baby solves the problem without any intervention. For example, if the baby is pressing on the umbilical cord and constricting the flow of oxygen-rich blood, he may shift his position so he moves off the cord, thereby restoring normal blood flow.

A baby with an indeterminate heart rate pattern needs to be monitored more closely, perhaps with internal EFM. Another way to monitor the baby is with fetal scalp stimulation. This procedure is reliable, simple, inexpensive, and can be repeated easily. During a vaginal exam, your caregiver lightly presses or scratches your baby's scalp. If your baby's heart rate speeds up, he's likely fine. If his heart rate doesn't react or slows down, he might not be tolerating labor well.

## Prolapsed Cord

During a normal vaginal birth, the umbilical cord stays high in the uterus as the baby descends through the birth canal and out the vagina. With a *prolapsed cord*, however, the cord slips below the baby so it's either in the vagina or lying between the baby and the cervix. Although a prolapsed cord is rare (about 1 in 400 pregnancies), it's a potentially serious complication because the baby's body can compress the cord, especially during contractions, and reduce the amount of oxygen available to her.

A prolapsed cord can occur when the membranes rupture with a gush of amniotic fluid and the cord slips toward the vaginal opening because the baby's body or head doesn't block its passage. This scenario can happen if the baby is premature or in a breech or transverse (lying sideways) presentation, or if her head isn't yet engaged in the pelvis and is still at a high station ("floating high") In a pregnancy with multiples, the risks of prematurity and malposition increase, which further raise the risk of prolapsed cord.

At your prenatal visits in late pregnancy, ask your caregiver to estimate your baby's position by using ultrasound scans or feeling your abdomen by hand. If your membranes rupture with a gush and you know that your baby is in a breech or transverse position, take the following steps to help ensure her well-being:

- Get into an open knee-chest position (see page 247) so gravity can help move your baby away from your cervix and possibly off the cord. You might or might not be able to feel the cord in your vagina, but get into this position even if you can't feel the cord.
- Arrange for immediate transportation to the hospital.
- Walk quickly to the vehicle or ambulance, and get into the knee-chest position for the ride to the hospital.
- When you arrive at the hospital, tell the staff that you may have a prolapsed cord. If a prolapsed cord is confirmed, a nurse will insert a hand into your vagina to keep your baby off the cord, and you'll have a cesarean section as soon as possible. If the cord isn't prolapsed, you can resume your plans for coping with a normal labor.
- If your baby's head is still unengaged but low in your pelvis, you probably can follow your caregiver's advice for managing ruptured membranes (see page 166).

If you don't know whether your baby's head is low or high in your pelvis, the risk of a prolapsed cord is less if the position of the head is unknown than if the head is known to be high. Regardless, you may wish to take the above steps as a precaution until you get to the hospital and confirm the position of your baby's head.

To improve the baby's heart rate, the mother is typically asked to change position and breathe deeply on her own or through an oxygen mask. These measures are often enough to restore a baby's heart rate to normal. If the heart rate is abnormal, then one of several interventions is necessary. If the mother is receiving Pitocin and it's causing contractions that are too intense, the dose can be reduced to slow or stop contractions. If the mother isn't receiving Pitocin, she can receive a *tocolytic* (anticontraction) medication to slow or stop contractions. Having fewer, milder contractions allows oxygen levels (and thus the baby's heart rate) to improve. If the volume of amniotic fluid is too low to cushion the umbilical cord, the caregiver may use *amnioinfusion*, a procedure that replaces enough water in the uterus to remove the pressure on the cord caused by the baby's head or body.

If these interventions don't resolve the problem and the baby's condition worsens, a cesarean section may be necessary (see page 304).

# Prolonged Second Stage of Labor

The second stage of labor begins when your cervix is fully dilated and ends with the birth of your baby. In this stage, labor progress may slow or stop for the same reasons that can cause a prolonged active phase (such as exhaustion or a malpositioned baby). In those cases, the same measures used to resolve a prolonged active labor can be tried to resolve a prolonged second stage (see page 284). Sometimes, receiving an epidural prolongs the second stage. (See page 189 for information on pushing with an epidural.)

One problem that's unique to the second stage is a baby that doesn't descend through the birth canal, despite hours of pushing. In this situation, try the measures described below. In rare circumstances, a prolonged second stage is more difficult to resolve than usual. For example, the baby can fit through the upper part of the pelvis (pelvic inlet), but she can't rotate and descend through the lower part (pelvic outlet).

A second rare problem is a short umbilical cord, which can cause the baby's heart rate to slow during contractions or limit her descent because the cord can't stretch enough for her passage through the vaginal opening. Sometimes, a cord that's long enough can pose the same problem if it's wrapped around the baby; however, in most cases the cord remains loose enough to prevent such a problem. In both of these examples, a cesarean section may be required if time and the measures taken to resolve the problem aren't successful.

2nd stage

2nd stage
(typical descent = ½–3 hours)

Shoulder dystocia is a rare but potentially serious complication that occurs when the baby's head has been born, but the birth of her shoulders is delayed because they're too broad to fit through the pelvis. It becomes critical for the baby to finish being born quickly, because her oxygen supply from the cord may be reduced. The caregiver may ask the mother to change position, which may resolve the issue. The caregiver may also use skilled maneuvers to rotate the baby and deliver the shoulders. Often an episiotomy is necessary (see page 292), and sometimes the baby's collarbone breaks in the effort to get her out quickly. A newborn's collarbone is flexible and usually heals quickly.

## WHAT YOU CAN DO IF THE SECOND STAGE IS PROLONGED

If your baby isn't descending, a change in position can help resolve the problem, as long as your baby is handling labor well. Try squatting, lap squatting, the supported squat, or the dangle (see pages 238–240). These positions may be the best aids to help your baby descend and rotate because they use gravity and allow for maximum enlargement of the pelvic outlet.[33] You may also try the standing, semi-sitting, and hands-and-knees positions. Sometimes, rocking forward and back while on hands and knees gives the baby enough room to find her way. If you don't have apparent progress after twenty to thirty minutes in one position, change to another one.

If you can't use these positions because of your caregiver's preference or because an epidural limits your movements, or if you try them but they don't work, your caregiver may ask you to try the exaggerated lithotomy position, in which you're flat on your back with your knees drawn up toward your shoulders. This position may help your baby move beneath your pubic bone.[34]

If tension in your perineum seems to interfere with your ability to effectively bear down—even after receiving warm compresses and reminders to relax—try sitting on the toilet to encourage the muscles of your perineum to release (assuming you don't have an epidural).

If trying various positions doesn't enhance your labor progress, your caregiver may suggest that you use prolonged directed pushing (see page 252). In this situation, the advantages of prolonged pushing may outweigh the drawbacks.

## MEDICAL CARE FOR PROLONGED SECOND STAGE

With a prolonged second stage, the caregiver carefully monitors the baby's heart rate. If your baby seems to be tolerating labor, expect your caregiver to encourage you to continue your efforts to speed up labor, such as using various positions. However, your caregiver may recommend using a medical procedure if you experience any of the following:

- You're exhausted and can't push effectively.
- You've received medications that restrict your efforts and slow your labor.
- Pitocin augmentation isn't helping (see page 282).
- Your baby is no longer tolerating labor.
- You've been pushing for more than three hours (if a first-time mother) or more than two hours (if you've given birth before) without progress. If you've had an epidural or your baby is malpositioned, you may be allowed to push for a longer time.[35]

Medical procedures include manual rotation (see page 138); vacuum extraction, forceps delivery, and episiotomy (see page 292); and cesarean delivery (see chapter 15). Visit our website, http://www.PCNGuide.com, to learn more information.

## Routine Episiotomy

The use of episiotomy was once standard practice in maternity care, but well-designed studies performed in the 1990s found no benefit and some risks to routine episiotomy.[36] As a result, the practice has declined greatly over the years.

Caregivers who continue to perform routine episiotomies (some of whom have rates as high as 80 percent) hold on to two outdated, disproven beliefs. The first is that a spontaneous tear is always worse than an episiotomy. In fact, spontaneous tears are almost always smaller—and heal faster—than episiotomies. The second is that an intact perineum has been over-stretched and is therefore more damaged than one that has had an episiotomy. However, an intact perineum is rarely over-stretched, especially if the woman uses spontaneous bearing down techniques and doesn't lie on her back to push and give birth.

Other skilled caregivers reserve episiotomies for situations in which problems arise with the birth. These caregivers usually have episiotomy rates between 5 and 15 percent. (Many midwives' rates are less than 10 percent.) They point out that most spontaneous tears (which occur in half of all vaginal births) are smaller than the average episiotomy; furthermore, serious large tears are more likely to occur with an episiotomy than without one.

If avoiding an episiotomy is important to you, discuss it at a prenatal visit. Ask for your caregiver's opinion on the practice and on when it's necessary. If you're uncomfortable with the answers, you may want to consider changing caregivers (see page 18). In addition to choosing the right caregiver, follow the measures on page 193 to help safely avoid a tear or an episiotomy.

*Note:* Be aware that if your baby is in distress in the late second stage, your caregiver may decide that an episiotomy is necessary for your baby's well-being.

## *Episiotomy*

An *episiotomy* is a surgical incision of the perineum that enlarges the vaginal outlet. When necessary, the procedure is performed just before the baby's head is born, as the perineum is stretching. An episiotomy has been found to shorten the time to birth by five to fifteen minutes, which may be necessary  for the baby's well-being if he's in distress. A caregiver also may recommend an episiotomy if forceps are used to deliver the baby or if shoulder dystocia is suspected (see page 290).

After the birth, an episiotomy is repaired with sutures, and the mother may experience moderate to severe pain during the first few days. The pain gradually lessens over the next few weeks. See page 326 for more on information on healing and comfort after an episiotomy or a spontaneous tear.

## *Vacuum Extraction and Forceps Delivery*

A *vacuum extractor* is a silicone suction cup, and *forceps* are long steel tongs. Either instrument can be applied to the baby's head to help make a vaginal birth possible, although vacuum extraction is used more often than the forceps. Both instruments are used much more frequently on women who have received epidural pain medication than on women who haven't. Overall, vacuum extraction is used for 3 percent of births, and forceps for less than 1 percent.[37]

To use either instrument, the caregiver pulls on it as the woman pushes during contractions. When used according to established safety protocols, both instruments are generally safe for babies, although bruising, swelling, and scraping of the baby's head often occur. To protect the baby, the caregiver discontinues use of the instruments if it's obvious the baby isn't descending. At that point, a cesarean section becomes necessary.

# Problems after the Birth

The following sections describe complications that can occur after the birth, including problems with the third stage of labor. Also discussed are what to expect if your baby has a health problem or worse, as well as care options you may want to consider now, before labor begins.

## COMPLICATIONS IN THE THIRD STAGE OF LABOR

The third stage of labor begins with the birth of your baby and ends with the delivery of the placenta. The following sections describe complications that may arise during this stage.

### Postpartum Hemorrhage

*Postpartum hemorrhage* is the excessive loss of blood (more than 500 milliliters or 2 cups) during the first twenty-four hours after the birth. It occurs in 2 to 4 percent of women.[38] Treatment may require IV fluids or a blood transfusion if the bleeding is severe. Also, the excessive loss of blood may lead to symptoms of shock, such as rapid pulse, pale skin, trembling, faintness, feeling cold, and sweating.

The treatment of postpartum hemorrhage depends on its cause. The three main causes are uterine atony; vaginal, cervical, or perineal lacerations; and retained placenta or placental fragments. The following sections describe these conditions and their treatments.

#### Uterine Atony

*Uterine atony* is poor uterine muscle tone, and it's the most frequent cause of postpartum hemorrhage. To prevent atony, many caregivers routinely use Pitocin (intravenous or intramuscular) as the baby is being born—a practice that has significantly reduced postpartum hemorrhage. Some caregivers use Pitocin only if the need becomes clear, especially with women in excellent health and at very low risk for hemorrhage. Other treatments a caregiver or nurse might try include massaging the uterus to encourage contractions and having the mother nurse the baby or lightly stroke her nipples to stimulate the release of oxytocin and help contract the uterus.

#### Lacerations

Lacerations (or tears) of the cervix, vagina, or perineum may occur spontaneously during birth or as an extension of an episiotomy. If you have lacerations, they'll be sutured to control bleeding. Your vagina also may be packed with sterile gauze to further stop blood flow. (See page 326 for comfort measures that you can take to ease the pain of a laceration.)

#### Retained Placenta or Placental Fragments

If the placenta or fragments of it aren't expelled from your uterus, they interfere with postpartum contractions and allow blood to flow freely through vessels at the site where the placenta attached to your uterine wall. To stop the blood flow, the placenta or fragments are removed and you receive Pitocin to contract your uterus. You can promote further contractions by massaging your uterus (fundal massage—see page 199) and by breastfeeding your baby (which stimulates the release of oxytocin).

Very rarely, the placenta doesn't separate from the uterine wall (placenta accreta). The only safe treatment for this serious complication may be a hysterectomy (removal of the uterus).

# PREMATURE OR SERIOUSLY ILL NEWBORN

Although most babies are born healthy and normal, others regrettably are not. Some babies are born prematurely; some have health problems (congenital problems) or birth defects. In these situations, parents experience a great deal of anxiety and despair. The following sections describe what to expect if your baby has a health problem, as well as care options you may want to think about. By learning about and discussing these issues during pregnancy, you can have peace of mind that you won't have to make uninformed decisions when grief or worry is affecting your ability to think clearly.

## Care of the Premature Baby

If your baby is born prematurely, expect your caregiver and the hospital staff to take the following measures:

- If your baby is born before her lungs matured on their own or before the corticosteroids have had enough time to mature her lungs, treatment for respiratory distress syndrome (RDS) becomes necessary. Treatment may include administering oxygen, mechanical assistance with breathing, or instilling *surfactant* into the lungs. This substance allows the lungs to expand during an inhalation and remain partially inflated during an exhalation.[39]
- Depending on your baby's condition, you might not be allowed to hold her right after the birth.
- If your baby is very premature, you may need to transfer to a hospital with an intensive care nursery and highly trained nurses and neonatologists. Because your baby is at high-risk, her heart rate may require continuous monitoring. Most premature babies stay in a nursery until they can breathe on their own, stay warm at room temperature, and breastfeed or take a bottle.

## Seriously Ill Newborns and NICU

If your baby has a serious health problem and is placed in a *special care nursery* or a *neonatal intensive care unit (NICU)*, you can help by contributing to his care whenever possible. If your baby is transferred to a hospital that specializes in the care of seriously ill babies, you may be able to arrange for an early discharge from your maternity hospital so you can visit your baby. (If an early discharge isn't possible, your partner may need to divide time between visiting you and being with your baby.) Because of the special nutritive qualities of colostrum and breast milk (see chapter 19), you may want to nourish your baby by breastfeeding him or by bottle-feeding him your expressed milk. If your baby can't suck or swallow, he may still be able to receive your colostrum by tube feeding.

The number of people and machines involved in your baby's care may worry and exhaust you. You may become impatient with staff if you feel that they're not fully answering your questions about your baby's condition, treatment, and prognosis. To help you feel more in control of the situation, consider keeping a notebook with you so you can jot down your questions as they arise and record the answers as you receive them. You can also keep track of your baby's treatment and progress.

## Kangaroo Care

Kangaroo care is a method of treatment in which newborns are kept in skin-to-skin contact with one of their parents as much as possible. It also allows parents to offer something very special to their baby that no one else can provide.

As soon as the newborn's condition is stable, he's placed nude on his mother's bare chest or abdomen (or that of the other parent or loved one, if the mother is unavailable). A blanket covers both of them. With kangaroo care, the baby spends more time in deep sleep, more time in the quiet-alert state (see page 377), and less time crying. He has fewer episodes of apnea (suspension of breathing) and fewer episodes of brady-cardia (slow heart rate). His temperature stabilizes, and he gains weight more rapidly, which can lead to a shorter hospital stay if he's ill or was born pre-maturely. Although all babies benefit from kangaroo care, a premature baby's health particularly improves. The skin-to-skin contact—during which he can smell his parents' familiar scent, hear their heartbeats,[40] and absorb their body heat—often helps ease any anxiety he may have from being connected to the various monitors, IV lines, and tubes for oxygen and food. Parents are encouraged to give kangaroo care for extended peri-ods several times a day, which results in faster growth and earlier discharge of the baby.[41] Singing to your baby may also help keep him calm and focus his energy on growing, not crying.

## *Coping with a Seriously Ill Newborn*

If your baby has a health problem, you and your partner will need to support each other and rely on supportive family, friends, and community resources to help you with the care of other children, transportation, food preparation, housecleaning, and notification of events to extended family, coworkers, and others. You may want to join a support group for parents in a similar situation.

Your baby may require prolonged hospitalization. Most hospitals recognize that having parents participate in their baby's care benefits both the child and the adults. Expect the hospital staff to encourage you to spend as much time with your baby as you can. They may even provide you with sleeping arrangements.

# INFANT DEATH

Some babies are born dead (stillbirth) or die around the time of birth from genetic abnormalities, birth trauma, or infection. These tragic events are uncommon, but they do occasionally occur. If you have a stillbirth or your baby dies soon after birth, you'll have to make several tough decisions. The emotional grief and sadness will consume you, making it difficult to think clearly. To ensure that everyone knows your preferences for care, it's helpful to think about them in advance and note them in a special birth plan (see page 151).

To help you begin thinking about your options, ask your caregiver or childbirth educator how families are typically cared for after a stillbirth or infant death. Then begin thinking about your specific preferences. For example, if your baby dies before labor begins, do you want your labor induced? If so, when? Do you want to be awake and participate in the birth? Do you want the support of a doula or someone other than your partner (who will also need support during this difficult time)?

After the birth, do you want to recover in an area that's separate from other mothers and babies on the postpartum floor, or somewhere else in the hospital? Do you want to have an early discharge from the hospital? Do you want to have an autopsy done to help find the cause of death?

What may make your memories of your baby more meaningful? You may want to hold your baby so you can physically acknowledge her existence. You may want to name your baby or have a religious ceremony for her, such as a baptism. You may want to photograph her, have her footprints taken, or obtain a lock of her hair. You may want to have a funeral or memorial service to provide an opportunity for family and friends to grieve together, say good-bye to your baby, and express their love and concern for you.

## Coping with an Infant Death

If your baby is stillborn or dies after the birth, you and your partner will need the opportunity to grieve. Although grieving is inevitable and necessary for coming to terms with your loss, it's a painful and exhausting experience. You feel often overwhelming numbness, sadness, shock, disbelief, fear, anger, blame, and guilt. Make sure you and your partner frequently discuss what each of you is feeling; your reactions during the grieving process may differ at times. Rely on any emotional and practical help that family, friends, and community resources can provide. Also consider joining a group for parents who have experienced an infant death. While nothing can take away the pain of losing a baby, such a group can offer support at an extremely difficult time. (See appendix C for a list of resources.)

To help you accept the death of your baby, at some point in the grieving process you'll need to review the birth experience and reflect on it. Recall the events with your partner, caregiver, doula, attending nurse, or childbirth educator. Use their recollections to help you write a record of your birth experience. Because remembering these events can be overpowering, consider asking a counselor, therapist, hospital chaplain, or spiritual leader to help you work through your emotions.

Take plenty of time (months to years) to heal emotionally and physically. Eventually, you and your partner will reach a level of acceptance, although the sorrow may always remain. Allow yourselves to acknowledge your baby's life and savor the good memories from pregnancy, the birth, and the special time you had with this special child.

# Key Points to Remember

- Although most labors are normal, complications sometimes arise. Many problems are anticipated because of conditions such as a pregnancy with multiples, a preexisting illness in the mother, malposition, or developmental problems in the baby. Other problems are unexpected, such as a premature birth, post-date pregnancy, prolonged labor, distress in the baby, or postpartum hemorrhage.
- When a complication in childbirth arises, numerous medical and nonmedical interventions are available to increase the chances of fixing the problem and improving the well-being of both you and your baby. By becoming fully informed about these interventions, you can decide whether they're right for you and can participate meaningfully in your care.
- Although rare and often unexpected, tragedies in childbirth—such as injury to the mother, serious health problems for the baby, or even death of the baby—can occur. To help you cope should such a misfortune happen to you, it's wise to think about your care preferences and make any practical decisions during pregnancy, when you can think about them clearly.

# CHAPTER 15

# All about Cesarean Birth

A *cesarean birth* (also called a "cesarean section," "C-section," "cesarean delivery," or simply "cesarean") is a surgical procedure used to deliver a baby through incisions in the mother's abdomen and uterus. It's the most common surgery performed in hospitals in the United States. In high-risk situations, a cesarean can be a lifesaving procedure, vital for preserving the health of mothers and babies. While a cesarean is a relatively safe and routine procedure, it's still major surgery and should be used only when its potential benefits outweigh its possible risks.

# Cesarean Birth Trends[1]

In 1970 about 5 percent of birthing women in the United States had a cesarean. From 1985 to 2001, the overall cesarean birth rate ranged from 20 percent to 22 percent. Then the rate began increasing dramatically. From 2007 to 2013, 32 to 33 percent of *total births* were by cesarean. For women who hadn't had a previous cesarean, the chance of a having one for the first time, or a *primary cesarean*, ranged from 22 percent to 24 percent.

Cesarean rates vary greatly by location: One state's rate averages 23 percent, while another state's rate averages almost 40 percent. Rates also vary among hospitals, ranging from 7 percent to nearly 70 percent of deliveries. Studies have examined whether this variation is because of the types of women who gave birth in each hospital (for example, if a hospital admitted only very high-risk patients, the expectation is that it'd have a higher cesarean rate than a hospital that admitted only very low-risk patients). However, a hospital's high cesarean rates typically don't apply only to its high-risk patients; they apply to *all* women giving birth at that facility. In other words, no matter a woman's age, weight, ethnicity, or socioeconomic status, her risk of having a cesarean at that hospital is higher than at a hospital with low cesarean rates. These studies suggest that the way caregivers practice medicine at a given hospital has a clear impact on the hospital's cesarean rates.

The reasons for the increase in cesareans have been debated. When compared to pregnant women of just a generation ago, more of today's pregnant women are older, obese, or carrying multiples—factors that can increase the risk of cesarean. However, cesarean rates have increased for *all women*. The majority of cesareans are for somewhat subjective diagnoses, such as indeterminate or abnormal fetal heart rate, failure to progress, and suspected macrosomia (big baby). It's possible that the rates of these problems haven't changed much; rather, caregivers have begun to lower the threshold at which they decide a cesarean is needed. As cesarean birth has become safer, caregivers may be more likely to consider it sooner.

Many experts believe that too many babies are born by cesarean. In 2014 the American Congress of Obstetricians and Gynecologists (ACOG) and the Society for Maternal-Fetal Medicine released this statement: "The rapid increase in cesarean birth rates from 1996 to 2011 without clear evidence of concomitant [simultaneous] decreases in maternal or neonatal morbidity or mortality [injury or death in the mother or baby] raises significant concern that cesarean delivery is overused." They recommended several ways to safely reduce the cesarean rate, including increasing the use of continuous labor support, changing how failure to progress and fetal heart rates are evaluated, changing how induction is used, and changing how breech presentation and multiples are cared for. Those recommendations have been incorporated throughout this book, although some might not yet be common practice with caregivers.

# Risks and Benefits of Cesarean Birth

Cesareans may be planned, unplanned, or emergency surgeries. With a *planned cesarean*, you may have weeks or months to learn the procedure's benefits and risks, explore whether vaginal birth is an option, and prepare a cesarean birth plan.

With an *unplanned cesarean*, you begin labor expecting a vaginal birth, then a problem arises (such as failure to progress) and you must make an unexpected decision. It may seem difficult to ask questions and make choices while coping with the challenges of labor, but there's usually time to discuss your options.

Despite the widespread use of the term *emergency cesarean*, this procedure is fairly rare. It occurs when a life-threatening situation arises and a physician must deliver a baby within minutes. Time for questions may be limited, and the mother must emotionally process events later.

When preparing your birth plan (see chapter 8), you may choose to write a "Plan B" to be used in case of an unplanned or emergency cesarean.

When considering a cesarean birth, you should weigh the surgery's possible risks against its potential benefits and against the risks and benefits of a vaginal birth.

## RISKS OF CESAREAN BIRTH[2]

Why does a high cesarean rate concern maternity care experts? At first glance, cesarean birth seems to be a quick, safe, and easy way to deliver a baby without the pain and uncertainty of labor. A closer look at the procedure, however, reveals major risks, leading experts to recommend limiting cesareans to only those cases in which vaginal birth is unsafe or impossible.

The following effects are more likely to happen with a cesarean birth than a vaginal birth. They're listed in order of most common side effects to rare complications.

### Effects on the mother

- longer hospital stay
- pain from the incision
- increased blood loss
- infection
- rehospitalization and/or admission to the intensive care unit (ICU)

## Reducing Your Chances of Having a Cesarean Birth

Read Ten Steps to Improve Your Chances of Having a Safe and Satisfying Birth on page 26. After reviewing those recommendations, also follow these guidelines:

1. If your baby is breech at thirty-five weeks, attempt to turn her using positions, sound, acupuncture, or chiropractic techniques. Ask your caregiver about external version (see page 138).

2. If labor progress is slow, try various positions and movement to speed it up. Or try self-help techniques, including nipple stimulation, relaxation techniques, eating or drinking, and emotional support to reduce fear and anxiety (see chapter 12). If your caregiver recommends a cesarean for failure to progress, ask these questions: "How much time do we have to decide? Can I labor for another hour before having a cesarean?" Look at the guidelines for failure to progress (see page 304). If your labor doesn't meet those guidelines (for example, if failure to progress is diagnosed before your cervix has dilated more than 6 centimeters), ask for clarification.

3. If your caregiver recommends a cesarean for concerns about your baby's heart rate, ask the following questions: "What else could help my baby's heart rate? Should I try changing positions? Using oxygen? Having amnioinfusion (see page 289)? Stopping medications? Can we use fetal scalp stimulation to check my baby's response?"

4. If you're uncomfortable with your caregiver's response, ask for a second opinion. Continue to ask questions until you feel that you understand your caregiver's answers. Once you do, you can make an informed decision.

Be prepared for the possibility that a cesarean may still be necessary for a safe birth. See page 320 for information on how to have the best possible cesarean birth.

- injury to the bowel, bladder, or ureter (a muscular tube which connects the kidney to the bladder)
- hysterectomy

- blood clots
- complications from anesthesia
- death (very rare)

### Effects on the baby

- less immediate contact with his mother
- more likely to have trouble breastfeeding
- breathing problems at birth
- admission to the neonatal intensive care unit (NICU)

- asthma
- scalpel injury during the surgery
- death (rare)

### Effects on future pregnancy and birth

- adhesions (excess scar tissue that binds together tissues in the abdomen)
- higher probability of cesarean birth
- higher rates of the potentially life-threatening conditions of placenta previa, placenta accreta, placental abruption, and ectopic pregnancy

- infertility or reduced fertility
- increased risk of uterine rupture
- doubled risk of stillbirth

## BENEFITS OF CESAREAN BIRTH (REASONS FOR A CESAREAN)

The benefits of a cesarean depend on why your caregiver has recommended the surgery. Below are reasons caregivers recommend a cesarean.

### Cesareans planned for clear medical reasons[5] (benefits outweigh the risks)

- placenta previa (see page 132) or a uterine tumor that blocks the cervix
- malformed or injured pelvis
- severe preeclampsia (see page 134)
- genital herpes, if the infection occurs in late pregnancy

- human immunodeficiency virus (HIV), if the viral load is over 1,000 copies per milliliter[6]
- transverse lie, in which the baby lies horizontally in the uterus
- twins if the first baby is breech; triplets or more
- certain birth defects, problems with the baby, or medical problems with the mother

### Cesareans planned for less clear medical reasons (some caregivers recommend a cesarean; others don't)

- prior cesarean (see page 315)
- recurrent genital herpes with active lesions at the beginning of labor

- breech presentation (see page 136)
- twins if the first baby is presenting head down
- large baby (see page 277)

### Cesareans planned without medical reason

- fear, convenience, and so on (see below)

**Unplanned cesareans for situations that arise in labor**

- failure to progress/cephalo-pelvic disproportion (see page 304)
- variations in the baby's heart rate that indicate possible distress (see also page 305)

**Emergency cesarean**

- placental abruption (see page 133)
- prolapsed cord (see page 289)
- uterine rupture (see page 315)
- urgent health problems with mother or baby

## Cesareans without Medical Reason

Some women request a cesarean birth because they fear vaginal birth, want to avoid labor pain, believe the surgery will prevent damage to their pelvic floor, want to schedule the birth for convenience, want to feel more in control of the birth, or have some other nonmedical reason. These planned cesareans are considered "maternal request cesareans" or "elective cesareans."

Elective cesareans have raised concern with maternity care experts because of the surgery's risks. In 2013 the ACOG stated that without a medical reason for cesarean delivery, "vaginal delivery is safe and appropriate and should be recommended." In particular, elective cesarean isn't recommended for women desiring several children because the risks of future problems (such as placenta previa and placenta accreta) increase with each cesarean. If an elective cesarean *is* chosen, it shouldn't be performed before thirty-nine weeks.[7]

If considering a cesarean, it's important to make an informed decision. Be sure to learn about both vaginal and cesarean birth. If your reason for requesting a cesarean is convenience (because of your circumstances, support needs, or your schedule or your caregiver's schedule), be aware of the long-term impact of the surgery. If your goal is to avoid labor pain, remember that although a planned cesarean may eliminate labor pain, it may result in weeks of painful recovery.

If your goal is to avoid sexual function problems and prevent urinary incontinence (preserve your pelvic floor), know that within a few months after the birth, there's no difference in sexual function between women who birthed vaginally and those who had a cesarean, and there's no difference in incontinence by one year after the birth. To limit your chances of developing perineal pain, tears, and incontinence in a vaginal birth, use side-lying or hands-and-knees position during the second stage of labor, don't hold your breath or strain for long periods, and avoid an episiotomy and forceps delivery. To limit your chances of incontinence throughout life, do Kegel exercises and squats, don't smoke, and maintain a healthy weight.

If fear of pain, fear of vaginal birth, or a need to feel in control is driving your desire for a cesarean, you can take steps to make vaginal birth seem more manageable. Take childbirth classes to better understand the reality of labor and learn pain-coping techniques; plan for an epidural; hire a doula for support; talk with women who have had positive birth experiences; and consider seeking counseling to address your fears.

In rare circumstances, these measures aren't enough and a cesarean may be appropriate for preserving your psychological well-being.

## Fact or Fiction?

*Because a planned cesarean is more predictable and controllable, it's safer for mothers and babies.*

**Fiction.** While cesarean surgery is a vital tool for coping with high-risk situations, it's not safer than a vaginal birth and shouldn't be used without a clear medical reason. Studies show that low-risk mothers who had planned cesareans are nearly three times more likely to suffer from severe complications or die than those who had vaginal births.[3] Likewise, babies born by planned cesareans are more likely to be admitted to the neonatal intensive care unit (NICU). In one study, the chance of infant death was 1.77 per 1,000 for babies born by cesarean. By comparison, the chance of death was 0.62 per 1,000 for babies born vaginally.[4]

# HOW COMMON IS EACH REASON FOR A CESAREAN?

The following is a rank-order list of the most common reasons caregivers give for a primary cesarean:

1. Failure to progress in labor (see below)
2. Concerns about the baby's heart rate (see page 305)
3. Baby that's breech or in another unfavorable position
4. Multiple gestation
5. Suspected macrosomia

About 40 percent of cesareans are planned, and about 60 percent are unplanned and occur because of problems or concerns that arise during labor.[8] The factors that lead to planned and emergency cesareans are typically beyond your control. For an unplanned cesarean, several choices could have been made that might have prevented the need for cesarean (see page 301). However, at the point in labor when cesarean is recommended, options are generally much more limited. If your caregiver recommends an unplanned cesarean, ask whether you might first try any alternatives before consenting.

## Understanding Failure to Progress

*Failure to progress* is the most common reason caregivers recommend a cesarean for first-time mothers. The term can mean two things:

- Labor is taking longer than expected for the cervix to dilate to 10 centimeters.
- The pushing stage is taking longer than expected.

A long labor or delivery isn't necessarily harmful, and if both mother and baby are doing fine, it's not automatically a reason for a cesarean. Some people call failure to progress "failure to wait long enough."

Sometimes caregivers diagnose failure to progress as macrosomia or *cephalo-pelvic disproportion (CPD)*, which means the caregiver believes the baby's head is too large to fit through the mother's pelvis. Even if you had ultrasound scans to check the size of your pelvis and your baby, they aren't always accurate. CPD is impossible to predict, because the position or angle of the baby's head—and not the baby's size—has a big influence on how the baby fits through the mother's pelvis. To help a baby of any size be in the best position for birth, mothers should move and change positions frequently in labor (see page 238).

A caregiver can't reliably diagnose failure to progress during the early phase (before your cervix is 6 centimeters dilated), because this phase can progress very slowly and still be normal (see pages 172–176). If you become exhausted during the early phase, medications may help you rest (see page 221).

Once you have moved into active labor (after 6 centimeters dilation), your labor should progress more rapidly. Some labors remain slow. As long as labor is progressing, slow labor isn't a reason for a cesarean. "Failure to progress" or "arrest of labor" should be diagnosed only if your cervix has dilated beyond 6 centimeters *and* you've had no cervical progress after four hours of strong contractions or six hours of contractions augmented with Pitocin.[9] If your caregiver is concerned about slow progress, ask what you can try to get labor moving (see page 290).

If progress is very slow during the pushing stage, ask your caregiver about using different positions, warm compresses, manual rotation of your baby's head, vacuum extraction, or forceps delivery to help birth your baby vaginally (see page 292).

Although trying these options may help labor progress, if they don't work—or if there are other factors, such as concerns about your baby's heart rate or your ability to continue pushing—your caregiver may recommend a cesarean.

## Understanding Concern about the Baby's Heart Rate

Concern about the baby's heart rate is the second most common reason for a primary cesarean. The baby's heart rate is put into one of three categories, according to the degree of concern. Category 1 is "normal." Category 2 is "indeterminate" (formerly called "nonreassuring"), which means the baby requires close monitoring and possibly further testing to ensure well-being. Category 3 is "abnormal" (formerly called "fetal intolerance of labor" or "fetal distress"), which means the baby requires prompt evaluation and possible treatment.[10]

Monitoring the baby's heart rate is how caregivers monitor his well-being (see page 182), but interpreting this heart rate is challenging. A change in fetal heart rate patterns may indicate that the baby is having problems. But a short-term change in the heart rate might just be a temporary problem that will fix itself. The heart rate can be affected by several factors, including pain medication, Pitocin, cervical exams, the mother's blood pressure, and fever in the mother. Monitoring the baby's heart rate electronically gives caregivers clues about the baby's *current* well-being. However, the following are reasons why electronic fetal heart rate monitoring isn't a reliable tool for determining a baby's *long-term* well-being:

- Interpretations of heart rate patterns vary widely among caregivers. When analyzing the same heart rate pattern, one caregiver may determine the baby is fine, while another may diagnose fetal distress.
- Heart rate monitoring has a high rate of *false positives*, in which the heart rate pattern appears abnormal but the baby is fine.
- While indeterminate and abnormal fetal heart rate patterns have led to an increased rate of cesareans, the surgery hasn't reduced the number of birth injuries or infant deaths.[11]

If a caregiver is concerned about your baby's heart rate, ask questions to learn how worrisome it is. Ask whether another caregiver would make the same interpretation. Ask about trying options to improve your baby's heart rate, such as changing position, using oxygen, amnioinfusion, reducing the Pitocin, or taking medications to slow contractions (see page 289). You can also ask your caregiver to do fetal scalp stimulation (see page 288).

# The Cesarean Procedure

Whether a cesarean is planned, unplanned, or an emergency, knowing the procedure demystifies the surgery and helps you prepare for having a cesarean birth.

## PREPARATION FOR A PLANNED CESAREAN

You'll be instructed not to eat anything for the eight hours before the surgery (in case you need general anesthesia) and to arrive at the hospital two hours before the procedure.

## PREPARING FOR THE SURGERY

First, a hospital staff member asks you to sign a consent form stating that you understand the reasons for the cesarean and its risks and benefits. A nurse shaves your abdomen and the upper portion of your pubic hair, then you're given a liquid antacid medication. The nurse starts an intravenous (IV) drip for fluids and medications, then inserts a catheter to drain urine from your bladder (to reduce the risk of bladder injury). You can request that the nurse insert the catheter after you've received anesthesia.

## ANESTHESIA

For a planned cesarean, most women have spinal blocks because of their ease of administration, rapid onset, and degree of anesthesia. Twenty percent of women have epidural anesthesia.

For an unplanned cesarean, if you already have an epidural catheter in place, the anesthesiologist increases the dosage of medication to numb you completely from chest to toes. If you don't, the anesthesiologist administers a spinal block. Epidurals and spinal blocks let you stay awake and alert, but prevent you from feeling pain during the surgery.

General anesthesia, which makes a woman unconscious for surgery, is used only for these rare situations:

- emergency cesareans, when the baby must be delivered within minutes
- unplanned cesareans in small hospitals with limited anesthesia services
- instances in which an anesthesiologist can't successfully place an epidural or spinal, or a woman can't tolerate a regional anesthetic

If you have general anesthesia, hospital policy might not allow your partner to be in the operating room. For more information on pain medications, see chapter 13.

## THE OPERATING ROOM

In the operating room (OR), the staff includes the primary obstetrician, an assisting physician or midwife, an anesthesiologist, a surgical nurse who handles sterile instruments, a nurse for your baby, and an assisting nurse. Others may be present if there are concerns about your baby's health. The anesthesiologist is next to your head throughout the surgery. Let this person know if you feel any pain, nausea, or other discomfort. To remain calm and relaxed, use the visualizations, slow breathing, and relaxation techniques that you learned in childbirth class or on pages 234–237.

During surgery, you're on your back, usually with a foam wedge under your left hip to reduce supine hypotension (see page 83). The nurse washes your abdomen with an antiseptic, drapes a sterile sheet over your body, and places a surgical screen at your chest to prevent you from viewing the surgery or touching the surgical area.

## Seeding and Feeding the Microbiome

Your microbiome is the collection of bacteria, fungi, and other organisms that live in and on your body. A balance of microbes establishes best health by helping with digestion, regulating the bowels, and protecting you from infection. Pregnancy, vaginal birth, skin-to-skin contact after birth, and breastfeeding help create a healthy microbiome for your baby. Antibiotics, cesarean birth, routine hospital procedures, and formula feeding can disrupt this process and affect a baby's long-term health. For example, babies born by cesarean aren't exposed to vaginal bacteria and are at increased risk for asthma, allergies, obesity, diabetes, and bowel disease. Here are steps you can take to build a healthy microbiome:

- **During pregnancy,** the following actions can increase your exposure to diverse healthy bacteria:
  - taking probiotic supplements (such as lactobacillus acidophilus and bifidobacteria)
  - eating probiotic foods that introduce healthy bacteria (fermented foods and foods with live cultures, such as yogurt, sour cream, sauerkraut, tempeh, miso, soy sauce, kimchi, sourdough breads, and kombucha)
  - eating prebiotic foods that feed healthy bacteria (onions, garlic, legumes, asparagus, and starchy vegetables, such as sweet potatoes, squash, turnips, carrots, parsnips, beets, and plantains)
- **During pregnancy and labor,** minimize your exposure to antibiotics. If they're needed, ask your caregiver about consuming probiotics or prebiotics while taking antibiotics or after the course of antibiotics has been completed.
- **If your baby will be delivered by cesarean,** ask to have him exposed to vaginal bacteria by swabbing his mouth, face, and hands with sterile gauze that was placed in the your vagina before the surgery.[12]
- **After the birth,** encourage the development of your baby's microbiome by taking the following actions:
  - Have immediate skin-to-skin contact with your baby. In the first few hours, a baby should be held primarily by his parents. Encourage others to look at your baby, but not touch him. Wait twenty-four hours to bathe your baby.
  - Feed your baby only breast milk for as long as possible.
  - Consider giving your newborn probiotics to help build gut flora (for all babies, but especially those who were exposed to antibiotics, delivered by cesarean, or formula-fed, probiotics may reduce diarrhea, ear infections, recurrent colds, eczema, colic symptoms, and obesity in later life).

*Note:* People who are critically ill or immune-suppressed should consult with a caregiver before taking probiotics. To learn more, visit our website: http://www.PCNGuide.com.

## THE SURGERY

First, the obstetrician cuts through your abdominal wall (skin, fat layer, and a fibrous layer of connective tissue called "fascia"), using a *transverse incision*, or horizontal cut, 4 to 6 inches across and 1 inch above your pubic bone (a bikini cut). Rarely, in unfavorable conditions (such as placenta previa or a transverse baby), for obese women, or in an emergency, this cut may be a vertical incision between the navel and pubic bone (a classical incision).

The obstetrician then manually separates your abdominal muscles and cuts through a fibrous tissue (the peritoneum) that encases your abdominal cavity. A low transverse incision is then made in your uterus. In some cases, it's a low vertical incision or a classical incision.

After making a small incision, the obstetrician stretches the opening wide enough for your baby's head to fit through. To control bleeding, the ends of cut blood vessels are cauterized, and you may smell a burning odor. If needed, your membranes are broken, and you soon hear the suctioning of amniotic fluid.

Then the obstetrician reaches in to lift out your baby as the assisting physician presses on the top of your uterus to help push out your baby. You may feel intense pulling and tugging while they work on you, but you shouldn't feel pain. The obstetrician first lifts out your baby's head (or, if breech, his buttocks), then may cup a hand around your baby or apply vacuum extraction to his head. Then fluids are suctioned from your baby's nose and mouth before the obstetrician lifts him completely out, clamps and cuts the umbilical cord, then holds him up for you to see.

## Immediate Baby Care

The operating room staff may care for your baby at a warming table or they may take your baby to the nursery. During a vaginal birth, contractions squeeze fluids out the baby's airway, but a baby born by cesarean doesn't have that advantage. For this reason, your baby's mouth and nose may need additional suctioning.

The staff evaluates your baby with Apgar scores and a newborn assessment and may do other procedures, including administering eye ointment, injecting vitamin K, and measuring height and weight (see pages 363–364).

If your baby is having trouble breathing (which is more likely after a cesarean than a vaginal birth), she may need assistance, supplemental oxygen, and extra observation in the nursery. If she's premature, she may be given surfactant medication, which makes breathing easier.

A cesarean surgery takes about one hour, but your baby is born just ten to fifteen minutes after surgery begins. As soon as possible after the birth, a nurse or your partner should bring your baby close to you. That person can hold your baby so you can get to know her while the obstetrician repairs the incisions. Or, ideally, your baby should be placed skin-to-skin on your chest.

## *During the Repair*

At the beginning of the repair, Pitocin is added to your IV to make your uterus contract and prevent excessive bleeding. Then the obstetrician manually removes the placenta and inspects it.

The obstetrician may lift out your uterus completely for repair or may do the repair internally. Some physicians feel they can do a better repair if the uterus is outside the abdomen; however, external repair can cause nausea and vomiting.[13] To close the incision in your uterus, the obstetrician uses stitches that will dissolve. Most experts recommend obstetricians use the double-layer suturing method,[14] which requires suturing both the inner and outer layers of the uterus, thereby creating a stronger scar that's less likely to reopen in future labors. The obstetrician then repairs your abdominal muscles, closes your skin with staples or stitches, and bandages the area.

During or after the surgery, you may feel nauseated, anxious, or panicky. You may tremble all over. Medications can help ease these discomforts, but may make you so drowsy that you sleep through your baby's first hours. Instead, try slow, deep breathing and ask for a cool cloth on your forehead to help ease nausea. Warm IV fluids or blankets over your shoulders can help reduce trembling. If you decide you need medications, ask for those that let you stay awake and alert.

After the surgery, you may return to the room where you labored, or you may go to a surgical recovery room. Then staff will transfer you to a postpartum room a few hours after the surgery.

## In Their Own Words

While they were finishing the surgery, I started shaking. I wanted to hold my baby, but I was worried the trembling would disturb her. They gave me medication for the shaking, but then I fell asleep for the next hour. I wish I had just put up with it and snuggled my baby. Instead, I slept for her first hour—and no one even thought to take a photo of her during that time, so I feel as though that part of her life was lost to me.
—*Maria*

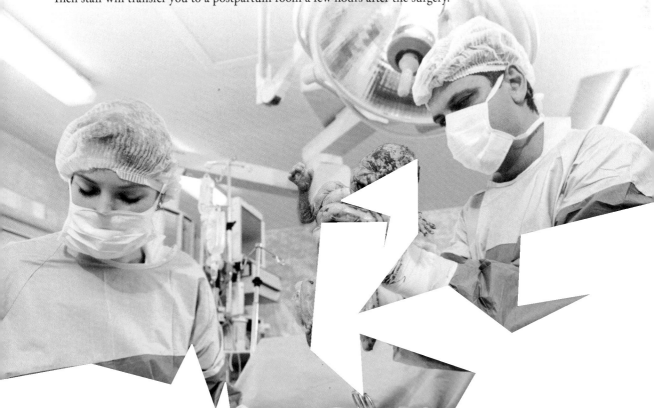

## Common Q & A

**Q:** My wife and I just found out she'll need a cesarean. I want to support her in the OR, but I'm worried I'll pass out when I see blood. What can I do?

**A:** Ask ahead of time if you can bring an extra support person (doula, friend, or family member) into the OR in case you need to leave. Be sure to let the anesthesiologist know about your concerns. That person will have good ideas for what you should do. Plan to stay close to your wife's head, where the surgical screen will prevent you from seeing the surgery, and focus on her face, giving encouragement and reassurance.

# A Note to Fathers, Partners, and Other Support Partners

When the surgery begins, you may feel pushed to the side as the experts do their work. But you have an important role to play. Your job is to support your partner and be the primary caregiver for your baby while the surgery is completed.

During the surgery, you'll sit by your partner's head, behind the sterile area. If you're interested, you may stand and watch the surgery, but you must stay behind the screen and out of the staff's way.

Whether you sit or stand, hold your partner's hand, talk to her, stroke her hair, and rub her shoulders. Help her with relaxation techniques and visualization. The medication may make her feel as though she can't take a deep breath. She may panic and say, "I can't breathe." Coach her through slow breathing and remind her that she's breathing well—otherwise, she couldn't talk!

After your baby is born, go where your partner directs you. Most likely, she'll want you to stay with your baby, but she may want you close by her side. If hospital policy allows for two support people in the OR, one of you can stay with your baby and the other can remain with your partner.

If you're with your baby in the OR, tell your partner everything you notice about your baby and describe all the details of what's happening to him. As you talk, your familiar voice will soothe your baby. Usually, you can touch and hold your baby shortly after birth. In that case, your main goal is to bring him to your partner as quickly as is safely possible so you can begin to bond as a family. During the time immediately after birth, your baby will benefit from being skin-to-skin with a parent. This close contact helps the baby regulate his breathing and temperature. If possible, hold him on your partner's bare chest while surgery is completed. If not, open up your surgical gown and tuck the baby inside under your shirt so he's skin-to-skin with you. Sing to your baby. Your familiar voice may soothe him.

If you go with your baby to the nursery, or if medication and the stress of the surgery makes your partner fall asleep, pay attention to all the events so you can tell her about them later. Take lots of photos. Think of other ways you can capture these moments for her. For example, you may ask visitors (even grandparents) to wait to hold your baby until after your partner has had a chance.

Remember that it's important for your partner and baby to begin breastfeeding as soon as possible after the birth. Babies often become sleepy an hour or two after birth, so it's best if the first feeding happens before then. Some mothers can begin breastfeeding in the OR while their surgeries are completed, but others begin nursing in the recovery room. If your partner is groggy from medication, she may need your help holding your baby as he nurses. If she has trouble latching him onto her breast, ask a nurse, doula, or lactation consultant for help. You may be tempted to help her rest by feeding your baby by bottle, but introducing a bottle at this time may make breastfeeding challenging. Get the contact information of a local lactation consultant or breastfeeding hotline you can call if you have breastfeeding questions when you're back home.

# Recovery

After you've had a cesarean birth, you experience all the normal parts of postpartum physical recovery (see chapter 16), and you're recovering from major surgery!

For the first twenty-four hours, you need help doing everything—holding your baby, rolling over, sitting up, walking, and using the toilet. For the first two weeks, you're sore, move slowly, and need help with baby care and household tasks. At six weeks, your body should feel back to normal.

The following sections provide more detail on the recovery process.

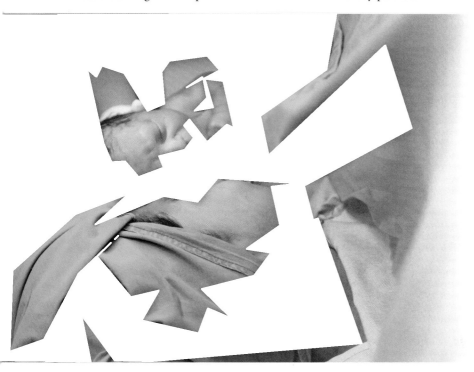

## YOUR HOSPITAL STAY

A cesarean birth requires a hospital stay of two to four days. During that time, your nurses regularly monitor your vital signs, check vaginal bleeding (lochia), ask if you're urinating and moving your bowels, and check that your incision is healing well.

## PAIN MEDICATION

During the surgery, you may be given epidural or spinal narcotics that provide many hours of pain relief. Alternatively, after the surgery you may be given patient-controlled analgesia (PCA). PCA lets you push a button to release a narcotic into your IV when you need more pain relief. (The amount of the narcotic is controlled so overdose isn't possible.)

Take enough medication to be comfortable. (Only low concentrations of the medication reach your baby through your breast milk, so the effects on your baby are slight.) When you're in pain, it's hard to move around, bond with your baby, learn parenting skills, and relax for breastfeeding. Don't let medications wear off completely. Take your next dose when it's due, even if you're not hurting yet.

Itching and nausea are frequent side effects. Other medications counteract these side effects, but they may cause drowsiness or diminish pain relief. If your medications make you groggy, ask to have the dosage decreased or medication changed.

After about twenty-four hours, you're given oral pain medications, which you may need for several days to a week. As the pain subsides, reduce the dosage or switch to regular acetaminophen or ibuprofen. If you don't need pain relief, you may stop using pain medications, even if you haven't taken all of them.

## Supporting Your Belly (Splinting)

When you first get up after a cesarean, it may feel as though your belly is sagging and needs support. It may even feel as though your insides are shifting around. Your belly may hurt whenever you change positions, cough, or laugh. To support the area, try using your hand, a pillow, or a rolled-up towel to press gently against your incision area. A cesarean support band (an elastic band that supports your abdomen) can be helpful as well.

# PHYSICAL ACTIVITY

Moving as soon as possible after the surgery boosts blood circulation, which lowers the risk of blood clots, and improves digestion and lung function. But don't overdo it. For the first two weeks, minimize lifting heavy objects and climbing stairs. These activities strain your abdominal muscles.

## *Rolling Over, Sitting, Standing, and Walking*

Within a few hours after a cesarean birth, you're encouraged to sit on the side of the bed. If you're on your back, roll onto your side by "bridging": Bend your knees, press your feet into the bed, and lift your hips. With your hips elevated, rotate them to one side so one hip is directly above the other. Rest your bottom hip on the bed, then use your arms to push yourself to a sitting position with your legs dangling over the side of the bed. Rest for a moment; this move may make you dizzy, especially the first few times you do it.

With the nurse's help, stand up by pushing down with your hands. Stand as tall as you can—you won't harm your incision even though it may hurt and feel as though it's pulling apart.

Within eight hours of the surgery, you should be able to walk to the bathroom with help. Within twelve hours, you should be able to walk short distances independently; within twenty-four hours, you should be able to walk the hospital hallways.

## *Exercises and Physical Activity*

The following exercises are recommended to help your body recover from a cesarean.

### First day after surgery

*Deep breathing:* Take a few deep breaths down into the lower part of your lungs. This movement in your belly gently exercises your abdominal muscles.

*Coughs:* Hold your hands or a pillow over your incision, inhale deeply, and exhale with either a gentle huffing cough or a forceful short puff. This movement dislodges any accumulated mucus from your respiratory system.

*Ankle pumps:* Flex and point your feet and rotate your ankles to help circulation and prevent blood clots in your legs.

### Days two to four

*Knee bends:* While lying on your back in bed, flex your feet, bend one leg while sliding your heel toward your bottom, then straighten the leg. Repeat with your other leg. This motion helps prevent blood clots in your legs.

*Tension relievers:* While sitting, roll your shoulders and rotate your ankles.

*Abdominal pull-ins:* Pull in your belly to your spine, hold for five to ten seconds, then relax.

### For the first two to four weeks

- Rest and take it easy. Don't lift anything heavier than your baby and don't drive. Limit climbing stairs, reaching into high cabinets, doing laundry, vacuuming, entertaining visitors, and so on.
- Wait to resume sexual activities.
- Ask your caregiver when to begin the postpartum exercises described in chapter 16.

# Digestion, Elimination, and Gas

Abdominal surgery can slow digestion and lead to problems with gas, gas pains, constipation, and urination. As soon as you can walk to the bathroom, your bladder catheter is removed.

In the past, women were told to consume only clear liquids until day three. Research has shown, however, that women who are allowed to eat when desired (within four to eight hours after surgery) have more satisfactory recoveries. They experience less gas, start moving their bowels sooner, require less IV fluid, and can expect an earlier discharge from the hospital.[15]

During the first few days after the surgery, take the stool softeners that your nurses give you, drink lots of water, and gradually add high-fiber foods to your meals. To minimize gas, avoid consuming iced drinks, carbonated beverages, and very hot or cold foods. To help digestion, walk, change positions often, and rock back and forth in a chair.

# Incision Care

After the surgery, you're shown how to clean the incision area and check for swelling and infection. (It's normal for the area to itch and ooze a watery yellow or pink discharge.) Gently clean and dry the wound daily. Avoid touching the incision without first washing your hands. Twenty-four hours after the surgery, you can shower or bathe as usual. Dry thoroughly, and then wear loose, comfortable clothes. If you're overweight, make sure air can circulate around the incision area so it stays clean and dry.

If tape was used to close your incision, it eventually comes off on its own. If staples or clips were used, your caregiver removes them and applies tape to the incision before you leave the hospital.

After six weeks, your scar shouldn't cause you discomfort, although it may still feel stretched or pulled. It may also feel numb for three months or more. When the feeling returns, you may experience some "zinging" or prickly sensations, due to the healing of damaged nerve pathways. After the incision has healed, you may notice a hard ridge along it. This is scar tissue, which tends to shrink and attach to the soft tissue underneath. Massage the scar tissue in different directions (along and across the scar) and roll it between your thumb and index finger. These motions ensure the different layers of skin, tissue, and muscles can move freely underneath. If the massage is painful, do it more gently. Massage your scar one to three times every day (ten to fifteen minutes each time) until all the layers in the abdomen move without restriction. A women's health physical therapist can teach you how to massage this area as well as guide you in abdominal strengthening appropriate to your level of healing.

See page 329 for warning signs of an infected incision.

# BREASTFEEDING

Some research suggests that, when compared to women who had vaginal births, fewer women who had cesarean births start breastfeeding, or they quit breastfeeding sooner. With education and support, however, initial breastfeeding rates and breastfeeding duration are similar for both mothers who had cesareans and those who didn't.[16]

After your surgery, finding a comfortable position to breastfeed may be problematic. To protect your incision from your baby's weight and wiggling, lie on your side or use the football hold (see page 400). If using the cradle hold or cross-cradle hold, first place a pillow on your incision.

Your baby may be quite sleepy, depending on what medications you had. Have patience as she figures out how to latch onto your breast and feed. Also, if your baby needed extensive suctioning of her nose and throat after birth, she may have trouble latching on during the first days. Skin-to-skin contact helps calm her and promotes a good latch.

The surgery may delay when your milk comes in. Frequent feedings and lots of skin-to-skin contact between feedings is the best way to increase your milk supply. The sooner you initiate breastfeeding after the birth and the more often you breastfeed your baby, the more milk she takes, and the more milk you make.

After the surgery, you may have a higher chance of acquiring a bacterial or yeast infection, which can cause sore nipples (see page 423).

# EMOTIONAL REACTIONS TO HAVING A CESAREAN BIRTH

Women have all sorts of feelings about having a cesarean. Reactions often depend on prior hopes and expectations. If you learn you need a planned cesarean, you may feel relieved that you don't have to go through labor. Or you may feel disappointed that you don't get to experience childbirth. You may worry about your medical condition or the surgery and its risks. Or knowing exactly what to prepare for may reduce your anxiety.

If the need for an unplanned cesarean arises during labor, you may be disappointed or you may be relieved that labor is about to end. You may feel frustrated that you worked so hard for all those hours only to have your baby delivered surgically. Or you may be frightened about facing something you never expected to happen. You may worry about your baby's well-being.

## Coming to Terms with Your Feelings about the Cesarean

When the surgery is over and you know your baby is fine, you may feel acceptance (if you felt the surgery was necessary), anger (if you didn't feel part of the decision making), disappointment, guilt, resentment, or relief. Sometimes women don't feel any particular emotions right away, but do eventually.

For some women, a cesarean leads to low self-esteem. They don't feel confident about their mothering skills because of their failure to birth "normally." They have trouble connecting emotionally to their babies because the birth wasn't what they'd wanted. They may feel emptiness or sadness when recalling the birth, instead of feeling fulfillment and joy.

If your cesarean birth depresses you, you may feel guilty and upset. You may feel as though you should "just be happy" to have a healthy baby. Know that it takes time to let go of the birth you envisioned, and it's perfectly normal to grieve for one thing as you celebrate another. If possible, talk honestly and openly about the birth with people who understand your feelings.

Sometimes, understanding the reason for the surgery can help you better accept the birth. Your recollection of the experience might not be complete, especially if labor was exhausting or the cesarean was an emergency. Ask your caregiver to discuss with you the events that led to the cesarean, or review your hospital chart together.

Also consider talking with your childbirth educator, doula, or a counselor about your birth experience. Look into joining a support group, such as the International Cesarean Awareness Network (ICAN), or search online for discussion groups. Continue using these resources until you come to terms with your birth experience.

# Vaginal Birth after Cesarean (VBAC)

If you've had a cesarean and are pregnant again, you need to decide between planning another cesarean birth and planning a *trial of labor after cesarean (TOLAC)*, in which labor is allowed to begin and to progress with the hope of having a *vaginal birth after cesarean (VBAC)*.

## Making the Choice between VBAC and Repeat Cesarean

After reading the following information, discuss with your caregiver the benefits and risks specific to your situation. Because caregivers' views on VBAC vary widely, you may want to consult with multiple providers. Also consider the emotional and practical issues unique to your situation that may affect your decision. For example, you might have lingering fears of labor that may stall a TOLAC, or there might not be a caregiver or hospital near you that permits VBAC.

## Medical Benefits and Risks of VBAC versus Repeat Cesarean

In 2010 the ACOG and a panel of experts called together by the National Institutes of Health agreed that attempting VBAC is a safe and appropriate choice for most women. [17] In general, the benefits and risks between TOLAC or VBAC and repeat cesarean balance out. TOLAC or VBAC is better for the mother but a little riskier for the baby. A repeat cesarean is a little safer for the baby, but has more risks for the mother. Therefore, women and their caregivers should work together to decide between these often medically equivalent options, and the woman's preference should be respected.

When analyzing the benefits and risks, you need to examine the relatively rare but real risk of *uterine rupture*, the separation or opening of the scar from the uterine incision. *If rupture occurs*, it can result in a hysterectomy for the mother and can lead to the death of the baby.[18] However, the vast majority of women *won't* experience uterine rupture. With TOLAC, the risk of rupture is 325 in 100,000, or about one-third of 1 percent; with a planned repeat cesarean, the risk of rupture drops to 26 in 100,000.[19]

Even with the increased chance of rupture, vaginal birth carries fewer overall risks for the mother than surgical birth. For example, when compared to repeat cesarean, TOLAC carries a lower risk of hysterectomy, blood transfusion, and deep vein thrombosis; it also involves a shorter hospital stay. The overall risk of maternal death is less than 4 in 100,000 for TOLAC and more than 13 in 100,000 for repeat cesarean.[20]

## What Influences My Chance of Uterine Rupture?

Although the thought of uterine rupture is scary, the chance of its occurrence is relatively small (one-third of 1 percent for TOLAC).[23] Here are some general guidelines of the risk:

- The chance of rupture is lowest for a woman who has had only one prior cesarean with a low transverse scar and who hasn't been induced.
- The chance of rupture is higher if the woman has had more than one prior cesarean, had an infection after a prior cesarean, had a cesarean less than eighteen months ago, or has had labor induced.
- The chance of rupture is highest (and VBAC is too risky) for a woman who has had a vertical incision or an inverted T- or J-shaped incision for a prior cesarean, had a rupture from a previous labor that caused problems, or has had an ultrasound scan that found the uterine scar to be less than 2½ millimeters thick.[24]

Improving Your Chances of Having a Successful VBAC

- Choose a caregiver who proves support of VBAC by having a high VBAC attempt rate and a success rate of 70 percent or more. You may have to interview several providers. Discuss your goals and preferences and ask questions about how you can work together toward a successful VBAC experience. If your current caregiver doesn't support your goals, consider finding a new one.
- Consider hiring a doula who has had a VBAC herself or has worked with women who have had one.
- Take a childbirth refresher class or a VBAC class.
- If your cesarean birth was traumatic or you feel anger, mistrust, or fear about your next birth, talk with a birth counselor, childbirth educator, or doula to help you deal with these feelings. You may also contact your local branch of the International Cesarean Awareness Network (ICAN). This organization's mission is to prevent unnecessary cesareans through education, provide support for cesarean recovery, and promote VBAC. They're a good source of local information and emotional support. You can find abundant information on their website, http://www.ican-online.org, including the paper "My Hospital Is Not Allowing VBAC."[25]
- Avoid induction with Pitocin or prostaglandins. One study showed the risk of uterine rupture was less than one-half of 1 percent for spontaneous labor, just over 1 percent if labor was induced with Pitocin, and just under 1½ percent with prostaglandins.[26] If induction is necessary, nondrug methods, balloon catheters, and rupture of membranes may be safer for a VBAC (see pages 280–282).
- Try to minimize medications for pain relief and use other interventions only if necessary.
- Review Ten Steps to Improve Your Chances of Having a Safe and Satisfying Birth on page 26 and Reducing Your Chances of Having a Cesarean Birth on page 301.

By following these suggestions, you'll have done all you can to ensure a vaginal birth. But always remember that there's no guarantee a cesarean won't become the wise option if serious problems arise during labor. Consider writing a VBAC birth plan as well as a "best possible cesarean" plan to use if a repeat cesarean becomes the safest option (see page 320).

After balancing the rare chance of rupture against all other factors, the overall risk of the baby's death is 130 in 100,000 for TOLAC and 50 in 100,000 for repeat cesarean.[21] Although this risk may seem alarming, it's similar to the risk of the baby's death for a first-time mother laboring with an unscarred uterus (about 100 in 100,000). We summarize the risk this way: If you were brave enough to have your first baby, you can be brave enough to have a TOLAC with this one.

Weighing the benefits and risks of a VBAC against those of a repeat cesarean can be challenging, and it's best to closely consult with your caregiver to better understand your options. If your risk of uterine rupture is high or your chances of other complications in labor are high, a planned cesarean may be best. A planned cesarean has fewer risks than an unplanned cesarean that occurs after a failed TOLAC. If your risk of uterine rupture is low and your chances of VBAC success are favorable (see page 316), your best option may be a TOLAC.

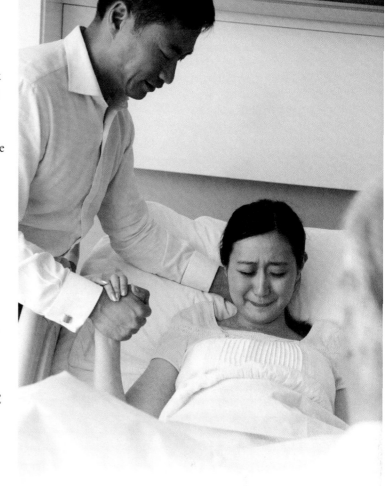

## Monitoring for and Managing Uterine Rupture

During a TOLAC, the caregiver closely monitors both mother and baby for uterine rupture, which can be diagnosed by carefully observing the baby's heart rate, the shape of the mother's abdomen, and the mother's blood pressure. If a caregiver suspects a rupture, the mother has an emergency cesarean to prevent excessive bleeding and distress to the baby. With careful monitoring and quick intervention, the majority of babies are fine at birth after a rupture.

## Likelihood of VBAC Success

Most women who plan a TOLAC have a vaginal birth (60 to 94 percent).[22] VBAC is more likely if a woman is younger than forty and has had a prior vaginal birth, and if the reason for her previous cesarean hasn't recurred and her labor is progressing well. VBAC is less likely in the following situations:
- The mother has had multiple prior cesareans, has complicating medical conditions, or is obese.
- Gestation is over forty weeks and the baby is estimated to weigh over 9 pounds.
- Labor is induced or augmented.

## Two Views on VBAC

I gave birth to my daughter by unplanned cesarean. I was disappointed for quite a while afterward, because I'd had my heart set on delivering vaginally. When I got pregnant again, I didn't waste any time learning all I could about VBAC. I know there's no guarantee I'll deliver vaginally this time, but I want to do all I can to better my odds.

—*Jana*

When my first labor failed to progress, I ended up needing a cesarean. I remember thinking at the time, "Thank goodness! I'm sick of this pain!" Now I'm pregnant again, and I'm not keen to repeat that labor experience. Part of me wants to skip it all together, but another part realizes that recovering from a C-section is no piece of cake, either. I think I need to learn how to better handle the labor pain so I can avoid the pain of cesarean recovery.

—*Samantha*

# AVAILABILITY OF VBAC

Before 1980, common thought was "once a cesarean, always a cesarean." From the 1980s to 1999, experts recommended VBAC because they believed it was safer than repeat cesarean. However, in 1999 and again in 2008, the ACOG recommended that hospitals permit VBAC only when a physician, staff, and anesthesia were immediately available to provide an emergency cesarean.[27] As a result, due to staffing and liability concerns, hospital policies turned against VBAC. By early 2010, one-third of hospitals no longer permitted VBAC and one-half of physicians stopped offering it as an option.[28]

Many maternity care experts disagreed with the ACOG recommendation.[29] In July 2010, ACOG changed their stance, stating that if a laboring woman arrived at a hospital that didn't support TOLAC, she shouldn't be forced to have a repeat cesarean against her will. However, during prenatal care, a physician who is uncomfortable with VBAC may refer the patient to another physician. Some women who want to try for a VBAC but can't find a caregiver who supports that decision have relocated for the end of pregnancy to a friend's or relative's home near a hospital and caregiver that support VBAC.

# Emotional Reactions When Deciding between a Repeat Cesarean and a VBAC

Some women may have emotional challenges during pregnancy when choosing whether to plan for a VBAC or a repeat cesarean. Emotional challenges, or "second thoughts," can also arise during a TOLAC. Because anxiety can slow labor, it's best to address these emotional issues during pregnancy.

## Fear

The thought of laboring again may seem more frightening than the risks of major surgery. You may fear labor pain, a long labor, uterine rupture, complications, another cesarean, failure to deliver "normally," or simply the unknown. Discuss your fears with your caregiver, childbirth educator, doula, or cesarean support group. These people can reassure you and support your decision. They can help you identify the most distressing parts of your previous birth and help you plan how to avoid or address them. For example, if you dread laboring for hours and then having a cesarean, you may set a time limit after which you'd opt for a cesarean.

## Shame or guilt

You may feel ashamed that you might have done things that led to a prior cesarean birth, or you may feel guilty for having agreed to a cesarean. Talk with others who understand your feelings so you can forgive yourself and approach this birth from a fresh perspective.

## Lack of confidence

You may doubt your ability to give birth vaginally and hesitate to invest time and effort in a VBAC because you don't want to be disappointed. Remember that each pregnancy and birth is different. Get to know women who have had a successful VBAC. Ask what helped them become confident enough to birth vaginally.

## Feeling pressured

You may feel pressured by caregivers, friends, or family to make one decision or another. Always remember that you have the right to make an informed decision. Others can provide information and opinions, but only you can make the choice that's best for you and your family.

## Stress in labor

In addition to the emotional hurdles that arise in most labors (see graph on page 173), specific events in a VBAC labor may raise your stress level:

- When early labor is underway, you may suddenly second-guess whether a VBAC is such a good idea. Be prepared for this "moment of truth" beforehand by thinking of ways to deal with it.
- Particular events in labor may trigger flashbacks of your previous labor that ended in a cesarean. Don't suppress them, even if they're unpleasant. Acknowledge them openly and note how things are different this time.
- A big hurdle may be reaching the point in labor that led to a previous cesarean. Until you pass that point, you may continue to question your ability to birth vaginally. After you've passed it, you can breathe a sigh of relief and enjoy a boost of optimism.

## Common Q & A

**Q:** I've heard of "natural cesareans" or "slow cesareans." What are they?

**A:** Historically, cesareans were emergency procedures that emphasized rapid delivery and immediate access to the baby for resuscitation. As cesareans have become more commonplace, some obstetricians have begun doing the surgery more slowly and encouraging immediate skin-to-skin contact between the mother and baby. This woman-centered, baby-friendly way of doing cesareans is not yet commonplace, and your caregiver might not be aware of it. Learn more about family-centered cesareans and find articles to share with your caregiver by visiting http://tinyurl.com/la83t2 and http://tinyurl.com/family-centered-cesarean.

# Having the Best Possible Cesarean Birth

Whether or not a cesarean birth is what you want, you can have a satisfying experience. The following steps will help you make your cesarean birth the best it can be.

### Educate yourself.

- Learn about the cesarean procedure from books, classes, and discussions with your caregiver.
- Find out your birthplace's policies and regulations for cesareans.

### If a planned cesarean is necessary, prepare in advance.

- Take care of yourself in pregnancy. Eat well and exercise regularly if possible. The more physically fit you are before the surgery, the quicker you recover afterward.
- Tour the hospital, including the special care nursery. Ask to have any lab work, tests, and paperwork done before the day of surgery. Meet with an anesthesiologist to learn what medications will be used.
- If hospital policy allows for two support people in the OR, ask a friend or family member to join you for the surgery. Or consider hiring a doula. Her calm, familiar presence and knowledge can reassure you. Plus, after your baby is born, she can remain by your side while your partner stays with your baby.
- Take a breastfeeding class with your partner so you both know ways to help make nursing after a cesarean easier.

### Wait for labor to begin (or at least until week thirty-nine of pregnancy).

If your caregiver recommends scheduling a cesarean before your labor begins, be certain that it's for clear medical reasons. Ask that your caregiver schedule the surgery as close to your due date as possible, and ask about amniocentesis to verify your baby's lung maturity before surgery.

- Labor benefits babies. Babies born by scheduled cesarean without experiencing labor are four times more likely to develop persistent pulmonary hypertension, a rare but potentially life-threatening situation.
- Severe complications, including breathing difficulties, infection, and other problems that require admission to the neonatal intensive care unit (NICU), are twice as likely for babies born at thirty-seven weeks than are babies born at thirty-nine weeks.[30]
- A planned cesarean can lead to accidental prematurity if the estimated gestational age is wrong. Knowing the exact date of conception, having an ultrasound scan early in pregnancy that documents a gestational age, or having the baby's lung maturity verified are ways to better estimate an accurate gestational age.

### Prepare a cesarean birth plan.

Even if you're planning a vaginal birth, consider writing a cesarean birth plan (see chapter 8). Here are questions to consider asking at a prenatal appointment:

- Can I have two support people in the OR with me?

- What will be the atmosphere in the OR? Can I choose music to play? Will the staff narrate what's happening? Will they chat with me to keep me relaxed during the procedure? Will they stop chatting if I request it?
- Will staff lower the screen or use a mirror so I can see my baby's birth? Are there restrictions on photographing and video-recording the birth?
- Can my partner announce our baby's sex? Will you do minimal suctioning of my baby's nose and mouth? Can I have skin-to-skin contact with my baby after birth? Will newborn exams be done where my partner and I can see our baby? If possible, can my baby stay in the OR during my repair? Will breastfeeding be initiated as soon after the birth as possible?
- Will you do internal repair and double-layer suturing (see page 309)?
- If I experience anxiety, trembling, or nausea, will I be offered nondrug options for coping or medications that will keep me alert?

If the options and answers don't satisfy you, consider switching to a different caregiver or birthplace.

### Understand the reasons for a cesarean.

If you're having a planned or unplanned (but not emergency) cesarean, ask your caregiver as many questions as you need to fully understand the benefits, risks, and alternatives before consenting to surgery. If you have an emergency cesarean, talk with your caregiver after the birth about why it was needed. This information may help you feel that the decisions made during the birth were necessary at the time, which can help you accept the events.

### Insist on early, frequent contact with your baby.

Cesarean delivery, narcotic pain medications, and high levels of stress at birth may delay breastfeeding and affect breast milk production. The more time you spend nestling with your baby and the more frequently you nurse, the sooner your milk supply increases. Skin-to-skin contact also enhances the emotional bond between you and your baby.

### Develop a postpartum plan.

The postpartum period is more challenging when you're recovering from major surgery, so plan ahead for the extra support you'll need (see page 152).

## Key Points to Remember

- More than 30 percent of women giving birth in the United States have cesareans. Although a cesarean is a relatively safe surgery, vaginal birth has fewer overall risks. For this reason, birthing women and their caregivers should consider a cesarean only when the potential medical benefits clearly outweigh the possible risks.
- You can take steps to increase your chances of a vaginal birth, and you can ask important questions if your caregiver recommends a cesarean.
- VBAC is a viable option for many women with prior cesareans; however, policies at your local hospital may limit access to a VBAC.
- Preparing a cesarean birth plan helps ensure that if you need a cesarean, you'll have a positive birth experience that lets you feel nurtured and cared for.

# CHAPTER 16

# What Life Is Like for a New Parent

The days, weeks, and months that follow your baby's birth are a time of major physical, emotional, and social readjustment and recovery.

After the birth, your reproductive organs return to their pre-pregnant state (usually within six weeks). You begin to lose the extra weight you gained during pregnancy. Your breasts begin to produce milk. These physical changes are normal, but they can seem more difficult than you expected.

During the first weeks, most new parents experience sudden mood changes. You may feel joyous and energetic one moment, then exhausted, let down, or even disappointed the next. Caring for your baby may also upset the balance within your family until you can adjust your roles and schedules.

This chapter describes the typical changes that can affect the lives of a new mother and her family, and offers ways to help smooth your adjustment to parenthood.

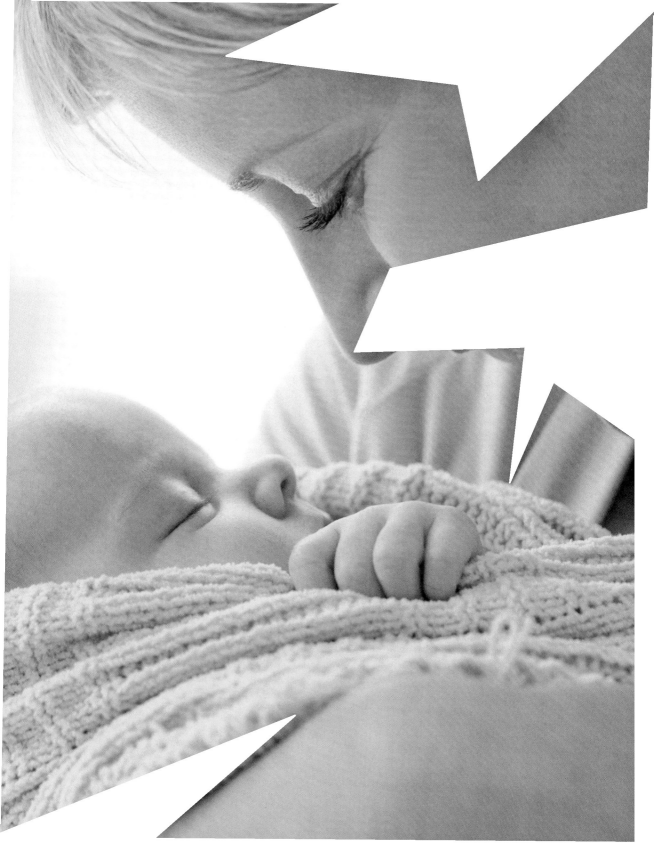

# Your Care in the Days Following the Birth

If you have a vaginal birth in a hospital, your postpartum stay is typically one to two days (unless a medical reason necessitates a longer stay). If you have a cesarean birth, your stay is usually two to four days. At a freestanding (unaffiliated with a hospital) birth center, your stay is typically three to six hours. At a home birth, your midwife leaves about three to four hours after the birth.

Before leaving the hospital or birth center (or your midwife leaves your home), ask your caregiver for information on newborn care and postpartum recovery. If you're birthing at a hospital, attend classes offered on these topics during your stay.

Ideally, your caregiver and your baby's caregiver (or a mother/baby nurse) should examine you and your baby on the third or fourth day after the birth, to detect jaundice, dehydration, or excessive weight loss in your baby and to check your physical recovery, help you with any feeding challenges, assess and treat pain, and answer your questions about baby care. If you develop pain or a fever before this scheduled visit—or if your baby looks yellow (see page 383), has trouble feeding, or seems sleepy or listless—request an appointment for as soon as possible.

Learn about possible warning signs that indicate problems with your health or your baby's health (see pages 329 and 386). Contact your caregiver and your baby's caregiver with any health concerns. For nonmedical concerns, your childbirth educator, a breastfeeding counselor, doula, or experienced parents may provide helpful advice and information.

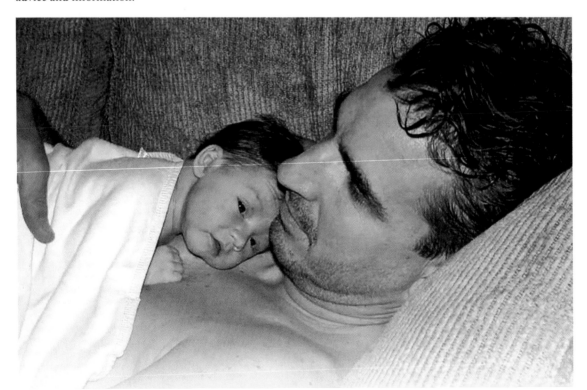

# Your Physical Recovery: Early Postpartum Period

Immediately after the birth, your caregivers will closely observe your physical condition. They'll frequently check your temperature, pulse, respiratory rate, and blood pressure. They'll monitor vaginal bleeding; your uterus's size, firmness, and position; and the functioning of your bladder and bowels. If you had anesthesia, they'll monitor the return of feeling and movement in your legs.

## UTERUS

Over the first six weeks after the birth, the uterus returns to its pre-pregnant size—a process called *involution*. On the day of the birth, the top of the uterus (fundus) can be felt behind the navel. It drops (involutes) about the width of one finger each day.

Soon after the birth, you or your nurse will massage your uterus, stimulating it to contract. Breastfeeding your baby will also stimulate the uterus to contract. Keeping the uterus firm and tight helps prevent heavy blood loss from the site where the placenta attached to your uterus.

As your uterus contracts, you may experience discomfort or pain. These *afterpains* often occur during breastfeeding and are more common if you've given birth before. To ease the pain, relax and use slow breathing patterns (see page 243). Ibuprofen or prescribed medications may also help. Afterpains typically disappear after the first week.

*Lochia* is the bloody, fleshy-smelling discharge that flows from your uterus and out your vagina for up to six to eight weeks after the birth. For the first few days, the flow looks like heavy menstrual flow. Passing jellylike clots is normal, especially in the first days. Lochia is heavier when you change positions, are overactive, breastfeed, or have a bowel movement. If flow increases, remind yourself to slow down and rest. Within ten days, lochia diminishes and becomes pale pink or rust in color. Over the next several weeks, it becomes white, yellowish white, or tan. (See page 329 for warning signs.)

If you're not breastfeeding, you'll probably resume menstruation four to eight weeks after the birth. If you're breastfeeding, you might not menstruate for several months or until you wean; however, you can become pregnant, because you may ovulate before your period returns. Your first few periods may be heavier and longer than usual or they may be lighter than usual, but they'll eventually return to normal.

## CERVIX AND VAGINA

As your uterus approaches its pre-pregnant size, so does your cervix. After the birth, your vagina gradually regains its tone, and your labia remain somewhat looser, larger, and darker than before pregnancy.

# PERINEAL CARE

Your perineum needs special care after a vaginal birth, especially if you're bruised or swollen, or had stitches for an episiotomy or a tear. (See below to learn how to care for your perineum.) Stitches dissolve in two to four weeks, and the tissue usually heals within four to six weeks, although you may feel discomfort for some time. Discomfort during intercourse may persist for months. See your caregiver if the discomfort worsens or continues beyond several months.

## *Recommendations for Perineal Care*

Follow these recommendations to relieve perineal pain, promote healing, and prevent infection:

- Apply ice to your perineum to reduce swelling. Soon after the birth, your nurse or midwife will apply an ice pack to your perineum. For the next several days, continue to use ice intermittently to soothe pain from a tear, episiotomy, or hemorrhoids. To make an ice pack, put crushed ice or a frozen wet washcloth in a zip-close plastic bag and wrap it in several layers of paper towel. Hold it in place with your perineal pad. Or dampen a maxi pad with witch hazel and freeze it before use.
- Begin doing Kegel exercises immediately after the birth (see page 90). Frequent pelvic floor exercises increase circulation, promote healing, and reduce swelling. They also help restore strength and muscle tone. Don't be discouraged if you can't do Kegels as well as you could before the birth. Your strength should improve quickly.
- After urinating, clean yourself by pouring warm water over your perineum from front to back (to prevent infection from organisms in the rectal area). If you birth in a hospital, you may be given a "peri bottle" (squirt bottle filled with warm water) to wash yourself. Use toilet paper to gently pat yourself dry from front to back.
- Don't use tampons before your postpartum checkup.
- Don't douche.
- Take a sitz bath to help relieve perineal soreness: Sit in a clean tub of warm water for ten to twenty minutes. After the bath, lie down for fifteen minutes to decrease swelling caused by the warm water. If you like, use cold water. It can be as soothing as a warm bath and doesn't increase swelling.
- Sit on a plastic donut pillow to lift your perineum off the surface you're sitting on. If you don't have a donut pillow, make your own by rolling a bath towel lengthwise and shaping it into a horseshoe shape. Sit on the pillow with both buttocks supported.
- Sit on a firm surface if your stitches are causing pain. You may find sitting on a firm surface more comfortable than sitting on a soft one or on a donut, either of which can separate the edges of your incision. To help keep your incision pressed together and avoid pain, sit down on one buttock first, then ease onto the other buttock.
- Lie down and rest as often as you can in the first weeks after the birth. When sitting or standing, gravity can increase swelling and cause the pelvic floor to ache.

# Bowel and Bladder Function

After the birth, you may have trouble urinating because of a tear near your urethra or swelling around it (from the birth or a bladder catheter). To help start the flow, try to relax your perineum, drink lots of liquids, or pour warm water over your perineum (or try urinating in the shower or bathtub). If you still can't urinate, call your caregiver.

The birth may cause you to become constipated because of loose abdominal muscles, episiotomy, hemorrhoids, or a sore perineum. Iron supplements and narcotic pain medications may also cause constipation. Prevent constipation by eating lots of fresh and dried fruits, vegetables, and whole-grain cereals (to increase your fiber intake) and by drinking plenty of water. Adding a tablespoon of flax meal to your food also may help. When you're able, walking and exercising your abdominal muscles help restore normal bowel function, as does moving your bowels when you have the urge (instead of waiting until later). If your caregiver prescribes a stool softener, follow the instructions for use.

When moving your bowels, support your perineum by gently pressing toilet paper against your stitches to prevent the tissue from bulging and stretching.

If these suggestions don't help and you remain uncomfortable, your caregiver may prescribe a laxative, suppositories, or an enema.

# Hemorrhoids

*Hemorrhoids* are swollen varicose veins in the rectal area that may be as small as a pea or as large as a grape. They may itch, bleed, sting, or ache, especially during a bowel movement. Many women develop hemorrhoids during pregnancy; some develop them after a vaginal birth. Most hemorrhoids disappear in the first postpartum month. To prevent hemorrhoids or to reduce discomfort and promote healing, follow these suggestions:

- Take steps to prevent constipation (see page 114).
- Do your Kegel exercises (see page 90), with emphasis on the anal muscles.
- Use witch hazel on the area.
- Take sitz baths (see page 326).
- Avoid heavy lifting. If you must pick up a heavy object (such as an older child), do a Kegel (see page 90) and hold it as you lift.

If these measures don't help prevent hemorrhoids or reduce their discomfort, see page 347.

# Breasts

For the first twenty-four to seventy-two hours after the birth, your breasts secrete colostrum (highly nutritious fluid that's your baby's first milk). Mature breast milk appears between the second and fifth day. At that time, your breasts may become engorged, which may present feeding challenges (see page 410).

## If You're Not Breastfeeding

If you decide not to breastfeed (or can't), your breasts typically undergo the same initial changes as breastfeeding mothers. To reduce milk production and increase comfort, apply ice packs and avoid breast stimulation. On the second or third day after the birth, wear a snugly fitting sports bra or wrap an extra wide elastic bandage across your breasts and around your chest to compress your breasts and decrease the swelling that occurs as your milk comes in. Rewrap the elastic bandage every few hours. Keep your breasts bound for twenty-four to forty-eight hours.

Once your milk comes in, apply ice to your breasts for twenty minutes every four hours or so to decrease the pain from inflammation and swelling. Use ice packs or an elastic bandage to hold several bags of frozen peas or corn in place over your bra or shirt. Consider taking ibuprofen or acetaminophen (Tylenol) for pain relief.

If you're not breastfeeding because you gave your baby up for adoption or because your baby has died, suppressing your milk may cause you to experience a "second grieving" for your baby who can't have the milk. Know that you don't have to immediately suppress lactation if you don't want to. Some mothers express and donate their milk in honor of their babies. (See page 296 for more information on newborn death.)

# HORMONAL CHANGES

When you deliver the placenta, your estrogen and progesterone levels drop rapidly and remain low until your ovaries begin producing these hormones again. If you breastfeed, your production of prolactin and oxytocin increases, while estrogen and progesterone levels remain low until you wean your baby.

# CIRCULATORY CHANGES

During pregnancy, you accumulate extra blood and fluid. When giving birth, bleeding naturally occurs as the uterus contracts to compress the blood vessels that flowed to the placenta. During an uncomplicated vaginal birth, the average blood loss is about 1 cup. If you had an episiotomy or a sizable perineal tear, you may lose more blood. You continue to lose blood in your lochia for a few weeks. See page 293 for signs of excessive blood loss.

In the early postpartum period, you urinate often and sweat heavily (especially at night) to lose the extra fluid accumulated during pregnancy. You may lose as much as 5 pounds of fluid during the first week after the birth.

# ABDOMINAL AND SKIN CHANGES

After giving birth, your abdominal muscles are loose, and take several months to regain firmness. Exercise speeds up the process. Your stretch marks fade from red to silver but don't completely disappear. If your skin darkened during pregnancy, the pigmentation will fade. Any increased hair growth also disappears gradually.

If you pushed hard for a long time during the birth, the rapid changes in blood pressure during and between pushes may have caused broken blood vessels in your eyes and on your face and neck. They typically disappear within a week or two of the birth.

## Warning Signs after the Birth That Require Medical Attention

Report any of the following warning signs to your caregiver.

| Warning signs | Possible problems |
|---|---|
| Fever (oral or temporal artery temperature of 100.4°F/38°C or higher) | Uterine infection |
| | Breast infection (mastitis) |
| | Infection of episiotomy or tear |
| | Infection of cesarean incision |
| | Other illness |
| Burning with urination; blood in urine | Bladder or kidney infection |
| Inability to urinate | Swelling or trauma of the urethral sphincter |
| Swollen, red, painful area on the leg (especially the calf) that's hot and tender to the touch | Thrombophlebitis or deep vein thrombosis (blood clot in the blood vessel—see page 124); do not rub or massage the area. |
| Sore, reddened, hot, painful area on breast(s), along with fever and flu-like symptoms | Breast infection (mastitis—see page 425) |
| Passage of blood clot larger than a lemon followed by heavy bleeding, or any bleeding heavy enough to soak a maxi pad in an hour or less | Passage of some (but not all) of a retained placenta |
| | Uterine infection |
| | Late postpartum hemorrhage (see page 348) |
| Vaginal discharge that has an extremely foul odor (like spoiled fish); vaginal soreness or itching | Uterine infection |
| | Vaginal infection |
| Increased pain at site of episiotomy or tear; may be accompanied by foul-smelling or pus-like discharge | Infection of episiotomy or tear |
| | Reopening of incision or tear |
| Opening of cesarean incision; may be accompanied by pus-like discharge or blood | Infection of cesarean incision |
| Appearance of rash or hives; may be accompanied by itching | Allergic reaction to medication |
| Severe headache that begins after the birth and is worse when upright and less painful when lying down | Spinal headache following regional anesthesia |
| Any sudden onset of pain that's new, such as abdominal tenderness or burning near perineal stitches when urinating | Uterine infection |
| | Reopening of perineal tear or incision |
| Pain and tenderness in front or back of pelvis, accompanied by difficulty walking and a "grating" sensation in pubic joint | Separation of pubic symphysis (cartilage between the pubic bones in the front of your pelvis—see page 349) |
| Feeling extremely anxious, panicky, or depressed; accompanied by rapid heart rate, difficulty breathing, uncontrollable crying, feelings of anger, or inability to sleep or eat | Postpartum mood disorders, including anxiety and panic attacks, obsessive thinking or worrying, or depression (see page 351) |
| Frightening relationship with your partner; being verbally or physically abused | Domestic violence increases during pregnancy and after the birth. If you need to talk or get help, call the National Domestic Violence Hotline, 800-799-SAFE (7233) or 800-787-3224 (TTY). |

## In Their Own Words

After my baby's birth, I struggled to get the time to feed myself and use the bathroom—and I had a lot of helpers! I found it helped to order groceries online and have them delivered. Small decisions like that kept me from feeling too overwhelmed.

—Paige

# Your Physical Recovery: Later Postpartum Period

Within three to eight weeks after the birth, your caregiver will give you a general physical examination (including a pelvic exam) to assess your recovery and to discuss any physical or emotional problems you may have. You also may discuss your family-planning preferences (see page 338).

If you notice any of the warning signs listed on page 329 before your checkup, call your caregiver immediately for an appointment.

Your caregiver may also recommend that you have regular physical exams as well as a Pap smear every three to five years.[1] For breast health, if you're younger than forty, you may be advised to have a clinical breast exam every three years. If you're older than forty, you may be advised to have a clinical breast exam and mammogram every year,[2] or you may be advised to begin mammograms at age fifty, unless you're at high risk for breast cancer.[3] Although routine breast self-exam is no longer recommended, breast self-awareness is advised. If you notice any unexplained changes to your breasts, report them to your caregiver.

# Caring for Yourself after the Birth

After giving birth, you can help your recovery by eating well, getting adequate rest, and asking others for help with household chores, meal preparation, and other tasks that you may find difficult to accomplish while caring for your baby.

## NUTRITION

In the postpartum period, continue eating healthful foods, as you did during pregnancy (see chapter 6). If you're breastfeeding, see page 407 for nutrition suggestions.

Don't drastically change or restrict your diet to lose weight. The maximum amount of weight you should lose per week is 1 to 2 pounds. Most new mothers lose pregnancy weight gradually over several months without special effort.

If you're anemic, your caregiver may recommend that you continue taking prenatal vitamins and iron supplements. To prevent constipation, ensure your diet contains plenty of fiber.

## REST AND SLEEP

When you first begin caring for your baby, finding time to sleep may seem impossible. If you're not tending to your baby's needs, you're trying to finish household chores or attempting to take a shower.

However, fatigue and sleep deprivation can greatly challenge your physical and emotional recovery, so make sleep a top priority and take every opportunity to nap. Even if you can't sleep, simply resting gives you the energy to meet your baby's often unpredictable needs.

You may notice that your baby sleeps as much during the day as she does at night. This sleep pattern is common and temporary for newborns. As you baby grows, she'll begin to sleep longer at night when you and your family do (see page 375). If you're used to sleeping only at night, or if your baby naps for short periods and wakes up frequently, the advice to "sleep when your baby sleeps" may frustrate you. In addition, constantly listening for your baby's cries may make you feel wired and unable to sleep.

You'll eventually adjust to being awake at night and learn how to rest and sleep when you can. But what can you do in the meantime? Try the following suggestions to help you relax and fall asleep:

- First, commit to making sleep a priority, right after meeting your baby's needs. Someone else can do household tasks, or they can wait until you're rested.
- Give yourself permission to do whatever it takes to be able to rest, such as turning off the phone, sitting outside, taking short walks, having a bath, eating and drinking particular food and beverages, having a massage, or taking pain medication.
- Limit visitors; don't worry about being a gracious host. If a visit lasts too long, ask the guests to leave or excuse yourself with your baby and retire to your bedroom.
- Try relaxation techniques, such as the relaxation countdown (see page 236).
- Keep your baby close to you so you don't strain to listen for her (which can interfere with your ability to rest).
- Conversely, you may find that your baby's sounds increase your anxiety and restlessness, especially if you're extremely tired. In that case, let someone else tend to your baby in another room while you rest. Once you're rested, anxiety usually decreases.
- If your partner is available, take turns caring for your baby throughout the night. Or try scheduling parenting shifts: One parent goes to bed early, while the other is responsible for caring for your baby during the night. The parent who went to bed first takes over care early the next morning, allowing the other parent to sleep in. If you're breastfeeding, you may need to adapt this schedule to accommodate feeding patterns.

## ASKING FOR HELP

After the birth, you may be upset to realize that you can't do things (such as manage your household) as well as you could before the birth. You may find it difficult to ask for help, but having support will speed your postpartum recovery.

Accept any offer that will make it easier for you to rest, shower, or otherwise care for yourself. Someone may offer to do the dishes and laundry, shop for groceries, vacuum and dust, or simply watch your baby. If you're concerned about meals, someone can cook and freeze meals in advance, or bring a meal every day for the first few weeks.

If you're unable or unwilling to ask friends and family for help, consider hiring part-time household help or a postpartum doula (see page 23) for a few weeks after the birth. Many communities have agencies that specialize in postpartum home care.

## Recipe for Sleep in the First Weeks after the Birth

Many first-time parents use the following approach to get an adequate amount of sleep until their babies begin to sleep for longer stretches.

1. Ask yourself how much sleep you needed before pregnancy to function well. Six hours? Eight hours? That's the amount of sleep you now require every day.

2. Because feedings and baby care prevent you from getting this amount of sleep in one stretch, you'll need more time in bed to meet your sleep requirement. Stay in bed until you've slept enough (meals and trips to the bathroom are obvious exceptions). Each time you wake up, keep a mental note of how long you slept.

3. Don't brush your teeth, shower, or dress until you've met your sleep requirement. If you require eight hours of sleep, it may take from 10 p.m. until noon (or later) the next day to get out of your pajamas!

*Note:* You may find that having your baby sleep with you (or in the same room) makes it easier to get enough sleep, because you can care for your baby quickly. Also, if you have other children, this approach may require the help of another adult who can care for them while you sleep.

# Postpartum Fitness

Immediately after giving birth, your body begins recovering from the event as your mind begins reordering your priorities to emphasize rest, healing, and caring for your baby. In the early postpartum period, there's little time, energy or need to resume or begin a vigorous exercise regimen. However, gentle activity, such as walking and conditioning exercises (see below), can help speed your recovery. You can begin doing these exercises when you feel ready, whether that's in a few days or a few weeks after the birth. Follow your caregiver's recommendations about exercise and other activities, such as driving, stair climbing, and lifting.

After several weeks to months, you may want to resume more vigorous exercise. Work with your body and increase the intensity of exercise gradually. Your uterine ligaments need time to shorten to effectively stabilize your uterus for physical activity. Many women push themselves too hard, too fast. You'll know you're overexercising if you become exhausted, experience any pain, pelvic floor heaviness, or have increased vaginal bleeding. (See page 329 for postpartum warning signs.) Adjust your activity by reducing the intensity or changing to a different type of exercise.

Very vigorous exercise, such as running, jogging and jumping, jar your uterus and are best postponed for several months until your ligaments can adequately support your uterus. Ignoring this can result in uterine prolapse or worsen a bladder or rectal prolapse. When you need guidance or are worried you're injuring yourself, consult with your physical therapist or caregiver before continuing the exercise.

As time passes and you gradually increase your fitness level, your energy, joint stability, motivation, and endurance will improve.

## EXERCISES TO CONDITION YOUR MUSCLES AND RELIEVE TENSION

In the postpartum period, your abdominal muscles require exercise and may need external support to recover their former shape and strength while avoiding further separation if you experienced a diastasis of the rectus abdominis (see page 334). Starting at six weeks postpartum, it's a good idea to have a women's health physical therapist assess your abdomen, as well as your pelvic floor for pain, strength, tone, coordination and scar mobility. The physical therapist can suggest exercises designed for your optimal recovery. These exercises increase circulation, reduce swelling and promote healing in the perineum, and restore vaginal and rectal muscle tone. When these muscle groups are in good condition, they provide core muscle support for your pelvic organs and entire body. (To find a women's health physical therapist, see appendix C).

You can do conditioning exercises throughout the day (as time permits) while caring for your baby. For example, each time you change a diaper, you can contract your pelvic floor muscles or do pelvic tilts. Before or after feeding your baby, you can adjust your posture by doing head tilts and shoulder circles. During a feeding, try doing transverse abdominal contractions.

### Core and Postural Exercises

Every day or so, try working in some the following conditioning exercises:

**Pelvic Floor Strengthening (Kegel Exercises)**

See page 90 for instructions. You can do Kegels as soon as you'd like after the birth (vaginal or cesarean) to start toning your pelvic floor and supporting your pelvic organs. If these exercises cause pain, give yourself more time to heal before trying again.

*Sustained contractions:* The goal of sustained contractions is to hold each one for ten seconds. Do ten repetitions, with a five-second rest between each one.

*Pulsed contractions:* These contractions are done more rhythmically and faster than sustained contractions. Every two seconds, alternate between contracting and relaxing your pelvic floor. Each time you contract and relax is a pulse. Do up to fifteen pulses. The goal is to train your pelvic floor to react quickly when you sneeze or laugh to prevent incontinence (leaking urine).

*Note:* If you know your pelvic floor is hypertonic (has high muscular tension), Kegels aren't the exercise for you. If you're unsure whether your pelvic floor is hypertonic, signs include pain during sexual intercourse or difficulty having a bowel movement without straining. The best way to know for certain is to work with a physical therapist who specializes in internal pelvic floor care. (To find a women's health physical therapist, see appendix C).

### Pelvic Tilts I, II, and III

See page 92 for instructions. You can contract the pelvic floor when performing these exercises.

### Transverse Abdominal Contractions

See page 91 for instructions. This exercise helps close a separation of the rectus muscles while toning your abdominals and flattening your stomach. It becomes progressively easier to do over time. Begin with three sets of fifteen contractions per day and increase the number of sets as you like.[4]

### Head Lifts

*Aim:* To help close a separation of your rectus muscles while toning your abdominals and flattening your stomach.

*Exercise:* Lie on your back with your knees bent. Cross your hands over your abdomen, placing them on either side of your waist. Inhale; as you exhale, raise your head. At the same time, use your abdominal muscles to pull your bellybutton toward your spine and use your hands to pull the side abdominal muscles toward each other (see photo below). Avoid contracting your oblique muscles (the muscles along the sides of your abdomen) as they can further pull apart your diastasis. Hold for a slow count of five. Slowly lower your head and rest.

*Repetition:* To close any separation, repeat twenty times each day. The separation should regain its normal 1-inch (or smaller) width within several weeks. Progress to more advanced abdominal work only after the separation is within this normal range.[5]

## Common Q & A

**Q:** I know I should exercise to help my recovery, but I just can't find the time. What can I do?

**A:** As your baby grows and begins to need your care and attention less frequently, you'll have more time for exercise. In the beginning, exercising outside the home might not appeal to you. If you'd rather avoid the hassle of having to look presentable and getting to a class on time, exercise at home with your baby by dancing with him or doing postpartum exercises with him next to you. No matter how long it's been between showers, you're the best thing your baby has seen!

When you feel ready, schedule walks with other new mothers or take a postpartum exercise class to motivate you to get moving and reconnect with the outside world. Just remember to adapt any exercises to your current fitness level.

**Bridge Pose**

*Aim:* To tone your hamstrings and buttocks.

*Exercise:* Lie on your back with your knees bent and your arms resting on the floor along your sides. Inhale; as you exhale, lift your tailbone off the floor, then each vertebra, until your weight is resting on your shoulders.

Push your heels into the floor and keep your thighs parallel to each other (not rolled outward). To protect your neck, don't use a pillow and avoid turning your head. If you like, clasp your hands together under your back and press your arms into the floor to lift your chest.

*Repetition:* Hold the position for several breaths, then roll back into the starting position. Repeat the exercise five to ten times each day.

## Reducing the Separation of Your Rectus Abdominis Muscles

Before you begin doing any abdominal muscle exercise other than head lifts, transverse abdominal contractions, and pelvic tilts (see pages 91–92), check your rectus abdominis muscles for separation. These are the muscles from the bottom of your ribcage to your pelvis. As your abdomen grew and stretched during pregnancy, the midline connective tissue between these muscles may have separated painlessly and without bleeding to create more space for your baby. Separations are common and a variation of normal, but your attention is required to close the gap.

To check for separation, lie on your back with your knees bent. Press the fingers of one hand into your abdomen at your navel. Slowly raise your head and shoulder blades. The rectus muscles will tense, letting you detect any gap. Move your fingers up along this line from the navel to your sternum, noticing the width of the gap. Then move your fingers down from the navel to your pelvis. A slight gap (1 finger's width) indicates normal muscle separation after pregnancy; it doesn't need to be closed. A larger gap between the muscles (more than 1 finger's width) indicates that you need to close the gap before doing crunches and other conventional abdominal exercises. If you don't close the separation, your abdominal muscles can't support your body as effectively. Doing moderate to strenuous exercise—or even certain movements such as sitting up straight when getting out of bed—puts you at risk for widening a large gap further.

To help narrow any gap, do transverse abdominal contractions and head lifts (see page 91). Progress to more advanced abdominal exercises only after the gap has narrowed to the width of one finger throughout the length of your abdomen and when your abdominals can keep your rectus muscles closely aligned without your support.[6] If the gap is the width of two fingers or more, work with a women's health physical therapist. An abdominal binder will likely be recommended to help support your muscles for proper healing.

### Squats

*Aim:* To strengthen your buttocks, hamstrings, and pelvic floor.

*Exercise:* Stand with your feet shoulder-width apart with your knees up against a couch or chair. Begin by bending your knees, slowly lowering your buttocks backward, as if you're preparing to sit back on a toilet. As you move down, your arms should extend in front of you for balance. Push through both of your heels equally as you rise, lowering your arms as you do.

*Repetition:* Do two sets of ten. Repeat the exercise two to three times each day.

### Pectoral Stretch, Hip Flexor Stretch, and Posture Check

See pages 93–94 for instructions.

## *Tension Relievers*

The following exercises relieve muscle tension and promote overall relaxation.

### Head Tilts

*Aim:* To relieve muscle tension in your neck caused by holding your baby.

*Exercise:* Look straight ahead and tilt your right ear toward your right shoulder and hold for ten seconds. Don't let your left shoulder rise. Repeat on your left side.

*Repetition:* Do this exercise once a day or as often as feels good.

### Chin Tucks

*Aim:* To strengthen your neck muscles to keep your head aligned for proper posture.

*Exercise:* Look straight ahead and imagine you have a crown on your head. Slowly move your chin straight backward, keeping the crown parallel to the floor. Return to the starting position by moving your chin straight forward. Don't move your chin up and down.

*Repetition:* Do this exercise five to ten times throughout your day.

### Shoulder Circles

See the instructions on page 94. This exercise relieves tension in your shoulders and upper back caused by holding your baby.

### Relaxation and Slow Breathing

*Aim:* To relax and rejuvenate your body and to release mental stress that accompanies baby care.

*Exercise:* Use the same relaxation techniques you found helpful during pregnancy and birth. For example, try five minutes of slow breathing (see page 243), passive relaxation (see page 234), relaxation countdown (see page 236), or the five-minute meditation (see page 97).

*Repetition:* Do this exercise whenever you have a moment. Use the time to recognize what a phenomenal job you're doing as a new parent!

## Peekaboo Yoga

Here's a fun way to stretch your body and bond with your baby. Start on your hands and knees. Place your baby on his back underneath you so your eyes are level with his. Then follow this sequence of poses, which are described on pages 95–97:

1. Cat pose
2. Child's pose (Stretch your arms above your head with your forearms cradling your baby.)
3. Opposite-limb extensions
4. Child's pose
5. Downward-facing dog
6. Child's pose
7. Downward-facing dog
8. Child's pose
9. Half-dog pose
10. Bridge pose (While you do this exercise, move your baby to the side, perhaps on his tummy. Or hold him on your abdomen)
11. Corpse pose with five-minute meditation (Your baby can be either on your abdomen or next to you.)

## POSTPARTUM FITNESS AFTER A CESAREAN BIRTH

If you've had a cesarean birth, see chapter 15 for activities that are appropriate for the first few days after surgery, such as deep breathing, knee bends, and abdominal pull-ins. Pelvic floor exercises are also fine to do.

Your caregiver will probably recommend that you wait at least six weeks before doing any strenuous activities, including the postpartum exercises described on pages 332–335. Consult with your caregiver before starting an exercise regimen.

## POSTPARTUM FITNESS AFTER A CHALLENGING PREGNANCY OR BIRTH

If you were pregnant with multiples, were on bed rest, or had a difficult pregnancy or birth, your recovery may be more challenging than other women's. Conserve your energy initially, until you can do things more normally. As you resume your daily activities, your strength will return. When you're able to exercise, begin gently and try not to get frustrated that you can't do more. Set reasonable expectations and try not to compare your progress with other women's. Be patient with yourself and celebrate every accomplishment.

## A NOTE TO FATHERS AND PARTNERS

When your partner is ready, gently encourage her to exercise, but don't pressure her. Help her make time for exercise, and consider exercising with her so you can spend some time together while improving your health.

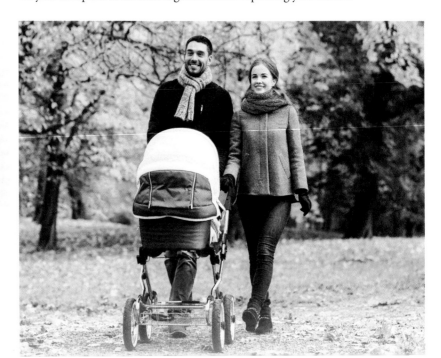

# Adapting to Postpartum Life

As a new parent, you may sometimes yearn for the simpler, more predictable life you had before you began tending to your baby's seemingly never-ending needs. You may wonder how long it'll take you to physically recover from the birth and to balance the interests and demands of your former life with the joys and needs of your new life with your baby. A common question asked by new parents is: "When will my life ever get back to normal?" In one informal survey, when parents of four- to twelve-week-olds were asked, "Do you feel confident about your ability to parent well," only 11 percent agreed strongly.

At some point after your baby's birth, you'll find a "new normal" (also called *postpartum adaptation*), and your life will return to more predictable patterns. You can take care of daily demands, feel rested most of the time, and begin to enjoy previous interests again. Your body is healing, and you can meet your baby's needs with growing confidence. In the same informal survey mentioned earlier, when parents of six-month-olds were asked if they felt confident about their parenting abilities, 99 percent either agreed or strongly agreed. (See page 340 for factors that influence your adjustment to postpartum life.)

The following sections describe areas of your life that will be affected by your baby's arrival and may require special attention as you adapt to your new role. Visit our website, http://www.PCNGuide.com, to download a work sheet to help you prepare.

## LEARNING TO PARENT

Parenting is learned skill; it's not instinctive. Your ability to parent depends on several factors, including how your parents raised you; parenting styles you've seen; experiences you've had with young children; knowledge of the physical, emotional, and intellectual abilities and needs of children; and the temperament and needs of your baby.

Your baby is your best teacher. You can learn about her abilities, needs, and development by observing her behavior and responses to your care, reading baby-care books, or attending parenting classes.

The early weeks of parenting aren't always easy, but if you (and your partner) are nurtured and receive help, you'll have the time and energy to care for your baby and build strong family bonds.

## PARENTING WITH A PARTNER

If you're parenting with a partner, you both don't need to do things the same way to appreciate each other as parents. If you have different approaches, discuss your views and arrive at a comfortable solution together so you both feel respected, supported, and involved. Consult with your baby's caregiver, a parent educator, a postpartum doula, or a baby-care book for ideas. Let the small problems go (such as a diaper put on backward) so you can work out the large issues together (such as how to respond to crying). Try not to interfere with each other's parenting or protect each other from the realities of baby care.

## Parenting Groups and New-Parent Classes

Connecting with other new parents is one of the most helpful ways to ease the transition to parenthood. (See appendix C for information on specialized support groups for complicated circumstances.) By attending a parenting group or new-parent class, you can learn about other parenting styles, hear new solutions to common parenting problems, see other babies' development, and discover that you're not the only one overwhelmed by postpartum life.

Hospitals, churches, community colleges, and community organizations may offer parenting groups and classes. Many of these target mothers, but most welcome fathers and partners. Plan ahead by learning about local groups and classes before your baby's birth.

# Your Sex Life after the Birth

Many caregivers recommend that new mothers don't have intercourse for the first six weeks, but this time frame is arbitrary. If you and your partner want to resume intercourse as soon as possible after the birth, it's probably safe to do so after any stitches have healed and the amount of lochia has decreased. But be gentle; you may be sore at first. In addition, after giving birth (and for as long as you breastfeed), hormonal changes reduce vaginal lubrication. A water-soluble lubricant can help.

If you'd rather wait until well after the birth to resume your sex life, that's perfectly normal. Having a sore perineum, a demanding baby, little help, and extreme fatigue can affect your ability to enjoy sex. You may even fear it. Cuddling with your partner and gently enjoying each other's bodies (with or without orgasm) can help you both relax and show your love.

If you find even touching undesirable, express those feelings honestly but respectfully, especially if your partner has an interest in sex. Discuss other ways you can show your love for each other until you're ready to resume a physical relationship.

Whenever you choose to have intercourse, remember that you can become pregnant whether or not you've begun to menstruate. Your caregiver can help you choose a family-planning method. For example, using a condom in combination with spermicidal foam, cream, or jelly is safe and effective contraception soon after the birth. To learn more options, visit http://www.plannedparenthood.org/health-info/birth-control.

If you're breastfeeding, you may leak breast milk during intercourse, especially when you have an orgasm. The hormone oxytocin plays a strong role in both orgasm and milk ejection (let-down). Some women wear a bra and nursing pads when having sex. Others choose to ignore the leaking or find humor in the situation. As one woman said, "When the milk starts flowing, my partner and I know I'm having a good time!"

# A Note to Fathers and Partners

Once the excitement of having a new baby has faded, your baby's constant demands and frequent crying may begin to tax everyone's endurance. You may feel frustrated that your partner can soothe your baby and meet his needs better than you, especially if she's breastfeeding.

Despite your feelings, your family needs your continued support and care. By acknowledging that both parents are under a lot of stress and by sharing the parenting duties, you'll strengthen your relationship with your partner and your family.

To learn more about baby care and soothing skills, read chapters 18 and 19.

# Changes in Family Relationships

The birth of a baby can bring many emotional and social changes to immediate and extended family. Relatives, especially grandparents, are often eager to be a part of your baby's life. Think about what role they want to play—and the role you want them to play. Then try to discuss ideas and expectations with them before the birth. The sample letter on page 339 may help you express your thoughts.

If you have other children, a new sibling might or might not be a welcome addition. See chapter 21 for information on preparing an older child for a new baby.

Some new parents find that the demands of baby care challenge their relationship, especially if it was strained before the birth. If your relationship with your partner is troubled after the birth, see page 355 for help.

If you're a single parent, you may want (or need) the help of your family. See page 356 for a discussion on single parenthood.

# Returning to Work

Returning full-time to work or school is a big adjustment for any new parent and his or her family. See page 25 for information about child-care options. If you plan to continue breastfeeding, see page 412 to learn about pumping and storing your breast milk and about ways to keep up your supply. If you're struggling with the return to work or school, see page 430 for suggestions on ways to cope.

## A Letter to Grandparents

*Although grandparents are the focus of this letter, you can adapt it to suit another family member or friend and to reflect your circumstances.*

Dear Grandparents,
Congratulations on the birth of your new grandchild! This arrival continues your family for another generation. If you're wondering how you can best help the new parents' transition to parenthood, we have some suggestions.

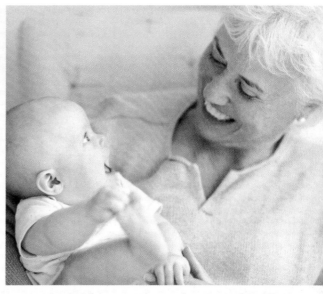

The new parents need to know that you think they're the best parents your grandchild can have. They need to hear that parenthood is challenging, tiring, and one of the most import-ant and rewarding experiences they'll ever have.

You'll find that some things have changed since you raised children, and some have remained the same. You need to honor the new parents' decisions and parenting style, even if their ways differ from your own. Please offer advice only when asked and help the new parents find up-to-date answers to their questions. Reading the same books they're reading about newborn care and feeding may help.

If you're invited to help, recognize the request as an honor. While it may be tempting to tell the new parents how to take care of the baby or to do everything for them, ask them *how* they want you to help. Be willing to take care of *them*—cook meals, do laundry, shop, and clean the house—so they can mas-ter caring for their baby. New parents need hands-on experience to learn the skills that all parents need to develop.

If you can't be with the new family or if your relationship with them is strained, think of another way to support them. For example, you can help pay for a postpartum doula, diaper service, meals, or travel expenses for another family member to help them. The new parents will appreciate your gesture, and it can help reconcile a troubled relationship.

Remember your first weeks as new parents and try to have realistic expectations. For example, forgive the new parents if they forget to thank you for your help and gifts. Your care and concern will enhance not only your relationship with your grandchild, but also your relationship with her parents. With best wishes for joyful grandparenting,

*Penny Janet Ann*

Penny, Janet, Ann
Grandmothers and coauthors of *Pregnancy, Childbirth, and the Newborn*

# Factors That Influence
# Your Adjustment to Postpartum Life

Every parent adjusts to life with a new baby differently. Some parents seem to find a comfortable balance in their lives within weeks. Others take months to adjust, and some never do.

Why do some parents adjust to postpartum life more easily than others do? Numerous factors can influence the adjustment process. Some factors are internal, such as the health of the pregnancy. Others are external, such as the strength of a new family's support network.

The following are favorable or positive factors that can help ease your adjustment to parenthood. The more of these factors you have, the more likely your adjustment to postpartum life will be smooth. The fewer of these factors you have, the more likely your adjustment will take longer than the typical eight to twelve weeks. You might not be able to control some of these factors, but developing a postpartum plan can help improve others (see chapter 8). In addition, getting counseling may help you cope with past challenges, and finding extra support can help you manage current challenges, such as getting errands done and paying bills.

## Before pregnancy

- positive experience with how you were raised
- good mental and physical health (you and your family)
- minimal exposure to trauma
- positive experience with previous pregnancies, births, and baby care

## During pregnancy

- planned pregnancy
- no pregnancy complications
- pregnant with only one baby
- no need for prolonged bed rest or treatment for a high-risk pregnancy
- minimal financial worries
- physically undemanding job
- adequate sleep
- good relationship with the baby's father or your partner
- presence of other supportive people

## During labor and birth

- normal, uncomplicated birth
- presence of continuous, competent care and support from staff, your partner, and other support people
- feeling respected, informed, and empowered to make choices about your care

## Early postpartum period

- immediate contact with your baby (including breastfeeding)
- minimal postpartum pain
- good health (you and your baby)

## Later postpartum period

- delaying the return to employment until you feel ready
- your baby's easy temperament and continuing health
- no feeding problems
- adequate sleep for the whole family
- positive emotional state
- continuing supportive relationships with your partner, family, and friends

# Postpartum Emotional Challenges

After giving birth, your emotions will fluctuate, partly from extreme changes in your hormone levels and partly from fatigue, inexperience or uncertainty with baby care, loneliness or isolation, changes to your normal routine, and your baby's around-the-clock demands. Mood swings may also be caused by a disappointing or difficult birth, an unexpected illness or condition in your baby, a personally stressful situation (social, financial, or physical), or a personal or family history of mood disorders.

For most women, these emotional fluctuations are mild and decrease within a few weeks (see below). For others, the mood swings are overwhelming, long lasting, and may require treatment.

## BABY BLUES

About 80 percent of new mothers and many new fathers experience *baby blues* (or the "blues"), usually within the first week after the birth. Symptoms of baby blues include the following:

- crying easily
- feeling overwhelmed or out of control
- feeling exhausted, anxious, or sad
- lacking confidence as a parent

Baby blues are normal and rarely last longer than two weeks. You can diminish the condition by getting more rest, reducing any pain you're experiencing, and surrounding yourself with supportive family and friends. If you're feeling sad or upset, get support immediately. A few encouraging words may be all you need to feel better. Without support, you may have a tougher time shaking baby blues.

## POSTPARTUM MOOD DISORDERS

About 20 percent of new mothers develop postpartum mood disorders (PPMD), which are more serious than baby blues. See chapter 17 for a complete discussion of PPMD.

# Putting Parenthood into Perspective

The early weeks and months of parenting can seem all consuming and overwhelming. But when you think of how long your lifetime will be, parenting is just a small slice of the "pie of life" (see chart). Some parents find that this chart helps put the daily frustrations in perspective.

You live roughly the first third of your life before becoming a parent. During this time, you develop as an individual and may begin a relationship with someone and consider starting a family with that person.

You spend the next third of your life having and caring for your children. During this time, many couples are caught up with child care and careers, and they neglect to nurture their relationship. Make time with your partner for conversation and shared activities. Also make time for your own interests so you keep growing as an individual, as well as a parent and partner.

You spend the last third of your life with an "empty nest." Your children are grown and living elsewhere, and you and your partner are once again just a couple. This phase may come with reduced responsibilities or different duties, such as caring for your aging parents. You may have time to pursue interests—perhaps grandparenting! One of you will outlive the other at some point, and that person must draw on the support of family and friends, as well as on interests and passions, to find a new way in life.

From the moment your child is born, you'll be a parent for the rest of your life. However, your time spent as a parent of a baby is brief. Enjoy it!

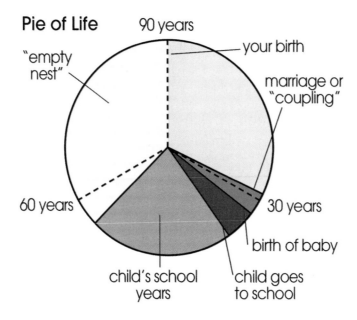

# *Key Points to Remember*

- The postpartum period is a time of physical and emotional readjustment and recovery. Everyone's adjustment is unique. Factors that arise before, during, and after pregnancy and birth all affect your recovery.
- Your body undergoes many normal changes in the postpartum period. You can help your recovery by eating well, exercising when ready, asking for help when needed, and getting adequate sleep. Be aware of any warning signs that may indicate a problem with your physical or emotional recovery (see page 329).
- Transitioning to parenthood can be frustrating and overwhelming at times, but most parents adjust well with help and support.
- Although you'll be a parent for a lifetime, the time you'll spend on baby care is brief.

# CHAPTER 17

# When Postpartum Becomes Complicated

Our culture embraces a joyous picture of new motherhood:
A stylish, slender mother tending to her beautiful, chubby
baby with minimal signs of stress or fatigue. But this depiction
doesn't represent reality. After the birth, many mothers just try
to get through the days and nights with a newborn as best as
they can. They may need months to become confident, comfortable, and happy with baby care and their new roles as mothers.

For some women and their families, postpartum recovery
is more challenging than usual because of a traumatic birth
experience, a physical condition that makes recuperation difficult, an emotional complication (such as postpartum depression), or a strained relationship. This chapter addresses some of
these unexpected and uncommon complications and troubling
situations that can challenge the postpartum period. It also
offers empathetic advice and solutions so you can learn how
to manage these complications and focus on enjoying life
with your baby.

# Physical Challenges after the Birth

Physical challenges can prolong postpartum recovery and make it more painful than usual. After giving birth, you may find it difficult to sit, walk, or carry your baby. You may be in constant pain and require frequent medical appointments or even hospitalization. If you're in this condition, you'll need extra help and support from family members, friends, or professionals, such as lactation consultants or postpartum doulas. These people can help take care of you, your baby, your family, and your household.

The following sections discuss common physical challenges after birth and comfort measures to help manage them.

## LARGE EPISIOTOMY OR SEVERE PERINEAL TEARING

To reduce the pain from a large episiotomy or severe perineal tearing (laceration), use the comfort measures discussed on page 326 and take any prescribed pain medication. Because constipation is a common side effect of narcotics such as Vicodin, see page 114 for tips to treat constipation. To reduce swelling, lie down as often as possible. If the pain worsens, contact your caregiver to detect problems that need further treatment.

## URINARY INCONTINENCE

For a short time after giving birth, you may have urinary *incontinence*, a condition that causes you to leak urine when you have a full bladder, exercise, cough, or sneeze. Leaking usually stops on its own within weeks of the birth.[1] To treat urinary incontinence, practice your Kegel exercises and squats (see page 90) frequently each day. Use maxi pads or incontinence pads to protect clothing.

Sometimes, leaking happens even without a full bladder or exercise, and it can persist for more than a month or two. This condition is more serious—and often embarrassing and depressing. Talk with your caregiver about treatment options. If necessary, consider asking your caregiver to recommend a physical therapist to evaluate the effectiveness of your Kegels and suggest other exercises and therapies.[2] In rare cases, caregivers recommend surgery if the condition persists for more than a year.

## FECAL INCONTINENCE

After giving birth, you may have fecal incontinence, an embarrassing and upsetting condition that causes you to uncontrollably pass gas or leak stool.[3] The condition may persist for the first few weeks after the birth. (If it persists for more than a month, contact your caregiver.)

To treat fecal incontinence, practice your Kegel exercises. Research shows that Kegels can help a woman regain bowel control.[4] Use incontinence pads to protect clothing. Consult with your caregiver about medications or changes to your diet that can help stop fecal incontinence. On rare occasions, caregivers recommend surgery to correct the problem.

# Persistent Hemorrhoids

Pregnancy often causes hemorrhoids (dilated veins in the anus and rectum that can cause pain or itchiness). Most hemorrhoids disappear in the first month following the birth; however, some persist for months.

To help prevent and treat hemorrhoids, follow the recommendations in on page 327. If these measures don't provide adequate relief, consult with your caregiver about any outpatient procedures that may help. In rare circumstances, a caregiver may recommend surgery to correct the problem.

# Persistent Breastfeeding Problems

In the first weeks after the birth, most breastfeeding women experience sore nipples and breast fullness. But some women have intense breastfeeding challenges that continue for weeks or months. If you find breastfeeding to be an ongoing painful, time-consuming challenge and you dread the next feeding, you may feel angry, sad, or even depressed because your breastfeeding experience isn't what you expected.

If breastfeeding problems make you think about quitting breastfeeding, contact a lactation consultant or other breastfeeding expert for support, information, suggestions, and tips. These professionals can tell you whether and how soon the problem can be fixed, and they can help you adjust your approach to nursing if necessary. If the problem requires medical attention, they can refer you to a physician who specializes in breastfeeding medicine, dermatology, or infectious disease. Some communities offer support groups for women with breastfeeding challenges.

Despite having excellent support and a commitment to breastfeeding, some women have problems that don't improve, causing exhaustion and despair. These women realize that stopping breastfeeding is the only solution—one that may cause great sadness or great relief. If you're in this position, a lactation consultant or your caregiver can help you sort out your feelings with the decision, acknowledge the hard work you put into breastfeeding, and show you how to feed your baby with formula. If you have strong negative feelings about your breastfeeding experience, consider talking to a counselor to help you come to terms with your decision.

For more information on breastfeeding challenges, see chapter 20.

# Thyroid Problems

Three to eight months after giving birth, 5 to 7 percent of women develop postpartum thyroiditis, a two-phase condition in which the thyroid gland first becomes inflamed and overactive (hyperthyroidism) and then returns to normal function or becomes underactive (hypothyroidism).

Symptoms of hyperthyroidism typically last a short time and include feeling overheated, muscle weakness, shakiness, anxiety, rapid heart rate, inability to concentrate, and weight loss. The thyroid may recover completely from hyperthyroidism, but if the inflammation damaged the gland, it may then become underactive.

Symptoms of hypothyroidism include tiredness, constipation, memory loss, intolerance of cold, muscle cramps, weakness, weight gain, and inadequate breast milk production. Hypothyroidism may disappear and the thyroid function may return to normal. If the gland remains underactive, caregivers typically prescribe thyroid hormone replacement medication.

## Advice from the Authors

### Asking for Help

When asking family members and friends for help during your postpartum recovery, you may find that people are more eager to help if given specific tasks, such as cooking meals, shopping, housecleaning, or holding your baby. This way, your loved ones don't have to worry their help is misdirected, unwanted, or duplicated by someone else. Plus, by letting people know what you'd like them to do, you ensure you get the kind of help you need when you need it.

## In Their Own Words

If you experience these symptoms, don't ignore them or blame them on sleep deprivation. Instead, call your caregiver. Because thyroiditis is a risk factor for developing postpartum depression (see page 352), it's important to diagnose and treat the condition or rule it out as the cause of your symptoms.

## GALLBLADDER PROBLEMS

The gallbladder is a small organ that receives bile from the liver and concentrates it before sending it to the digestive tract to aid with fat digestion. Pregnancy hormones slightly increase the risk of developing gallstones, caused by a slowdown in the passage of bile from the gallbladder. When the stones leave the gallbladder, they may clog the bile duct and cause sharp and extreme pain.

Symptoms of gallstones include nausea, vomiting, abdominal bloating, burping, gas, indigestion, and steady, increasing pain in the upper abdomen, under the right shoulder, or between the shoulder blades. The pain often occurs after eating fatty foods or at night and lasts thirty minutes to several hours. If you experience sweating, chills, fever, yellow skin, or clay-colored bowel movements, see your caregiver immediately. The treatment for gallbladder problems is laparoscopic surgery.

## LATE POSTPARTUM HEMORRHAGE

Late postpartum hemorrhage is a large loss of blood occurring between twenty-four hours to six weeks after the birth. Infection or retained fragments of the placenta usually cause the bleeding, which occurs in 1 percent of women. If a woman loses a significantly large amount of blood, she may develop anemia (see below).

To treat late postpartum hemorrhage, a caregiver removes the fragments of placenta using medications or a D&C (see page 122), or treats a uterine infection with antibiotics.

## SEVERE ANEMIA

*Anemia* is a condition in which the number of red blood cells is lower than normal. Many women are mildly anemic during pregnancy and after the birth, but 2 to 4 percent of women become severely anemic from postpartum hemorrhage. Anemia is also a risk factor for developing postpartum depression (see page 352).[5]

Symptoms of anemia include weakness, lightheadedness, shortness of breath, and overwhelming fatigue. A caregiver can diagnose anemia by analyzing a blood sample.

To treat anemia, caregivers advise women to take an iron supplement and eat iron-rich foods. (Visit our website, http://www.PCNGuide.com, for more information on iron-rich foods.). Caregivers rarely order a blood transfusion to treat anemia unless the blood loss is life threatening.

If you have severe anemia, you'll need extra help with baby care and housework. When getting up from sitting or lying down, move slowly. Have someone accompany you to the bathtub or shower to prevent falling if you become lightheaded.

# Postpartum High Blood Pressure (Hypertension)

Hypertensive disorders (high blood pressure) affect 6 to 8 percent pregnancies in the United States.[6] For most women with gestational hypertension (see page 133), blood pressure returns to normal after the birth. Some women, however, continue to have high blood pressure, and a few women develop the condition after the birth.

Little information exists on preventing or treating postpartum hypertension,[7] but complementary medical approaches (such as acupuncture, meditation, and yoga) may help augment traditional medical therapies.

If you develop postpartum hypertension, your blood pressure will most likely return to normal, but it may remain a continuing health concern. To monitor your blood pressure and find an effective medication for treatment, you'll need to see your caregiver frequently. While these appointments can complicate postpartum life, they're necessary to ensure your health. If breastfeeding, ask your caregiver or a lactation consultant if a blood pressure medication is safe for nursing.

# Back and Hip Pain

After giving birth, many women experience pain in the lower back or pelvic region. Sometimes, the pain results after a woman twists or overstretches her lower back or pelvic and hip joints while she's numb from epidural or spinal anesthesia. This pain may last for the first few days or weeks after the birth, and many caregivers recommend ibuprofen for relief. If you develop this pain and it interferes with your ability to walk or roll over, ask your caregiver to refer you to a physical therapist.

If you injured or broke your tailbone (coccyx) before the birth, your baby's passage through your pelvis may flex or even rebreak your tailbone, causing pain and bruising. Even if you didn't injure or break your tailbone before birth, it may break or become injured during birth if your baby is large. The tailbone will reset itself, but it may take weeks to months. Taking ibuprofen, applying heat or cold packs, and sitting on a firm surface can help relieve pain.

Sometimes in pregnancy or during birth, the pubic joint in the front of the pelvis (pubic symphysis) widens or separates, causing some women to experience mild to debilitating pain in the pubic region after giving birth. Because pubic pain isn't well documented, caregivers may underestimate the severity of the condition or even dismiss it as normal pain that will disappear with time.

To treat pubic pain, avoid lifting objects and making movements that cause pain, such as stair climbing, vacuuming, and spreading your legs or knees wide apart. Use a walker or a sturdy baby stroller if walking is especially painful. Working with a physical therapist can speed recovery.

# Numbness and Pain in Your Hands

After birth, you may experience numbness, tingling, weakness, or pain in your hands and wrists. These symptoms may stem from the swelling around the nerves in your wrists (for example, carpal tunnel syndrome), caused by extra fluid your body retained in pregnancy. After the birth, the swelling diminishes as the fluid level naturally decreases over time; however, until it does, repetitive activities—such as holding, lifting, and carrying your baby—can exacerbate these symptoms.

To treat numbness and pain, try to keep your wrists in a neutral position (not bent or curled) when handling or feeding your baby. Consider buying wrist splints if keeping your wrists in a neutral position is difficult. If symptoms don't improve, ask your caregiver to refer you to a physical therapist or hand specialist for ultrasonic therapy, custom splinting, exercises, or corticosteroid treatments.

# Traumatic Birth Experience

If birth was much worse than you'd expected, you may feel traumatized, sad, angry, and confused. In the weeks and months afterward, as your baby needs less immediate care and you have time to think about your experience, these feelings may intensify.

Sadly, you're not alone. Between 25 and 34 percent of women describe their births as traumatic, and up to 9 percent develop post-traumatic stress disorder (PTSD).[8]

When you share your birth story with others, you may receive responses such as, "But thank goodness you have a healthy baby!" or "But you're okay now!" These comments may make you feel ashamed of your feelings about the birth, and you may try to ignore them.

Ignoring feelings of extreme sadness, fear, loss, or anger won't make them go away. An event such as a new pregnancy or the birth of a friend's baby can unexpectedly bring up unresolved feelings you may have about your labor, birth, and postpartum experience.

To deal with these feelings, talk with your caregiver (or someone knowledgeable about birth) about your experience to help you understand how events unfolded. You may want to visit an online support group for parents who have experienced birth trauma, such as http://www.solaceformothers.org, to help validate your feelings. You may want to work with a therapist or counselor who can help you acknowledge the unusual difficulty of your experience and find healthy ways to express your feelings and be an advocate for yourself, your baby, and your family. For example, if you choose to have another baby, you can work with your caregiver on a plan for having a better birth experience. For more resources, visit http://pattch.org.

# Emotional and
# Mental Health Challenges

*Perinatal mood and anxiety disorders (PMAD)* —sometimes called prenatal or postpartum mood disorders (PPMD)— include the emotional conditions that can develop during pregnancy and in the first year after giving birth, such as anxiety and panic disorder, obsessive-compulsive disorder, postpartum depression, bipolar disorder, and post-traumatic stress disorder. Women can have multiple disorders at once. About 20 percent of women will experience one or more PMAD in the weeks or months after giving birth. About a third of those women say their symptoms developed during pregnancy.[9] About 5 percent of new fathers experience PMAD.

PMAD are more serious than "baby blues" (see page 341) and can complicate the postpartum period significantly. They can be emotionally paralyzing and cause feelings of hopelessness and isolation. In addition, our culture presents pregnancy and postpartum as times when an expectant or new parent should be blissfully happy, which may lead affected new mothers to feel ashamed and hide their symptoms and not seek the help they need and deserve.

The following sections describe PMAD and their risk factors. As you read about the conditions, know that the severity of the symptoms varies among individuals.

## In Their Own Words

I had preeclampsia and a very premature birth. Soon after the birth, my daughter was admitted to the neonatal intensive care unit, and I had two seizures. It was a frightening time. A year later, I became upset when I visited a friend in the same hospital. After leaving my friend, I sat in my car and cried for quite some time. I knew then that I needed to understand what had happened to me and to learn how to deal with the triggers (such as being in a hospital) that had caused me to feel deeply and inconsolably sad. I talked with my doctor, who helped me understand the events of my pregnancy and birth. I also found a therapist to help me deal with my feelings and reactions.
—*Elsa*

## POSTPARTUM ANXIETY AND PANIC DISORDER

About 10 percent of women have postpartum anxiety and panic attacks; however, those women with a history of anxiety and panic disorder have an increased risk of developing the condition after giving birth. Symptoms include shortness of breath, sensations of choking, lightheadedness, faintness, rapid heart rate, chest pain, nausea, and diarrhea. If you develop this disorder, an overwhelming fear of being alone, dying (you or your baby), or leaving your home may immobilize you.

## PERINATAL AND POSTPARTUM OBSESSIVE-COMPULSIVE DISORDER (OCD)

About 3 to 5 percent of women develop perinatal and postpartum OCD, a condition characterized by obsessive (uncontrollable) thoughts and compulsive rituals to protect the baby. Many report that symptoms started during pregnancy. All mothers typically have instincts to protect their babies, but these instincts are extreme in women with postpartum OCD. Examples of obsessive thoughts include a fear of being a "bad" mother, of hurting the baby, or of germs. Compulsive rituals can include constant hand washing (up to hundreds of times each day), frequent housecleaning, excessively checking on the baby, or constantly ensuring that doors are locked. Not surprisingly, these rituals interfere with normal daily living.

## Common Q&A

**Q:** What is placental encapsulation? Can it help with postpartum depression?

**A:** Placental encapsulation is the process by which a mother's placenta, after it's expelled, is dried, powdered, and put into capsules. The mother takes the capsules in the weeks after the birth with the belief that they'll help raise her energy level, increase her milk supply, and reduce the risk of PMAD or the severity of symptoms. The practice is traditional in some cultures, and it's becoming more common in North America. Although many women swear that the capsules helped them, the research on the efficacy and safety of placental encapsulation is limited.

# PERINATAL AND POSTPARTUM DEPRESSION

*Perinatal and postpartum depression* can occur in pregnancy or within the first six months after the birth. Depression in pregnancy appears in up to 20 percent of expectant parents—and rates are even higher among those with a lower income.[10] Postpartum depression occurs in 10 to 20 percent of new mothers. For a woman with a history of depression, the risk of developing the condition increases to 30 percent. For a woman with past perinatal depression, the risk increases to 70 percent.[11]

Depression can begin at any time in pregnancy, but it's most common in the late third trimester. Postpartum depression generally occurs between two weeks to one year after the birth, although the onset typically begins between the sixth week and the sixth month. Symptoms vary in severity among women and include the following:

- feelings of hopelessness, despair, and exhaustion
- feelings of extreme inadequacy and low self-esteem
- lack of energy
- loss of interest in everything
- inability to sleep, even when an opportunity arises
- overeating or forgetting to eat
- constant crying
- surprising and frightening outbursts of anger at loved ones
- recurring thoughts about hurting oneself (even committing suicide) or the baby

## BIPOLAR DISORDER OR MANIC DEPRESSION

Bipolar disorder (BD) occurs in 2 percent of the population. A woman diagnosed with BD before pregnancy will likely relapse if not treated during pregnancy and the postpartum period.

BD usually begins with extreme mood elevation, energy, and grandiose thoughts within a few days to weeks after the birth. A long-term period of depression may follow. Suicide is a risk during both mania and depression. A woman with BD needs the care of a psychiatrist or therapist with expertise in treating the condition.

## POSTPARTUM POST-TRAUMATIC STRESS DISORDER

After the birth, post-traumatic stress disorder (PTSD) may result from a difficult or frightening birth or from traumatic situations, such as an unexpected illness, sudden problems for the baby, or insensitive or hurtful care. PTSD can also occur when birth triggers memories of a traumatic event, such as a frightening hospital experience, physical or sexual abuse, or rape.

Common symptoms of PTSD include preoccupation with the trauma, flashbacks to the event or recurrent nightmares (both possibly accompanied by anxiety and panic attacks), anger or rage, and extreme protectiveness of oneself or the baby.

## RISK FACTORS FOR PMAD

While no one can predict who will have PMAD, the factors listed below increase your risk of developing one of the conditions. If you have several of these risk factors or are worried about developing PMAD, consider getting extra support during pregnancy, making a postpartum plan (see chapter 8) or learning about resources for support *before* the baby comes and your life becomes challenging for you.

### History of mental health challenges

- panic disorder, OCD, depression, or BD (or history of these challenges in an immediate family member)
- physical, emotional, or sexual abuse
- eating disorders
- substance abuse (or living with someone who's abusing drugs or alcohol)

### Challenges with menstruation, pregnancy, birth, or your baby

- history of severe premenstrual symptoms
- history of infertility or miscarriages
- unplanned and unwanted pregnancy
- traumatic pregnancy or birth
- high-needs baby or a baby with a chronic medical condition
- feeding problems with your baby

### Temperament

- low self-esteem
- high expectations to be perfect and in control

### Recent stressful life events

- death in the family
- moving to a new home
- changing jobs or losing a job
- getting married, separating, or divorcing
- financial pressures
- excessive sleep deprivation

### Lack of support

- unsupportive partner or no partner
- unsupportive friends or family
- poor or absent relationship with your mother

### Health issues

- thyroid disease
- anemia[12]
- inflammation

## TREATING PMAD

If you suspect that you're experiencing symptoms of PMAD, discuss them with your caregiver, a therapist, or other professional who's familiar with PMAD. Seek help early, before you start having trouble coping. Early treatment can shorten the duration of PMAD.

## Myths and Facts about PMAD

**Myth:** All women feel sad, anxious, or angry after giving birth. The feelings will go away if I just "tough it out" or ignore or deny them.
**Fact:** Acknowledging how you feel and getting help will speed your recovery. If your feelings are strong enough that they interfere with your ability to care for your baby or yourself, seek support.

**Myth:** Having PMAD means I'm a weak person.
**Fact:** Strong, intelligent women have PMAD. You didn't cause the condition by anything you did.

**Myth:** Feeling angry or having thoughts about hurting myself or the baby means I'm a bad mother.
**Fact:** Having these feelings and thoughts isn't unusual. Your life has just been upended, and you're trying to find your balance again. Although women with PMAD may have these harmful thoughts and feelings, they don't act on them.

**Myth:** If I take medication for PMAD, I can't breastfeed.
**Fact:** Check with your caregiver or therapist for medications that are compatible with breastfeeding.

## Advice from the Authors

### Inflammation and PMAD

Research shows that inflammation and a lack of omega-3 fatty acids in a woman's diet are major risk factors for PMAD (as well as for depression in the general population).

Consuming too many omega-6 fatty acids (found in vegetable oils and many processed foods) can cause inflammation. Late pregnancy and postpartum stressors (such as sleep deprivation, major life stress, and pain) also raise inflammation levels.

Consuming omega-3 fatty acids (found in fish, flax meal, and other foods and supplements) can lower high levels of inflammation and prevent or treat postpartum depression and possibly other PMAD.[13] For more information on omega-3 fatty acids, see page 108.

Appropriate treatment for PMAD depends on the severity of the symptoms. A mild case may resolve with just the self-care ideas listed below. Most parents, however, benefit from a combination of self-care, peer support, professional support, and/or medications.

### Self-care for PMAD

- Eat well and get regular exercise.
- Avoid alcohol, caffeine, and over-the-counter sleep medications.
- Get enough sunlight or use a light box to decrease the risk of developing seasonal affective disorder (SAD).
- Take time for yourself each day—even if it's just for five minutes.
- Get adequate rest and sleep.
- Get enough omega-3 fatty acids to reduce inflammation (see page 108).

### Other treatment options

- Attend a PMAD support group, which helps women and their families understand the conditions, recognize the causes, and learn about resources for support. Your caregiver, childbirth educator, local hospital, or health department can refer you to a support group in your area. You can also contact Postpartum Support International by phone (800-944-4773) or by visiting their website at http://postpartum.net.
- Get counseling or therapy. Choose a therapist or psychiatrist who specializes in PMAD.
- Take prescribed medication for anxiety, OCD, depression, and bipolar disorder. (Getting counseling along with medication can help with a more rapid recovery than medication alone.)

### *A Note to Fathers, Partners, and Relatives*

PMAD can affect the whole family. Parents with PMAD often worry about their ability to be physically and emotionally available to their babies. You may worry, too.

To help new parents with PMAD, encourage them to get treatment, provide support and care, gather information on interacting with a newborn, help with housework, and find ways to ensure they get rest and sleep.

Getting enough sleep may be the most important step to recovery, but it can also be the most challenging. Help with nighttime feeding and parenting so a new parent with PMAD gets two or more three- to four-hour stretches of sleep each night. Consider getting support from other family members, a postpartum doula (see page 23), or mother/baby support groups.

## POSTPARTUM PSYCHOSIS

*Postpartum psychosis* is a rare condition that occurs in about one woman out of a thousand soon after giving birth. It's more serious than PMAD. Symptoms include severe agitation, mood swings, depression, and delusions. Women with postpartum psychosis need immediate care and psychiatric treatment. Hospitalization is often necessary at the onset of the condition, at which time women take medications to treat symptoms. Once home, women continue taking medications (monitored by a psychiatrist) and receive ongoing psychotherapy.

# Relationship Challenges

The postpartum period can become more challenging than usual if there are problems in your relationship with your partner or if the relationship is abusive. You may also feel stress if you feel your partner isn't taking on a fair share of the parenting and housekeeping tasks.

If you're a single parent, you may have additional stress.

The following sections discuss these challenges and suggest ways to manage them.

## Your Relationship with Your Partner

Research finds that many spouses (especially women) become less satisfied with their marriages after the birth of their first babies.[14] Caring for a newborn disrupts family life and can cause chaos and confusion until the family establishes new comfortable patterns.

New parenthood can leave little time to nurture a couple's relationship. If a new mother believes her partner isn't as supportive as she expected, or if the couple's lifestyles and activities grow apart after becoming parents, the relationship can become strained.[15] Relationship problems may also arise if relatives are intrusive or unsupportive, or if the baby is high-needs or has serious medical needs.

How can relationships survive the strain of new parenthood? Having a good relationship before the birth is the best predictor that a couple will have continued satisfaction with the relationship after the birth. Also, if both parents wanted to have the baby, they're more likely to be happy with their relationship than if one of them had reservations about adding to the family.[16]

If your relationship with your partner becomes strained after the birth, improving matters will usually require a joint effort. First, you and your partner need to agree that a problem exists. Second, you need to agree to get the counseling that's critical to the relationship's survival and to your baby's healthy development. (If one of you refuses to get help, the other will still benefit from counseling.)

Professionals and resources that can help your relationship include marriage or couples counselors, religious counselors with professional expertise in helping families, or courses designed to provide practical, researched-based strategies for building strong relationships between couples, such as Becoming Parents Program, Inc. (http://www.becomingparents.com) and Bringing Baby Home (http://www.bbhonline.org).

## Two Views on Relationships after the Birth

I had an unexpected, frightening, and very premature birth. My son spent a month in the neonatal intensive care unit and another month in the special care nursery. Because my marriage was strong, my husband and I together faced the fears and challenges of having a baby born so early. It did take months for us to feel safe taking our son out in public, but now he's almost a year old, and we see he's a strong and hearty boy. I'm grateful my husband and I had each other to lean on during that first tough year.
—Morgan

The birth of our son was a frightening time. I worried that I might lose both my wife and my child. Over the next months, I came to be in awe of both my wife's and son's resilience. Yes, there were some tough days and weeks, but we just took one day at a time. Now we have a sturdy one-year-old, and we are talking about having another baby.
—James

# ABUSE AND DOMESTIC VIOLENCE

Abuse and domestic violence (any combination of verbal, psychological, emotional, sexual, economic, or physical abuse) affect women of all ages, physical abilities, and lifestyles and of all religious, ethnic, socioeconomic, and educational backgrounds in rural and urban areas. The only risk factor for abuse and domestic violence is being a woman,[17] and the risk increases during pregnancy and especially after the birth.[18]

If you're in an abusive relationship, you are *not* at fault. The goal of abuse is to leave you feeling confused, ashamed, powerless, hopeless, and out of control. National and local agencies can help you and your children. Memorize the phone number for the National Domestic Violence Hotline, 800-799-SAFE (7233), and call if you need to talk to someone or need resources, including help making an escape plan for you and your children.

# SINGLE PARENTHOOD

About 30 percent of new mothers are single parents, some by choice and others by circumstance. For some single mothers, money is tight, and they need to find affordable child care and return to work soon after the birth. Others have jobs that pay well and provide excellent maternity leave benefits. For still others, the father may provide financial support or family members may provide a home and help with child care.

If you're a single mother, you'll need support as you recover from the birth and gain confidence as a parent. New parenthood can be socially isolating, especially if there aren't adults to talk to in the days following the birth. Organizations and networks exist that provide single mothers with opportunities to talk with one another. Visit http://www.single moms.org or http://www.singlemothersbychoice .com to learn more information.

# Returning to Work

In the United States, 60 percent of employed first-time mothers return to work by three months after giving birth. During pregnancy, a three-month parental leave may have seemed reasonable; however, many new mothers feel that they're just getting to know their babies at three months.

The return to work can be manageable for many families, but overwhelming for others. Some challenges include: finding suitable and affordable child care (see page 25), commuting to and from child care and work, coordinating breastfeeding and working (see page 430), feeding difficulties, health complications for mother or baby, sleep deprivation, or PMAD. If you're returning to a stressful job or unsupportive coworkers, the adjustment is further complicated.

If your child-care options are unacceptable or your work situation is unbearable, try to negotiate with your employer to delay your return to work, or adjust your schedule. Or you may choose to leave work. See our website, http://www.PCNGuide.com, for questions to consider.

If you want to help improve maternity and family benefits in the United States, support political action groups, such as Moms Rising (http://www.momsrising.org), whose efforts seek to change public policy on maternity and family leave and other benefits for mothers and families.

## *Key Points to Remember*

- For some women and families, physical, emotional, or social challenges can complicate the postpartum period and prolong recovery and adjustment to life with a newborn.
- Acknowledging the difficult circumstances of your postpartum period and seeking help are essential for recovery.
- Women who anticipate a complicated postpartum period should explore their options and learn about supportive resources before birth. Having a plan for extra help in place can reduce postpartum complications.

# CHAPTER 18

# Caring for Your Baby

After months of waiting, meeting your newborn can be an overwhelmingly emotional experience. You rejoice at finally being able to hold your baby in your arms and begin to eagerly observe and memorize every detail about this new child. At the same time, though, you realize that you're now responsible for another human being. You appreciate how much there is to learn about your baby, and you begin to worry about keeping her healthy and happy.

In this chapter, we cover all the basics about how to care for your baby, from interpreting her cues to meeting her needs, from soothing her crying to settling her to sleep. We also give you resources for where to look for more information, including one of the best sources of support and advice: other parents. With this information—along with time, practice, and guidance—your ability to care for your baby will soon become second nature.

# Meeting Your Baby

Immediately after the birth, the best place for your baby is on your bare chest, with just a blanket covering you both. This skin-to-skin contact helps stabilize your baby's breathing, temperature, and blood sugar,[1] and it allows your new family to bond (see page 198). These first few moments together provide you with wonderful memories as you discover all the things that make your baby unique. The following sections describe what you can expect as you get to know your newborn.

*Note:* In some circumstances, additional time is necessary for mothers and babies to get acquainted. If you had a long and tiring labor, your recovery may delay the enjoyment of meeting your newborn. If your baby has trouble adjusting to life outside your womb, he may need to be separated from you so medical staff can care for him. Prioritize skin-to-skin contact with your baby when you're reunited.

## YOUR NEWBORN'S APPEARANCE

When you first meet your baby, her appearance may surprise you. Newborns don't look like the "perfect" babies you see in advertisements. Their features can make a strong first impression, but they're completely normal. You'll probably find that you can't take your eyes off your new baby.

### Body

The average full-term baby weighs 7 to 7½ pounds and measures about 20 inches in length. A newborn's shoulders and hips are narrow, his tummy is round, and his arms and legs are relatively short, thin, and flexed.

### Head

A baby's head is large in proportion to her body. Her head may be molded (that is, appear cone-shaped or longer than expected) from pressures within the pelvis during birth. Her head will return to a normal round shape within a few days. Her scalp or face may appear bruised and swollen, but bruising and swelling will disappear with time.

A baby's skull has two soft spots called fontanels (areas where the bones haven't completely fused together). The smaller, triangle-shaped fontanel at the back of the skull will close by two to six months. The larger, diamond shaped one at the front will close by eighteen months. A thick, tough membrane covers the fontanels, so gently brushing or washing a baby's hair and scalp won't hurt her.

### Hair

At birth, a baby may have a full head of hair or be nearly bald. He may also have lanugo (fine, downy body hair) on his back, shoulders, forehead, ears, and face—especially if he's premature. Lanugo usually disappears during the first few weeks after the birth.

## Eyes

Fair-skinned babies usually have gray-blue eyes at birth; dark-skinned babies have brown or dark gray eyes. If a baby's eye color is going to change, it usually does so by the time she's six to twelve months old. Her tear glands won't produce many tears until she's about a month old.

## Sucking Callus (Blister)

Intense sucking often causes a painless white callus on the center of a baby's upper lip. Sometimes the callus peels. It doesn't need treatment and gradually disappears as the lip toughens.

## Skin

At birth, a baby's skin is dusky blue, wet, and streaked with blood and varying amounts of *vernix caseosa*, the white creamy substance that protected his skin before birth. Within a minute or two after a newborn begins breathing well, his skin color changes to normal tones, beginning with his face and torso and soon reaching his fingers and toes. The vernix often remains in skin creases even after bathing. It can be gently rubbed into his skin.

A fair-skinned newborn baby often looks blotchy. After a few weeks, his skin has a more even color, although it may appear blotchy when he's cold. Also common on a fair-skinned baby's skin are stork bites and angel kisses, red areas formed by a collection of tiny blood vessels near the skin's surface. They often appear on the baby's eyelids, nose, forehead, or back of the neck. They usually fade or disappear within six to nine months; however, some may be permanent.

Mongolian spots (black and blue areas) commonly appear on the lower back and buttocks and occasionally on the thighs or arms of some babies, usually of Native American, Asian, African, or southern European descent. They gradually fade and usually disappear by the time the child is four years old. Parents should make sure those who care for their baby know that the spots aren't bruises.

Many babies have peeling skin, particularly on the hands and feet. Babies born after their due dates peel more than babies born at term. The peeling is normal and doesn't usually require treatment. If cracks on the wrists or ankles bleed, a skin ointment, such as A&D ointment, can be applied.

## Breasts

Pregnancy hormones may have caused the baby's breasts to swell. Some babies (male and female) leak milk from their nipples, which is normal and doesn't require treatment. Parents shouldn't try to express milk from a baby's nipples; doing so may cause infection. The condition typically disappears within a week or two.

## Genitals

Pregnancy hormones also may have caused a baby's genitals to swell. If the baby is a boy, he may have an unusually large, red scrotum. If the baby is a girl, she may have milky or bloody vaginal discharge called a "pseudo menstrual period." This discharge indicates that her uterus has had a healthy response to the mother's hormones and is now shedding its first lining. The conditions for both sexes are normal and temporary, and they don't require treatment.

## Umbilical Cord

Immediately after a newborn's umbilical cord is cut, it's bluish-white and 1 to 2 inches long. To stop the bleeding, a plastic cord clamp is applied or umbilical tape is tied around the cord. The cord clamp is removed when the cord is dry, usually within twenty-four to forty-eight hours after the birth. The tape doesn't have to be removed. Usually within one to two weeks, the umbilical cord will fall off.

# YOUR NEWBORN'S REFLEXES

When you observe your newborn, you may notice that loud noises, bright lights, or quick movements startle her or make her fling her arms and legs out and straighten her body, especially when she's on her back. This physical response (called the "Moro reflex") is one of the normal early reflexes that indicate good neurological health. (*Tip:* When trying to soothe a crying baby, hold her on her side or stomach. Laying her on her back can cause this startle reflex, which may upset her.)

Another early reflex is when your newborn firmly grasps your finger when you place it on her palm. (Reflex or not, this action is simply wonderful!) The stepping (or automatic walking) reflex occurs when your baby alternately moves each foot when she's held upright and her feet bear weight. Your baby's sucking and swallowing reflexes let her eagerly suckle milk from your breast or a bottle nipple. She also may suckle your breast or suck on her fingers or yours to soothe herself. Your newborn responds to a touch on her cheek or lips by turning toward it and opening her mouth wide. This rooting reflex is especially pronounced when she's hungry.

Whether awake or asleep, your baby may yawn, quiver, hiccup, stretch, or cry without apparent reason. Hiccups are especially common soon after feeding and don't require treatment.

Some reflexes are protective. Your baby coughs to help move mucus or fluid from her airway. She sneezes when she needs to clear her nose or when it's irritated, or when a bright light shines in her eyes. She blinks if something touches her eyelashes, and she pulls away from a painful stimulus, such as a blood draw from her heel. If lying on her stomach, she lifts her head and turns it to the side to avoid being smothered. If something is placed over her nose and mouth, she twists away from it, mouths it vigorously, or attempts to knock it away with her arms.

Your baby's caregiver checks these reflexes in the newborn exam (see page 363). As your baby matures, many of these early reflexes will disappear.

# YOUR NEWBORN'S BREATHING PATTERN

You may notice that your baby breathes more rapidly than you do (between thirty and sixty times per minute). You also may notice that he has periods of irregular breathing, which can seem worrisome to you but is normal. When your baby sleeps, he may snort, squeak, pant, groan, and even occasionally pause his breathing. These irregularities usually disappear a month or two after the birth, when you'll notice that his breathing is more regular.

If you're worried whether your baby's breathing patterns are normal, observe him as he sleeps. If you see the irregularities described in the previous paragraph, don't be concerned. However, if you observe signs of respiratory distress (such as blue lips, a struggle to breathe, flared nostrils, or a deep indentation of the chest with each breath), call your baby's caregiver immediately.

# HOLDING YOUR BABY

If you don't have much experience holding babies, ask your nurse or other caregiver to show you options. It's important to support your newborn's head for the first month or so, until her neck muscles are strong enough to hold up her head unassisted. Don't worry if you forget to support her head for a moment—the brief bobbling won't harm her.

# What Happens after the Birth

If you give birth at a hospital, your baby will typically stay in your room ("room-in"), and you and your family will provide basic baby care, including diaper changes. This arrangement allows you to get acquainted with your baby and discover questions you may have about his care. Your nurses, caregiver, and other hospital staff can help you find answers.

If you give birth at a birth center or at home, be sure to take advantage of the brief time you'll have with your caregiver to ask questions. (At birth centers, people typically go home three to six hours after the birth. At home births, caregivers usually leave three to six hours after the birth.) In addition to your caregiver, you may also consult with a doula, lactation consultant, or your childbirth educator with any questions you may have about newborn care.

Regardless of where you give birth, your caregiver will likely evaluate your newborn soon after the birth. The following sections describe common tests and procedures.

## NEWBORN TESTS AND PROCEDURES

The table below describes common tests and procedures that evaluate your baby's health and ensure she remains healthy. They're part of routine newborn care, and many are required by law. Find out which tests and procedures your state or province mandates by visiting the website for its public health department, or ask your caregiver for this information.

If you give birth at a birth center or at home, talk with your midwife about when and where these tests and procedures will be offered.

Protocols for tests and procedures vary somewhat among caregivers. Ask your caregiver which tests are routinely performed at your birthplace and which are used only if medically indicated. You can find further information on our website, http://www.PCNGuide.com.

| Test or procedure | What it is | Comments |
| --- | --- | --- |
| Apgar score | Immediately after the birth, your caregiver will evaluate your baby's well-being by a quick assessment of breathing, reflexes, and muscle tone. | See page 196 for a full discussion on this routine assessment. |
| Infant vital signs | Your caregiver assesses your baby's temperature, heart rate, and respiration to ensure she's adjusting well, to detect any problems with her heart or lungs, or to determine whether she needs to be warmed. | A normal heart rate for infants is 90 to 160 beats per minute; normal respiration is 30 to 60 breaths per minute. Your baby should appear pink and breathe easily. If there's a concern, your baby's caregiver may admit her to the hospital nursery. Normal axillary (underarm) temperature of newborns is between 97.4°F (36.3°C) and 99.5°F (37.5°C). If your baby has a fever, she'll be admitted to the nursery and may have a septic workup and antibiotics. If she's too cool, she'll be placed on your bare chest and covered with warmed blankets, or placed under a special warming light in your room or in the nursery. |
| Newborn eye ointment | Erythromycin is placed in your baby's eyes within an hour after the birth. The goal is to prevent infection and possible blindness if the baby was exposed to gonorrhea or chlamydia in the birth canal, although research indicates that screening and treatment of the mother during pregnancy is a more effective method of prevention.[3] | Can cause temporary blurring of vision. In the first hour after the birth, your baby is very alert and wants to gaze at you. Wait until after that hour before giving treatment. Ointment is currently required in most of the United States, but Canadian pediatricians say it shouldn't be routinely recommended.[4] Visit our website, http://www.PCNGuide.com, for more information. |

| Test or procedure | What it is | Comments |
|---|---|---|
| Vitamin K | Vitamin K is injected into your baby's thigh soon after the birth to enhance blood clotting and prevent a bleeding disorder.[2] | Although oral vitamin K is available, the injection is more effective at preventing bleeding for the first twelve weeks. |
| Infant security | At birth, babies are given wrist and ankle identification bands that match their mothers' wristband. All staff caring for babies should wear easy-to-read identification badges. | These procedures reduce the risk of kidnapping or accidentally switching infants—both very rare situations. Having your baby in your room and never leaving her unattended are the best ways to keep your baby safe. |
| Newborn hearing screening | Your baby's caregiver will assess her hearing in the first days after the birth using soft headphones for about 10 minutes while she's sleeping. | Hearing screening is recommended for all babies. If screening reveals potential problems, then diagnostic tests are done. The sooner treatment begins for hearing loss, the better for baby's language development. |
| Newborn screening | Your baby's blood is drawn by a heel prick when she's 24 to 48 hours old. (Sometimes an additional blood test before your baby is 2 weeks old is required.)[5] The blood is then screened for various rare conditions. | Although the conditions screened for are rare and most children don't have them, affected babies greatly benefit from early diagnosis and treatment. These conditions include sickle cell anemia, beta thalassemia, phenylketonuria (PKU), hypothyroidism,[6] and galactosemia. It's possible to screen for over sixty conditions; states and provinces vary widely in the number of conditions that they screen for. Visit http://www.babysfirsttest.org for more information. |
| Pulse oximetry test | A sensor is placed on baby's skin (usually on the hand or foot) to measure the oxygen levels in the blood. | This painless test takes minutes and can detect heart problems that can be corrected by surgery. |
| Hepatitis B vaccination | Your baby is given an injection (shot) to immunize her against hepatitis B, a blood-borne viral infection that can lead to liver infection, cirrhosis, or liver cancer. | Side effects are rare, other than localized pain and tenderness at the injection site. Some parents question the need for a baby to receive this vaccine unless the mother is carrying the virus, since a baby is highly unlikely to get hepatitis B from the usual modes of transmission (IV drug use or sexual encounters). Although the chance of infection may be small, if a child does contract the virus in the first year of life, there's a 25% chance it'll cause lifelong health issues. See pages 381–382 for more information on vaccinations. |
| Test for hypoglycemia or low blood sugar (only if medically indicated) | Your baby's blood is drawn from her heel to test for hypoglycemia. | Hypoglycemia is most common in babies that weigh more than 8 pounds 13 ounces or less than 5 pounds at birth, or in babies who had preterm or postterm births. It also can occur in babies whose mothers are diabetic or received large amounts of IV fluids with dextrose during labor. Hypoglycemia can lead to respiratory distress, lethargy, slow heart rate, and seizures. Treatment includes frequent feeding. In more serious cases, the baby may be given IV dextrose. |
| Septic workup (only when infection is suspected) | Your baby's blood is drawn and cerebrospinal fluid may be obtained and sent to laboratory to be tested for bacteria. Results are available in 48 hours. | Because infections can be dangerous for a newborn, if one is suspected (for example, if baby has a fever), the baby will be tested and may be admitted to the hospital nursery and treated with IV antibiotics while waiting for test results. |
| Test for jaundice (used only when there are concerns) | Your baby's blood is drawn from her heel and is sent to a laboratory, where the bilirubin level is determined. Sometimes, a jaundice meter is used first to estimate bilirubin levels by flashing a light onto your baby's forehead. If your baby's skin and the whites of her eyes are yellowish, an elevated bilirubin level is suspected. | Most jaundice is mild and disappears with little or no treatment. (See page 383 for more information on jaundice.) |

# Circumcision

*Circumcision* is the surgical removal of the foreskin covering the glans (tip) of the penis. It's done for social, cultural, religious, and medical reasons.

Some communities practice circumcision more often than others. For example, the Jewish and Islamic communities use circumcision as a religious ritual. It's a common procedure in North America, Africa, and the Middle East; however, it's uncommon in Latin America, South America, Europe, Australia, and the Far East.

The benefits and risks of circumcision are debated among health-care professionals. Parents of baby boys will need to gather information (preferably during pregnancy) so they can make an informed decision about circumcision.

## *Facts about Circumcision*

Think about the following facts as you consider circumcision:

- In 1979 65 percent of boys in the United States were circumcised. By 2010, the rate dropped to 58 percent nationwide. (In some regions, the rates were as low as 40 percent.[7])
- The American Academy of Pediatrics (AAP) states that the preventive health benefits of circumcision outweigh its risks, but not enough to recommend routine circumcision for all newborn boys.[8] AAP further advises parents to "weigh medical information in the context of their own religious, ethical, and cultural beliefs and practices."[9]
- Research shows that circumcision reduces, but does not eliminate, the risk of getting HIV and some STIs. The Centers for Disease Control and Prevention (CDC) say that in the effort to slow the HIV epidemic, all available options for preventing transmission of the disease should be used. Circumcision is simpler, safer, and less expensive for newborns and infants than for adults. However, delaying circumcision until adolescence or adulthood allows the teenage boy or man "to participate in—or make—the decision."[10]
- Circumcision reduces a man's risk of contracting HIV, genital herpes, and human papillomavirus (HPV) during vaginal sex; however, it doesn't reduce the risk of transmission to the female partner.[11] Circumcision doesn't reduce the risk of transmission during anal sex, and it doesn't reduce the risk of contracting other sexually transmitted infections.[12] For these reasons, everyone should be educated about correct condom use, whether circumcised or not.
- Studies find a connection between an intact (uncircumcised) penis and urinary tract infection (UTI) in the first year of life; however, the risk of infection is low (less than 1 percent).[13] Exclusive breastfeeding can reduce the risk of UTIs (by 300 percent).[14]
- About 1.5 percent of newborn circumcisions cause minor to serious complications, including irritation of the glans from rubbing against wet diapers, painful urination, bleeding, infection, and scarring of the urinary outlet.[15]
- Some medical ethicists oppose newborn and infant circumcision because it's an elective surgery done without the patient's consent. Some parents are uncomfortable with the idea of a surgical procedure to remove healthy tissue from their child.
- Opinions differ about whether newborn circumcision affects adult sexual performance. Some experts say it does, while others argue it doesn't.
- The full procedure (including prep time and aftercare) usually takes less than thirty minutes. Healing takes seven to ten days.

- A newborn will feel the pain caused by the procedure. Health-care providers recommend an injection of local anesthesia to reduce the pain of circumcision.[16] Applying local anesthetic creams to the penis also decreases pain, although less effectively than an injection.[17] Sucking on a special pacifier that delivers a small amount of sugar water during the procedure may reduce pain and can be used in combination with the other options.

- Health insurance might not cover the caregiver's fee for the procedure or the hospital's or clinic's fee for equipment use. Fees may total $500.

## The Circumcision Procedure

Before the procedure, you need to sign a consent form. Then your baby is placed either in a special chair or on his back on a rigid board, with Velcro straps holding his body and limbs firmly in place.[18] He then receives anesthesia. After it has taken effect, his penis is washed with an antiseptic. A sterile sheet with a hole in the center (to reveal the penis) is placed over his torso. The foreskin is separated from the glans and removed by one of three instruments: Gomco clamp, Plastibell device, or Mogen clamp. (The Mogen clamp procedure is the fastest and least painful method.[19]) Circumcision takes about five minutes, and you may be allowed to stay with your son during the procedure.

## Care of the Circumcised Penis

After the circumcision, ask the medical staff how to care for your son's penis. If a Mogen clamp or Gomco clamp was used, he'll usually have Vaseline-covered gauze applied to the circumcision site for twenty-four hours, at which time the gauze typically falls off. If the gauze doesn't fall off, wrap the area in a warm, wet washcloth. Once the gauze is soaked, gently remove it. Once the gauze is removed, apply an ointment or diaper cream on your baby's diaper where it touches his penis to prevent irritation.

If a Plastibell device is used, a small plastic ring will remain on his penis, with a suture thread tying the foreskin tightly to the device. The device and foreskin usually fall off seven to ten days after the circumcision. Don't pull the ring off.

At the circumcision site, you may see small yellow or white patches of normal, healing tissue. Report any swelling, bleeding, inability to urinate, or pus-like discharge to your baby's caregiver.

## Care of the Intact (Uncircumcised) Penis

During diaper changes and baths, "clean what can be seen." Don't force back your baby's foreskin to clean the glans. The foreskin will gradually loosen as your son matures. Most boys' foreskins are fully retractable when they're between four and eight years old. Once your son's foreskin can be easily retracted, the glans can be cleaned with soap and water.

# Caring for Your Baby at Home

If you give birth in a hospital or birth center, you may feel both excitement and anxiety when heading home with your newborn. If you give birth at home, your caregiver's departure after the birth may cause the same feelings. Once the anticipation of the birth is over, many new parents suddenly realize that they're responsible for this tiny person, and they wonder whether they're up to the challenge.

Caring for a baby becomes easier with practice. During the first days and weeks, you'll begin to master diapering, bathing, dressing, and comforting your baby. To learn about these tasks, take a newborn care class before the birth. If you give birth at a hospital, attend any predischarge classes offered and ask your nurses any questions that come up during your postpartum stay. If you give birth at home, ask your caregiver for advice on baby care. You can find numerous helpful how-to videos online (use common sense and reliable sources to verify online information). You may also consider hiring a postpartum doula to help with baby care (see page 23).

The following sections are an introduction to the basics of baby care.

## CAR SAFETY

It's the law in the United States and Canada that babies traveling in a vehicle must be restrained in a car seat that meets current federal safety standards.[20] Get your baby's car seat by the third trimester of pregnancy so you can practice installing it in your vehicle (rear-facing and in the back seat). Follow the instructions from the car seat manufacturer and your vehicle's manual to ensure correct installation, then have a car seat technician double-check it. Visit http://www .seatcheck.org to find a car seat technician near you.

Most car seats are used incorrectly. When placing your baby in the seat, refer to the instructions for correct adjustment of the harness. Don't add pads or cushions to the seat.

For the latest information on car seats, visit the National Highway Traffic Safety Administration's website, http:// www.safercar.gov/parents.

If your baby is premature or weighs 5½ pounds or less, the hospital staff will assess her ability to breathe well when seated in a car seat. They may recommend a special car bed to ensure safe transport.

## Two Views about Leaving the Hospital

The hospital stay was very pleasant. I didn't want to leave! I enjoyed getting spoiled with attention, and I was nervous to be on my own with a newborn.
—*Michelle*

Leaving the hospital felt like such a big, momentous event. Then we arrived home, and that was really exciting for the first few minutes. Then we sat down, looked at each other, and said, "Okay, now what?" We realized that we had to figure out what this parenting thing was all about.
—*Alice*

## In Their Own Words

# DIAPERING YOUR BABY

Today's parents have several options to manage their babies' waste, from cloth diapers to disposable diapers to no diapers at all.

**Cloth diapers** are usually used with a waterproof wrap to prevent leaks. Some kinds have the wrap sewn to the cloth diaper (all-in-ones); others require the diaper to be folded and placed inside the separate wrap. Both kinds have elastic around the leg holes and are fastened by either snaps or Velcro tabs. You can use a baby diaper service (if available in your area) to provide clean diapers and take away used ones. Or you can buy cloth diapers and launder them at home.

**Pocket diapers** have a diaper wrap on the outside and a fleece liner on the inside, which can keep your baby dry and reduce diaper rash. You can fill the pocket between the inner and outer layers with a cloth diaper, hemp, or other material. Launder pocket diapers at home according to the manufacturer's directions.

**Disposable diapers** come in various sizes and styles. Although they may be more convenient than other diapering options, they also may be more expensive. Buying in bulk may save money, but your child may outgrow the diapers before using them all. Used diapers must be disposed of properly.

**Ecologically friendly disposable diapers and biodegradable diapers** can be composted if wet with only urine. With some brands, a portion of the diaper can be flushed if it's poopy. (*Note:* diaper wipes are *not* flushable, even if they claim to be. They're notorious for clogging sewer systems.)

Expect a newborn to use fifty to seventy diapers a week. If you plan to use disposable diapers, be sure to have at least that many on hand before the birth. If you plan to buy cloth diapers, decide how often you want to do laundry and purchase the appropriate number of diapers. For example, if you expect to launder diapers daily, you may choose to buy a dozen or more. You can find helpful information online by using the search terms *diaper choices* to find websites that review cloth diapers and disposable diapers.

Some parents use a diaper-free method called **elimination communication (EC)** and avoid using diapers entirely or part of the time. EC is a common practice worldwide, where access to diapers and the ability to launder them is limited or unavailable. This method eliminates or reduces the cost of diapers and is ecologically friendly, but it requires paying close attention to a baby's cues to urinate or have a bowel movement. Parents dress their babies with the diaper area open and unrestricted. When they observe their babies' cues to urinate or have a bowel movement, they hold their babies over a sink or special potty.

## How and When to Change a Diaper

To learn how to diaper your baby, take a newborn care class, ask an experienced parent, or watch how-to videos online. Babies urinate often and have three to ten bowel movements a day. Whenever your baby urinates, change the diaper soon—no need to change it immediately (for example, if your baby is sleeping). Whenever your baby has a bowel movement, change the diaper as soon as possible to prevent diaper rash. An easy way to tell that your baby is pooping is to listen for it "in progress"; he may also grunt. Another way is to watch your baby's face for "poop cues." A serious, contemplative expression with a furrowed brow and pursed lips likely indicates he's pooping.

## Your Newborn's Bowel Movements

Your baby's first bowel movements (*meconium*) will be a sticky, green-black substance that was in her intestines before birth. By two to three days after birth, she'll produce brown or brown-green stools that are the consistency of cake batter. After that, the frequency and consistency of bowel movements depend on the food she eats.

Breastfed newborns may poop after each feeding, or have at least three yellow, green, or brown stools each day after their mothers' milk has come in. Stools will be wet and runny, and may have curds in them. Formula-fed babies may produce one to three tan putty-like stools each day. To learn more, search online for "diaper decoders," which show photos of normal and abnormal baby poop.

## Diaper Rash

If the skin on your baby's diaper area becomes irritated, he may have diaper rash. Many substances can cause diaper rash, including urine and stool, some laundry detergents, chemicals used in some disposable diapers, or inadequately laundered cloth diapers.

To prevent or treat diaper rash, change your baby's diapers frequently and rinse his skin with water at each change. Be sure to clean off your baby's bottom completely. Before putting on a new diaper, wait a few minutes to allow your baby's clean bare skin to air-dry (or blow-dry the area with a hair dryer set on no heat).

When laundering cloth diapers, use a milder detergent or run them through an extra rinse cycle. Try switching to a different type of wrap. You can also try adding a ½ cup of distilled white vinegar to the diaper pail or to the rinse cycle. Vinegar helps restore the acid pH in the cloth to neutral.

If these treatments don't work, you may consider applying a diaper rash cream to the irritated area after you clean and dry it. Ask experienced parents for recommendations on effective diaper creams. To learn about the safety of ingredients, see http://www.cosmeticsdatabase.com. If the diaper rash persists, consult your baby's caregiver.

## Constipation

Constipation is the production of small, hard, dry stools that can be painful to pass. The condition is more common in formula-fed babies than in breastfed babies, because formula is harder to digest than breast milk.

If you're breastfeeding your baby, about six to ten weeks after the birth you may notice that she has begun pooping only once a day or even once a week. This change doesn't indicate constipation; instead, the composition of your breast milk has changed. It no longer contains colostrum, which had a laxative effect on your baby. If you're still concerned, call her caregiver.

## Diarrhea and Vomiting

Diarrhea (frequent, watery bowel movements) and vomiting are serious conditions for babies because they can cause dehydration quickly. Formula-fed babies experience diarrhea and vomiting much more often than exclusively breastfed babies, probably because formula is harder to digest than breast milk and also may be exposed to more contaminants. (When formula-fed babies were given probiotic supplements, they had less diarrhea as well as fewer colds and ear infections.[21] See page 307 to learn more about probiotics and the microbiome.)

Signs of diarrhea include more frequent stools that may smell foul, look bloody, or contain mucus. An affected baby may appear ill, weak, or listless. If you see any of these signs, call your baby's caregiver for advice.

For more information on vomiting, see page 395.

## Common Q & A

**Q:** My son's diapers are always leaking. Is the kind of diaper I'm using to blame?

**A:** Try pointing your baby's penis straight down as you diaper him. That way, the urine will be directed toward the most absorbent part of the diaper. Also, be sure to fasten diapers tightly. If you're using cloth diapers, be sure all the cloth is tucked inside the waterproof wrap.

# BABY CLOTHES AND EQUIPMENT

As you prepare for your baby's arrival, you may wonder if you need all the items available in baby shops and department stores. The truth is, you need very little to effectively care for a newborn. See page 153 for a list of typical supplies.

# BATHING YOUR BABY

Newborns need bathing only once or twice a week.[22] In between baths, just a "spot clean" is needed—wiping spit-up off the neck, cleaning drool off hands, and so on.

You may choose a sponge bath or a full bath. For a sponge bath, have warm water ready in a warm bathroom. Undress your baby (except the diaper) and wrap him in a towel. First, dip a washcloth in the warm water and wipe his eyes. Put a small amount of mild baby soap in the water, dip the washcloth, then wipe his face and dry it with the towel. Bring one arm out from under the towel, wash it, then tuck it back in the towel to keep him warm. Repeat this process for the rest of his body.

A tub bath may be a more enjoyable experience for you both. Babies stay warmer and calmer when immersed in warm water than when given a sponge bath. A tub bath won't increase the risk of infection in the cord or a newly circumcised penis. Fill a sink or baby bathtub with comfortably warm water. Hold your baby securely with his head resting in the crook of your arm or the bend of your wrist, with your hand gently grasping his arm. Lower him into the water so it covers his body, but not his head and neck. Use only water to clean his eyes and face. Next, wash his hair with mild soap, massaging his head with your fingers or a soft brush. Wash his body with a mild baby soap. Rinse. Let your baby enjoy the warmth of the water. When the bath is done, make sure his skin and hair are completely dry before dressing him.

Many parents enjoy bathing with their babies as a way to relax together. Fill the bathtub with comfortably warm water. Get into the tub first and have someone hand you your baby. Lay him on his back on your thighs so the water covers his body but not his neck and head. Enjoy relaxing in the water together. Wash his body with a mild baby soap. When you're done, hand him to someone who can wrap him in a warm towel. *Note:* If no one is available to help, line your baby's car seat with a towel, undress him, and set him in the car seat next to the tub. Pick him up once you're in the water. At the end of the bath, place him back in his towel-lined car seat while you get out and dry off.

# CORD CARE

To promote the separation of the umbilical cord from your baby's abdomen while preventing infection, follow these tips:

- Wash your hands before touching the cord.
- To keep the cord dry and clean, fasten your baby's diaper or diaper wrap below the cord.
- If the cord is soiled, gently clean it with a cotton swab and warm water and let it dry thoroughly.

- If the cord area is red, emits a foul odor, oozes pus, or bleeds bright red blood in a spot larger than a quarter, call your baby's caregiver. (*Note:* When the cord falls off, some dark brownish-red blood or clear yellow sticky fluid at the separation site is normal.)
- If your baby leaves the hospital with a cord clamp attached, have her caregiver or the hospital staff remove it at a later date. (Or you can remove it if given clear instructions.) Don't cut off the cord clamp.

## DRESSING YOUR BABY

In general, dress your baby in the same amount of clothing that you're wearing, then add one layer, such as a hat or lightweight blanket. In the summer, your baby might wear a onesie (also called a bodysuit) and socks. In the winter, he might wear a onesie and a fleece one-piece ("footies") indoors, with a warm hat added when outdoors. (*Note:* Never bundle your baby in thick clothing before buckling him into a car seat or stroller. Cover him with a blanket *after* strapping him in. The bulky fabric can interfere with how effectively the harness holds him in an accident.) At night, your baby might wear lightweight footies or a sleep sack over lightweight clothing if his sleep space is 69°F to 72°F (20.6°C to 22.2°C) or heavier weight footies or a sleep sack over warmer clothing if sleep space is 64°F to 68°F (17.8°C to 20°C).

When your baby is dressed appropriately, his tummy will be warm and his toes may be a bit cool. If your baby is warm all over and flushed or breathing rapidly, he's overdressed. If your baby's tummy is cool or his skin is blotchy, he's not dressed warmly enough.

How much clothing you need to buy depends on how often you want to do laundry. Expect a newborn to go through two to four outfits a day (because of spit-up, diaper leaks, and so on). Don't buy many newborn-size clothes. Many babies outgrow them in the first weeks of life.

# Your Baby's Communication

Although your baby can't talk, he can communicate his needs, likes, and dislikes through *infant cues*. Your baby will show many of these cues ten to fifteen minutes before he starts to cry. If you respond to early cues, your baby is less likely to cry. If you don't respond, he may begin to fuss and cry. By the time you see this late cue, it may take longer to satisfy his needs because you must first calm him.

As you get to know your baby, you'll be better able to interpret his cues. Your baby may let you know he's hungry by rooting, sticking out his tongue, or sucking on his hand (see page 393). He may yawn and half-close his eyes to tell you he's sleepy (see page 377). He may grunt when pooping (see page 368). When gassy, he may look uncomfortable, squirm, and make creaky noises (see page 395).

## ENGAGEMENT AND DISENGAGEMENT CUES

When your baby is calm, quiet, and alert, she has subtle ways to get your attention and keep it. Her body relaxes, her eyes brighten and open wide, and she stares at you intently. If you ignore these engagement cues or look away, she may vocalize or move her arms to catch your attention. When you return her gaze, a quiet exchange begins as she explores your face. When she needs a brief rest to process what she has seen, she may turn or look away until she's ready to return her gaze to you. During these exchanges with your baby, be sensitive to her needs by returning her gaze when she wants your attention and by letting her rest when needed without coaxing her to look at you.

From birth your baby can imitate some of your facial expressions. For example, shape your mouth into an O and hold the expression for ten seconds where your baby can clearly see you; repeat this action several times. If your baby is quiet and alert, she'll shape her mouth into an O. You can also stick out your tongue or lower lip; your baby will mimic these expressions as well.

When your baby is around six weeks old, she'll begin to smile and coo to initiate an exchange and in response to your smile. (These endearing interactions make many parents fall deeper in love with their babies!) To help you learn more about your baby's cues and abilities, consider taking a newborn care class or consulting with your baby's caregiver or nurse, your childbirth educator, or other experienced parents.

Your baby can best teach you what calms or agitates her. When your responses to soothe your baby are effective, she becomes calmer and less fussy, and she relaxes into your body as you hold her. If your responses overstimulate her, or if the day's activities have overstimulated her, she'll show disengagement cues. At first, she may just look glassy-eyed or turn away. If the stimulation continues, she may stiffen, arch her back, squirm ("disorganized" movement), or spread her fingers wide as if trying to push something away. If you miss these disengagement cues, she'll cry. If the overstimulation is too intense, she may cry loudly for a long time.

## CRYING

Contrary to traditional thought, you won't "spoil" your baby by responding whenever he cries. When your baby cries, he's not manipulating you for your attention; he simply has no other way to tell you he needs something. Crying is often your baby's last attempt to communicate that he's hungry, overstimulated, tired, or uncomfortable. He may cry because he has gas and needs to be burped. He may cry because he has a wet or dirty diaper, a diaper rash, or sore circumcision site. He may cry if he's ill or simply because he wants to be held and rocked.

Responding to your baby's crying helps develop his trust in your ability to meet his needs. Try to respond before he becomes so upset that he can't calm himself easily. Your baby will become more agitated if you're upset, so try to stay as calm as possible by talking quietly to him and moving slowly and calmly around him.

It's important to remember that all babies cry at times. The fact your baby is crying doesn't make you a bad parent! It's not your job to make your baby stop crying—sometimes that's not possible. It's your job to care for your baby and create an environment where it's possible for him to calm down.

Soothing your baby is easier if you know why he's crying. You may be able to determine the reason from watching his cues or thinking back to recent events—for example, if it's been a few hours since he last fed, he's likely upset because he's hungry.

Occasionally, you might not immediately know the reason for his distress, which can be frustrating. The reason may be that his brain and nervous system are just too immature to handle the stimulation, and crying allows him a release. In those cases, try comforting him with any of the following calming techniques. Don't switch between techniques frantically, as that will further overstimulate him. Give each one several minutes to work before trying another.

- Try feeding your baby first.
- Try any or all of the Five S's (see at right).
- Take your baby for a walk in a sling, baby carrier, or stroller. Or sit on a birth ball with your baby cuddled to your chest, and gently bounce up and down.
- Take a bath with your baby. The warm water may calm him, and he may even breastfeed.
- Give your baby a gentle massage.

If nothing seems to calm your baby and you find yourself losing your temper, put him safely in his bed or car seat and take a short break. If after five to ten minutes your baby is still agitated and you still feel angry and frustrated, never shake or roughly handle him, no matter how upset you are. Instead, call your partner, a relative, a friend, or a neighbor to help you.

Although at first you may have trouble figuring out exactly why your baby is crying, let your instincts and feelings guide you. You'll become more comfortable in your ability to calm your baby with time, practice, and advice from your baby's caregiver, a supportive relative or friend, or a new-parent group.

## The Five S's

Dr. Harvey Karp suggests calming babies using a five-step method called the Five S's. This method provides babies with a familiar and comforting womb-like environment. Some babies need all five steps, while others are calmed by just a few.[23]

### Swaddling

Swaddling might not calm a baby by itself. However, if you swaddle your upset baby first then calm her, the swaddling may help her stay calm. Swaddling also increases how long your baby sleeps by preventing her from startling herself awake.[24] You can swaddle your baby in a large, lightweight blanket or a commercial swaddling blanket. Your nurse, midwife, or doula can show you how to swaddle your baby, or search online for how-to videos. You can also provide a swaddle-like environment by tucking your baby snugly inside a baby carrier, sling, swing, bouncy seat, or sleep sack with her arms tucked inside. Visit our website, http://www.PCNGuide.com, to learn an effective double-swaddle technique for older babies who can wiggle out of a basic swaddle.

### Side or stomach position

Hold your baby in your arms on her side, or on her stomach with gentle pressure against her tummy, or sitting up. Being held on her back may cause her to startle easily and upset her.

### Shushing

Make a shushing sound near your baby's ear or use white noise (continuous noise, such as a fan, radio static, or the clothes dryer) loudly enough so she can hear it over her crying.

### Swinging

Repetitive motion helps soothe babies. Swing your baby by swaying, rocking, jiggling, or gently bouncing with her on an exercise ball. Take a walk while carrying your baby in a sling. To give yourself a chance to eat or rest, consider using a baby swing.

### Sucking

Feeding is often the first thing you'll try to calm your baby. If she's fussing but not hungry, let your baby suck on a pacifier or your finger.

## Advice from the Authors

## *Colic or Fussy Periods*

When babies are between three and twelve weeks old, most have predictable fussiness in the evening (a time some parents call "fuss and feed"). Dr. T. Berry Brazelton, an expert in infant development, states that this fussy period is a normal "touchpoint" or parenting challenge.[25] His research reveals that an overload of stimuli (such as bright lights, loud noises, and feelings of hunger) throughout the day causes the predictable fussiness. As the day progresses, the baby's immature nervous system begins to cycle into shorter sleep periods, more frequent feeding, and more fussiness.[26]

Some parents feel that their babies are colicky, or unusually fussy. *Colic* is defined as three or more crying episodes each week for three or more weeks, with each episode lasting three hours or longer.[27] It usually starts around three weeks of age and ends around three months. It's more likely in premature babies, in babies exposed to nicotine or tobacco during pregnancy, or in babies whose daily interactions are overstimulating. (See page 372 for information about disengagement cues.)

Although all babies have gas, if your fussy baby seems especially gassy, use comfort holds that provide pressure against his tummy, such as those illustrated on page 373, to help alleviate the pressure. Some research shows reduced colic symptoms in babies given probiotic supplements. (Probiotics may also help treat or prevent diarrhea and reduce risk of infections.[28] See page 307 to learn more about probiotics and the microbiome.) In breastfeeding infants, colic symptoms *may* be reduced if the mother decreases or eliminates common allergens (especially dairy) from her diet.[29] You may have heard to give your baby simethicone (Mylicon) drops; however, research hasn't

found them to treat gas any more effectively than a placebo.[30] Some parents give "gripe water," which contains potentially gas-reducing ingredients, such as fennel, spearmint, and ginger.

Fussy periods can be stressful. You may want to ask your baby's caregiver, other parents of colicky babies, or members of a parent-baby support group for advice on coping with the stress. If you're spending several hours each day soothing your baby, take a break now and then. Let a trusted person relieve you so you can take a walk. Or take your baby on a walk with another new parent and baby. As with most parenting challenges, these fussy periods will end with time, your growing confidence as a parent, and your baby's increasing maturity.

Parents sometimes mistake colicky symptoms for those of gastroesophageal reflux (GER or reflux), in which the acidic stomach contents flow up into the esophagus, making the tissue inflamed and painful. Babies with GER often arch and stiffen during feedings, may spit up or cough, may have sour breath, and are especially uncomfortable when placed on their backs. The difference between colic and GER is that reflux symptoms are constant during the day and night. Also, GER can be treated with medication and by positioning the baby upright after feedings and for sleep.

If your baby isn't usually fussy but is constantly crying in addition to showing signs of illness (vomiting, fever, constipation, or having a cold), consult with his caregiver.

# Your Baby's Sleeping and Waking Patterns

After a period of wakefulness after the birth, many babies sleep for much of the first day. They rouse only briefly and might not be interested in feeding. After babies have adjusted to their new environment, they sleep twelve to eighteen hours in a 24-hour period; however, they don't sleep for long periods at a time. Instead, newborns cycle in and out of sleep all day and night, with short catnaps sprinkled with brief periods of alertness and lots of time spent feeding.

Babies typically don't have a noticeable sleep pattern in the early weeks. Some newborns sleep up to two to three hours at a time, but many don't. (Babies are more likely to sleep longer stretches if swaddled for sleep.) A newborn's immature brain hasn't yet learned how to regulate itself or to recognize the difference between day and night. While this behavior is normal and healthy for a newborn, it's challenging for new parents! (See self-care tips on page 330.)

Sleep patterns vary among babies and are based on temperament, environment, and maturity. Whatever your newborn's sleep pattern is, it'll become more predictable as he gets older. He'll be awake and playful for longer periods and sleep for longer stretches (a five-hour stretch overnight is considered "sleeping through the night"), and his sleep schedule will become more predictable. The more consistent and expected your responses and your day's routines are, the more likely he'll regulate his rhythms.

The illustration on page 376 shows that a newborn may have eight to ten sleep and wake cycles in a 24-hour period. By four to six months, many babies have settled into four to five cycles, with two daytime naps and one or more nighttime awakenings. By two years, many toddlers have one afternoon nap and sleep for a long stretch at night. One-third still wake up at night, but generally at a predictable time.

# RECORDING YOUR BABY'S SLEEPING AND ACTIVITY PATTERNS

By charting your baby's feeding, sleeping, quiet-alert, and crying or fussing periods for a week, you can see when and how long your baby typically sleeps, is awake and content, and cries. You may notice that she has a fussy period at a certain time. Or you may learn that she takes a long nap at roughly the same time every day. Visit our website, http://www.PCNGuide.com, for a sample chart that you can use to record your baby's patterns.

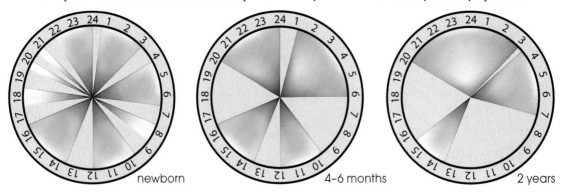

newborn    4–6 months    2 years

# SLEEP SPACE

Upon first learning they're pregnant, many expectant parents plan on creating a separate nursery filled with adorable decorations and a lovely crib. However, experts recommend that babies sleep in the same room as their parents in the early months to reduce the risk of sudden infant death syndrome (SIDS—see page 385). A baby may wake up slightly more often when in the room with his parents; however, his awakenings tend to be milder, as his parents can quickly respond to his needs before crying escalates.

Some parents choose to have their baby sleep in a cosleeper or in a basket, bassinet, or crib near their bed. Other parents find they get more sleep if they tuck their baby in bed with them. Because a newborn has long wakeful periods at night just as he did while in the womb, he may sleep better with his parents in their bed than by himself. Many parents put their babies in a crib at the beginning of the night and move them into their bed later. As your baby grows older and needs you less at night, you can move him to a crib in your room or another room. Or he can continue sleeping in your bed with you. It's your decision.

Wherever your baby sleeps, you need to place him in a safe space and position him on his back on a firm surface to reduce the risk of SIDS. See page 385 for more information on safe sleeping spaces.

# YOUR BABY'S SLEEP-ACTIVITY STATES

Experts have identified six states that babies experience as they move between sleep and wakefulness. Some babies move gradually from one state to another, while others make abrupt transitions. Understanding these states will help you give your baby appropriate care.

## Sleep States

In **deep sleep** your baby is still and relaxed; her breathing is rhythmic. She occasionally jerks or makes sucking movements, but rarely awakens. She doesn't need anything from you at this time, so use it as an opportunity to rest and take care of yourself.

**Light sleep** is the most common sleep state in newborns. Your baby's eyes are closed, but they may move behind her eyelids. She twitches, makes momentary mewing sounds, sucks, grimaces, or smiles. She breathes irregularly. She responds to noises and efforts to arouse or stimulate her. When your baby moves and makes sounds, wait a few moments to see if she's awakening to a drowsy state and needs care or if she's falling back to deep sleep. If your baby is stirring because she's hungry, she'll root, suck on anything close by, and wave her arms and legs vigorously. If you feed her promptly, she may fall back asleep.

## Awake States

When your baby is **drowsy**, he appears sleepy, he may rub his eyes or ears, and he may yawn or startle occasionally. His heavy-lidded eyes, which open and close for brief periods, lose focus or appear cross-eyed. He breathes irregularly and slowly reacts to sensory stimuli. If you hope he'll fall asleep, try shushing or patting him to help him settle down. If you hope he'll awaken, try picking him up, singing to him, or dancing with him.

**Quiet alert** is the most pleasing and rewarding state for parents. Your baby shows engagement cues, lying still and looking at you calmly with bright, wide eyes. He breathes with regularity and focuses attentively on what he sees and hears. By providing him something to look at, listen to, or suck on, you encourage him to spend longer times in this state. (See page 380 for information on playing with your baby.)

**Active alert** is the state that indicates your baby is starting to need something, although he might not know what it is yet. He can't lie still; he may be fussy. His eyes are open but not as bright and attentive as when he's in a quiet-alert state. He breathes irregularly and makes faces. Hunger, fatigue, noises, and too much stimulation readily affect your baby and may lead to fussing or crying.

When your baby reaches this state, try to determine what he needs. If he shows feeding cues, feed him. If he looks away (disengages), he probably needs less stimulation. If you act immediately, you may bring him to a calmer state before he begins to cry.

**Crying** is your baby's last attempt to tell you he can't cope any longer. If he's hungry, overstimulated, tired, sick, gassy, frustrated, wet, cold, hot, or lonely, he may have first tried communicating with subtle cues. If his needs continue to go unmet, he communicates his distress by crying. In this state, he also moves his body actively, opens or closes his eyes, makes unhappy faces, and breathes irregularly. Sometimes, crying is a way to let himself enter another state ("self-soothe"). More often, however, he needs you to feed or comfort him.

## Tummy Time

Because babies need to sleep on their backs and spend time in car seats, swings, and strollers, the back of their heads can become flattened from contact with a firm surface. To prevent your baby from developing a misshapen head and to give her an opportunity to lift her head and strengthen her neck muscles, frequently place her on her tummy when she's awake for as long as she's happy in that position. Also limit the amount of time your baby spends in baby equipment that puts pressure on the back of her head. Many babies fuss when they're first learning to lie on their tummies. Over time, they'll tolerate tummy time and eventually will begin to enjoy longer sessions. Here are ways to provide supervised tummy time:

- Lay your baby across your lap or on your chest.
- Lay your baby on the floor with a nursing pillow supporting her chest.
- Lay your baby on an exercise ball, hold her steady, and roll the ball gently forward and back.
- Hold your baby tummy-side-down on your chest while practicing postpartum exercises (see page 332).

In addition, holding your baby upright in your arms or in a baby carrier (such as a Moby Wrap or Ergobaby carrier) will provide tummy-time benefits.[32]

# Your Baby's Growth and Development

Your baby has a unique appearance, temperament, and personality. His activity level and sleeping and eating patterns differ from those of all other babies, as do his responses to pain, hunger, or boredom.

Some babies are easy to care for; others are more difficult. For example, you may need additional patience and flexibility if your baby reacts to stimuli intensely, adapts to changes in his environment slowly, has a high activity level, and has mostly unpredictable feeding, sleeping, and activity patterns. As you get to know your baby's temperament, you'll learn to care for him in an effective and satisfying way.

Although your baby's temperament will probably change little over time, his abilities will quickly change. Because normal development patterns vary widely from one baby to the next, don't worry if your baby develops later or earlier than another baby. If, however, you notice that your baby misses some developmental milestones (see below) or is consistently older than the typical age when he reaches a milestone, consult with his caregiver. Early detection and treatment of developmental delays may improve your baby's long-term development.

## DEVELOPMENTAL MILESTONES

Here's a list of developmental behaviors or characteristics and the age when your baby is most likely to begin showing them. If your baby was premature, these milestones may occur somewhat later.

| Behavior or characteristic | Approximate age |
|---|---|
| Looks or stares at your face for short periods | Birth to 4 weeks |
| Holds up his head for a few moments while lying on his tummy | Birth to 4 weeks |
| Pays attention to sound by becoming alert or by turning toward it | Birth to 6 weeks |
| Smiles or coos when you smile, talk, or play with him | 6 weeks to 2 months |
| Lifts head and shoulders while lying on his tummy | 2 to 3 months |
| Holds his head steady when upright | 2 to 3 months |
| Brings his hands to his mouth | 3 months |
| Laughs and squeals | 3 to 4½ months |
| Rolls over from front to back or back to front | 2 months to 6 months |
| Grasps a rattle placed in his hand | 3 to 4½ months |

## YOUR NEWBORN'S SENSES

While getting to know your baby over the first weeks, you may wonder what she can see, hear, and taste. For years, experts underestimated a newborn's abilities. After years of study, experts now know that newborns have amazing capabilities.[33]

### Vision

When your newborn is quiet and alert, he can focus on objects 7 to 18 inches away. His vision at birth is about 20/200 and will be about 20/20 by six months.[34] He prefers to look at human faces (especially eyes), round shapes, high contrast of dark and light colors, complex patterns, and slowly moving objects—especially shiny ones. He may be sensitive to bright lights and will open his eyes wider when the lights are dimmed. His eyes might cross or might not seem to focus. As his eye muscles strengthen and mature, his eyes will track together.

## Hearing

Your baby heard your heartbeat, your voice, your partner's voice, and other internal and external noises while inside you. After she's born, she responds to voices, especially higher pitched voices (this is why people "speak parentese"—they unconsciously raise their voices' pitch when talking to babies). She may become calm or alert when she hears familiar voices or sounds, or when she hears white noise (such as a dishwasher or a washing machine) or familiar music. She also startles at sudden, loud noises.

## Smell

Your baby has a refined sense of smell. Within the first week after the birth, he recognizes differences in smells and can even tell the difference between the smell of his mother's milk and another mother's milk. In fact, the smell of your milk when you hold him may excite him to root and suckle.

## Taste

Your baby can taste things that are sweet, sour, salty, or bitter; however, she prefers sweet tastes. When offered something that's bitter, salty, or sour, she turns away.

## Touch

Your baby enjoys being stroked, rocked, caressed, gently jiggled or bounced, and allowed to nestle into your body while being held. He also likes warmth. Infant massage is a great way to touch your baby (see below).

## Advice from the Authors

Wearing your baby in a wrap, sling, or carrier frees up your hands while keeping her happy. Learn more using the following resources:

- Read "Ten Reasons to Wear Your Baby," a great article by Laura Simeon. You can find it online by using the article title as a search term.
- Read *Babywearing* by Maria Blois.
- Learn about different types of slings and carriers at http://kellymom.com/parenting/parenting-faq/sling and http://www.midwiferytoday.com/articles/slings.asp
- Visit http://www.youtube.com and use "wear your baby" as a search term to find how-to videos.

# INFANT MASSAGE

Infant massage is an excellent way to calm and soothe your baby and to communicate your love and care. Many communities offer infant massage classes, or you can follow these instructions to give your baby a massage:

1. Make sure the room is comfortably warm. Undress your baby, lay her on her back on the floor, and kneel in front of her. Or lay her on her back on your lap.
2. Put a little vegetable oil on your palm, then rub your hands together to warm them. (Don't use baby lotion or oil. Baby lotion will soak into her skin too quickly, and baby oil and other petroleum products aren't healthy for babies.)
3. Keep at least one hand on her until the massage is over. Massage her arms, legs, and other areas that she enjoys having touched. Use as much pressure as she finds pleasurable. (If she relaxes, it's just right. If she tenses, it's too much pressure.) Tell your baby what you're doing or sing a song. Don't massage your baby's tummy if it's full, and stop the massage if she's not enjoying herself.

## Tips to Protect Your Baby's Health

- Before feeding her, and after diaper changes, wash your hands well with soap and water. If you can't wash your hands, use an alcohol-based hand sanitizer.
- Keep anyone with a cold, cough, sore throat, rash, fever, or other signs of illness away from your baby. If you're ill, wash your hands thoroughly before feeding and caring for your baby.
- If you participate in group activities, such as parent-baby groups, be sure all participants understand and respect that they should attend only if they and their babies are healthy.
- If your baby is premature or has a chronic health condition, ask her caregiver for additional wellness guidelines.

4. If she's enjoying the massage (and she probably is), here are some motions to try:
   - stroking with open palms
   - stroking with thumbs or fingers
   - "raking" with fingertips
   - tapping lightly with fingertips
   - massaging your baby's arms or legs with a gentle wringing motion
   - doing whatever makes your baby happy

## PLAYING WITH YOUR BABY

A newborn has as many brain cells (neurons) as an adult; however, the connections between brain cells (synapses) that allow him to process information quickly haven't yet been wired. Babies learn about the world by interacting with it and with their parents. To build a baby's brain, parents need to expose him to new things, letting him explore those things over and over until he's memorized every detail, then give him quiet time to process what he has experienced.

For your baby, play is how he learns about himself and the world around him. When your baby grabs and shakes a rattle or plays peekaboo with you, he's discovering that he can make things happen. When you talk, coo, laugh, hug, and kiss your baby, he's learning that his responses affect you.

There are many ways to play with your baby every day. Here are a few:

- singing and talking to him or dancing with him
- caressing, touching, and cuddling when changing or feeding him
- massaging him (see above)
- playing games such as peekaboo or playing with age-appropriate toys
- having him do exercises with you (see page 332).

Play doesn't always need to focus on your baby. He absorbs information from you no matter what you do together. For example, your baby will enjoy hearing you read aloud from a novel or even a newspaper's business section. Your baby will like to see all the colorful clothes in your closet and smell all the interesting scents in your kitchen. If you're meeting friends for coffee, your baby will enjoy experiencing new sights, sounds, and smells. Even when you're putting away silverware, your baby can begin to hear numbers if you count each fork out loud as you place it in the drawer. Wearing your baby keeps him close to you and allows him to experience your everyday activities.

# Medical Care for Your Baby

The following sections describe ways to monitor your baby's health, reduce her risk of catching diseases, and treat illnesses or conditions that she may have, including when to call for medical help.

## WELL-BABY CARE

To make sure your baby is growing well and developing normally, he should have periodic routine well-baby exams by his caregiver. Three to four days after the birth, the caregiver will assess your baby's feeding, check for jaundice, and discuss any concerns you may have. Your baby may have another checkup when he's a week or two old to assess his weight and feeding, give you a chance to ask questions, and possibly repeat newborn screening tests (see page 363). Going forward, your baby's caregiver will let you know when to schedule additional appointments.

## VACCINATIONS

Prepared in a laboratory, vaccines are biological agents that can protect people from specific diseases and their complications—including death. An administration of a vaccine is called a *vaccination*. The process by which someone becomes protected from a disease is called *immunization*. Health-care professionals recommend that babies receive vaccinations according to a schedule from the CDC (see page 382).

### How Vaccines Work

Vaccinations are usually done by injection (a shot), but a few are given orally or with a nasal spray. They introduce a small amount of a disease (in a weakened or killed form) into the body. The immune system then produces antibodies that "teach" how to fight off that disease if the immune system encounters it again in the future.

### Benefits of Vaccines

Having your child vaccinated against a disease significantly reduces the chance that she'll contract it. If she does contract the disease despite being vaccinated, the vaccine will weaken the strength of the disease and help speed recovery.

If most people in an area are immunized against a disease, an outbreak is unlikely to spread in that community. This "herd immunity" helps protect people who can't get immunized, such as infants or people whose immune systems are weakened by disease or medical treatments. Vaccinations have been one of the most significant health contributions in the last century, nearly eradicating diseases such as polio and diphtheria.

### Risks of Vaccines

Because vaccinations introduce a foreign substance to the body, each has potential side effects. The most common side effects are pain from the injection, mild fever, fussiness, or rash in the twenty-four to forty-eight hours after receiving a vaccination. The chance of more serious complications varies by vaccine, but the risk is rare—for example, the risk of allergic reactions is about one in a million.[35]

The CDC has determined that the benefits of vaccines to an entire population outweigh the risks to a small number of individuals. It's natural, however, for parents to worry about possible risks to their children. They may be concerned about thimerosal (a preservative with trace amounts of mercury) in vaccines. Thimerosal, though, hasn't been used in childhood vaccines since 2001, except in flu vaccines that come in multidose vials.[36] Parents may have heard that vaccines can cause autism, a neurodevelopment disorder. However, the original research that supported this claim has been discredited, and numerous studies have since failed to show a connection between autism and vaccines.[37]

When evaluating benefits and risks, get current facts from reliable sources (see page 382).

## Information on Vaccines

### Alternatives to Vaccines

Some parents wonder whether breastfeeding, a healthy diet, herbs, and supplements are effective alternatives to vaccines. Although they may boost your child's overall health and strengthen her immune system, they can't protect against specific diseases as effectively as vaccines can.

Some parents choose to have their child receive only some of the recommended vaccines; others choose to follow an alternative vaccination schedule, which spreads out the shots over more time. Work closely with your caregiver if making these adjustments. For each disease, consider the following: how common the disease is in your community and the places you travel to (many public health departments publish local data about infectious diseases), how likely your child is to contract the disease if she's exposed to it, and how severe the disease can be. Then weigh the risks of the disease against the risks of the vaccine.

### Getting Vaccinations

Vaccinations are typically given at well-baby visits. When your baby is getting a shot, hold her in your arms to comfort her; if possible, breastfeed her to reduce the pain she experiences. Plan for a quiet day at home after her appointment to soothe her. Ask her caregiver how to treat a mild fever or any discomfort she may experience.

Your baby's caregiver will give you a form that shows completed vaccinations. Many child-care centers and schools require proof of certain vaccinations before allowing a child to attend.

If your baby has a reaction to a vaccine, inform her caregiver. You may also contact the Vaccine Adverse Event Reporting System (VAERS) at http://vaers.hhs.gov/index or the National Vaccine Injury Compensation Program (VICP) at http://www.hrsa.gov/vaccinecompensation/index.html, which provides compensation to people who may have been injured by vaccines.

## TAKING YOUR BABY'S TEMPERATURE

If your baby seems sick (listless, weak, unusually fussy, loss of appetite, runny nose, and so on), compare the warmth of her chest or back to the warmth of the back of your neck. Both areas should feel about the same temperature. If your baby feels too warm, take her axillary (under arm) temperature with a digital thermometer. Center the bulb in her armpit, making sure her clothing doesn't touch the bulb. Lower your baby's arm and hold it firmly against her body for five minutes or until the thermometer beeps. Remove it and read the temperature.

You can also take your baby's temperature with a temporal artery thermometer by moving it across her forehead. (Read the manufacturer's instructions for correct use.) Or you can take a rectal temperature. (Visit http://www.healthychildren.org for directions.) Ear probe thermometers, pacifier thermometers, and strips placed on the forehead aren't accurate for young babies.

Your baby's caregiver will tell you when to call for further advice—typically, when your baby's temperature is below 97.4°F (36.3°C) by any method or when her axillary temperature is over 99.5°F (37.5°C) or her temporal artery or rectal temperature is over 100.4°F (38°C).

# When to Call for Medical Help

If you're worried about your baby's health, write down his temperature and any symptoms that worry you, then call his caregiver. Here's other information your baby's caregiver may wish to know:

- physical symptoms, such as abnormal temperature, breathing difficulties, coughing, vomiting, diarrhea, constipation, fewer wet diapers than usual, or rash
- behavioral symptoms, such as listlessness, weakness, loss of appetite, unusual fussiness or irritability, change in typical behavior and activity level (for example, loss of interest in surroundings or in feeding)
- any newborn warning signs (see page 386).
- home treatment you've provided and your baby's response to it, including any medications
- general considerations, such as any recent exposure to illness

Visit our website, http://www.PCNGuide.com, to download a work sheet to help you organize your thoughts. Keep a pad and pen handy to write down any advice and suggestions your baby's caregiver may have.

# Common Health Concerns

The following sections discuss conditions in newborns that can cause concern but often clear up with minimal treatment.

## Newborn Jaundice

After the birth, your baby has a normal excess of red blood cells that break down into a substance called bilirubin, which she excretes in her bowel movements. Frequent feeding helps with this process.

About half of all newborns develop *jaundice*, an excess of bilirubin that causes her skin to become yellow by the third or fourth day after the birth. Yellowness in the face is typical; however, if your baby's arms, legs, abdomen, or the whites of her eyes are yellow, call her caregiver. (To confirm that your baby's skin is yellow, press your fingers on her breastbone. If the skin looks yellow when you remove your fingers, jaundice may be a concern.)

To diagnose jaundice, your baby's caregiver may take a blood sample from your baby's heel, then measure the bilirubin level. If the level is high enough to warrant treatment, your baby's caregiver will first make sure your baby is getting enough milk. If necessary, your baby will receive *phototherapy*, which causes the bilirubin level to drop. Phototherapy can be done by shining special cool lights on your baby or wrapping her in a special blanket. Treatment may be done in the hospital or at home and usually continues for two to four days, until further blood tests show that the bilirubin has fallen to a safe level.

Jaundice that appears on the first or second day after the birth (early jaundice) is more serious than when it appears on the third or fourth day. It may require intensive treatment, such as phototherapy or a blood *exchange transfusion*, to prevent possible hearing loss or severe neurological damage. If your baby develops jaundice after the first two weeks, have her caregiver evaluate her.

Jaundice is more likely when there's inadequate feeding, prematurity, bruising during birth, exposure to certain drugs, liver or intestinal problems, sepsis (infection), and blood incompatibilities, such as Rh (see page 128) or ABO incompatibility (when the mother's blood type is O and the baby's is A, B, or AB).

## Rashes

Several types of rashes are common in newborns
- Eryhtema toxicum presents as red blotches with waxy yellow or white pimples in the middle. It appears on the torso, arms, and legs in the first week and usually disappears without treatment.
- Facial rashes are smooth pimples, small red spots, rough red spots, or small white spots (milia) on a baby's nose, cheeks, and chin. They appear and disappear in the first few months. Applying breast milk as a "lotion" may help reduce the rash.
- Prickly heat presents as clusters of tiny pink pimples surrounded by pink skin. Found most often on the shoulders, torso, and neck. As it dries, the rash becomes slightly tan. Prickly heat may look worse than it feels to a baby. It's caused by overheating, so parents should take care not to overdress their babies.
- Cradle cap is a yellowish, scaly, patchy condition on a baby's scalp. Daily washing or brushing of the scalp may help treat or even prevent cradle cap. First, baby's scalp is massaged with vegetable oil. Next, the scales are gently combed or brushed out with a baby comb or soft fingernail brush. Then baby's scalp is washed with mild soap.

## Colds

Although it's normal for a baby to have a slightly stuffy nose or make a snuffly noise when she breathes through her nose, she may have a cold if she has a very runny nose and goopy eyes, is fussier than usual, has trouble eating and sleeping, and perhaps has a slight fever.

To reduce your baby's risk of catching a cold, minimize the number of sick people she comes into contact with, especially when she's younger than three months. Make sure all those who want to handle your baby wash their hands thoroughly first.

When your baby has a cold, consult with her caregiver. Suggested treatments may include using a cool-mist vaporizer near your baby and putting her in a semireclined position (such as in a car seat) to sleep. You also can run a hot shower or bath, then take your baby into the steamy bathroom to help ease congestion. There's no need to clear your baby's nostrils if she can nurse well. If she's too stuffy to nurse, you can clear your baby's nostrils by dripping saline or breast milk into each one (breast milk soothes the mucous membranes and contains anti-viral and antibacterial properties), then "milking" her nose by gently squeezing it with your fingers. If that's not enough to remove the mucus, you can use a bulb syringe or nasal aspirator.[38]

Don't give your baby cold medications, such as decongestants and cough medicine; they aren't safe for infants.

## MEDICATIONS

Use the following guidelines if your baby's caregiver prescribes medications or vitamins:
- To dispense liquid medication, use a medicine dropper placed between your baby's cheek and gum; don't squirt it on his tongue. Hold your baby in a semiupright position and let him suck the medicine as you gently squeeze the dropper.
- Another option is to pour the medication into an empty bottle nipple, then have him drink it all. When the nipple is empty, fill it with water and have your baby drink it all as well.
- Don't mix medication into a bottle of breast milk, formula, or water. If your baby refuses to finish the whole bottle, you won't know how much medication he's received.
- Give only the medication your baby's caregiver specifies.

# Sudden Infant Death Syndrome (SIDS)[39]

*Sudden infant death syndrome (SIDS)* is the sudden death of a baby younger than one year that remains unexplained after a thorough investigation. Almost every parent worries about SIDS at some time. You may have read about the condition or even know of someone whose baby died of SIDS. Although there's no way to minimize the loss and grief caused by SIDS, the following facts may help put your fears and worries into perspective:

- SIDS is rare, occurring in about one in two thousand babies in the United States.
- SIDS deaths most commonly occur in babies who are between two and four months old.
- No one—including parents—is to blame for SIDS.
- Death occurs quickly and painlessly; it isn't the result of suffocation, asphyxiation, or regurgitation.
- SIDS isn't caused by vaccinations. In fact, SIDS deaths are statistically less common in babies who have been vaccinated.

For parents faced with a loss by SIDS, support groups can help. The baby's caregiver, a public health nurse, or a childbirth educator can help locate a group. Other resources include First Candle (800-221-7437 or http://www.firstcandle.com) and the American SIDS Institute (http://www.sids.org).

You can take steps before and after your baby's birth to help reduce her risk of SIDS. During pregnancy, eat a healthful diet, don't smoke and avoid exposure to secondhand smoke, have regular prenatal care to help reduce your baby's risk of prematurity, and don't use cocaine or heroin. After your baby is born, breastfeed her, don't expose her to secondhand smoke, and avoid overheating her. If you choose to use a pacifier, you may offer one to your baby to help her fall asleep. If it falls out of her mouth after she falls asleep, there's no need to reinsert it. (If breastfeeding, wait until it's well established—three or four weeks—before introducing a pacifier.) Place her in a safe position in a safe space to sleep.

## Safe Sleeping to Reduce the Risk of SIDS and Suffocation

Make sure that everyone who cares for your baby places him on his back to sleep. Placing him on his tummy or side to sleep increases his risk of SIDS. If your baby is unhappy on his back or wakens easily, try swaddling him in a lightweight blanket. (If he can wiggle out of the blanket overnight, it's unsafe to leave a loose blanket in the crib with him. Either stop swaddling or try using a double-swaddle technique—visit our website, http://www.PCNGuide.com, for more information.)

Also make sure your baby's sleep space is safe. Use a firm, flat surface and avoid waterbeds and couches. Don't place soft, loose materials—such as pillows, quilts, comforters, soft toys, sheepskins, and bumper pads—in a crib. Make sure there isn't space between the mattress and the headboard or walls, or between the crib mattress and the crib slats. These spaces may entrap your baby and lead to suffocation.

The American Academy of Pediatrics (AAP) recommends that to reduce the risk of SIDS, babies should sleep in the same room as their mothers, but not in the same bed (bed-sharing).[40] This recommendation has been disputed by other experts, who recommend bed-sharing for such benefits as frequent and convenient breastfeeding, reduced crying, and better sleep for both parents and babies.

Bed-sharing requires following safety guidelines in addition to laying babies on their backs on firm surfaces without loose bedding. A baby shouldn't share a bed with a parent who has consumed medication, alcohol, or any substance that causes extreme drowsiness or unawareness (increases the risk of rolling onto the baby and smothering him). A baby shouldn't share a bed if a parent also is a smoker or is very obese. It's important that everyone is aware of bed-sharing safety guidelines because parents who hadn't expected to bed-share often end up doing so. For more information on bed-sharing, read *Sleeping with Your Baby: A Parent's Guide to Cosleeping* by James J. McKenna or http://cosleeping.nd.edu/safe-co-sleeping-guidelines.

## Newborn Warning Signs

If any of the following signs appear in the first month after the birth, report them to your baby's caregiver.

| Warning signs | Possible problems |
| --- | --- |
| Fever (axillary temperature above 99.5°F/37.5°C) | Infection |
| Temperature below 97.4°F/36.3°C (whether taken axillary, by temporal artery, or rectally) | Infection caused by Group B streptococcus (GBS) or other bacteria |
| Your baby's face, chest, and the whites of his eyes are yellow. | Jaundice (see page 383) |
| Problems with feeding, including a breastfed baby who feeds fewer than 7 or 8 times in 24 hours or any baby who feeds poorly | Difficulty with breastfeeding, jaundice, illness, or prematurity (see chapter 19) |
| Fewer wet diapers than expected: In the first week, expect the number of wet diapers to at least equal the day of life (for example, at least 3 wet diapers on day 3). After day 7, expect 6 or more wet diapers in 24 hours. | Inadequate feeding or illness (see page 405 for signs that your baby is getting enough milk) |
| Problems with bowel movements, including no bowel movement in any 24-hour period in the first month after the birth. After your baby is a month old, it's normal from him not to have a bowel movement for a day or longer. | Inadequate feeding (see page 368 for description of normal bowel movements in newborns) |
| Problems with breathing, including blue lips, a struggle to breathe, flared nostrils, or deep indentations of the chest when breathing. | Prematurity, illness, or heart or lung problems |

**Call 911 if your baby can't breathe easily.**

# Babies with Special Circumstances

Babies who are born early or small for their gestational age may have needs that require special care.

## PREMATURE BABIES

A baby is *premature* if she's born before the thirty-seventh week of pregnancy and weighs less than 5½ pounds. (For more information on prevention and treatment of preterm labor, see page 129.) Thankfully, advances in care have increased the survival rates of very premature babies (even as young as twenty-four weeks) and have greatly reduced the long-term respiratory and neurological problems experienced by premature babies born just a decade ago.

If a baby is born before term, she looks different than a full-term baby does. She's small, limp, and frail. Her skin is reddish and appears tissue-paper thin, and she has little to no fat or muscle. Her head appears disproportionately large. Vernix caseosa and lanugo (fine, downy hair on her body) are abundant, her fingernails and toenails haven't grown out, and her tiny ears are soft and hug her head. Her cry is feeble, and she may be more difficult to soothe than a full-term baby.

A premature baby is physically vulnerable until she grows older. She sucks weakly, and her swallow and gag reflexes are unreliable. She may need to be fed by a tube into her stomach. Because her body temperature is unstable, she usually stays in a temperature-controlled isolette. Because her lungs are immature, her breaths are irregular, rapid, and often shallow; she may need oxygen to help with breathing. Her ability to absorb food is less efficient than a full-term baby's, although her need for nutrients—especially calories, protein, iron, calcium, zinc, and vitamin E—may be greater. Because her immune system is less developed, she may need to have extra precautions taken to protect her from infection.

If you give birth to a premature baby, the experience can be upsetting and frightening. Your baby will need special medical attention that may separate her from you, but she also needs to feel your touch and hear your voice, even when inside an isolette.

Your baby's nurse may encourage holding your baby skin-to-skin (also called *kangaroo care*—see page 295). Your closeness, breathing movements, and warmth will help regulate her breathing, keep her warm, comfort her, and help her grow faster.

If your baby is too immature to breastfeed, you can express milk and have it fed to her with a dropper or through a tube that passes from her mouth to her stomach (see page 414).

Feeding, touching, and caring for your premature baby will help you both cope as she grows stronger. For additional support, you may want to contact a group that provides information, assistance, emotional support, and perhaps preemie baby clothing to parents of premature babies. For more information, check with hospital staff.

## Babies Who Are Small for Gestational Age

Babies who are small for gestational age (SGA) are smaller in size and weight than expected at birth, given the length of time they were in the womb. This condition has several possible causes, including an inadequate transfer of nutrients across the placenta to the baby, the effects of some drugs (such as tobacco) taken during pregnancy, some congenital and genetic malformations, and certain infections, such as toxoplasmosis. Sometimes the cause is unknown.

SGA babies present challenges to parents that are similar to those of premature babies. SGA babies don't move easily from state to state (for example, from active to quiet alert or from drowsy to deep sleep—see pages 376–377). They're often fussy and difficult to soothe. Parents spend lots of time calming SGA babies; successful soothing techniques include frequent feeding, gentle rocking, quiet talking, and maintaining a calm environment. SGA babies can handle only one source of stimulation at a time. Too much stimulation—such as talking to the baby while jiggling or feeding him—overwhelms him.

If your baby is SGA, he'll become less intense and fussy as he matures. In the meantime, your sensitivity to his special needs will help you both cope.

## *Key Points to Remember*

- Every newborn has a unique appearance and temperament. Babies teach their parents what they need by giving cues. Crying is often your baby's last attempt to communicate that she's hungry, overstimulated, tired, or uncomfortable. Try to respond to your baby's early cues so you meet her needs before she cries.
- The Five S's method (see page 373) can be an especially effective tool for calming a crying baby.
- Learn about vaccinations, circumcision, and other newborn procedures so you can make informed decisions about your child's health care.
- You can significantly reduce the risk of SIDS by breastfeeding, not smoking and avoiding second-hand smoke, having your baby sleep in the same room as you, and always placing your baby on her back to sleep.
- Be aware of newborn warning signs (see page 386) to know when to seek medical help.
- As a parent, you're going to have days when everything goes great, and you feel very successful. You'll have other days when everything is hard, and you feel like a failure. That's normal! Just try the best you can every day, and hopefully in the end, you'll have more good days than bad.

# CHAPTER 19

# Feeding Your Baby

During pregnancy, your body nourishes your baby as he grows from an amazingly tiny fertilized egg to a fully developed newborn who weighs several pounds. After the birth, you continue to nourish him with breast milk, formula, or both. Although either type of nourishment helps your baby triple his birth weight and grow 10 to 12 inches during his first year, only breast milk provides valuable substances, such as hormones and human growth factors, that enhance the development of your baby's immune system, digestive tract, brain, and nerves throughout his body.

Whether you feed your baby breast milk or formula, *how* you feed him is also important to his growth and development. The way your baby is fed influences his physical, social, and emotional well-being.[1] Feeding him with care and love whenever he shows he's hungry helps foster his emotional development and encourages bonding and attachment.

# What to Feed Your Baby

Before deciding what and how you'll feed your baby, it's important to become well informed about breastfeeding, feeding expressed breast milk from a bottle, and formula feeding. Each method of feeding may have advantages and drawbacks, depending on your circumstances.

## WHY HEALTH-CARE PROVIDERS RECOMMEND BREAST MILK AND BREASTFEEDING

Except in certain rare instances (see page 392), almost all health-care providers recommend breastfeeding because of its health benefits for both babies and mothers.

Breast milk's nutritional composition is ideal for babies. Unlike formula, breast milk adapts to meet your baby's changing nutritional needs. It contains more than two hundred nutrients and components not found in formula, which may explain why breast milk can (and formula can't) boost the development of your baby's immune system. Breast milk also enhances the development of your baby's brain and may contribute to a higher IQ and better cognitive test scores.[2]

Babies who are exclusively breastfed have fewer and less severe allergies than formula-fed babies.[3] Breastfed babies are much less likely to be hospitalized for infections; overall, they have fewer ear infections, respiratory infections, urinary

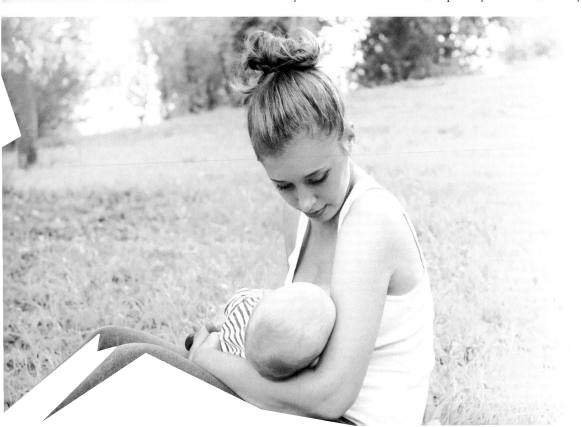

tract infections (UTIs), and infections from bacterial meningitis.[4] Breastfed babies also experience less diarrhea and vomiting. In addition, studies show that breast milk can lower a baby's risk of sudden infant death syndrome (SIDS).[5]

Looking ahead to your baby's future, breastfeeding can reduce the risk of diseases, such as diabetes, asthma, obesity, leukemia, lymphoma, and multiple sclerosis.[6]

For you, breastfeeding reduces postpartum bleeding and helps your uterus shrink to its normal size faster. Breastfeeding reduces your lifetime risk of some diseases, including premenopausal breast cancer, ovarian cancer, and osteoporosis.[7]

Your family will likely find breastfeeding to be both economical and convenient. (It's virtually cost free and always available.) It also promotes a close, nurturing relationship between you and your baby.

## ADDRESSING YOUR CONCERNS ABOUT BREASTFEEDING

Despite health-care providers' endorsement of breastfeeding, you may doubt its advantages or wonder about your ability to breastfeed successfully. These concerns may lead you to decide that breastfeeding won't work for you. Before making a decision, talk to your caregiver, a lactation consultant, your baby's caregiver, or a childbirth educator. You may discover that your concerns, such as the examples that follow, are unfounded or can be addressed:

- If you had trouble breastfeeding in the past, talk with a lactation consultant during pregnancy to discuss how it can be different this time. If you remain unsure, give breastfeeding a try. You can stop if it's unsuccessful.
- If you doubt that breastfeeding can be more convenient than formula feeding, talk with families who breastfeed and those who formula feed to get an idea of how the effort and costs compare.
- Returning to work can present challenges to breastfeeding, but they can be overcome or minimized. See page 430 for further information.
- The baby's medical condition can affect breastfeeding. A lactation consultant can show parents special techniques for feeding a baby with physical challenges. Breastfeeding or providing expressed breast milk can be an excellent way to help a premature or special-needs baby grow and stay healthy. See page 414.
- A breast reduction might or might not affect your ability to breastfeed. If you've had this surgery, get the support of a lactation consultant before giving birth.

## Common Q & A

**Q:** Does breastfeeding work as a birth control method?

**A:** Breastfeeding does reduce the chance of becoming pregnant. For as long as you exclusively breastfeed your baby, you have less than a 2 percent chance of becoming pregnant if the following is true:

- Your baby is less than six months old.
- You don't menstruate until after fifty-six days postpartum.
- You're nursing frequently (at least every four hours during the day and every six hours at night).
- You rarely supplement your baby's feedings and give him tastes of foods or fluids only occasionally.[8]

After your baby begins eating table foods, you can extend some of breastfeeding's contraceptive benefits by nursing before offering table foods and by continuing to breastfeed throughout the day and night. You can use fertility awareness methods to monitor your body's fertility signs. Identifying these signs is trickier when you're nursing because of the fluctuating hormone levels required for breastfeeding, but it can be done.

After giving birth, you may ovulate before you have your first menstrual period. If preventing pregnancy is essential or desirable, talk to your caregiver about contraception. Barrier methods (condoms and diaphragms), intrauterine devices (IUDs), and progestin-only pills and injections (minipill and Depo-Provera) don't interfere with breastfeeding. Birth control pills containing estrogen, however, can reduce your milk supply.[9]

## Advice from the Authors

When you have breastfeeding questions, concerns, or need encouragement, consider these sources of support:

- your caregiver or your baby's caregiver
- hospital staff (ask if they have a breastfeeding hotline or if it's okay to call the labor and delivery unit with questions)
- lactation consultant
- physician specializing in breastfeeding medicine
- La Leche League group or any new moms' support group
- someone who has success-fully breastfed her baby
- National Women's Health Center: http://www.womens health.gov/breastfeeding
- websites on breastfeeding support, including http://www.llli.org, http://www.breastfeeding.com, and http://www.breastfeeding online.com
- online forums on breastfeeding, including http://forums.llli.org, http://www.mothering.com/discussions, and http://www.kellymom.com

- If you have twins, triplets, or more, breastfeeding may be challenging. Even if you can't always nurse your babies, you can still provide them breast milk by expressing it. See pages 412 and 428 for more information.
- If your partner or others worry that breastfeeding will eliminate an opportunity for them to care for your baby, point out several other ways they can actively parent. They can cuddle and soothe her, bathe her, and change her diapers. They can observe how your baby latches onto your breast and give suggestions if needed. They can also bring you something to drink or eat while breastfeeding—feeding you helps feed your baby.

After considering your circumstances, if you decide not to breastfeed, see pages 418–419 to learn about formula feeding. If you want to breastfeed but discover that you can't, seek the support of your caregiver or a lactation consultant to help you adjust to a different method of feeding.

## WHEN HEALTH-CARE EXPERTS RECOMMEND FORMULA-FEEDING

In a few cases, health-care providers do recommend formula feeding over breastfeeding or breast milk. For example, if a baby has galactosemia (a rare condition in which the baby can't digest the sugar in breast milk), formula becomes necessary. In most cases, however, the mother's health is the reason for the recommendation. Formula-feeding is best if the mother is HIV positive (and lives in a developed country),[10] has untreated tuberculosis, takes certain medications that may harm the baby (such as radioactive drugs), uses street drugs (such as heroin, cocaine, or methamphetamines), is receiving high doses of methadone, or has had extensive breast surgery.

Some women's concerns about breastfeeding are psychological. For example, some are overly anxious about nursing in public; others chronically worry that they might not produce enough milk or that breastfeeding may damage their breasts' appearance. For most women, these concerns are mild and talking with a lactation consultant, obstetrician, or midwife may help overcome them. For other women, however, these concerns are overwhelming anxieties, especially if a woman is a survivor of sexual abuse. If you have serious concerns, talking with a lactation consultant or a caregiver can help you decide whether formula feeding is appropriate. If formula-feeding is recommended, see page 418 for further information.

# When to Feed Your Baby

Your baby shows she's hungry by giving *feeding or hunger cues*. Knowing these cues and watching for them makes it easier on all of you. Typical feeding cues include the following:

- Your baby "roots" (opens her mouth and turns toward anything that touches her cheeks or lips).
- She brings her hand toward her mouth.
- She thrusts out her tongue often or makes lots of mouth movements.
- She makes lots of body movements.
- She awakens from a drowsy state and seems to want something.

Most babies show these cues to signal hunger long before beginning to fuss or cry, which are last-ditch attempts to communicate their needs. Trying to feed a crying baby is difficult, so watch for your baby's feeding cues and promptly feed her whenever she's hungry. Expect to see these cues every few hours (see below for more on feeding patterns).

Continue the feeding until you see *full cues*. Your baby may do one or more of the following:

- fall asleep
- let go of the nipple
- slow her sucking and pause often between sucks

When you see these cues, burp your baby, then offer the second breast or reoffer the bottle.

Later in this chapter, we discuss how many minutes a breastfed baby typically nurses and how many ounces on average a bottle-fed baby takes at each feeding. This information will help ensure that your baby is getting enough milk.

## YOUR BABY'S FEEDING PATTERNS

During the first days, weeks, and months of your baby's life, the frequency and duration of his feedings change to facilitate his growth. A nursing mother's breasts adapt to these changes to meet her baby's changing needs. Parents who bottle-feed add more breast milk or formula when their babies consistently want more after finishing a feeding. This section describes typical feeding patterns.

### The First Days after the Birth

After feeding vigorously during the first few hours after the birth, many healthy newborns show less interest in feeding until they're twenty to twenty-four hours old. By that time, most babies perk up and are eager to feed again. However, mothers should try to feed their babies every two or three hours throughout the first day.

As your newborn becomes more awake after the birth, she may want to feed more frequently.[11] When breast-feeding, your baby may feed in clusters (five or more times in three hours followed by deep sleep) or seem to feed constantly until your milk supply increases.

To help ensure your baby gets enough milk, feed her whenever you see hunger cues (see above). Newborns need to feed at least eight times every twenty-four hours (about once every three hours), but many babies feed ten to twelve times a day.

## *The First Weeks after the Birth*

As your baby gets older, she begins to eat every one to three hours. As the weeks pass, she consumes more milk at each feeding, which may reduce the number of feedings. She also begins to feed less at night and more during the day and evening. Because babies don't always eat on a regular schedule, your baby may want to cluster her feedings, eating four to five times in five to six hours and then sleeping for several hours.

When your baby is two to three weeks old, she begins to fuss and fret for about an hour (or longer) every evening as a way to cope with new stimulation. During this time, your baby cries, feeds frequently, takes brief rests, then cries and feeds again. When you're breastfeeding, this frequent feeding stimulates your breasts to make more milk. Although common and normal, this fussiness can frustrate new parents. See page 373 for ways to soothe a fussy baby.

## *The First Months after the Birth*

Your baby also may experience fussy and challenging stages at ages six weeks, three months, and six months. At these times, babies are acquiring new skills. At three weeks old, your baby awakens to his world. (see page 378). At about six weeks old, he starts to interact with others by smiling. At three months old, he's very alert to his surroundings, recognizes one parent from another, and is learning to roll over. At about six months old, he masters sitting unaided.

The acquisition of new skills can affect feeding and sleep patterns until your baby masters them. For example, when he's around three months old, his environment may so distract him that he eats less frequently during the day, only to wake more at night to feed. Feeding your baby in a quiet, dimly lit place can help him feed more during the day. Usually within a few days to a week, your baby returns to a more predictable pattern.

# Burping Your Baby

When your baby feeds (or cries), he may swallow air that travels to his stomach, causing fullness and possible discomfort. Burping releases the swallowed air, and until he can burp on his own (around two weeks old), he needs help doing so. Even then, he still may need help.

If breastfeeding, try burping your baby after he's done nursing at each breast. If bottle-feeding, burp him after he takes two ounces. Place him in one of the following positions to burp him:

- *Over-the-shoulder*: Place your baby high on your chest with his head peeking over your shoulder. Support him well across his back and buttocks.
- *Over-the-lap:* Lay your baby on his tummy across your lap.
- *Sitting on your lap:* Your baby can be sitting upright or you can lean him backward or forward before sitting him up. Place your thumb and index finger under his chin with your palm supporting his chest and your other hand supporting his back.

Have your baby's head above his stomach to allow air bubbles to rise up and out of his stomach. You can gently pat or rub your baby's back to help bring up the bubbles. If after a minute or two he hasn't burped, stop trying. He might not need to burp.

# When Your Baby Spits Up

During or after feedings, many babies *spit up* a dribble or more of milk (up to 2 to 3 tablespoons). A newborn has an immature sphincter muscle at the top of the stomach, which lets milk and swallowed air back up. Spitting up usually isn't harmful if it occurs only occasionally and the baby is otherwise healthy and growing well. Babies typically outgrow spitting up at around six months old.

Your baby may spit up if she cries hard before a feeding. If you're breastfeeding, your baby is more likely to spit up if you have a strong let-down reflex (see page 397) and an abundant milk supply, causing her to eat too much too quickly or swallow more air. Try leaning back when nursing or sitting your baby up during feedings, to help her manage the rapid milk flow (see page 401).

You can reduce spitting up by burping your baby. To help keep milk in your baby's stomach after a feeding, try to gently position her upright or on her side in your arms or sitting in a car seat or swing with her head elevated.

If your baby spits up continuously or vomits with force (projectile vomiting) frequently, she may have a more serious condition. Call your baby's caregiver if you see the following signs:

- Your baby seems in pain when spitting up (may be gastroesophageal reflux—see page 374).
- Your baby vomits after every feeding and doesn't poop frequently.
- Your baby vomits after each of two to three consecutive feedings and seems weak, limp, or lethargic.

## Nipple Types and Treatment for Flat or Inverted Nipples

Knowing your nipple type lets you know what (if anything) you can do to help make breast-feeding go more smoothly.[12] To determine your nipple type, place your thumb and index finger above and below your areola at its edge and gently squeeze them together.

- **Typical nipples** elongate or protrude (stick out) when squeezed. They're the most common type.
- **Flat nipples** flatten or move inward (retract) when squeezed.
- **Inverted nipples** are tucked into the areola. When squeezed, some protrude while others remain inverted, probably because tiny bands (adhesions) bind the tissue.

If you have flat or inverted nipples, some correction often occurs naturally during pregnancy,[13] as hormonal changes enlarge the nipples and improve their ability to protrude. If your nipples remain flat or inverted, you may have trouble starting breastfeeding. In that case, here are a few suggestions:

- Contact a lactation consultant to help with early breastfeeding.
- Consider using a nipple shield, an ultrathin silicone device that you place over your nipple. When your baby sucks on it, he pulls your nipple and milk into his mouth. Don't use a nipple shield without a lactation consultant's help; you may need her expert advice to transition to breastfeeding without it.
- Your baby's sucking also helps *evert* (draw out) your nipple. But if your baby has difficulty latching on, consider using a breast pump before each feeding to draw out your nipples. A lactation consultant or maternity nurses can show you how and may suggest other ideas, such as using commercial "nipple enhancers" designed to draw out nipples. (Evert-it and Avent Niplette are two brands.)

# Breastfeeding

The following sections first discuss breastfeeding preparation and explain the composition of breast milk and how a woman's hormones and anatomy make breastfeeding possible. Knowing this information can help you trust that breastfeeding is working and well worth doing. Next, they cover *how* to breastfeed a baby, including positions for holding the baby, ways to help him get an effective latch, signs that he's getting plenty of breast milk, and more.

## PRENATAL PREPARATION FOR BREASTFEEDING

To prepare for breastfeeding, learn as much as you can before the birth. Read breastfeeding books, attend a breastfeeding class, and seek the support of groups such as La Leche League, Nursing Mothers Counsel (NMC), new mothers' groups, or WIC (the US government program for low-income women, infants, and children). Spend time around women who breastfeed so you can see how they nurse their babies and learn how they make breastfeeding part of their busy lives.

Choose caregivers who are committed to supporting breastfeeding. While pregnant, ask your caregiver to assess the changes to your breasts and evaluate your nipples. Many caregivers haven't had training to assess breasts for breastfeeding, so you may need a referral to a lactation consultant.

A prenatal visit with a lactation consultant is recommended if you've had breast surgeries, are expecting multiples, have had a previous unpleasant breastfeeding experience, or have specific concerns about your health, nipples, or breast anatomy. Together, you can determine what steps to take during pregnancy and the postpartum period to create a positive experience.

Arrange for help during the first weeks after the birth. Enlist family, friends, or a postpartum doula (see page 23) to help with meals and household tasks so you can focus on feeding and caring for your baby and yourself. Keep the contact information of a lactation consultant and breastfeeding support groups handy. Lastly, know that with time and experience, breastfeeding becomes much easier and more enjoyable.

# How Breastfeeding Works

Your body began preparing for breastfeeding long before you became pregnant. When you were in your early teens, increasing amounts of the hormone estrogen stimulated the growth of your breasts, including your mammary (milk) glands and fatty tissue.

During pregnancy, your breasts prepare for lactation (breast milk production) through a complex interaction of hormones that causes rapid growth of your milk glands. These glands contain the small round sacs (lobules) that make milk and the pathways (ducts) for milk to flow out the nipple. Blood supply to your breasts supports this growth and delivers the nutrients in breast milk.

As early as the sixteenth week of pregnancy, the hormones *prolactin* and *human placental lactogen (HPL)* stimulate your breasts to produce and provide *colostrum* (the first milk). After you give birth, progesterone levels fall and prolactin levels increase, triggering breast milk production. These amazing changes occur naturally during pregnancy and after birth.

## Anatomy of Your Breasts

Your breasts are well designed to make milk. Each breast contains fifteen to twenty milk-producing units called lobes. Each lobe contains branches of *alveoli* (cells that make milk) and milk ducts. Milk flows from the alveoli through the ducts and leaves your breast through six to ten nipple openings.[14] As your baby compresses the *areola* (the darker skin around each nipple) with her lips, gums and tongue, she pulls milk into her mouth. *Montgomery glands* are the small bumps on the areola that secrete a lubricating substance, which keeps the nipple supple and helps prevent infection. (Use only water to clean your breasts; scrubbing with soap removes this special lubrication.)

Your breasts likely look different during pregnancy. They're probably larger with more visible veins and stretch marks. Your areolae may appear larger and darker; these changes help your newborn see your nipples. Your Montgomery glands also appear larger. Colostrum may leak from your breasts or dry into a crust on your nipples. These changes show that your breasts are responding to pregnancy hormones and preparing to make milk.

Of all women, 2 to 6 percent have *accessory mammary tissue*, extra breast tissue under the arm or below the breast that may have a nipple.[15] This tissue may swell during pregnancy and as milk comes in. If left alone, the tissue diminishes, but placing cold packs on the area may decrease discomfort.

Contrary to popular belief, your breast size doesn't determine the quality or quantity of the milk you produce. Bigger breasts simply have more fatty tissue surrounding the milk-producing structures than smaller breasts have. Breasts, areolae, and nipples of all sizes and shapes are usually perfect for breastfeeding.

## How Your Breasts Make Milk

Prolactin and oxytocin are two hormones that play a significant role in milk production and milk ejection (flow). When your baby suckles, the action stimulates the nerve endings in your areola and tells the anterior pituitary gland to release prolactin. This hormone causes the cells in the alveoli to draw water and nutrients from your blood to make milk. Your baby's suckling also prompts the posterior pituitary gland to release oxytocin. Oxytocin makes the muscles around milk-producing cells contract and expel milk. It also makes the ducts widen and shorten, helping with milk flow. This process is called the *let-down reflex*.

You have several let-downs from each breast during each feeding.[16] During the first weeks, let-down might not occur until several minutes after your baby has begun suckling. Later on, let-down occurs within seconds.

Let-down sensations vary widely. After their milk comes in, many women feel a tingling, itching, or flowing sensation during the first let-down. If you don't feel your milk let-down, you'll know it has occurred when you hear your baby swallow, see milk in his mouth, or feel uterine cramping.

The frequency and duration of feedings strongly affect your milk supply. The more your baby suckles and drains your breast, the more milk you produce. Conversely, you make less milk if you delay or limit feedings, use a pacifier, offer supplements (formula, water, or other liquids), or schedule your baby's feedings to every three to four hours. The reason is a protein in breast milk called *feedback inhibitor of lactation (FIL)*. When your breast is full of milk, FIL slows milk production. When your baby frequently drains your breast, there is less FIL and milk production increases.[17]

To develop a good milk supply, feed your baby frequently in response to his feeding cues and let him feed until he shows full cues (see page 393).

## Composition of Breast Milk

**Colostrum.** The first milk you produce is colostrum, a yellowish or clear syrupy fluid that's ideally suited to your newborn's needs. Colostrum helps speed the passage of meconium (first bowel movement) and establish the proper balance of healthy bacteria in your baby's digestive tract. Because colostrum is rich in antibodies, it protects your baby from infection. It's also higher in protein than mature milk. On average, you make just over an ounce in the first twenty-four hours after birth, which is exactly what your baby needs. The volume increases over the next few days.[18]

**Transitional milk.** After making only colostrum, your breasts produce transitional milk, which is higher in fat, calories, and volume than colostrum but lower in protein. It's yellowish white because it contains colostrum and milk.

**Mature milk.** Usually by the end of the first week, you produce mature milk. This bluish white liquid looks like nonfat milk and contains more calories than transitional milk. The volume of milk production increases substantially. By the fifth day postpartum, you make about 16½ ounces of milk a day. By three to five months, you make 25 ounces a day; by six months, 27 ounces.[19]

The composition of mature breast milk varies from the beginning of each feeding to its end. The milk produced early in the feeding is called *foremilk*. The milk released with let-down is called *hindmilk*, which provides most of the calories and contains more fat and protein. Also, your breast milk contains more fat when your breasts are less full.[20] As your baby grows, your breast milk changes to meet her nutritional needs.

## Components of Breast Milk

Vitamins, minerals, enzymes, hormones, and other components make up breast milk. Here are the main ones:

### Nonnutritive qualities

These components protect against disease and promote healthy development. They include anti-infective properties, anti-inflammatory factors, enzymes, hormones, and growth factors.[21]

### Water

About 87 percent of breast milk is water, which helps newborns maintain their body temperature. Even in very warm climates, breast milk contains all the water a baby needs.

## Fats

Cholesterol, essential fatty acids, docosahexaenoic acid (DHA), and other fats account for half the calories in breast milk and are necessary for normal development of a baby's nervous system and brain. Fats also aid visual development and enhance the growth of a special coating on nerves as they grow (myelinization).[22]

## Carbohydrates

Lactose (milk sugar), the primary carbohydrate, helps a baby absorb calcium. It's metabolized into two simple sugars (galactose and glucose) necessary for rapid brain growth.

## Proteins

Whey, the primary protein in breast milk, becomes a soft curd when a baby digests it, letting her bloodstream readily absorb the nutrients. (Casein, the primary protein in cow milk and cow milk formula, forms a rubbery curd that babies digest less easily than whey, sometimes contributing to constipation.)

## Vitamins and minerals

Breast milk provides almost all the vitamins and minerals your baby needs. Your caregiver or your baby's caregiver may recommend a few supplements.
*Vitamin D*
Vitamin D is essential for your body to absorb calcium. Adequate calcium is necessary for bone growth and the normal functioning of your nervous system. You make vitamin D when you expose your skin to sunlight, or you can obtain it by eating foods with added vitamin D or taking vitamin D supplements. Since appropriate levels of sun exposure are difficult to determine and hard to get in northern climates, your caregivers may recommend vitamin D supplementation.

The Institute of Medicine recommends 600 IU of vitamin D each day in pregnancy. Taking more vitamin D (1,000 to 4,000 IU) when you're breastfeeding may help increase the amount in your breast milk. To ensure babies have sufficient levels, the American Academy of Pediatrics (AAP) recommends that a breastfed baby consume 400 IU of vitamin D daily;[23] the Canadian Paediatric Society (CPS) also recommends this amount except for during the winter months, when 800 IU is advised.
*Iodine*
The AAP recommends that breastfeeding women take a daily 150-mcg iodine supplement and use iodized table salt to taste.[24] (The salt used in processed food isn't generally iodized.) Iodine deficiency can interfere with normal brain development.
*Iron*
Although in the past iron supplements were recommended to breastfeeding women, research shows that a full-term, healthy, breastfed baby rarely needs iron supplementation before six months.[25] During the final months before birth, a baby stores up iron. In addition, the iron in breast milk is highly absorbable.
*Fluoride*
Fluoride is a mineral that protects against tooth decay. Only small amounts are present in breast milk. The natural water resources in some regions contain fluoride. Some communities add fluoride to their water supply; others don't. The American Academy of Pediatric Dentistry recommends that parents have a dentist assess their babies' teeth before giving them supplemental fluoride.[26]

## Common Q&A

**Q.** My baby lost 10 percent of her body weight in the first few days. Does that mean breastfeeding will never work for me?

**A.** In general, an initial weight loss of 10 percent isn't a reason to panic, and it doesn't mean that breastfeeding won't work in the long term or that you need to supplement with formula. But it does tells you that you need to pay close attention now and must work toward solving this problem in the short term.

It's helpful if you know how much your baby weighed at twenty-four hours. A big drop in the first twenty-four hours typically isn't cause for concern. It usually means a loss of "fluid weight" (especially if you had a lot of IV fluids during labor).

# FIRST FEEDINGS

The first feedings are a special time for you and your baby to get to know each other. Most newborns are alert and interested in feeding or nuzzling in the first hour after birth. Research shows that frequent and unrestricted feedings help prevent engorgement (painful swelling of the breasts) and promote an abundant milk supply.[27]

Here are some tips for the first feedings:

*   Breastfeed as soon as possible after the birth.
*   Make sure your caregiver and nurses know that you want to breastfeed your baby within the first hour. If you have a cesarean, the surgery may delay the first feeding. In this case, you need extra help establishing breastfeeding (see page 427).
*   Keep your baby with you, preferably skin-to-skin, and let her suckle frequently. (Skin to skin leads to increased milk production.)
*   Try to nurse in a calm, peaceful environment so you and your baby can relax and focus on feeding.
*   Don't hesitate to ask some or all visitors to leave the room, or have your partner or a nurse ask them to leave.
*   Take advantage of the breastfeeding knowledge of experienced staff or your doula. They can offer you invaluable reassurance, encouragement, and support.

# BREASTFEEDING POSITIONS

If you've never breastfed before, the techniques may seem awkward and difficult at first. With experience, time, guidance, and support, your skills should improve.

There are several breastfeeding positions, and each has special advantages. Whichever position you choose, try to get comfortable and use our basic guidelines to help your baby's get a good latch and take plenty of milk.

Bring your baby to your breast with his nose near your nipple and his ears, shoulders, and hips in a straight line. Nestle him close to your body and support his body from his neck to his hips. When you stabilize his body, he can easily move his head and help with the latch. You can use a pillow to support your arm while feeding.

## Cradle Hold

Cradle your baby's head in the crook of one arm and have her facing your breast. Use your forearm to support her body and your hand to support her buttocks.

These are the advantages of this hold:

*   It's usually the easiest and most comfortable position for you once your baby is nursing well.
*   Many mothers use it after learning to breastfeed, because it's convenient for a bigger baby.

## Cross-Cradle or Alternate Cradle Hold

Hold your baby with the arm opposite of the breast from which you're feeding, with his tummy against your chest. Support his head with your fingers and thumb on the nape of his neck behind his ears. (Don't press on his head; he may pull away from your breast.)

These are the advantages of this hold:

- Supporting your baby's neck and shoulders with your hand instead of your forearm allows you and your baby to have more control of his head.
- It's usually the easiest position to learn how to latch him onto your breast.
- It's especially helpful for a premature baby or a baby who's having difficulty latching onto your breast.

## Football or Clutch Hold

Tuck your baby beside your body. Support her body with your arm and cradle the nape of her neck with your fingers and thumb. Bring her up toward your breast as needed so she can easily latch on—she may be lying on her back or side or be sitting up against your chest.

These are the advantages of this position:

- It's easy to see that your baby has latched on effectively.
- It may be the most comfortable if you had a cesarean, because your baby isn't pressing on your incision.
- It's helpful if you have large breasts, because your baby's chest helps support your breast.

## Lying Down

Lie on your side with your lower arm tucked around your baby. Lay your baby on his side, tucked alongside your body facing your lower breast. Use pillows for your comfort. To feed from the top breast, lean over slightly to bring your nipple toward your baby's mouth.

These are the advantages of this position:

- It's easy to rest during feedings.
- It's comfortable if you have hemorrhoids or are recovering from an episiotomy or tear.

These are the disadvantages of this position:

- It often takes practice to learn.
- It may be difficult to see if your baby has latched on well. Have someone check.

## Baby Sitting Upright

Seat your baby on your lap (or on a pillow on your lap) so she faces you and her legs straddle your leg or body. Support her back with your forearm, and support her shoulders and neck with your hand.

These are the advantages of this position:

- It's easy to see if your baby has a good latch.
- It's helpful if your baby has gastroesophageal reflux or if you have a very active let-down and a large volume of milk. Sitting upright helps your baby swallow the rapidly flowing milk.

# DOES YOUR BABY HAVE A GOOD LATCH?

Your baby's latch affects the amount of milk he receives and your comfort while breastfeeding. Getting a good latch may occur naturally or you may need to help your baby latch on well. The following sections can help you with breastfeeding challenges.

## Challenges with the Latch during the First Days

Some babies seem to know how to nurse right from birth, while others seem sleepy or uninterested or have difficulty latching on.

During the early feedings, your baby may immediately *latch* onto your breast, tugging and sucking energetically. She may grasp and pull on the nipple so firmly, the discomfort surprises you. Or she may tentatively lick and mouth your breast, struggling to get a good latch. Try not to worry if your baby doesn't nurse on the first try or if every feeding seems to take a lot of work before she latches on well. If your baby's nose was suctioned at

## Helping Your Baby Latch onto Your Breast

1. **Use a comfortable breastfeeding position.** The cross-cradle hold is used in the following example.
2. **Hold your baby close to you.**
   - Have his body touch your chest and his arms near your breast instead of tucked between the two of you. (You may need to lay your other breast over his diaper.)
   - Support his head with your fingers and thumb behind his ears—don't put your whole hand on his head. Light support allows him to move his head, which will help him latch on more easily.
   - If you lean back with your feet up on a footstool, it's easy to keep him near you.

3. **Bring your baby to your breast.** If you hold your breast with your hand, keep your fingers and thumb away from the areola. Allow your breast to remain where it naturally falls and avoid moving it.
4. **Help your baby have a good, deep latch.**
   - Have his nose and upper lip near your nipple.
   - Press on his upper back so his head tilts back slightly.
   - Place his chin on your breast and his lower lip on the outer edge of areola. This position encourages him to open his mouth and grasp the areola and nipple.
   - Wait for him to open his mouth wide (as if yawning), then bring his upper lip over the nipple.

5. **Look for signs that your baby has a deep latch on the breast.**
   - His chin indents your breast and his nose is near or barely touching your breast.
   - He has more areola in his mouth near his lower jaw, and you see more areola above his lips.
   - You hear and see him swallowing (you hear an "ugh" sound and see a pause in suckling).
   - After feeding, your nipple should be evenly rounded or the same shape as before feeding. It should not looked compressed or have a ridge in the middle or on one side.

6. **Keep your baby close during the feeding.** Press on his upper back with your palm, tuck his bottom in close to you, or lean back. Use pillows to support your arm.

To help visualize a baby latching on, visit our website, http://www.PCNGuide.com, for links to recommended videos.

birth, she may need time for the stuffiness to clear before latching onto your breast successfully. A long labor can tire babies, and some medications can make them drowsy or uncoordinated. If your baby is drowsy, try the suggestions on page 409.

You, too, may need rest and nourishment to combat the fatigue of a long, difficult labor. In addition, you may have painful uterine contractions (afterpains) when nursing (see chapter 16).

Whether your baby nurses well or not, the stimulation of her nuzzling, licking, and closeness to your body encourages milk production. With patience, perseverance, and the help of a knowledgeable lactation consultant, your baby can learn to nurse well.

If you have trouble getting a good latch when your breasts are very full, use hand expression to make the areola more graspable. Breast pressure or compression can increase the milk flow, which encourages sucking and swallowing (see pages 407 and 412.)

## *When Your Baby Latches Well*[28]

When your baby latches effectively onto your breast, she can get the milk she needs easily. Signs of a good latch are easy to spot. Just before your baby latches on, she opens her mouth as wide as a yawn, with her tongue down and forward. She then draws your nipple and much of the areola into her mouth, giving her a deep latch. Her chin indents your breast and her nose is close to your breast. Her lower lip is flanged outward and her tongue is extended over her lower gum.

Your baby begins feeding with short, rapid sucks, her jaw moving rhythmically as she suckles. After the milk has let down, she settles into a slower pattern, with bursts of sucking and short pauses. You can hear her swallow. In the first few days, she may need to suckle five to ten times before she has enough colostrum to swallow. Once the milk has come in, you can hear her swallow after one or two sucks. The more she swallows, the more milk she's gotten. A swallow may sound like a "huh" rather than a loud gulp.

## How to Find a Qualified Lactation Consultant

*Lactation consultants* are breastfeeding experts who recognize the value of breastfeeding and dedicate their work to its promotion, support, and protection. An International Board Certified Lactation Consultant (IBCLC) is someone who has successfully passed an exam administered by the International Board of Lactation Consultant Examiners (IBLCE). Look for a lactation consultant who has earned these internationally recognized credentials.

- Ask your childbirth educator or your local La Leche League group to refer you to an IBCLC.
- If you're birthing in a hospital, ask your caregiver or nurse whether the hospital has a breastfeeding service that employs lactation consultants.
- To find referrals, contact the International Lactation Consultant Association (ILCA) (http://www.ilca.org) or United States Lactation Consultant Association (http://www.uslca.org).

If you can't find an IBCLC, find a nurse trained in breastfeeding support, a doula, midwife, La Leche League Leader, childbirth educator, experienced breastfeeding mom, or another breastfeeding expert in your area to help you.

## In Their Own Words

At three months old, my daughter didn't cue for feedings as clearly as she had when she was younger. When she did feed, it was a social event. She'd suck, pull back, smile at me, pat me, suck some more and gaze at me. Feedings took a very long time until I learned to nurse her in a quiet, low-lit (or even dark) place, where she was less distracted.
—Tara

## *When Your Baby Doesn't Latch Well*

When your baby doesn't latch effectively onto your breast, he might not get enough milk and breastfeeding may become difficult. Like the signs of an effective latch, signs of an ineffective latch are easy to spot:

- Your baby's lips are pursed as though sucking on a straw.
- His cheeks appear sunken, because there's not enough breast tissue to fill his mouth.
- You hear clicking noises during a feeding.
- You don't hear him swallow.
- He slips off your breast and roots frantically.
- You may feel nipple pain that continues after the first minute of feeding or you don't feel much pulling or tugging on your nipple.

To correct an ineffective latch, see the tips on page 402. If needed, contact a lactation consultant for help. If your baby doesn't latch well in the first day or two, you can hand-express colostrum and feed it to him with a spoon or syringe. (One to two teaspoons is considered a "full meal" of colostrum.) Expressing colostrum encourages milk production. If your baby can't latch on well after a couple days, use a pump to express breast milk for your baby and maintain your milk supply while working with your baby to improve the latch.

## GETTING BREASTFEEDING OFF TO A GREAT START

If your baby nurses well soon after the birth, breastfeeding has gotten off to a great start. Watch for your baby's feeding cues (see page 393) and feed him when he's hungry, or at least once every three hours.

Let your baby nurse from the first breast for as long as he likes (ten to thirty minutes on average in the early days). When he comes off the breast on his own, offer the other breast. (He might or might not take it.) Begin the next feeding with the breast you offered second. If you can't remember, press your fingertips against your breasts and offer the one that feels most full. By alternating the breast you offer first, you make sure your baby's suckling stimulates both breasts to make milk.

If your baby remains with you after the birth, watch for his feeding cues and feed him when he wants. If your baby spends time in the hospital nursery, you must rely on the nursing staff to let you know when he's hungry. Request that the staff bring your baby to you for feeding, day or night. Ask the staff not to give your baby any bottles. When full-term, healthy babies breastfeed frequently in response to their feeding cues, they don't need supplemental bottles of formula, sugar water, or plain water. Supplemental bottles can increase problems with breastfeeding by diminishing your baby's hunger and interfering with his desire to nurse. When your baby spends less time at your breast, your milk supply might not increase enough to meet his needs.

Generally, it's wise to wait to give your baby a bottle until you have a good milk supply and your baby consistently latches onto your breast. Breastfeeding is typically well established about a month after birth.

Additionally, sucking on a bottle nipple is entirely different from suckling at a breast. A newborn who feeds from both a bottle and a breast may develop *nipple confusion* (trouble adapting to different sucking patterns and differences in flow). He may find feeding from a bottle easier and begin to refuse the breast.[29] Pacifiers can also cause problems with breastfeeding (see page 406). Wait to offer a pacifier until after breastfeeding is well established.

If your baby hasn't nursed well in the first twenty-four hours, get help from a lactation consultant right away to prevent your baby from becoming dehydrated or losing too much weight. Ask about using a breast pump to ensure that your baby is fed with your expressed milk and to stimulate your breasts to make more milk.

If your baby is nursing frequently, you can expect the amount of milk you make to increase on the second to fifth day after the birth. At that time, your body gradually stops making only colostrum and begins to make mature milk. When your milk "comes in," your breasts become heavy, full, and tender. Your nipples may appear flattened because of the swelling. See page 410 for ways to relieve breast fullness.

After a few weeks, your baby will feed every one to three hours. As she gets more milk at each feeding, she may feed less frequently, although she still may feed in clusters before or after sleeping. This frequent nursing stimulates your breasts to make more milk.

## MAKING SURE YOUR BABY IS GETTING PLENTY OF MILK

By the third or fourth day after birth, most babies lose between 5 and 8 percent of their birth weight. Once their mothers' milk is in, babies steadily gain weight. Full-term babies usually regain the weight they lost and return to their birth weight by ten to fourteen days postpartum.

After the fifth day, watch for the following signs to ensure that your baby is getting enough milk.

### Suckles frequently

Your baby feeds vigorously at least eight to twelve times in twenty-four hours.

### Swallowing

You hear your baby swallow often. Sometimes during a feeding, he swallows after every suck. Sometimes he sucks a few times before swallowing. He fully extends his jaw when swallowing.

### Softer

Your breasts feel softer after feeding.

### Satisfaction

Your baby seems satisfied after most feedings.

### Soaking

For the first week, expect the number of wet diapers to at least equal the day of your baby's life (for example, three or more wet diapers on day three). After your milk comes in, expect at least six to eight wet cloth diapers in twenty-four hours. If using disposable diapers, it's difficult to tell when they're wet. Place a tissue or small piece of paper towel in your baby's diaper where his urine will wet it.

### Stools

After your milk comes in, your baby produces at least three poopy diapers every twenty-four hours. The stools usually are yellow and seedy. For the first month or so, many babies poop after almost every feeding, up to twelve times per day. Later on, they usually poop less often.

## Signs That Your Baby Isn't Getting Enough Milk

When your baby doesn't get enough to eat, her risk of dehydration or problems with weight gain increase. If you observe any of these signs, schedule an appointment with your baby's caregiver to have your baby assessed:

- Your baby feeds fewer than eight times in twenty-four hours.
- She doesn't produce at least one poopy diaper in twenty-four hours.
- She has few wet diapers or produces urine that appears to have reddish "brick dust" in it.
- Your baby seems constantly hungry and is seldom content after feedings.
- Your baby's feedings worry or concern you.

Some signs are serious. If you notice these signs, call your baby's caregiver immediately:

- Your baby is lethargic and has no interest in nursing.
- The inside of her mouth doesn't glisten with moisture. (It's normal for a baby's lips to appear dry).
- When you gently pinch the skin on her arm, leg, or abdomen and then let go, her skin stays "tented."
- Her eyes, face, chest, and abdomen are yellow (see page 383 for more on jaundice).

## Advice from the Authors

*How others can help a breastfeeding mom*
A father, partner, or other person provides a breastfeeding mom with extra pairs of eyes, ears, and hands. Sometimes a mom has trouble seeing if the baby is latching on well. You can help check the latch by looking at it from a different view. If necessary in the first week, you can hold a baby's hand out of the way until he has latched on.

You can also help evaluate how much milk your baby consumes by watching for rhythmic jaw movements and periodic pauses and listening for swallowing noises that sound like "huh."

### Scales

Your baby should gain ½ to 1½ ounces per day. If your baby's weight doesn't return to his birth weight ten to fourteen days postpartum, there are two possible explanations:
- Your baby has trouble getting enough milk.
- You might not be producing enough milk and need to take measures to increase your milk supply. (see page 425).

To increase your milk supply, try to breastfeed more often rather than making each feeding longer. Also, try using breast pressure or compression (see page 407).

## WHEN YOUR BABY DOESN'T GET ENOUGH MILK

The following are common reasons why a baby can't get enough milk and tips to improve supply. If supply issues continue after the first few weeks, see pages 414.

### Ineffective latch

If a baby can't latch on well, she can't get enough milk. See our tips on page 402 and get help from a lactation consultant. Most latch problems can be corrected; the sooner you get help, the sooner you can fix the problem.

### Feeding on a schedule

Breastfed newborns, especially ones who gain weight slowly, need to feed more frequently than once every three hours. All newborns need to feed at night; feeding shouldn't be postponed until the morning. Feed your baby whenever she shows an interest in nursing, day or night. (See page 393 for feeding cues.) Let her nurse for as long as she wants.

### Feeding from only one breast

If you offer your baby only one breast, you risk inadequate milk production and may limit the amount of milk she gets. Always offer the second breast. For the first week, she may nurse very little from the second breast, but she may want to nurse from both breasts as she grows over the next month or so. When your baby is a month or two old, she may nurse from only one breast at most feedings if you have a good milk supply.

### Pacifiers

Giving babies pacifiers can lead to faulty sucking patterns and may shorten the overall duration of breastfeeding.[31] In the first few weeks, if you try to soothe your baby or delay a feeding by giving her a pacifier, she may develop an inability to suckle effectively at the breast, which may slow her weight gain. It may also interfere with establishing a good milk supply. For breastfeeding success, avoid using pacifiers, especially when your baby is learning to breastfeed.

### Sleepy baby

Most parents appreciate a baby who sleeps a lot, but long periods between feedings may prevent your baby from getting enough milk. For the first few weeks after the birth, try waking her every two to three hours during the day and every three to four hours at night. (See page 409 for suggestions on how to wake a sleepy baby.) If she remains sleepy or lethargic and you can't get her to nurse, call her caregiver.

*Note:* After a baby has returned to her birth weight (usually ten to fourteen days postpartum) and is growing well, she doesn't need to be awakened for feedings. If she isn't gaining weight well, her caregiver may recommend that parents continue to wake her to eat.

### Jaundice

If your baby has a yellowish tint on her face, chest, and the whites of her eyes, she may have jaundice (see page 383). Not getting enough breast milk increases the risk of jaundice. Frequent breastfeeding helps relieve jaundice, but a baby with jaundice is often sleepy and uninterested in feeding. (See page 409 for tips on waking sleepy babies.) Avoid giving your baby bottles of water. Bilirubin isn't excreted in urine, and supplementing with water may reduce the amount of breast milk she drinks.

## YOUR NUTRITION WHILE BREASTFEEDING

During pregnancy, your body prepares for lactation by storing 5 to 7 pounds of extra fat to support milk production. In the first month after the birth, you lose a large amount of the weight you gained during pregnancy, but you may maintain this extra fat for the entire time you breastfeed.

Your body also draws on your vitamin and mineral reserves to make milk. Although your body can produce plenty of healthy breast milk regardless of what you eat, eating a poor diet may deplete your nutritional stores over time. Eating poorly also affects your health and your overall well-being.

### *What to Eat*

Make sure your diet consists of a variety of healthy foods and includes additional protein (which helps produce milk) and calcium. Many women's diets don't include enough calcium, vitamin B, thiamine, folic acid, vitamin D, zinc, and magnesium.[32] This deficiency reduces a

## Enhancing Milk Flow with Breast Pressure and Compression

When your breasts are very full, pressing on your breast helps the milk flow toward your nipple and into your baby's mouth, causing a burst of suckling. Although this method is sometimes called "breast massage," you don't rub your breast in circles.

### Breast pressure

1.  When your baby takes long pauses or stops suckling, put your palm or your fingers on your chest near the outer edge of your breast.
2.  Slide your palm on your breast until you feel the firm milk glands.
3.  Press gently from the outer breast toward the nipple. If you move your hand down your breast, stop before you get close to the areola. Pressing near the areola can affect your baby's latch.
4.  When your baby begins to suckle less, move your hand to another part of your breast and repeat these steps.

This technique helps relieve breast fullness, helps empty plugged ducts, and provides more high-calorie hindmilk for your baby.[30]

### Breast compression

1.  Cup your breast with your hand, placing your thumb and one to two fingers near the outer part of your breast.
2.  Compress your breast by squeezing your finger(s) and thumb together and slightly pressing into your breast then out toward your nipple.
3.  When your baby begins to suckle less, cup your breast in another position and compress again.

This technique helps babies eat more, especially those who are gaining weight slowly, and entices sleepy babies to continue feeding.

mother's nutritional stores and poses health risks for both her and her baby.[33] Your caregiver may recommend that you take a vitamin and mineral supplement.

During pregnancy, you may have avoided certain foods that might have posed a health risk to your baby, such as soft cheeses, raw fish, and luncheon meats. Happily for you, eating these foods—and generally all foods—doesn't harm your breast milk and doesn't harm your baby when he consumes it. An old wives' tale warns that nursing women should avoid eating cabbage, broccoli, and spicy foods to prevent their babies from developing colic, but no evidence supports this theory. (See page 409 for information on food sensitivity.)

Instead, the foods you eat flavor your breast milk, which benefits your baby by introducing the flavors of foods he'll eventually eat at the family table. For example, researchers found that babies drank more breast milk when their mothers took garlic capsules.[34] Researchers also found that breastfed babies ate peas and beans more readily than did formula-fed babies,[35] likely because they recognized the flavors of these vegetables in their mothers' milk.

Contrary to myth, increasing the volume of fluids you drink doesn't increase your milk production. Having a well-hydrated body simply keeps you from feeling thirsty and maintains your overall well-being. You know you're drinking enough fluids when your urine is pale yellow.

## What about Caffeine?

If you drink caffeinated beverages or eat foods with caffeine, know that less than 1 percent of the caffeine you consume appears in your breast milk. Consuming a serving or two a day doesn't affect your baby. If, however, you limited caffeine consumption during pregnancy, you may find you're sensitive to it postpartum.

## What about Alcohol?

When you drink an alcoholic beverage, the concentration of alcohol in your blood equals the alcohol content in your breast milk. This means that the effects of the alcohol on your baby when he consumes your milk correspond to the amount of alcohol you drank. Although research hasn't shown that consuming the occasional drink is harmful, it's generally best to avoid drinking alcohol or drink only occasionally until after your baby is weaned. Researchers found that babies consumed less breast milk after their mothers drank alcohol than did babies whose mothers didn't drink before nursing.[36]

If you drink alcohol, consume it in moderation. Don't drink more than 8 ounces of wine, two beers, or 2 ounces

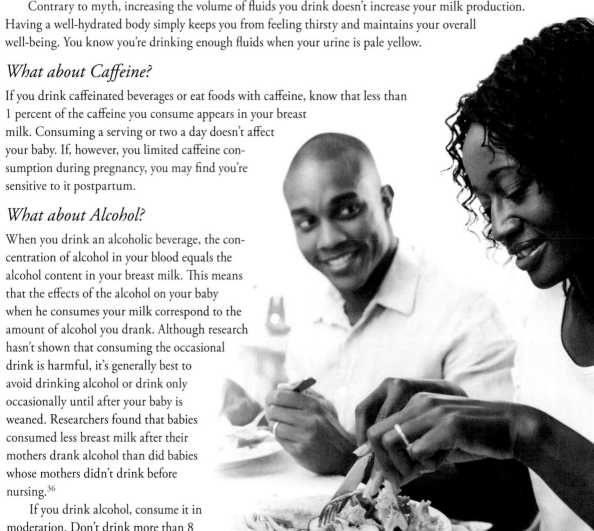

of liquor per day.[37] In addition, wait to have your drink until just after baby has nursed. That way, you allow time for the reduction of the alcohol in your bloodstream (and breast milk) before he needs to nurse again.

## What about Dieting?

By three months after the birth, some women have lost the weight gained during pregnancy. After you've reached your pre-pregnancy or desired weight, consume enough calories to maintain your weight. Compared to the number of calories you required before pregnancy, you may need only about 300 more calories per day while breastfeeding. (If you're breastfeeding multiples or a newborn and a toddler, you need more calories.)

If, however, you haven't shed the extra weight and find those extra pounds frustrating, limit your weight loss to 1 pound per week. Be sure to consume at least 1,500 calories a day and avoid liquid diets and diet medications. Severely restricting calories compromises your nutritional health and may make you produce less breast milk.[38]

## Food Sensitivity

In rare cases, a mother eats a food that adversely affects her baby. For example, the baby may become excessively fussy or develop eczema (patches of dry skin), a rash, bloody stool, or diarrhea after consuming breast milk containing protein from certain foods. A baby born into a family with a history of food allergies may react to some of the foods her mother eats. The most common food allergens include cow milk, soy, wheat, eggs, fish, shellfish, and nuts.

If you think a certain food bothers your baby, eliminate it from your diet for a week or so and see if your baby improves. (If you eliminate cow milk, be sure to get enough calcium from other foods or a supplement.) Discuss your concerns with a lactation consultant or your baby's caregiver. This person can help you identify the food causing your baby's problem and provide you with nutritional guidelines.

Some babies react negatively when their mothers eat large quantities of certain foods. For instance, if you eat an entire bowl of cherries, drink a pitcher of juice, or consume an enormous amount of chocolate, your baby may become fussy or otherwise bothered. The solution is prevention: Eat all foods in moderation.

Some foods (such as kelp, seaweed, or those containing artificial colors) and vitamin and mineral supplements can tint the color of breast milk or a baby's stools, but they don't pose problems for babies.

## How to Wake a Sleepy Baby

Once newborn babies are twenty-four hours old, they need to feed at least eight times in a 24-hour period. If your baby doesn't awaken from a light sleep to feed, try these suggestions to wake him:

- If he's swaddled, unwrap him. Remove his clothes (leaving just a diaper).
- Dim the lights so he can open his eyes. Talk to him.
- Hold him in a supported standing or sitting position.
- Massage his arms, legs, and chest.
- Rub expressed colostrum or milk onto his lips. Be patient; if he only nuzzles at first, that's a good start.
- Press on your breast to enhance milk flow and entice him to suckle more vigorously (see page 407).
- Change his diaper or burp him (see page 395).
- Change to another feeding position or switch to your other breast.

After you've tried for about fifteen minutes to wake your baby, let him sleep in your arms and try again when he starts to waken. Your baby might not get much milk if she's very drowsy during feedings, pauses for long intervals, or falls asleep even though she spends a long time at the breast.

If you continue to have trouble feeding a sleepy baby, get the help of a nurse or lactation consultant.

# Common Breastfeeding Concerns

Almost every woman has questions or challenges with breastfeeding at first. Many are common, predictable, and can be handled easily. Some are serious and require more information and assistance. See chapter 20 for more information about these challenges.

## BREAST FULLNESS AND TENDERNESS

When your milk comes in, it's normal for your breasts to become bigger. This initial fullness also comes from the retained fluid (edema) caused by your breasts' response to the increased milk supply. Feeding frequently in the first days may help prevent discomfort. Breast fullness and tenderness usually lasts for a couple days and can be relieved by using the suggestions on page 410. After several days, you may notice your breasts appear smaller, but you're still producing plenty of milk.

If a woman had an epidural or IV fluids in labor, she may notice fluid retention in her legs, arms, and breasts. This edema goes away in a week or so, but it can affect the baby's ability to get a good latch. Using "reverse pressure softening" before a feeding can help decrease swelling of nipples and areolas. See page 424 for instructions.

## SORE NIPPLES

During the first week, it's normal to have sore nipples for about a minute when your baby first latches on. As your baby learns to breastfeed, his mouth tugs, compresses, and rubs your nipple and areola. The resulting discomfort may make you stiffen in pain and breathe rapidly. As the feeding progresses, the pain lessens or ends. After the feeding, your nipples may appear slightly reddened, bruised or swollen. To reduce early tenderness, help your baby get a deep latch (see page 402). A deep latch means more milk to your baby and less nipple pain for you. See also the other tips to prevent sore nipples on page 422.

Research shows that most women's nipples are tender at the beginnings of feedings, but the tenderness usually lasts only a few weeks.[39] If the pain continues throughout the entire feeding and between feedings, seek help from a lactation consultant.

At the beginning of a feeding, some women experience a sharp, deep pain *behind* the nipple and areola that goes away when the milk begins to flow. This pain doesn't indicate a problem and usually disappears over time without treatment. Oxytocin is probably the cause; the release of this hormone shortens and widens the ducts, thereby increasing pressure as milk flows through them. If you had breast surgery, let-down may stretch scar tissue and cause pain. Slow breathing may help relieve pain (see page 243).

### Leaking

During the first few months of breastfeeding, your breasts may leak milk. As your breasts "learn" how much milk to make and when to let down, the leaking usually subsides. Leaking typically occurs when your breasts are very full, when you hear your baby cry, or when you're sexually aroused. Here are suggestions for minimizing leaking:

- When you start to feel your milk let down, discreetly press your hands or forearms firmly against your breasts to slow the milk flow.
- Compress your nipple between your thumb and index finger to stop the flow.
- To keep your clothes dry, wear washable cotton or wool nursing pads or disposable pads in your bra and change them when they become damp. Avoid using nursing pads with plastic liners; they retain moisture, which contributes to nipple soreness. Some mothers like using silicone pads that exert gentle pressure over the areolae to stop leaking. (Lilypadz is a popular brand.)

# Weaning

You may have heard that it's okay to wean your baby when she's six months old (or has teeth) because breast milk is most beneficial up to that time—but this information is incorrect. Breast milk benefits your baby for as long as you decide to breastfeed. In fact, the American Academy of Pediatrics (AAP) recommends breastfeeding babies for the first year or longer.

Making the decision to wean is complex; don't make your decision based on other's opinions. You may decide to wean because you're ready to have another child (see page 428). Or you may decide that demands at work make it difficult to continue nursing. Or you may have other reasons you're ready to stop. Sometimes, the decision to wean isn't the mother's: perhaps the child is no longer interested in nursing.

When you decide to wean your child, here are some practical tips to make the transition easier:

- Wean slowly to help gradually reduce your milk supply and decrease breast soreness. Also, if you change your mind and want to resume breastfeeding, you can rebuild your milk supply.
- First cut out the feeding you and your baby enjoy least. After your baby and you have adjusted to that change, continue to slowly cut out feedings one at a time, leaving the best-loved feeding (such as the first feeding of the day or the one that's part of the bedtime ritual) for last.
- When preparing bottles, gradually replace breast milk with formula or whole cow or goat milk, depending on your baby's age.
- Use the comfort measures discussed on page 410 to treat swollen breasts.
- If you're thinking of weaning your child in the winter, consider waiting until spring to give her the best chance of staying healthy during the cold and flu season.
- Think of the ways you cuddled with your baby before or after you breastfed her. For example, you may have read a book together, sang to her, rocked in a rocking chair, or bathed together. You can still do these special things while weaning your baby and afterward.
- Honor the time you nursed. Write your baby a letter about what nursing her meant to you.
- As you wean, your hormone levels change, bringing about the return of your menstrual cycle. Expect your emotions to fluctuate as your body adjusts.
- After weaning, some milk remains in your breasts. It gradually disappears over the following weeks to months.

## Fact or Fiction?

*You should continue to breast-feed your baby after he has begun to eat other foods.*
**Fact.** The American Academy of Pediatrics recommends that mothers exclusively breastfeed their babies for the first six months. When their babies are around six months old, parents can gradually begin introducing table foods, including foods rich in iron. However, breast milk is still the most important food in a baby's diet for the rest of the first year. (If babies are weaned before their first birthdays, they should consume an iron-fortified cow milk formula.) After the first year, mothers and babies can continue breastfeeding for as long as they desire.

## *When You Need to Wean*

Sometimes, weaning is necessary after an unexpected event, such as the death of a baby or a serious medical condition in the mother. These events bring sadness, grief, and uncertainty. (For more on infant death, see page 296.) In many cases, if a mother must wean, she can wean gradually or can help stop milk production by wearing a snug-fitting bra, applying ice packs, and taking ibuprofen. For more information, see page 327.

## Softening Your Areola by Hand Expression

To soften your nipples to make them easier for your baby to grasp, follow these steps before he latches on.

1. Place your thumb at the top edge of your areola (where it meets your skin) and your fingers on the bottom edge.

2. To keep your fingers and thumb from slipping to the end of your nipple, gently press your breast toward your chest.

3. Gently squeeze your breast for five to ten seconds. Then move your fingers and thumb to other locations at the edge of your areola. Continue squeezing and pressing your breast against your body until milk releases.

4. Stop when you see a few drops of milk or when the areola is smaller in diameter.

# Expressing and Storing Breast Milk

When your baby isn't available or able to nurse, you need to *express* your milk to relieve fullness and maintain your milk supply. Although expressing your milk by hand or by pump may seem daunting, both become easier with practice. All you need are clean hands, clean equipment, and clean containers for storing your milk.

## HAND EXPRESSION

This method is effective, inexpensive, and always available (see left). When you first learn to express by hand, you may get only drops of milk. You soon express a steady spray of milk after a little practice. Collect your milk in a measuring cup or special milk-collecting device. Using breast pressure or compression helps increase milk flow while expressing your milk. (See page 407 and watch "The Basics of Breast Massage and Hand Expression" on this website: http://bfmedneo.com/our-services/breast-massage/)

## WHEN PUMPING IS HELPFUL OR NECESSARY

In the following situations, using a pump to express your milk is more efficient and desirable than hand-expressing:

- You must leave your baby because of travel or work outside your home.
- You're trying to build or rebuild your milk supply.
- Your baby is in the neonatal intensive care unit (NICU) or special care nursery and can't breastfeed or can't yet feed frequently or vigorously.
- Your baby can't get enough milk by breastfeeding alone and must have supplemental breast milk.
- You're having a medical procedure that requires you to take a medication that's unsafe for your baby. You may need to temporarily stop breastfeeding, but you can still maintain your milk supply by pumping until breastfeeding is safe to resume. In this case, you don't save the pumped milk for your baby to drink later.

## FINDING AND USING A BREAST PUMP

A lactation consultant, La Leche League Leader, or your caregiver can help you select a pump. (Visit http://www.kellymom.com for a discussion on pump selection.) If your baby needs only an occasional bottle, hand expression or a manual pump is sufficient. If you need to pump several bottles a day or if you're building or maintaining your milk supply, you may need an electric pump. Hospital-grade electric double breast pumps are the most efficient and effective; they're available to rent. Or you can purchase a personal-use double-pump model, which is almost as effective. Check with your health insurance plan to find out which pumps are covered.

Be sure to follow the directions for use. When using a pump, always center your nipple in the pump cup (also called a flange or breast shield). When the nipple isn't centered, friction on the areola causes soreness. Use only enough suction to make milk flow well. Too much suction stretches the areola and pulls it too deeply into the pump cup, possibly injuring the tissue and causing nipple soreness. Many pumps come with different-size pump cups to best fit breasts. Some have a soft silicone insert to increase comfort. If your pump's cup seems too large or too small, check with the manufacturer to find the right size for you.

If you want to multitask, you can buy a bustier or other device to hold an electric pump's cups in place so you can use your hands for other tasks. To make your own "hands-free" device, buy an inexpensive sports bra and cut slits in the center of each bra cup that are wide enough to hold the pump cups snugly against your breasts.

The following suggestions may help increase milk flow when pumping:

- Find a private, warm environment that's free of interruptions and distractions.
- Before pumping, cup your breasts and gently but firmly stroke them from your chest toward your areola. You can also jiggle or gently shake your breasts, or stroke them lightly with your fingertips to simulate the nerves on your areola and skin to encourage let-down.
- Use pressure or compression on your breasts while pumping, especially if your let-down reflex isn't as effective as it could be.
- Develop a pumping ritual, such as having a cup of tea or listening to relaxing music.
- Imagine you're nursing your baby or look at photos of your baby and visualize your milk flowing.

## STORING BREAST MILK

You can store expressed breast milk in clean glass bottles or jars, plastic bottles, or feeding bags designed for breast milk storage. Experts debate whether glass or plastic is the safest container; see page 415 for further information. See right for guidelines on storage time.

## USING STORED BREAST MILK

Use stored breast milk in the following order:
1. Freshly expressed milk
2. Newly refrigerated milk, then all other refrigerated milk
3. Frozen milk (use oldest container first, to keep your entire supply as fresh as possible)

Breast milk does lose some (but not all) of its anti-infective and nutritional properties over time and with freezing and heating. Regardless, it's still far more nutritious than formula.

For information on how to thaw frozen milk, or warm refrigerated milk see page 416. You can safely store thawed breast milk in the refrigerator for up to twenty-four hours, but don't refreeze it.[40]

## How to Store Breast Milk

The following guidelines explain where and how long to store breast milk for healthy, full-term babies. (Mothers whose babies are ill or premature may need to follow other guidelines.) Always label the container with the collection date. For expressed milk collected under very clean conditions, the Academy of Breastfeeding Medicine recommends these guidelines for maximum storage time:[41]

- eight hours at room temperature (60°F to 85°F or 16°C to 29°C)
- eight days in a refrigerator set at 39°F (4°C)
- six to twelve months in a freezer set at 0°F (-17°C) (Place the milk at the back, where the temperature remains coldest. Also, before freezing breast milk, leave room at the top of the container for expansion.)

# Feeding Your Baby Expressed Breast Milk or Supplemental Formula

Whenever a breastfed baby can't nurse or needs extra milk, providing your expressed breast milk is best. When that's not possible, you might use donor breast milk or an appropriate formula. Talk with your baby's caregiver to find out how you can access safe donor milk or which formula is recommended.

How you feed your baby expressed breast milk or formula depends on many factors, including your baby's age and maturity, how long you're apart from her, and whether the supplementation is permanent or temporary. In complicated situations, a lactation consultant can help you figure out how best to feed your baby. Your options include:

## Tubes

For this method, you put milk into a syringe, bottle, or bag that you hold, pin on your shirt, or hang from a cord around your neck. Attach the tube that's connected to the milk container onto to your breast along your areola and nipple using paper tape. (A lactation consultant can show you how.) As your baby nurses, she draws milk from the container through the tube. Some devices have two tubes—one for each breast. A tube device may be for temporary use, but if you persistently can't produce enough milk during a feeding, you can use the devices for as long as necessary.

## Droppers, spoons, and small cups

You can use these items to feed your baby small amounts of supplemental milk. They provide a temporary solution for supplementation and help avoid an early introduction to bottles, which may cause nipple confusion.

## Bottles

If your baby needs help feeding or gaining weight, you can use bottles to provide supplemental breast milk or formula. If you're gone for a long time (such as returning to work), your baby will probably use a bottle.

If possible, wait to introduce a bottle until you're certain your baby is nursing well and gaining weight steadily (usually four weeks or so after you've begun breastfeeding). Begin introducing a bottle about two weeks before your baby will need to feed from it while you're away. The first bottle-feeding may be challenging for you or your partner, friend, or child-care provider. Some babies learn quickly; others suck only once then stop. It may take a while for your baby to learn to accept a bottle. See page 417 for more information.

# Choosing Bottles and Nipples

Bottles come in many shapes, styles, and materials. Glass bottles are stain-proof and easy to clean but are heavy and can break. Because plastic bottles are lightweight and don't break easily, they may seem the more practical choice. Some parents use a feeding-bag system, which consists of a disposable plastic bag inside a plastic container. These can be more expensive to use, and it's not as easy to mix formula in a bag as it is in a bottle.

Nipples also come in various shapes and sizes. Try buying two or three types, then select the one your baby likes and stay with it. Before feeding your baby a bottle, check that the breast milk or formula drips adequately from the nipple. If it flows in a stream, the nipple hole is too big and your baby may consume too much too fast and she may spit up. Discard the nipple. If the milk drips very slowly or not at all, your baby may tire of sucking and not consume enough (or any) milk. Remove any dried breast milk or formula that may be clogging the hole or enlarge the hole with a clean needle, then check the drip again.

As long as your water supply is safe for drinking, you don't need to sterilize bottles and nipples. You can wash bottles by hand or in the dishwasher. Clean nipples with a nipple brush and hot soapy water; rinse them with hot water and dry.

## Common Q&A

Q: Is it true that some plastic bottles can release chemicals that are bad for my baby?

A: Yes. The major concern is clear plastic bottles made of polycarbonate (which contains the chemical bisphenol A, or BPA) because of its reported harmful effects on the neurology and behavior of exposed babies and children. Because of these concerns, BPA is no longer used in new baby bottles, sippy cups, and infant formula containers in the United Stated or Canada. (However, BPA continues to be used in other food packaging. In 2014 the FDA stated that BPA exposure from these food containers is below the levels that may harm children.)

Using glass bottles for storing and serving breast milk and formula will minimize your baby's exposure. If you choose plastic, here are your options. Those at the top of the list are believed safest, while those at the bottom of the list should be avoided.

- **polypropolene bottle**, which are softer, semicloudy plastics (may be marked with the number 5 recycling symbol or the letters PP)
- **polyethylene for breast milk storage bags** (marked number 1 or number 2), although polyethylene may reduce the antibacterial properties of breast milk
- **BPA-free clear plastic bottles** (however, the bisphenol S used in manufacturing these bottles may also have some harmful effects[42])
- **phthalate-free bottle liners** (phthalates have been linked to numerous health problems)
- **bottles labeled number 3** (contains phthalates and may contain BPA—avoid them)
- **older bottles labeled number 7** (avoid them unless also labeled BPA-free)

When using plastics, heat them with warm water (not boiling)—don't heat them in the microwave. Wash with warm water (not hot) and mild soap. Heat and harsh cleaners can cause the plastic to break down more quickly.

# PREPARING A BOTTLE

To thaw frozen breast milk, or to warm refrigerated breast milk or formula, never use a microwave or a stove. Using either appliance to heat the milk can destroy many important anti-infective properties in breast milk and may heat the milk unevenly, increasing the risk of hot spots that can burn your baby. Instead, place the milk container in a bowl of warm water. As the water cools, replace it with more warm water. To check if it's warm enough, test a few drops of water on the inside of your wrist. Your baby can drink breast milk that's at room temperature or slightly warmer. As he grows, he may begin to prefer a bottle that's cool or at room temperature.

*Note:* The fat in breast milk rises to the top during storage. Before giving the bottle to your baby, swirl the warmed milk gently to mix the fat back in.

# HOW MUCH MILK SHOULD YOU OFFER IN A BOTTLE?

To find out how much milk to give your baby, ask his caregiver for advice that's specific to your baby's age, weight, and health. Here are some general guidelines:

- **At each feeding:** A newborn may take only 1 to 2 ounces of breast milk or formula at a feeding. At one to two months, a baby may take 3 to 4 ounces per feeding. At two to six months, a baby may take 4 to 6 ounces per feeding.[43]

- **For a baby who is only bottle-fed:** Over the course of a 24-hour day, most infants drink 2 to 2½ ounces per pound of their weight (150 to 200 milliliter per kilogram). For example, a 10-pound baby has 20 to 25 ounces a day. Fed eight times per day, the baby drinks *an average* 2.5 to 3.2 ounces per feeding. However, you may find that your baby drinks more than that amount at some meals and less at other meals. This variation is fine, as long as the total amount eaten is within the guidelines. As you start giving solid foods to your baby at age six months or older, you'll gradually decrease the amount of milk you offer him.

- **For a baby who is fed from the bottle and the breast:** When breastfeeding, let your baby nurse for at least ten minutes per feed or until he gives cues that he's full. Follow the guidelines on page 405. If you're giving only an occasional bottle, offer as much milk as much as your baby wants to drink. Don't be too concerned about the total amount he consumes, because he's getting most of his milk at the breast. If your baby has many bottles each day, do the math to figure out how much milk he needs to get from the bottle. For example, a 10-pound baby who each day is fed four bottles and breastfeeds four times is getting eight meals. To get 20 to 25 ounces per day, each feeding would average 2.5 to 3.2 ounces.

For signs that your baby is getting plenty of milk, and warning signs that your baby isn't getting enough, see page 405.

# Tips for Bottle-Feeding

You can make your baby's feedings consistently successful and happy by doing the following:

- Cuddle your baby during feedings—this closeness helps him feel secure and promotes bonding.
- Hold your baby so he's semireclined. This position is more comfortable for him than lying on his back and prevents him from swallowing too much air.
- To promote normal development of your baby's eye muscles and symmetrical development of his neck muscles, hold him sometimes in your right arm and sometimes in your left.
- Burp your baby about halfway through a feeding. Babies that gulp air need to burp more often. See page 395 for tips on burping and spit up.
- Trust that your baby knows how much he needs to eat. For the first few days after the birth, full-term babies feed eight to twelve times in twenty-four hours. As they grow, they consume more at each feeding and eat less often. Your baby might not want to consume the same amount at each feeding. If he doesn't finish a bottle, don't coax him to do so if he seems satisfied. When your baby rapidly and consistently finishes a bottle at each feeding, add more breast milk or formula (typically 1 ounce more) to the bottle for the next feeding.
- Never prop a bottle to feed your baby. Interacting with you and others during feedings helps him thrive emotionally and develop trust.
- You may hear advice to add something sweet to the milk to get your baby to take a bottle, or to dip a pacifier in honey to encourage him to take it. Babies don't need this additional sugar, and honey shouldn't be given to babies younger than twelve months because it can contain spores that can develop into botulism in immature digestive systems.

## When Your Breastfed Baby Refuses a Bottle

If your baby is reluctant to take a bottle, consider these suggestions:

- Let your baby learn to suck from a bottle when he's calm.
- Choose a bottle and nipple brand that seems durable and easy to clean, then stick with it until your baby becomes familiar with it.
- Introduce a bottle gradually. At first, offer ½ to 1 ounce of milk after feeding at the breast. Then start offering it at the beginning of a feeding.
- Warm the bottle and nipple with running warm water.
- Your baby may accept a bottle if you hold him as you do for breastfeeding. Or he may accept it if you sit him more upright. You may try distracting him by talking, singing, or doing something else that you don't do while breastfeeding.
- If your baby absolutely refuses the bottle, don't force him to take it. Use a dropper, cup, or spoon to feed him enough milk to take the edge off his hunger, then try again later with the bottle. Until he accepts this method of feeding, engage the help of someone experienced with bottle-feeding.
- If you want to continue breastfeeding, make sure your baby has more opportunities to breastfeed than bottle-feed.

# Formula-Feeding

When breastfeeding isn't possible or desired, or when breast milk isn't available, parents typically feed their baby formula from a bottle. The American Academy of Pediatrics (AAP) recommends using formulas that are iron-fortified and commercially prepared to feed babies younger than one year.[44] They're fortified with vitamins and minerals, so formula-fed babies don't require a vitamin or mineral supplement. Parents should avoid using evaporated-milk mixtures, cow milk, goat milk, soy milk, and other products instead of infant formula. They lack many important and necessary nutrients and are difficult to digest for babies younger than one year.

Your baby's caregiver can give you guidelines on how much to feed your baby. Generally, in a 24-hour period a baby needs 2 to 2½ ounces for every pound he weighs (see page 416).

## TYPES OF FORMULAS

Be assured that all brands of commercially prepared formula must meet the same standards to ensure they meet a baby's nutritional needs. Here are some factors to consider when deciding which formula to use:

**Iron-fortified formula.** Many formulas are fortified with iron to reduce a baby's risk of becoming anemic (having a lower number of red blood cells than normal). Also, research suggests that babies who consumed low-iron formula have lower cognitive test scores at age five than do their peers who didn't consume low-iron formula.[45] Contrary to myth, consuming iron-fortified formula doesn't increase the incidence of colic, constipation, diarrhea, fussiness, or vomiting. The best formula for a baby's overall health is one fortified with iron.

**Cow milk formula versus soy formula.** For most babies, cow milk formulas are best. Your caregiver may recommend a soy formula only if your family eats a vegan diet (no animal proteins) or if your baby has a milk allergy or galactosemia (a rare disorder in which the baby can't digest lactose.) *Note:* Up to 25 percent of babies with a milk allergy are also allergic to soy.[46]

**Gentle and sensitive formulas.** If your baby has trouble digesting formula, you may consider trying a "gentle" or "sensitive" formula. These formulas differ from standard formulas in that they're either lower in lactose or are specially made so the proteins are broken down for easier digestion (or both).

**Hypoallergenic formula.** Sometimes, formulas truly don't agree with babies. If your baby shows signs of an allergy—such as eczema, diaper rash around the anus, diarrhea, bloody stools, vomiting, or wheezing—talk with your baby's caregiver. You may be encouraged to try a hypoallergenic formula, which is more expensive than other formulas.

**Organic and non-GMO formulas.** If your family regularly chooses organic foods or non-GMO foods, you may prioritize an organic or non-GMO formula in your grocery budget to minimize your baby's exposure to pesticides and other chemicals or to genetically modified organisms (GMO). Organic formulas are widely available. Non-GMO formulas were once difficult to find, but brands are beginning to enter the marketplace.

Some parents switch brands of formula after noticing one brand seems to make their baby gassy or fussy. Switching formulas, however, does *not* decrease gas or reduce fussiness. All babies—breastfed and formula-fed—are gassy and fussy at times, and parents should stick with the brand of formula that their baby tolerates. To learn more about formula, visit https://www.healthychildren.org and http://www.consumerreports.org/cro/baby-formula/buying-guide.htm.

# Preparing Formula

Formulas are available in ready-to-feed bottles or cans, canned liquid concentrates, and powdered forms. When prepared as directed, all three forms have equal nutritive value. Powdered formula is least expensive and ready-to-feed formula is most expensive, with concentrated formula slightly less so.

When preparing formula, carefully follow the package directions. Make sure your hands and all equipment are clean. Always use the correct amount of water to mix powdered or concentrated formula. If you use too little water, you can cause diarrhea, dehydration, and other problems for your baby. If you use too much water, you dilute the formula and your baby doesn't receive enough calories and nutrients to thrive. Formula-fed babies don't need extra water until they begin eating table foods.

If your water supply is fluoridated, be aware that the American Academy of Pediatric Dentistry reports that using fluoridated water can permanently discolor teeth.[47] The Centers for Disease Control and Prevention (CDC) says that fluoridated water can be used when mixing formula, but to reduce exposure in children who are exclusively formula fed, low-fluoride bottled water should be used to mix some of the bottles.[48]

## *Key Points to Remember*

- Feeding your baby has greater significance than simply providing nourishment. Consistently responding to her feeding cues develops her sense of trust, security, and well-being. Cuddling your baby during feedings promotes emotional development and offers an opportunity for her to express affection to you.
- Under most circumstances, breastfeeding is the best way to feed babies. With more than two hundred nutrients, breast milk is easily digestible, promotes your baby's overall health, and helps prevent some illnesses and diseases. Breastfeeding also offers unique health benefits to you.
- Breastfeed your baby whenever she shows feeding cues (typically eight to twelve times a day for a newborn). Let her feed for as long as she wants on the first breast (ten to thirty minutes), then offer the second breast. In the first weeks, count the number of wet and poopy diapers and monitor her weight gain to know she's getting plenty of milk.
- Common breastfeeding problems have several effective solutions. Getting help from a qualified lactation consultant or specialist can help you overcome most breastfeeding challenges.
- In most cases when using formula, you should feed your baby an iron-fortified cow milk formula.
- When bottle-feeding your baby, feed her whenever she shows feeding cues and always hold her to provide the emotional interaction and love she needs.

# CHAPTER 20

# When Breastfeeding Becomes Challenging

Although most women are able to successfully breastfeed, certain situations or conditions can make breastfeeding more difficult. Whether a complication begins before or during pregnancy, at birth, or while breastfeeding, in most cases you can find a solution to your problem. This chapter helps explain potential challenges and provides some possible ways to overcome them. Getting help from a lactation consultant or breastfeeding specialist can help you explore your options.

# Breastfeeding Problems and Solutions

Almost every woman has questions, concerns or challenges with breastfeeding in the first months. Many problems are common and predictable, and they can be solved easily (see chapter 19). Some are complicated or serious and require more information and assistance. See page 403 to find a breastfeeding specialist who can help.

## PERSISTENT SORE NIPPLES

Sore nipples are most common during the first weeks, when your baby first latches on. If the soreness lasts throughout the entire feeding and between feedings, or if you have intense pain, you need help to solve the problem. Common causes for persistent nipple pain include poor latch, infection, and improper pumping. Each is discussed below.

### Poor Latch

If your nipples remain sore throughout the feeding (and possibly afterward) or they begin to crack and even bleed, a poor latch is likely the cause. Another sign of a poor latch is a white ridge across the middle of your nipple when your baby comes off the breast. It might also be a flat area on one side of the nipple, making your nipple look like a new tube of lipstick.

You may need the help of a lactation consultant to help your baby get a better latch. Possible causes of a poor latch are too-full or engorged breasts (see page 410) or flat or inverted nipples (see page 396). Other causes are a baby who bites instead of suckles, whose mouth is only slightly open (not wide open), or who latches onto only the nipple or has an unusual sucking style.

Premature or ill babies may latch on poorly. A neurological or anatomical condition may prevent otherwise healthy babies from latching on and sucking well. An example is a "tongue tie," in which the frenulum (a thin membrane that extends from the bottom of the tongue) is too short to let the tongue stick out from the mouth.

Having sore nipples can make you dread breastfeeding. Here are suggestions for prevention and treatment:

- Correct the latch (see page 402), which relieves most soreness instantly, even if the nipple is cracked and bleeding.
- Nurse frequently. Delaying feedings leads to fuller breasts, making it more difficult for your baby to latch on. Also, frequent feedings may be shorter and less painful.
- Start on the least sore breast, because babies feed vigorously at the beginning of a feeding.
- To soften the areola and make latching on easier, hand-express some milk before feeding (see page 412).
- If the pain affects your let-down reflex, try using breast pressure to increase milk flow, which can shorten the feeding (see page 407).
- If you're sore where your baby's bottom lip rests on your breast, she may be tucking the lip inward over her gum. Try waiting to have her latch on until her mouth is wide open, or use your finger to gently roll her lip out during the feeding.
- Keep your baby close throughout the feeding. Newborns need extra help to maintain a good latch and not slip down the nipple. Leaning back helps keep your baby close to you. Also, when learning to breastfeed, support her with your arm and hand rather than having her rest on a pillow.
- Before pulling your baby from the breast to reposition her, first slip your finger into her mouth and break the suction so your nipple comes out easily.

- If you use nursing pads, change them whenever they become wet.
- To help heal sore nipples, express some milk after the feeding and rub it on your nipples. You also may want to use a special nipple cream or a hydrogel dressing (a gel-like pad) to help increase comfort and speed healing.
- Take a pain relief medication, such as ibuprofen.
- See a lactation consultant to help with your baby's latch and suggest treatments. She may recommend using a nipple shield during feedings to protect your nipple, help with the latch, and encourage a flat nipple to stick out. (Because of potential problems when using a nipple shield, use them only with the guidance of a lactation consultant.) She may show you nursing positions that are more comfortable. If infection or allergy may be the cause, she may encourage you to see your caregiver, a physician who specializes in breastfeeding medicine, or a dermatologist. If a tight frenulum is an issue (see page 422), she may refer your baby to a physician skilled in breastfeeding medicine, who may suggest a minor procedure to clip the frenulum and free the baby's tongue.

## Infection

Persistently sore nipples (often cracked and bleeding) can be caused by an infection—typically a bacterial infection (most often *Staphylococcus aureus*) but sometimes a fungal (yeast) infection or a viral herpes infection.

If the infection is herpes, you *must* discontinue breastfeeding on that breast until the herpes sore heals.

To determine whether the infection is bacterial, physicians may first take a culture of the area, then prescribe a topical antibiotic cream or suggest using a combination cream to treat bacterial and yeast infections and reduce inflammation. Occasionally, an oral antibiotic is recommended.

Yeast infections cause soreness less often than other infections. If you have a yeast infection, your nipples may look dark pink, shiny, and irritated, or they may look normal. Small blisters may appear. Stress and taking antibiotics can increase your risk of yeast infections, and a vaginal yeast infection can lead to an infection of the nipples. Yeast infections also occur when a baby has a yeast diaper rash or has a yeast infection of the mouth (thrush).

For a yeast infection, both you and your baby need treatment. Consult with your caregiver or a lactation consultant. Taking probiotics or acidophilus pills and eating yogurt with live cultures, particularly acidophilus and bifidus, help restore the delicate balance of microorganisms in your body.

Your caregiver also may prescribe an oral medication for you and may suggest a topical over-the-counter anti-fungal cream to treat your nipples and your baby's diaper rash. Your baby's caregiver may prescribe a liquid medication, such as nystatin suspension, to apply to your baby's mouth.

## Improper Pumping

A common cause of nipple soreness is overly vigorous or incorrect pumping. To fix this problem, carefully read the information about correct pumping on page 412.

# BREAST PAIN

Many women have some breast tenderness when first breastfeeding their babies. The tenderness typically fades after a few days. However, if it lasts for several days or makes you very uncomfortable, you can take steps to ease or get rid of the pain. The causes of breast pain are discussed below.

## Breast Fullness and Engorgement

Full breasts can lead to swollen, flattened nipples and areolae, which your baby may have trouble latching onto. You can soften your nipple and areola by hand-expressing a few drops of milk (see page 412). Applying warm packs or standing in a warm shower may also start milk flow, making the areola softer and easier to latch onto. Before feeding, some women find it helpful to use "reverse pressure softening," which involves lying flat on your back and putting pressure on the areola to decrease the amount of fluid in the tissue (edema) and move it back and up into the breast. You may need help from a lactation consultant to perform this technique successfully.

Once your baby is feeding, you can press on your breasts (see page 407) to enhance milk flow. Let your baby feed for as long as she wants on the first breast. If she doesn't feed from the other breast, hand-express or use a pump to reduce fullness. If your baby can't nurse even after you've expressed milk, seek a lactation consultant for support.

If your breasts are tender after feeding, apply a cool, moist pack or an ice pack. If you use ice, first wrap it in a dishtowel or apply it over lightweight clothing. Some women find applying cool cabbage leaves to their swollen breasts reduces tenderness and swelling. Although science hasn't confirmed the effectiveness of cabbage leaves, they do no harm and may be soothing.[1] You may take ibuprofen to reduce discomfort and relieve inflammation.

The fullness and tenderness you experience when your milk comes in is sometimes called engorgement. True engorgement, however, is a more serious condition, caused by unrelieved breast fullness and may produce a fever higher than 101°F (38°C), acute breast pain, tingling and numbness in the arm and fingers,[2] and difficulty removing milk from the breasts even with a pump. True engorgement may require the help of a lactation consultant.

## Plugged Ducts

If your breast gradually develops a tender, swollen lump or a sore area (but you don't have a fever), you probably have a plugged duct. The area near the plugged duct may be reddened. Plugged ducts are usually caused by milk stasis (poor milk drainage) in one portion of a breast. These suggestions help relieve discomfort and encourage milk flow from the affected area:

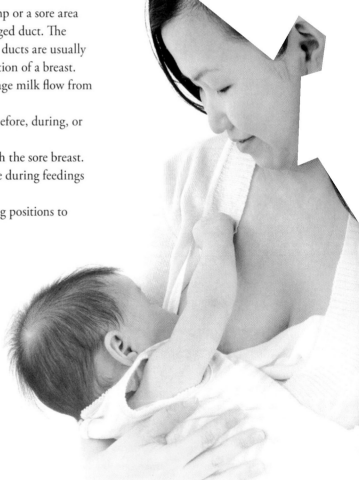

- Apply a warm, moist washcloth to the sore area before, during, or after feedings.
- Feed frequently and try starting each feeding with the sore breast.
- Press from behind the sore area toward the nipple during feedings (see page 407).
- If sore area is near the nipple, try different nursing positions to reduce pain.
- While showering, massage your breast, pressing from the plugged duct toward the nipple.
- Avoid wearing poorly fitting bras and check the fit of your baby carrier. Either item may block milk ducts.
- Pay attention when using a breast pump. Pressing the flange unevenly on your breast can reduce milk flow in one area.

It often takes a few days to clear a plugged duct, but have your caregiver evaluate any lump that doesn't disappear within a week or two.

## *Mastitis*

*Mastitis* is an infection of the breast that appears suddenly. It may follow a plugged duct or can occur any time. Besides a painful, reddened area of your breast, symptoms include fever, chills, fatigue, headache, and sometimes nausea and vomiting. If a breastfeeding woman is experiencing these symptoms, caregivers typically consider them signs of mastitis and prescribe antibiotics. Additional treatment instructions include the following:

- Continue to nurse from both breasts. The milk isn't infected and doesn't harm your baby.
- Take all the prescribed antibiotics. If you stop taking the antibiotics when you start to feel better, the infection will return.
- Drink plenty of fluids. Rest in bed until you feel better.
- During feedings, use gentle pressure behind the sore area to increase milk flow and decrease milk stasis (see page 407). This light pressure may help reduce breast pain when nursing. If not, don't do it.
- Apply a warm, wet washcloth on the painful area to help increase blood circulation to the breast.
- Take ibuprofen or acetaminophen to reduce fever, pain, and inflammation.
- Avoid wearing constricting bras and clothing so milk can flow easily.

If you don't feel better within twenty-four hours after starting an antibiotic, call your caregiver. You may need a different antibiotic.

# INADEQUATE MILK SUPPLY

The reasons for low milk supply are numerous. The most common causes come from infrequent feedings and ineffective milk removal. The following suggestions can help increase your milk supply:

- Feed frequently, at least eight to twelve times in twenty-four hours. Increased frequency leads to increased milk supply.
- Never limit feedings. Let your baby feed for as long as he likes. (Usually ten to thirty minutes at each breast.)
- Make sure that your baby latches well onto your breast and that you can hear him swallow as he suckles. If you don't, detach him and have him latch on again. If your baby can't get a good latch after trying all the suggestions on page 402, seek help.
- Rent a hospital-grade electric double-breast pump or purchase a double-breast electric pump. Pump after each feeding for ten to fifteen minutes. (More milk out means more milk made.)
- If you need to supplement your baby's feedings, use a syringe or feeding device to feed your expressed breast milk (or prescribed formula) to him through a tube attached to your breast (see page 414). That way, your baby receives all his milk from your breast and stimulates it to make more milk.
- To reduce your stress and increase breast stimulation, have a "babymoon." Spend a full twenty-four hours in bed with your baby. Pick a time when you can have a postpartum doula (see page 23), family, or friends help with meals, household chores, and other children so you don't have to leave the bed except to use the bathroom. Spend the day nursing as often as possible, snuggling skin-to-skin with your baby, eating and drinking well, sleeping, nurturing yourself, and letting others nurture you.
- Get help from a lactation consultant. She can help determine why you aren't making enough milk and may have suggestions for treating the problem. She can evaluate your breasts and know if you have issues with insufficient glandular tissue or challenges because of the anatomy of your nipples. She can also evaluate your baby's suck and examine his mouth and tongue.

- Low milk supply may result from medical issues such as a retained placenta, being anemic, or having a hormonal imbalance. These issues may require help from a medical professional.
- Some drugs may be suggested or prescribed. Here are some examples:
  - An herbal medication (such as fenugreek or blessed thistle) may increase your milk supply. Your lactation consultant or caregiver can tell you how much to take and let you know when you shouldn't take an herbal medication (for example, if you're diabetic).
  - A prescribed medication, such as Reglan or Domperidone, may be helpful. Domperidone isn't available in US pharmacies, but a lactation consultant can help you obtain it when appropriate. It has fewer side effects than Reglan, and the American Academy of Pediatrics (AAP) has approved it for nursing mothers.[3] Because of the potential risks of Reglan (for example, postpartum depression), try using other measures before taking it.

For further information, read *The Breastfeeding Mother's Guide to Making More Milk* by Diana West and Lisa Marasco (2008) to help you find the cause for your low milk supply and learn the most effective ways to make more milk.

## *When Your Milk Supply Dwindles*

You've had an adequate milk supply and your baby has gained weight well, but lately your milk supply has decreased. What's the problem? Consider these possibilities:

- You've begun to take birth control pills containing estrogen.
- You've begun using a prescribed estrogen cream to treat vaginal dryness.
- You're taking a substance that can inhibit milk production, such as a prescribed medication, over-the-counter drugs (for example, decongestants), herbs, cigarette smoke, or alcohol.
- You've recently returned to work or other activity, which has made you nurse less frequently.
- You're offering your baby more supplemental bottles and not breastfeeding as often.
- You're pregnant.

If you can determine the reason for your dwindling milk supply, take the steps on page 425 to increase it. If you don't produce more milk, seek a lactation consultant for help.

## *When You Have a Problem with Let-Down*

Extreme stress, inadequate nipple stimulation, and excessive amounts of alcohol, caffeine, and tobacco may delay or inhibit the let-down reflex.[4] Try to reduce your stress, let your baby touch your nipples and breasts as she latches on, and eliminate or limit alcohol, caffeine, and tobacco. To help your milk flow well even without let-down, use breast pressure or compression while feeding (see page 407). If the let-down reflex continues to give you trouble, contact a lactation consultant for help.

# Situations That May Make Breastfeeding Challenging

Sometimes circumstances require more support and persistence than usual to establish or continue breastfeeding.

## CESAREAN BIRTH OR DIFFICULT LABOR AND BIRTH

After a cesarean or a difficult birth, you may be exhausted and require more medical and nursing care. Repairing your incision, episiotomy, or lacerations or resolving any medical emergency (such as hemorrhaging) may delay your first breastfeeding, which in turn may delay when your milk comes in.[5] If you had a cesarean without labor, the smaller and less frequent releases of oxytocin and minimal rise in prolactin levels may also delay your milk.[6]

Despite the challenges, studies show that women who had cesareans or difficult labors and births—and who have a solid commitment to breastfeeding—tend to breastfeed for as long as women who had uncomplicated vaginal births.[7]

To help establish breastfeeding, ask to see, hold, and nurse your baby as soon as possible. Breastfeeding before the anesthetic wears off helps reduce any pain you may feel. Nurse your baby frequently while lying on your side and take advantage of any help offered.

When you're back home, concentrate on rest, comfort, and feeding your baby. Arrange for help with household chores. You may find it most comfortable to breastfeed leaning back, sitting upright with your back supported and a pillow on your lap, or lying down when someone can help you position your baby.

Continue to take your pain relief medication, which appears in breast milk in only trace amounts. Unrelieved pain can make breastfeeding more difficult.[8]

Sometimes a baby is born with a sore neck or crooked jaw (torticollis), which makes it difficult for him to breastfeed comfortably. This problem is similar to someone with a whiplash injury, and it usually goes away in a few weeks. A lactation consultant can help you find nursing positions that are most comfortable for your baby. Use them until he feels better. A physical therapist can help treat your baby's sore neck.

## PREMATURE, ILL, OR HOSPITALIZED BABIES

If your baby is premature, ill, or hospitalized, you may feel sad and worried about her well-being. Breastfeeding lets you care for your baby in an important way by giving her the closeness and comfort she needs, and your breast milk helps bolster her immune system and protect against infections.

When compared to mothers of full-term babies, mothers of premature babies produce milk that's higher in protein, nitrogen, sodium, calcium, fat, and calories. Because hospitalized premature babies are at risk for infection, breast milk's protective components are especially important. Breastfed premature babies have lower rates of infection and serious bowel problems than do formula-fed premature babies.[9] Also, breastfed premature babies have higher IQ scores at age eight.[10]

Breastfeeding is more difficult for a premature baby or one with a congenital condition, such as Down syndrome or a cleft lip. A lactation consultant can show parents special techniques for feeding a baby with physical challenges.

If your baby can't nurse or can't yet suckle well, express your colostrum or milk with a pump. As soon as your baby can take nourishment by mouth, feed her the expressed colostrum and milk by tube or dropper until she can nurse. Spend time in the hospital nursery with your baby to expose yourself to some of the organisms that can cause infection in her. Your mature immune system can make antibodies to protect you from these organisms. All your antibodies go in your breast milk and protect your baby from infection when she consumes it. Your ability to make antibodies increases when you hold your baby skin-to-skin. (See page 295 for information on kangaroo care.) Also, holding you baby next to your skin helps you produce more milk.

To establish and maintain your milk supply and to overcome obstacles you may encounter, get the continuing support of your partner, the nursing staff, or a lactation consultant. Other parents of premature or hospitalized infants can help immensely by giving advice on breastfeeding and other practical matters.

## BREASTFEEDING MULTIPLES

Breastfeeding multiples is more complex than breastfeeding one baby, especially if the babies were born prematurely. However, nursing twins or triplets is possible, even exclusively.

As soon as you discover you're pregnant with multiples, begin seeking the help you'll need after the babies are born. Contact a lactation consultant to learn about the special challenges of feeding multiples and about useful equipment that makes feeding easier (such as breastfeeding pillows). Arrange for support in the early days and weeks after the birth. Postpartum doulas are especially helpful to mothers of multiples (see page 23) as are parent support groups.

In the beginning, it may be easier to feed one baby at a time. As you become comfortable with breastfeeding, nursing two babies at once (if they're willing) saves you time.

Make sure to eat well and eat enough; your caloric needs are greater than those of mothers feeding one baby (see page 407).

## NURSING WHILE PREGNANT

Although your fertility is reduced with exclusive breastfeeding (see page 391), pregnancy is possible. If you become pregnant, you need to decide whether to continue breastfeeding or to wean your child. Breastfeeding doesn't harm a pregnancy; at birth, babies whose mothers nursed through pregnancy are of similar size to babies whose mothers weaned before becoming pregnant.[11]

Early pregnancy symptoms, especially sore nipples and fatigue, may affect breastfeeding. In addition, the hormones produced during pregnancy decrease the volume of your milk and cause its flavor to change. As a result, your child may become less interested in nursing. But generally, if you're healthy and well nourished, you may have no difficulty nursing through your pregnancy.

If you choose to wean, see page 411.

## TANDEM NURSING

When a mother breastfeeds a newborn and older child at the same time, it's called *tandem nursing*. Sometimes, the older child's desire to nurse is temporary as she adjusts to the new baby; sometimes, she just wants to nurse occasionally. In these situations, tandem nursing provides an opportunity for the mother, older child, and baby to bond.

When you tandem nurse, feed your newborn first to satisfy his needs for colostrum and breast milk. Encourage your older child to wait until the baby has finished feeding. Once your mature milk is in and you're breastfeeding your newborn without problems, you can nurse both children at the same time.

Tandem nursing is challenging when your older child nurses frequently and can't wait to feed. Get support from La Leche League, a lactation consultant, or parent educator to help and reassure you.

# Breastfeeding When You're Ill or Hospitalized

Depending on your condition and the treatments you're receiving while hospitalized, you may have several options. Speak with the hospital's lactation consultant for guidance. If your baby can stay with you, you can breastfeed her or pump your milk and cuddle her. Many hospitals let your partner stay in your room and care for your baby. If separated from your baby, you may be able to pump your milk so your baby can have it at home.

# Taking Medications and Drugs during Lactation

With few exceptions, any medication or drug you take is present to some degree in your breast milk. Some medications do affect your baby, but most don't. For example, pain relief medications used soon after birth are generally safe, and it's important to take them for your comfort. Likewise, stool softeners and hemorrhoid medications don't significantly affect breast milk.

Before taking any prescription or over-the-counter medications or any herbal remedies, consult with your and your baby's caregivers or a lactation consultant about the safety of taking the medication or drug while breastfeeding. Avoid taking street drugs (cocaine, heroin, methamphetamines, and so on), because the effects of these drugs pose serious health risks for you and your baby.

Most vaccinations—including influenza and MMR (measles, mumps, and rubella)[12]— are safe for breastfeeding mothers, except the smallpox vaccination. This vaccine causes a sore to develop at the vaccination site. If a baby is exposed to it, sores may develop on his skin.

If you take oral contraceptives, avoid those containing estrogen, which can decrease your milk supply. Progestin-only contraceptives, including the mini-pill and Depo-Provera, don't interfere with milk production.

Smoking affects babies in two ways: by ingesting breast milk containing nicotine and other chemicals in tobacco and by breathing in smoke. Even though smoking can create problems for a baby (such as increased fussiness[13]), a mother who smokes should breastfeed her baby. Breast milk produced by a smoker better protects a baby's health than formula does. Formula-fed babies of smoking mothers are seven times more likely to develop respiratory illnesses than are breastfed babies of smokers.[14]

If you smoke, try to quit or at least cut down the number of cigarettes you smoke each day. When you do smoke, avoid doing so around your baby. Secondhand smoke increases a baby's risk of sudden infant death syndrome (SIDS) and incidences of respiratory infections and ear infections.

## Questions about Medications and Breastfeeding

Before taking any medication or herbal remedy, ask your caregiver or lactation consultant the following questions:

- Does this medication go into my breast milk? Will it affect my baby?
- Do I absolutely need this medication now? Can I delay taking it until my baby is more mature and can better handle its effects?
- Is there a safer alternative?
- Can I take the medication topically (rubbed on the skin) instead of orally? (Usually, lower levels of topical medications pass into your bloodstream and breast milk.)
- Can we schedule the timing of the medication or the feedings so the smallest amount of the drug is in my breast milk when feeding?
- When I take medications that are unsafe for breastfeeding, should I temporarily stop nursing? (If the answer is yes, you can pump and discard your milk until the treatment is complete and the medication is out of your system.)
- What symptoms and possible side effects from medications should I watch for in my baby?
- Do you have access to the most accurate information about medication use during breastfeeding? (For example, *Medications and Mothers' Milk* by Thomas W. Hale is a regularly revised book on the subject that's well respected in the medical community.)

# Working Outside the Home

When you go back to work, breastfeeding your baby is more challenging, but it's easier with good planning and support. The extra effort to nurse your baby during the workday, or to express and store your milk, pays off in the following ways by

- maintaining your milk supply;
- providing your baby with nourishment that can protect him from acquiring infections while in child care;
- preserving the closeness with your baby that comes with breastfeeding; and
- helping you emotionally, because you can give your baby something that no one else can.

In general, a lengthy maternity leave and a flexible job make it easier to combine breastfeeding and work. Breastfeeding while working is less difficult when a maternity leave lasts at least until the baby nurses less frequently and on a more predictable schedule (for example, when he starts eating table foods).

Most industrialized countries provide mothers with maternity leaves that last a year or more. In the United States, however, maternity leaves are often very short (usually no longer than twelve weeks). Before returning to work, research your workplace's policy and attitudes toward breastfeeding as well as your legal rights.

When planning a return to the workplace, explore options for combining work and breastfeeding. For example, consider switching to part-time employment or telecommuting part- or full-time. Either option will make you available to nurse your baby regularly.

If your workplace is close to where your baby is during the workday, you may choose to arrange to work longer hours so you can take one to two long feeding breaks during the day. Either your baby can come to you (if your workplace supports that option) or you can go to your baby. If your baby is in child care, choose one that supports breastfeeding and won't mind if you stop by to nurse your baby.

If feeding your baby during the workday isn't an option, speak with your employer to arrange for time and privacy to pump at work. Mother-friendly workplaces often provide a room other than a restroom for working mothers to pump. Follow the guidelines on page 413 to store your milk. To maintain your milk supply, plan to pump as many times as your baby feeds in the hours that you're gone.

Mothers who can't pump at work can still breastfeed by feeding frequently when at home. Sometimes these babies go on a "reverse feeding" schedule; that is, they feed infrequently during the day and nurse more in the evenings and at night.

Some working mothers decide to breastfeed while at home and supplement with formula while away. As long as you continue to nurse frequently when you're with your baby, you should produce enough milk for those feedings. If your milk supply begins to dwindle, increase the number of feedings to stimulate your milk production.

For more information, visit http://www.withinreachwa.org/what-we-do/healthy-communities/breastfeeding. You can also contact La Leche League or check if a local hospital, clinic, or health department offers a class on breastfeeding and returning to work. In addition, talk with women who have returned to work and breastfed successfully.

# Relactation

If breastfeeding has been interrupted long enough to stop your milk production, it's possible to restart it—but it requires persistence, commitment, and a baby interested in nursing.

Frequent, around-the-clock nursing is the most effective method to reestablish lactation. Using a tube-feeding device at the breast encourages your baby to suckle at an empty or near-empty breast while receiving supplemental formula (see page 414). The suckling stimulates milk production while the device provides your baby with nutrition. Using an electric breast pump after a feeding may also increase your milk supply, as may taking herbal medications and prescribed medications (see page 425). Contact a lactation consultant for support and advice.

Mothers of adopted babies can use these same methods to try to produce milk, even if they've never been pregnant or nursed a baby. Although these mothers usually don't produce a full supply, they may produce some milk. Feeding a baby even a small amount of breast milk is beneficial and rewarding. If a mother can't produce milk to feed her adopted baby, she can still experience breastfeeding to a large degree by using a tube-feeding device to feed her formula.

# Sometimes, It's Okay to Quit

What if a mother has tried everything and breastfeeding just isn't working? She may have one or more reasons for wanting or needing to quit. For example, breastfeeding challenges may have begun to interfere with her relationship with her baby. Or she may have discovered that trying to breastfeed worsens her postpartum depression. The decision to quit breastfeeding is difficult for most mothers. They often feel sad, angry, guilty, inadequate, or rejected by the baby. Some mothers also feel relief.

If you decide not to breastfeed, try to have a plan that helps you cope with your decision. It may be helpful to share your feelings with your caregiver or a breastfeeding specialist. It's also good to learn how other mothers coped with their decision to quit. After you've made the decision, try to remember the good times you shared with your baby, congratulate yourself for your hard work, and think about the benefits that breastfeeding gave her. Then move on, giving her all your love when feeding and caring for her. You'll show her that you're a wonderful mother.

## *Key Points to Remember*

- At first, breastfeeding is challenging for many mothers. But when problems persist or become serious, your desire to breastfeed helps you persevere and work toward finding alternatives, answers, and solutions.
- Many breastfeeding challenges have several effective remedies. Lactation consultants, physicians who specialize in breastfeeding medicine, and your caregiver can help you solve most problems.

# CHAPTER 21

# When You're Pregnant Again

When you find out that you're expecting another child, you may feel just as you did after confirming your first pregnancy, or you may have a completely different reaction. You may be happy with the news or surprised by it. You may feel confident that you can handle pregnancy and birth again, or you may wonder how this pregnancy and birth will differ from your previous experience. You may have many questions and concerns about caring for another child. You may be unsure how your older child will adjust to a baby brother or sister. This chapter describes what you can expect emotionally and physically from another pregnancy, and it offers suggestions for preparing your child for your growing family.

# What to Expect with This Pregnancy and Birth

After you've been pregnant once, you may think that you'll know exactly what to expect when you're pregnant again. But every pregnancy is unique; a second pregnancy won't be exactly like your first.

Subsequent pregnancies, however, do share some predictable characteristics that make them different from a first pregnancy. Physical changes may occur sooner, but you might or might not notice them. For example, you may feel the baby's movements about a month earlier, because you recognize the sensation sooner. Or you may miss the early flutters because you're not as preoccupied with this pregnancy. Your abdominal muscles relax more easily, so your belly enlarges sooner and your pregnancy becomes noticeable earlier. Your pelvic ligaments may soften sooner, and you may feel that you're carrying the baby lower. Braxton-Hicks contractions may be more noticeable and numerous, especially toward the end of pregnancy, which can make it difficult to know when they indicate the start of labor.

On average, subsequent pregnancies are a few days shorter than a first pregnancy. Labor is typically faster, and pushing is much faster.[1] Most women report that the first stage of labor is less painful than they experienced the first time (possibly because they're less anxious), but that second-stage pushing is as painful or more so (possibly because it's faster). Despite these general observations, it's impossible to predict how labor will go in subsequent pregnancies. Each labor may be virtually identical to a previous one, or it may be completely different.

If your previous birth was a positive experience, you'll of course hope that this birth will be, too. But if your previous birth was difficult or disappointing, you naturally may worry that problems will arise again. It's common to feel anxious about labor, regardless of how many times you've given birth. Talking about your concerns with your partner, caregiver, or childbirth educator can raise your confidence and help make this birth a positive experience. If you have a specific concern, work with your partner and caregiver to create a birth plan that addresses it. For example, if a problem arose during your first birth or an intervention was needed, a birth plan can help reduce the chance of reoccurrence, and it can give you a clear plan for how you'll manage if the problem does happen again.

Even if you had excellent childbirth classes for your first birth, it may be helpful to take another series. These "refresher" classes will not only review coping techniques for labor, but they'll also prepare you for how this labor may differ from your first. In addition, classes provide updated information about maternity care, offer ideas for preparing your older child for the birth and managing your growing household, provide opportunities to talk to other parents, and give you time to bond to your new baby before the birth.

If you choose not to attend classes, refresh your memory by reading chapters 9 through 14. If a previous birth ended in a cesarean section, see pages 315–319 to learn about having another baby after a cesarean.

# Your Emotional Reactions to Having Another Baby

Compared to your first pregnancy, you may find that this pregnancy isn't as emotionally exhilarating. Pregnancy discomforts may seem more annoying, or you may be too busy to notice them. You may think less about being pregnant, partly because your older child requires your attention. Instead of thinking about your developing baby, you may think ahead to her as a newborn, because you already have a clear picture of yourself as a new parent. Your partner may be less attentive to you, possibly because of greater confidence in your well-being this time around.

Like many parents expecting a second child, you may worry that you won't have enough love for your new baby. Or you may wonder if your love for your older child will lessen with the new arrival. It's helpful to know that you can never run out of love. Think of all the people you care for. Your love expanded to include each of them, and it will continue to do so to include all your children.

You also may worry that there isn't enough time in the day to care for another child. It's true that your growing family will keep you busy, but you'll be surprised to discover that caring for a baby while parenting an older child isn't as hard as you may have imagined. With your first child, it took a while to learn about baby care and time management. With your second child, these skills will come quickly, allowing you to adapt to parenting two children more easily.

## Two Views on Being Pregnant Again

With my first pregnancy, we took all the classes, read all the books, and prepared the nursery—everything! With this pregnancy, I've barely had any time to think about it at all. I worry that this baby is getting shortchanged.
—*Mary*

I'd heard that it's easier to care for a new baby and a toddler than it is to take care of a toddler while pregnant. I agree. I'm not so tired and sore now that the baby is here, and taking care of a newborn isn't nearly as stressful as I remembered.
—*Heidi*

# Including Your Child in Your Pregnancy

When you're pregnant again, it's best to prepare your child for the pregnancy, birth, and new baby in a realistic and age-appropriate manner. The following sections offer ways to get your child ready for your family's new addition. Use the suggestions that best match your personal preferences and your child's maturity level.

One main question you may have is, when's the best time to tell my child that I'm pregnant? Some parents choose to announce a pregnancy after the first trimester, when the likelihood of miscarriage is reduced. They also delay the announcement to shorten the wait for a young child who doesn't understand the length of time until the birth. Other parents choose to announce the pregnancy earlier in the first trimester, especially if there's frequent vomiting, in order to reassure the child that his mother isn't ill. If you choose to delay announcing the news to your child, be careful not to wait *too* long, as he may hear about the pregnancy from someone else.

Another question you may have is, what's the best way to tell my child about the pregnancy? Once you decide to tell your child that you're pregnant, first talk to him about families, babies, and big brothers and sisters. When you see a family with two children, point them out to your child. Discuss families he knows who have a new baby. For example, you may say, "Did you see Cole's new sister, Maya, when his mommy picked him up at preschool?" or "Pretty soon, Aunt Heidi will have a new baby, and Amelia will be a big sister." Comments like these will help your child realize that it's normal for families to have more than one child.

To help make the wait for the birth more understandable to your child, try linking your due date to a special event or season. For example, you may say, "The baby will arrive sometime when there's snow on the ground." Also consider making a calendar so you can count down the days together.

Use the time until the birth to include your child in the pregnancy by helping him develop positive feelings and realistic expectations about the baby. Here are some suggestions:

- Talk to your child about pregnancy and birth. Depending on his age, find out what he already knows, correct any misconceptions, fill in gaps in his understanding, and answer his questions. Use appropriate terms, such as by saying that the baby is in your uterus, not in your stomach. At the same time, avoid overwhelming your child with too much information.
- Attend a sibling preparation class, if available in your community. This class may discuss the birth process or include a demonstration of a birth using a doll, which can help your child understand the process.

- Read together children's books about pregnancy and birth, about families having another baby, and about becoming a big brother or sister (see right and page 441).
- Show your child where you'll give birth. Let him know where he'll be when you're in labor. Talk about the possibility of his visiting you there after the baby is born.
- Let your child feel the baby move. Point out when the baby has the hiccups. Talk about how the baby can suck his thumb, wiggle, kick, and hear voices. Encourage your child to rest his cheek on your belly and talk or sing to the baby. Bring your child to a prenatal visit to hear the baby's heartbeat.
- Show your child photos or videos of him as a baby—especially ones showing you caring for him as a newborn. Help him make a picture book about families with two or more children.
- Talk about the care a newborn needs. Have your child interact with a friend's baby to see how small a baby is and what a baby can and can't do.
- If the baby's arrival will change where your child sleeps, move him to his new room or make new sleeping arrangements months before the birth to prevent your child from feeling suddenly displaced. Also, because accidents can happen with your child when you're busy with the baby, safety-proof your home if you haven't already done so.
- Help your child learn independence skills, such as how to get himself a snack, so he can take care of some of his own needs when you're busy with the baby.

## IF YOUR CHILD IS YOUNGER THAN TWO

If your child is younger than two, she can't easily tell you how she's feeling—but she probably understands more than you think. Use simple terms to talk about babies and to explain to her about becoming a big sister. You also may try the suggestions on page 436 and above, or simplify them.

A younger child's adjustment to a new baby usually occurs more rapidly than an older child's adjustment. In fact, a younger child may have trouble remembering her life without the baby. However, when the baby is older and begins playing with her sibling's toys, you may notice a period of adjustment, especially if your older child is still younger than three and has trouble sharing toys.

Although caring for multiple young children can be challenging and exhausting, the upside is that the overall duration of the babyhood phase will be shorter for your family than for families with siblings who are many years apart in age.

## Books for Children about Pregnancy and Birth

- *Waiting for Baby* by Rachel Fuller (2009). For ages 1 to 4. This wordless board book tells of a sibling's trip with mom to the doctor, helping prepare for the baby, and meeting the baby at the hospital.
- *Hello Baby* by Lizzy Rockwell (2000). For ages 3 to 7. This book touches on all aspects of the baby-to-come, from prenatal development and doctor appointments to meeting baby at the hospital.
- *Baby, Come Out!* by Fran Manushkin (2014). For ages 3 to 6. A silly book about a baby who wants to stay in utero and the family's humorous attempts to get her out.
- *Hello Baby* by Jenni Overend (2008). For ages 3 to 6. A beautifully illustrated story of a home birth. Originally released in 1999 with the title *Welcome with Love*.
- *We're Having a Homebirth!!* by Kelly Mochel (2012). For ages 3 to 6. A small paperback book with simple illustrations and brief details about home birth.
- *How You Were Born* by Joanna Cole (1994). For ages 4 to 8. Filled with vivid full-color photos, this book helps siblings understand a baby's prenatal development, birth, and early days.
- *There's a Baby* (DVD) by Penny Simkin (2013). For ages 3 to 8. A children's film about a baby coming to Maia's family.

# Including Your Child at the Birth

Many parents feel that a birth is a family event. They believe that including their older child at the birth will help him bond to his new sibling and encourage positive, healthy attitudes about birth.

Other parents feel that birth is a process that's too complicated or too disturbing for their child to witness. They worry how their child would react to seeing his mother's discomfort in labor or the blood from the birth. They wonder about the logistics of his care during the event. What if he became bored? What if he needed a nap? What if he began to disturb the staff? Who would care for him?

Some hospitals allow children to attend births. Most home birth providers and birth centers welcome children at births. They support the idea that having a child spend time with his mother and sibling soon after the birth will reduce separation anxiety and help him adjust to the change in the family structure.

Only you and your partner (and your child, if he's old enough to have a say) can decide whether your child *should* attend. To help you make your decision, assess your child's physical health, emotional readiness, personality, and maturity. The following sections offer suggestions for preparing your child for the event.

## IF YOU PLAN TO HAVE YOUR CHILD ATTEND THE BIRTH

If you decide to include your child at the birth, following these guidelines can help ensure a positive experience for everyone:

- Take childbirth classes or review what you learned in previous classes. To make your child feel comfortable at the birth, you'll need to be confident in your ability to cope with labor.
- Choose a birth setting that easily allows for your child's inclusion. An ideal setting is one that provides ample space and flexibility to come and go if your child becomes bored or uncomfortable. To reduce stress, set clear guidelines for your child's participation and familiarize your child with the birth setting, your caregivers, and any equipment that may be used at the birth. Make sure to bring your child's favorite toys and comfort items, such as a special blanket, to the birth.
- Arrange for someone to look after your child during the birth and help explain what's going on to her. This person should not be your partner or other labor support person—whom you're counting on to tend to *your* needs.
- Let your child know what to expect at the birth. Tell her what labor and birth are like (long and boring, yet exciting at times). Prepare her for the sights and sounds (such as the presence of blood and your groans, grunts, and cries). Suggest things that she can do during labor, such as bring you juice or a cool cloth, walk with you, play music, take photos, be quiet when asked, and so on. Prepare her for the baby's appearance and behavior immediately after the birth (see chapter 18). If you plan to breastfeed the baby, explain the process to your child. If your child is also breastfeeding, see page 428 for information on tandem nursing.
- Children's books or DVDs on birth also can help prepare your child for the event. During the birth, your child's support person can refer to them to help explain what's happening. For example, this person may say, "Your mommy's working hard to push the baby out. She's making noises just like those we heard on the DVD!"
- Avoid making promises about the birth that you might not be able to keep. For example, don't say, "You will be there to see your new brother being born." Instead, say, "We hope you can be with us when our baby is born."

- Let your child know what will happen if circumstances prevent her from attending the birth (for example, she's at school, asleep, or ill), if she changes her mind about attending, or if complications develop in your pregnancy or during labor or birth. See below for more information.
- Expect that your child will behave as usual during your labor. Don't expect the experience to change her character or suddenly make her more mature. She'll still fuss at times, need to be taken to the restroom, say no to requests, and want you to cuddle her.

# If Your Child Won't Be at the Birth

The following guidelines will help you plan for your child's care while you're away and prepare him to meet his new sibling:

- During the last weeks of your pregnancy, let your child know you'll be leaving when it's time to have the baby. Unless you're having a scheduled induction or cesarean, explain that the exact time will be a surprise—it may happen during the night or day. Tell your child whether he'll be at home or stay at another person's home while you're away. Let him know who'll care for him. Your child will be less anxious if he knows and trusts this person.
- If your child will be staying at someone's home, help him pack a bag with his favorite clothes, toys, and comfort items. If you like, have him help you pack your suitcase or the baby's bag to involve him in the birth preparations.
- When labor begins, tell your child when you'll be leaving and where you'll be going. Let him know that you may leave while he's asleep so he'll be prepared for your absence when he awakens.
- Prepare for the possibility of separation anxiety if you'll be giving birth in a hospital. A one- or two-day stay after a vaginal birth is typical, as is a three- or four-day stay following a cesarean birth. During that time, your child's ability to tolerate the separation will depend on his age, how often he's been separated from you before, how long this separation will last, how comfortable he is with the person caring for him, how comfortable he is with the place of care (if not cared for at home), and how well he understands what's happening. Separation anxiety may lead to fretting, crying, sadness, clinging, irritability, sleeping difficulties, and tantrums. Let the person who'll care for your child know about these normal reactions.
- Plan to have your child visit you and the new baby. Birth centers and most hospitals allow children to visit after the birth.
- Have realistic expectations when your child visits. Seeing you and the baby will probably reassure him and let him respond in a positive way. But it's possible that he may ignore you and the baby, cling excessively, or cry uncontrollably when it's time to leave. If he responds in this manner, you may feel that it'd have been easier to avoid the visit entirely. However, it's healthier for your child to see you briefly than to be separated from you for a longer period.
- Consider having a gift for your child to open when he visits you or when you phone him to announce the baby's arrival. Tell him the gift is from the baby.
- If your hospital stay lasts longer than expected or if your child can't visit, try to talk to him by phone or video chat. You also may want to send photos of you and the new baby.

# Helping Your Child Adjust to the New Baby

After the arrival of a new sibling, your child may have mixed feelings. Sometimes she may show fondness for the baby. Other times, she may express jealousy and resentment toward this tiny person who requires almost constant care, especially if your child had your undivided attention for several years.

If your child is angry and distressed by the baby's arrival, she may react by having tantrums, seeking attention, becoming excessively preoccupied with the baby, withdrawing, showing aggression toward you or the baby (hitting, biting, throwing things, and so on), changing her eating and sleeping patterns, or reverting to outgrown behavior, such as thumb sucking, wanting a pacifier, feeding from bottle or breast, or wetting herself. This behavior will typically be new for your child and may catch you by surprise.

How and when your child expresses this negative behavior (if she does) depends on her age. A child younger than three tends not to fully resent a new arrival's presence until the baby begins crawling and interfering in her play. A child who's at least three years old often immediately recognizes the impact a new baby has on her relationship with her parents, and she typically has little difficulty showing her displeasure. Even preteens can feel resentment toward a new sibling, although they usually feel guilty about it and may successfully hide their feelings from their parents.

What can you do if your child isn't adjusting well to her new position in your family? Because it's difficult to avoid your child's feelings of displacement, focus instead on helping her deal with the stress. Try to accept her behavior as a normal reaction to the changes in her life. The following are tips to ease your child's adjustment:

- Give your child a doll so she has a "baby" to care for, too.
- Have a party to celebrate both the birth of the baby and the "birth" of a big sister or brother. Provide a cake or treats and give a gift to your child. Encourage her to make a gift for the baby or choose one to buy. When visitors bring gifts for the baby, let your child open them for the baby, or delay opening the gifts until she's not around.
- Before the birth, have your partner provide more of your child's daily care, such as giving her a bath or reading her a bedtime story, to help establish a routine that won't be disrupted by the baby's arrival.
- Schedule time to be alone with your child and let her decide what you'll be doing together.
- Respond to your child's requests, comments, and actions. Ignoring her when you're busy may upset her at this vulnerable time. If you can't respond right away, try not to blame the baby. Don't say, "We can't go to the park now because the baby is eating." Instead, say, "We'll go to the park later, because I think it will be sunnier then."
- Correct negative behavior as you always have. Familiar rules and routines reassure young children. If you suddenly become permissive, the change may confuse your child.

- Help your child express her feelings by saying what you think she's feeling. For example, "New babies make a lot of noise" or "Sometimes it's hard to have a tiny baby around." Reading books about new siblings may help her find words to describe her emotions (see right).
- If your child wants to avoid the baby, let her. If she wants to help with baby care, include her in age-appropriate tasks. If she's older, she can hold the baby and help with diapering, dressing, or burping. Children of all ages can entertain the baby by smiling, singing, talking, and making funny faces. Teach your child how to recognize engagement cues that show the baby wants to play and disengagement cues that show the baby is overwhelmed (see page 372).
- Use the time when you're feeding the baby to read, talk, or share a snack with your child. Consider providing special toys, books, or snacks that are just for feeding times.
- Think of stimulating activities that you and your child will enjoy doing together, such as planting seeds, blowing bubbles, or making cookies. Spending time together may help remind her that she's still important to you.
- While your older child is listening, talk about her to the baby. For example, say, "Lily, today we're going to the zoo with your big sister, and she's going to show you all her favorite animals." Also, praise your child within her hearing. You may say something such as, "Grandma, did you see how Adelyn smiles when Kate talks to her? Kate is such a big help when she plays with her baby sister."

Although adjusting to a new baby may be difficult for your child, it's an opportunity for her to learn healthy ways of handling stress. With time and guidance, your child will adapt to the new family structure and eventually develop a lasting bond with her sibling.

## Books for Children about Babies and Siblings

- *My New Baby* by Annie Kubler (2000). For ages 2 to 4. This wordless board book tells the story of a family. The mother breastfeeds, and the father helps with housework and baby care.
- *I'm a New Big Brother/Sister* by Nora Gaydos (2010). For ages 2 to 4. This positive story is about what it's like to be a big brother or sister.
- *I'm a Big Brother/Sister* by Joanna Cole (2010). For ages 4 to 8. This story talks about what babies are capable of and what they need.
- *Tenemos un bebé / We Have a Baby* by Cathryn Falwell (2008). For ages 2 to 6. A simple bilingual board book about loving a new baby.
- *I Used to Be the Baby* by Robin Ballard (2002). For ages 4 to 8. This book positively portrays sibling relationships and their common problems and solutions.

# *Key Points to Remember*

- Every pregnancy and birth are unique. A second pregnancy won't be just like your first, and a second birth won't unfold exactly as your first did.
- After you've told your child that you're pregnant, use the time until the birth to help him develop realistic expectations about the baby and to include him in the preparations.
- The decision to include your child at the birth is one that's best made by you, your partner, and your child. Whether your child attends the birth or stays with someone else, preparing him for the event will help him understand and accept the new addition to your family.
- The arrival of a baby will forever change your child's life. Help him adjust by accepting any negative reactions to the change and helping him find new, positive coping skills.

# Appendixes

# Summary of Normal Labor

## Prelabor (see chapter 9)

| What physical changes and events occur | How you may feel and how you may respond | What you can do to cope | What your partner or doula can do to help you |
|---|---|---|---|
| Your cervix begins to ripen, efface, and move forward.<br><br>You may have nonprogressing contractions (change very little in length, intensity, or frequency over time).<br><br>You may have restless back pain, soft bowel movements, and menstrual-like cramps.<br><br>May last for a few hours or may last for days. | Feel tired, discouraged, and anxious. May be unable to sleep through contractions.<br><br>May overestimate labor progress, start rituals, and go to birthplace (or call home birth midwife) too early.<br><br>May focus more than necessary on the contractions. | Engage in distracting activities and projects.<br><br>Alternate distracting activities with restful ones, such as taking a bath, listening to music, lying down, having a massage, and so on.<br><br>Use labor-stimulating measures (only if you feel pressured to get into labor).<br><br>Eat if you're hungry (mostly carbohydrates).<br><br>Drink to quench your thirst. | Enhance emotional security and reduce stress by creating a soothing, safe, private, and loving atmosphere.<br><br>Ensure that you aren't left alone. Help make this time pleasant for you.<br><br>Encourage you to eat and drink.<br><br>Time your contractions (five or six at a time) every few hours or when your labor seems to have changed.<br><br>Alert your doula to be ready to come when you need her.<br><br>Review the route to the birthplace.<br><br>Pack the vehicle; be sure there's enough fuel in it. |

## First Stage of Labor: Early Labor (see page 172)

| What physical changes and events occur | How you may feel and how you may respond | What you can do to cope | What your partner or doula can do to help you |
|---|---|---|---|
| Denotes the time from the onset of labor until your cervix is dilated to about 4 to 5 cm.<br><br>Contractions are progressing, usually mild at first, then becoming longer, stronger, closer together.<br><br>Your cervix continues ripening, effacing, and begins to dilate.<br><br>You may have bloody show.<br><br>Your membranes may rupture (10 percent chance), but this usually happens later in labor. May have back pain with contractions. | Same as for prelabor, plus:<br><br>Have mixed feelings—excitement, confidence, and optimism; or anxiety and distress—often all at the same time.<br><br>As contractions intensify, you can no longer be distracted during them.<br><br>May begin to feel as if there's no going back. You're on a one-way street to the birth of your baby. Get out your Road Map (see page 444)! | Continue distracting (but not exhausting) activities, such as a taking a walk, eating a snack, cooking or other home project, and doing relaxation techniques or visualization.<br><br>Begin using planned rituals (relax, breathe, and focus through each contraction) when the intensity of contractions stops you from doing distracting activities.<br><br>Use slow breathing, releasing tension with each exhalation.<br><br>Ask your doula for help.<br><br>Contact your caregiver or birthplace as instructed, typically when your contractions have reached the 5-1-1 or 4-1-1 pattern (see page 177).<br><br>Use comfort measures to relieve back pain (see page 247.) | Continue timing your contractions periodically.<br><br>Call caregiver or birthplace when your contractions reach designated intensity, frequency, and length, or if your membranes rupture.<br><br>Focus on you during contractions as soon as you begin doing a planned ritual.<br><br>Give you constructive feedback, not false praise.<br><br>Help you release tension in a selected area of your body with each exhalation.<br><br>Remind you of positions and comfort techniques (see chapter 12). |

## First Stage of Labor: Getting into Active Labor (see page 178)

| What physical changes and events occur | How you may feel and how you may respond | What you can do to cope | What your partner or doula can do to help you |
|---|---|---|---|
| Your cervix is dilated 4 to 5 cm.<br><br>Your contractions intensify and occur every 3 to 4 minutes, lasting 1 minute or longer.<br><br>Your labor progress should begin to speed up when your cervix is 6 cm dilated. (Getting from 4 to 6 cm takes 2 hours on average for a first-time mother, but can take up to 9 hours.) | You probably head for your birthplace or call your home birth midwife.<br><br>May struggle to remain "in control" and worry that labor is too hard and long.<br><br>May become serious, withdrawn, and focused on your labor.<br><br>You may recognize that labor isn't within your control, leaving you feeling trapped.<br><br>You may weep.<br><br>You can no longer be distracted during contractions; you need your partner's or doula's undivided attention during them.<br><br>Find unnecessary conversation annoying.<br><br>Can release control and accept your labor if you can move freely, feel safe and uninhibited, and have good support.<br><br>May want pain medications. | Remember your 3 Rs.<br><br>Relax as much as you can (at least between contractions). Continue slow breathing if you find it restful.<br><br>Maintain a rhythm with your breathing and movements, letting your partner or doula help.<br><br>Try to release your need to be in control; let labor happen as you discover your spontaneous ritual to help you cope.<br><br>Remember that labor progress should speed up soon.<br><br>If you planned for an early epidural, you can probably receive it during this phase.<br><br>If you have an epidural, see chapters 11 and 13 to learn about pain medication procedures and how your partner or doula can support you. See also the "Epidural Highway" on the Road Map of Labor (see page 444). | Drive to the birthplace carefully!<br><br>Use comfort measures such as showers, massage, slow dancing, and a birth ball (see chapter 12).<br><br>Rhythmically murmur soothing, encouraging words to you.<br><br>Help you keep a rhythm in your breathing, moaning, swaying, or tapping. Guide you with visualizations, rhythmic talk, or breath-counting.<br><br>Help with your ritual (for example, stroking you, holding you, or talking to you through contractions) or simply stay by you if that's all you require.<br><br>Refrain from asking questions during contractions, and ask only simple yes-or-no questions between contractions.<br><br>Help you follow your preferences on pain medications (see page 241). |

## First Stage of Labor: Active Labor (see page 178)

| What physical changes and events occur | How you may feel and how you may respond | What you can do to cope | What your partner or doula can do to help you |
|---|---|---|---|
| Your cervix dilates from 6 to 8 cm.<br><br>Lasts on average 3 to 4 hours.<br><br>If your baby is occiput posterior or her head is tilted to one side, dilation of your cervix may pause as your baby corrects her position.<br><br>May have back pain (30 percent chance). | Become calmer than before, now that you've discovered how to get through contractions.<br><br>May enter the "birth zone" and become aware of little other than your labor.<br><br>May find it hard to cope if you're having irregular or coupling contractions, or lots of back pain. This is the "detour for back pain" on the Road Map (see page 444)—a longer, rougher road for labor. | Same as for early labor and getting into active labor, plus:<br><br>Take a bath, use a birth ball or rocking chair, take frequent sips of water, and rest between contractions.<br><br>For tips on coping with back pain or for a prolonged labor, see page 247. | Same as for getting into active labor, plus:<br><br>Stay by your side.<br><br>Offer you liquids.<br><br>Remind you to empty your bladder.<br><br>For back pain, try using positions that encourage the baby to rotate, massage techniques such as counterpressure and double-hip squeeze, and other techniques found on pages 247–249. |

## First Stage of Labor: Transition (see page 184)

| What physical changes and events occur | How you may feel and how you may respond | What you can do to cope | What your partner or doula can do to help you |
|---|---|---|---|
| Your cervix dilates from 8 to 10 cm.<br><br>Your baby begins to descend toward your vaginal opening.<br><br>Contractions are long and very close together.<br><br>Pain and intensity of labor is probably at its maximum.<br><br>Likely lasts less than 2 hours if this is your first birth, or less than 1 hour if you've given birth before.<br><br>As your cervix completes dilation, you may have a "lip" that remains. | May feel scared or lost in labor; may be angry or frustrated.<br><br>May want more help from others.<br><br>May feel that you've reached your limit.<br><br>May lose your rhythm and ritual.<br><br>May cry out, tense, weep, or protest.<br><br>May feel hot, then cold; may tremble.<br><br>May feel nauseated; may vomit.<br><br>May still experience some of these symptoms if you have an epidural, even though you don't feel the pain. | Keep a rhythm.<br><br>Follow your partner's or doula's lead with Take Charge Routine.<br><br>Hang in there! Remember that you're almost ready to push and will feel better soon. If you can keep a rhythm and follow a ritual now, you're better able to continue laboring without medications (if that's your wish and if your labor progress remains normal).<br><br>If you want an epidural, you can get it at this time as long as your labor isn't moving too fast (see chapter 13). | Maintain a confident, calm, optimistic manner; keep eye contact with you.<br><br>Use the Take Charge Routine (see page 186) if you're panicky or if your eyes are clenched shut and your expression is anguished, or if you can't maintain a rhythm.<br><br>Remind you that transition means you're almost ready to push out your baby (This encouragement may be especially helpful if your prelabor preference was to birth without pain medications, but you're now asking for them).<br><br>Hold you tightly (but not rub your body), if that's what you want.<br><br>Keep encouraging you and never give up.<br><br>Let you weep, if you must, while acknowledging your pain. |

## Second Stage of Labor: Resting Phase (see page 191)

| What physical changes and events occur | How you may feel and how you may respond | What you can do to cope | What your partner or doula can do to help you |
|---|---|---|---|
| Denotes the time from complete dilation to when you begin to push.<br><br>For up to 20 minutes, you may have few noticeable contractions (if any) or have no urge to push.<br><br>After your baby's head has slipped through your cervix, your uterus may need time to tighten around the rest of your baby's body before you can begin to push.<br><br>Not all women experience this phase. | Feel relief, optimism, confidence, and pain-free.<br><br>Get your "second wind." Have renewed energy, enthusiasm, hope, even if you don't experience a pause in contractions.<br><br>No longer in the "birth zone"—you're clearheaded, talkative, and more aware of your surroundings. | Rest or doze, if you can.<br><br>If you want to push spontaneously when you have the urge, remind your nurse or caregiver of this preference.<br><br>Review positions; review how to push and how to relax your pelvic floor muscles.<br><br>If the resting phase lasts more than 20 minutes, change to upright positions to encourage an urge to push. | Should match your enthusiasm (but not overly so).<br><br>Use this lull to renew energy (drink a beverage, close eyes and rest for a moment, use the restroom, and so on). If leaving the room, return promptly.<br><br>Help you change positions, if necessary or desired. |

## Second Stage of Labor: Descent Phase (see page 191)

| What physical changes and events occur | How you may feel and how you may respond | What you can do to cope | What your partner or doula can do to help you |
|---|---|---|---|
| Your baby rotates and descends into your birth canal.

Oxytocin surges cause an urge to push, which may be mild at first, but becomes compelling and irresistible.

You begin to push reflexively with contractions.

Contractions aren't as close together as they were in transition, and they may be shorter.

May last for a few minutes or up to 2 hours (or longer if you have an epidural).

At first, your baby's head can't be seen, then it appears at your vaginal opening when you push and retreats between pushes. | May feel inadequate in pushing until you get the hang of it.

May find this phase rewarding, but you may find it painful and tedious. Either way, you're working hard.

May find the pressure in your vagina alarming and fear it will worsen, making you "hold back" from pushing (see page 194).

May feel less pain as your baby's head repositions.

Might or might not feel the urge to push if you have an epidural. Ask your caregiver about delayed pushing (see page 189). | Hold your breath and strain when the contraction makes you feel that you can't avoid pushing. You may yell or cry out with the effort.

Consider touching your baby's head or watching her progress in a mirror.

If you're holding back, or if pushing is painful, try to push into the pain and through it. Doing so will feel better than stopping when it hurts.

Change your position every 30 minutes for comfort or to speed up labor progress.

Consider directed or prolonged pushing if your labor isn't adequately progressing with spontaneous bearing down.

If using directed pushing, follow the directions for when and how long to hold your breath and strain. | Encourage and praise your efforts. (Should not yell, "Push!").

Apply cool, damp cloths to your forehead, cheeks, neck, and chest.

Report on your progress (as soon as your baby's head is visible).

Remind you to release tension in your perineum and bulge your pelvic floor (see page 91).

Remind your caregiver of your feelings about episiotomy, if appropriate.

Support your position and help you change positions.

If pushing is ineffective, remind you to open your eyes and look toward where your baby is emerging (may use a mirror). |

## Second Stage of Labor: Crowning and Birth (see page 192)

| What physical changes and events occur | How you may feel and how you may respond | What you can do to cope | What your partner or doula can do to help you |
|---|---|---|---|
| Your baby's head emerges; it no longer retracts into your vaginal opening between contractions.

Your perineum and area around your urethra are most vulnerable to tearing in this phase.

Your caregiver either supports your perineum (often with warm compresses) or does an episiotomy (unlikely). | Feel excited because your baby's birth will be very soon.

May feel a burning sensation from vaginal stretching.

May have mixed feelings: May be tempted to push hard to get the birth over with, despite the burning. Or may fear the burning feeling and become reluctant to push. | Recognize the burning as a sign that labor is almost over.

Use your partner's help with positions.

To slow the birth of your baby's head and protect your perineum, stop pushing and pant or blow when your caregiver tells you to do so.

Rejoice in your baby's birth! | Support you as you change positions.

Refrain from rushing you; help you keep from pushing as needed.

Say little or nothing when your caregiver is directing you to slow the birth of your baby's head.

Rejoice in your baby's birth! |

## Third Stage of Labor (see page 196)

| What physical changes and events occur | How you may feel and how you may respond | What you can do to cope | What your partner or doula can do to help you |
|---|---|---|---|
| Lasts up to 30 minutes. | Feel relief that labor is over. | Move away clothing so your baby can lie skin-to-skin with you. | Help you get your baby onto your bare abdomen. |
| Your baby's umbilical cord is clamped and cut. | Become engrossed with your baby. | Don't rush breastfeeding. Your baby needs time to acclimate before she's ready to feed. Let her show you she's ready to start suckling (see page 400). | Help you breathe and focus through any painful procedures. |
| Your baby's condition is evaluated using the Apgar score. | Feel concern over trembling. | | Get you a warm blanket if you're trembling. |
| If your baby is fine and hospital policy allows, your baby is placed on your bare abdomen or chest. | Feel alarm if contractions are still painful. Feel surprise at the discomfort when your caregiver examines your birth canal or massages your uterus after the placenta is expelled. | Ask for a warm blanket to stop trembling. | Open shirt and snuggle skin-to-skin with your baby, if you can't hold her right away. |
| Your uterus contracts and shrinks, the placenta separates from your uterine wall. You expel the placenta with a few pushes. | | Use light breathing and focus on your partner or doula during uterine massage and the examination or stitching of your perineum. | Request that routine newborn procedures (such as weighing your baby or giving her a bath) be delayed for at least an hour so you can bond with your baby. |
| You may briefly tremble uncontrollably. (This is a normal reaction after giving birth.) | | Try to be patient during postpartum procedures. You'll have time to focus on your baby soon. | Enjoy this time with your new family! |
| Your caregiver checks your uterus to confirm it's contracting and checks your birth canal for tears. | | | |

# Recommended Resources

The following is a list of the best books, websites, and DVDs about topics discussed in this book. You can find additional resources on specific topics within the chapters. Visit our website, http://www.PCNGuide.com, to find many more resources.

## GENERAL PREGNANCY AND BIRTH INFORMATION

*The Official Lamaze Guide: Giving Birth with Confidence* by Judith Lothian and Charlotte DeVries (2010).

*Our Bodies, Ourselves: Pregnancy and Birth* by Boston Women's Health Book Collective and Judy Norsigian (2008).

*Ina May's Guide to Childbirth* by Ina May Gaskin (2003).

Childbirth Connection: http://www.childbirthconnection.org for information on maternity care options.

March of Dimes: http://www.marchofdimes.org for information on pregnancy and preventing preterm birth and birth defects.

*Healthy Birth Your Way: Six Steps to a Safer Birth* videos by Lamaze International and Injoy (2010)—visit http://www.mothers advocate.org to watch them.

*Orgasmic Birth* DVD or streaming video directed by Debra Pascali-Bonaro (2008).

Visit http://www.lamaze.org/YourPregnancyWeekByWeek to sign up for a weekly pregnancy e-newsletter from Lamaze International.

Visit http://text4baby.org to sign up for weekly texts about pregnancy and baby's first year.

## CHOOSING A BIRTHPLACE AND CAREGIVER

Visit http://www.childbirthconnection.org or download *The Great Starts Guide* (http://www.parenttrust.org/web-store/books) to see a discussion of maternity care options.

*The Doula Book: How a Trained Labor Companion Can Help You Have a Shorter, Easier, and Healthier Birth* by Marshall H. Klaus, John H. Kennell, and Phyllis H. Klaus (2012).

See page 15 or http://www.PCNGuide.com for a list of websites that allow you to search for birthplaces and caregivers in your area.

## HEALTHY LIFESTYLE DURING AND AFTER PREGNANCY

*Essential Exercises for the Childbearing Year: A Guide to Health and Comfort Before and After Your Baby Is Born* by Elizabeth Noble (2003).

*Lose Your Mummy Tummy* by Julie Tupler and Jodie Gould (2004).

Visit http://www.fitpregnancy.com for exercise and nutrition information.

Visit http://choosemyplate.gov for information on nutrition recommendations based on dietary guidelines for Americans.

Visit http://www.acog.org/Patients and http://www.marchofdimes.org for information on prenatal testing and maternity care.

United States Food and Drug Administration: 888-INFO-FDA (888-463-6332) or http://www.fda.gov.

*Yoga for Pregnancy, Labor and Birth* DVD directed by Colette Crawford (2005).

# Information on Hazards to Avoid during Pregnancy

**Alcohol:** Alcoholics Anonymous (AA): 212-870-3400 or http://www.aa.org.

**Domestic violence:** National Domestic Violence Hotline: 800-799-SAFE (7233) or http://www.ndvh.org.

**Drugs:** United States Substance Abuse and Mental Health Services Administration (SAMHSA): 800-662-HELP (800-662-4357) or http://www.samhsa.gov.

**Infectious Diseases:** United States Centers for Disease Control and Prevention: 800-CDC-INFO (232-4636) or http://www.cdc.gov/pregnancy.

**Narcotics:** Narcotics Anonymous (NA): 818-773-9999 or http://www.na.org.

**Teratogens** (medications, illnesses, and substances that can cause birth defects): MotherToBaby website, http://www.mothertobaby.org/fact-sheets-parent.

**Tobacco:** Smoking cessation: 800-CDC-INFO (232-4636) or http://www.smokefree.gov.

**Workplace hazards:** The National Institute for Occupational Safety and Health (NIOSH): 800-CDC-INFO (232-4636) or http://www.cdc.gov/niosh/docs/99-104.

# Special Circumstances in Pregnancy and Birth

**Multiples:** *Twins! Pregnancy, Birth, and the First Year of Life* by Connie Agnew, Alan H. Klein, and Jill Alison Ganon (2006).

**Pregnancy after loss:** *Trying Again: A Guide to Pregnancy After Miscarriage, Stillbirth, and Infant Loss* by Ann Douglas and John R. Sussman (2000).

**Survivors of childhood sexual abuse:** *When Survivors Give Birth: Understanding and Healing the Effects of Early Sexual Abuse on Childbearing Women* by Penny Simkin and Phyllis Klaus (2004).

**Teenage pregnancy:** *Your Pregnancy & Newborn Journey: A Guide for Pregnant Teens* by Jeanne Warren Lindsay and Jean Brunelli (2004).

**Lesbian families:** *The New Essential Guide to Lesbian Conception, Pregnancy, and Birth* by Stephanie Brill (2006). Also visit http://www.therainbowbabies.com.

# Labor and Birth

*The Labor Progress Handbook: Early Interventions to Prevent and Treat Dystocia* by Penny Simkin and Ruth Ancheta (2011).

*Listening to Mothers III: New Mothers Speak Out Survey and Report* by Eugene R. DeClercq, Carol Sakala, Maureen P. Corry, Sandra Applebaum, and Ariel Herrlich (2013); http://childbirthconnection.org/article.asp?ck=10394.

*Pathway to a Healthy Birth* by Childbirth Connection (2015); a research-based booklet on how hormonal interactions enhance normal physiological birth; http://childbirthconnection.org/pdfs/CC.NPWF.Booklet.Pathway.HealthyBirth.2015.pdf.

# Coping with Labor Pain

*Birthing from Within: An Extra-Ordinary Guide to Childbirth Preparation* by Pam England and Rob Horowitz (1998).

*Comfort in Labor: How You Can Help Yourself to a Normal Satisfying Childbirth* by Penny Simkin (2007); http://childbirthconnection.com/pdf.asp?PDFDownload=comfort-in-labor-simkin.

*Comfort Measures for Childbirth*, a DVD by Penny Simkin (2009). Visit http://www.pennysimkin.com to order a copy.

# Medical Interventions: Evidence-Based Resources

Childbirth Connection: http://www.childbirthconnection.org.

Cochrane Collaboration: http://community.cochrane.org.

PubMed: http://www.pubmed.gov.

Preventing Cesarean: *Safe Prevention of the Primary Cesarean Delivery,* ACOG/SMFM Statement (2014); http://tinyurl.com/CSPrevention.

Vaginal birth after cesarean (VBAC): *NIH Consensus Panel Statement* (2010); http://consensus.nih.gov/2010/vbac.htm.

# Postpartum Complications

**Cesarean support:** International Cesarean Awareness Network (ICAN): http://www.ican-online.org.

**Postpartum mood disorders:** Postpartum Support International: 800-944-4773 or http://www.postpartum.net.

**Traumatic birth:** http://solaceformothers.org; http://pattch.org.

**Loss of a baby:** *Mending Invisible Wings: Healing from the Loss of Your Baby* by Mary Burgess and Shiloh Sophia McCloud (2009).

# Fathers and Fatherhood

*The Birth Partner: A Complete Guide to Childbirth for Dads, Doulas, and All Other Labor Companions* by Penny Simkin (2013).

*The New Father: A Dad's Guide to the First Year* by Armin A. Brott (2015).

# Newborn Care

*The Baby Book: Everything You Need to Know About Your Baby from Birth to Age Two* by William Sears and Martha Sears (2013).

*The Happiest Baby on the Block: The New Way to Calm Crying and Help Your Newborn Sleep Longer* by Harvey Karp (2008). Available in paperback or DVD.

American Academy of Pediatrics: http://www.healthychildren.org.

**Health and safety topics:** http://www.seattlechildrens.org/safety-wellness.

# Breastfeeding

*Breastfeeding Made Simple* by Nancy Mohrbacher and Kathleen Kendall-Tackett (2010).

*The Nursing Mother's Companion, Revised* Edition by Kathleen Huggins (2015).

*The Breastfeeding Mothers' Guide to Making More Milk* by Diana West and Lisa Marasco (2008).

Kelly Mom: http://www.kellymom.com.

La Leche League: http://www.llli.org.

# Relationships after the Birth

*And Baby Makes Three: The Six-Step Plan for Preserving Marital Intimacy and Rekindling Romance After Baby Arrives* by John Gottman and Julie Schwartz Gottman (2008).

Notes

## Chapter 1: You're Having a Baby!

1. Penny Simkin, "Just Another Day in a Woman's Life?" *Birth* 18 (December 1991); P. Simkin, "Just Another Day in a Woman's Life? Part II: Nature and Consistency of Women's Long Term Memories of Their First Birth Experiences," *Birth* 19 (June 1992): 64–81.

## Chapter 2: So Many Choices

1. Glyn Elwyn et al., "Shared Decision Making: A Model for Clinical Practice," *Journal of General Internal Medicine* 27, no. 10 (2012): 1361–67, doi:10.1007/s11606-012-2077-6.

2. Truven Health Analytics Marketscan Study, *The Cost of Having a Baby in the United States: Executive Summary* (Ann Arbor, MI: Truven Health Analytics, 2013), http://transform.childbirth connection.org/wp-content/uploads/2013/01/Cost-of-Having-a -Baby-Executive-Summary.pdf.

3. American Congress of Obstetricians and Gynecologists and the Society for Maternal-Fetal Medicine, *Obstetric Care Consensus: Levels of Maternal Care* (Washington DC: American Congress of Obstetricians and Gynecologists, 2015), http://www.acog .org/-/media/Obstetric-Care-Consensus-Series/oc002.pdf ?dmc=1&ts=20150906T2311196878.

4. Kenneth C. Johnson and Betty-Anne Daviss, "Outcomes of Planned Home Births with Certified Professional Midwives: Large Prospective Study in North America," *BMJ* 330, no. 7505 (2005): 1416, doi:http://dx.doi.org/10.1136/bmj.330.7505.1416; Ank de Jonge et al., "Perinatal Mortality and Morbidity in a Nationwide Cohort of 529,688 Low-Risk Planned Home and Hospital Births," *BJOG* 116, no. 9 (2009): 1177–84; Patricia A. Janssen et al., "Outcomes of Planned Home Births versus Planned Hospital Births After Regulation of Midwifery in British Columbia," *CMAJ* 166, no. 3 (2002): 315–23; Melissa Cheyney, "Outcomes of Care for 16,924 Planned Home Births in the United States: The Midwives Alliance of North America Statistics Project, 2004 to 2009," *Journal of Midwifery & Women's Health* 59, no. 1 (2014): 17–27, doi:10.1111/jmwh.12172; Ank de Jonge, "Severe Adverse Maternal Outcomes among Low Risk Women with Planned Home versus Hospital Births in the Netherlands: Nationwide Cohort Study," *BMJ* 346, no. 7912 (2013): 3263, doi:http://dx.doi.org/10.1136 /bmj.f3263; Ole Olsen and Jette A. Clausen, "Planned Hospital Birth versus Planned Home Birth," *Cochrane Database of Systematic Reviews*, no. 9 (September 2012), doi: 10.1002/14651858. CD000352.pub2; Patricia A. Janssen et al., "Outcomes of Planned Home Birth with Registered Midwife versus Planned Hospital Birth with Midwife or Physician," *CMAJ* 181, no. 6–7 (2009): 377–83, doi:10.1503/cmaj.081869.

5. See note 4 above.

6. See note 4 above.

7. See note 4 above.

8. See note 4 above.

9. Ellen D. Hodnett et al., "Continuous Support for Women during in Childbirth," Cochrane Database of Systematic Reviews, no. 7 (July 2013), doi:10.1002/14651858.CD003766.pub5.

10. See note 4 above.

11. Childbirth Connection, "The Rights of Childbearing Women," http://www.childbirthconnection.org/article.asp?ck=10084& ClickedLink=0&area=27 (2006).

12. See note 9 above.

## Chapter 3: Common Changes and Concerns in Pregnancy

1. Kerstin Uvnäs Moberg, *The Oxytocin Factor: Tapping the Hormone of Calm, Love, and Healing* (Boston: Da Capo Press, 2003).

2. American Congress of Obstetricians and Gynecologists and the Society for Maternal-Fetal Medicine, *Obstetric Care Consensus: Safe Prevention of the Primary Cesarean Delivery* (Washington, DC: American Congress of Obstetricians and Gynecologists, 2014), http://www.acog.org/Resources-And-Publications/Obstet-ric-Care-Consensus-Series/Safe-Prevention-of-the-Primary -Cesarean-Delivery.

3. Aaron B. Caughey and Jennifer R. Butler, "Postterm Pregnancy," *Medscape*, http://emedicine.medscape.com/article/261369 -overview#showall.

4. Barbara Luke and Morton B. Brown, "Elevated Risks of Pregnancy Complications and Adverse Outcomes with Increasing Maternal Age," *Human Reproduction* 22, no. 5 (2007): 1264–72.

5. Janice H. Goodman, "Becoming an Involved Father of an Infant," *Journal of Obstetric, Gynecologic, and Neonatal Nursing* 34, no. 2 (2005): 190–200.

6. Sandra J. Berg and Katherine E. Wynne-Edwards, "Changes in Testosterone, Cortisol, and Estradiol Levels in Men Becoming Fathers," *Mayo Clinic Proceedings* 76, no. 6 (June 2001): 582–92, http://dx.doi.org/10.4065/76.6.582.

7. Penny Simkin and Phyllis Klaus, *When Survivors Give Birth: Understanding and Healing the Effects of Early Sexual Abuse on Childbearing Women* (Seattle: Classic Day Publishing 2004).

## Chapter 4: Having a Healthy Pregnancy

1. American Congress of Obstetricians and Gynecologists, *Committee Opinion: Cell-free DNA Screening for Fetal Aneuploidy* (Washington, DC: American Congress of Obstetricians and Gynecologists, 2015), http://www.acog.org/Resources-And -Publications/Committee-Opinions/Committee-on-Genetics /Cell-free-DNA-Screening-for-Fetal-Aneuploidy.

2. See note 1 above.

3. Diana W. Bianchi et al., "DNA Sequencing versus Standard Prenatal Aneuploidy Screening," *The New England Journal of Medicine* 370 (2014): 799–808, http://www.nejm.org/doi/full/10.1056 /NEJMoa1311037#Results=&t=articleResults.

4. "Stress and Pregnancy," March of Dimes Foundation, last modified January 2012, http://www.marchofdimes.org/pregnancy /stress-and-pregnancy.aspx.

5. Nicole M. Talge et al., "Antenatal Maternal Stress and Long-Term Effects on Child Neurodevelopment: How and Why?" *Journal of Child Psychology Psychiatry* 48, no. 3–4 (2007): 245–61.

6. American Congress of Obstetricians and Gynecologists, *Frequently Asked Questions: Tobacco, Alcohol, Drugs, and Pregnancy* (Washington, DC: American Congress of Obstetricians and Gynecologists, December 2013), http://www.acog.org/-/media /For-Patients/faq170.pdf?dmc=1&ts=20150927T1531353101.

7. Elisa K. Tong, Lucina England, and Stanton A. Glantz, "Changing Conclusions on Secondhand Smoke in a Sudden Infant Death Syndrome Review Funded by the Tobacco Industry," *Pediatrics* 115, no. 3 (2005): e356–66, http://pediatrics.aappublications.org /content/115/3/e356.full.pdf.

8. Eric Jauniaux and Graham J. Burton, "Morphological and Biological Effects of Maternal Exposure to Tobacco Smoke on the Feto-placental Unit," *Early Human Development* 83, no. 11 (2007): 699–706, http://www.earlyhumandevelopment.com/article/S0378-3782(07)00126-0/abstract?cc=y=.

9. American Congress of Obstetricians and Gynecologists, *Committee Opinion: Smoking Cessation during Pregnancy* (Washington, DC: American Congress of Obstetricians and Gynecologists, 2010), http://www.acog.org/Resources-And-Publications/Committee-Opinions/Committee-on-Health-Care-for-Underserved-Women/Smoking-Cessation-During-Pregnancy.

10. Organization of Teratology Information Specialists, *Marijuana and Pregnancy* (January 2015), http://www.mothertobaby.org/files/marijuana.pdf.

11. International Food Information Council Foundation, *Healthy Eating During Pregnancy* (2009), http://www.foodinsight.org/Content/3651/RevisedHealthyEatingPregnancy809.pdf.

12. Xiaoping Weng, Roxana Odouli, and De-Kun Li, "Maternal Caffeine Consumption during Pregnancy and the Risk of Miscarriage: A Prospective Cohort Study," *American Journal of Obstetrics and Gynecology* 198, no. 3 (2008): 279.e1–8; Laura M. Grosso et al., "Caffeine Metabolites in Umbilical Cord Blood, Cytochrome P-450 1A2 Activity, and Intrauterine Growth Restriction," *American Journal of Epidemiology* 163, no. 11 (2006): 1035–41; Fumihiro Sata et al., "Caffeine Intake, CYP1A2 Polymorphism and the Risk of Recurrent Pregnancy Loss," *Molecular Human Reproduction* 11, no. 5 (2005): 357–60.

13. Verena Sengpiel et al., "Maternal Caffeine Intake during Pregnancy Is Associated with Birth Weight but Not with Gestational Length: Results from a Large Prospective Observational Cohort Study," *BMC Medicine* 11, no. 42 (2013), http://www.biomedcentral.com/1741-7015/11/42.

14. Colin G. Rousseaux and Howard Schachter, "Regulatory Issues Concerning the Safety, Efficacy and Quality of Herbal Remedies," *Birth Defects Research Part B: Developmental and Reproductive Toxicology* 68, no. 6 (2003): 505–10; C.H. Chuang et al., "Herbal Medicines Used during the First Trimester and Major Congenital Malformations: An Analysis of Data from a Pregnancy Cohort Study," *Drug Safety* 29, no. 6 (2006): 537–48.

15. J.G. Silverman et al., "Intimate Partner Violence Victimization Prior to and during Pregnancy among Women Residing in 26 U.S. States: Associations with Maternal and Neonatal Health," *American Journal of Obstetrics and Gynecology* 195, no. 1 (2006): 140–48.

16. Judith McFarlane et al., "Abuse during Pregnancy and Femicide: Urgent Implications for Women's Health," *Obstetrics and Gynecology* 100, no. 1 (2002): 27–36.

17. National Institute for Occupational Safety and Health, *The Effects of Workplace Hazards on Female Reproductive Health* (CDC/NIOSH, February 1999), http://www.cdc.gov/niosh/docs/99-104.

18. Linda M. Frazier, "Reproductive Disorders Associated with Pesticide Exposure," *Journal of Agromedicine* 12, no. 1 (2007): 27–37; Anneclaire J. De Roos et al., "Parental Occupational Exposures to Chemicals and Incidence of Neuroblastoma in Offspring," *American Journal of Epidemiology* 154, no. 2 (2001): 106–14; G.R. Bunin et al., "Parental Heat Exposure and Risk of Childhood Brain Tumor: A Children's Oncology Group Study," *American Journal of Epidemiology* 164, no. 3 (2006): 222–31; Wojciech Hanke and Joanna Jurewicz, "The Risk of Adverse Reproductive and Developmental Disorders Due to Occupational Pesticide Exposure: An Overview of Current Epidemiological Evidence," *International Journal of Occupational Medicine & Environmental Health* 17, no. 2 (2004): 223–43.

# Chapter 5: Feeling Good and Staying Fit

1. American Congress of Obstetricians and Gynecologists, *Frequently Asked Questions: Exercise during Pregnancy* (Washington, DC: American Congress of Obstetricians and Gynecologists, 2011), http://www.acog.org/~/media/For%20Patients/faq119.pdf.

# Chapter 6: Eating Well

1. Allison Aubrey, "The Full-Fat Paradox: Whole Milk May Keep Us Lean," *The Salt* (blog), http://www.npr.org/blogs/thesalt/2014/02/12/275376259/the-full-fat-paradox-whole-milk-may-keep-us-lean; Patty W. Siri-Tarino et al., "Meta-analysis of Prospective Cohort Studies Evaluating the Association of Saturated Fat with Cardiovascular Disease," *American Journal of Clinical Nutrition* 91, no. 3 (2010): 535–46, http://ajcn.nutrition.org/content/91/3/535.full.

2. "All 48 Fruits and Vegetables with Pesticide Residue Data," Environmental Working Group, accessed September 20, 2015, http://www.ewg.org/foodnews/list.php.

3. The US Department of Health and Human Services and the US Department of Agriculture, *Dietary Guidelines for Americans* (2010), http://www.cnpp.usda.gov/dietary-guidelines-2010.

4. International Food Information Council Foundation, *Healthy Eating During Pregnancy* (2009), http://www.foodinsight.org/Content/3651/RevisedHealthyEatingPregnancy809.pdf.

5. American Congress of Obstetricians and Gynecologists, *Committee Opinion: Weight Gain during Pregnancy* (Washington, DC: American Congress of Obstetricians and Gynecologists, 2013), http://www.acog.org/Resources-And-Publications/Committee-Opinions/Committee-on-Obstetric-Practice/Weight-Gain-During-Pregnancy; Joan M.G. Crane et al., "The Effect of Gestational Weight Gain by Body Mass Index on Maternal and Neonatal Outcomes," *Journal of Obstetrics and Gynaecology* Canada 31, no. 1 (2009): 28–35; Mufiza Zia Kapadia et al., "Can We Safely Recommend Gestational Weight Gain Below the 2009 Guidelines in Obese Women? A Systematic Review And Meta-Analysis," *Obesity Reviews* 16, no. 3 (2015): 189–206.

6. Jennifer A. Hutcheon, "Pregnancy Weight Gain Charts for Obese and Overweight Women," *Obesity* 23, no. 3 (2015): 532–35, http://onlinelibrary.wiley.com/doi/10.1002/oby.21011/epdf; American Congress of Obstetricians and Gynecologists, *Committee Opinion: Weight Gain during Pregnancy* (Washington, DC: American Congress of Obstetricians and Gynecologists, 2013), http://www.acog.org/Resources-And-Publications/Committee-Opinions/Committee-on-Obstetric-Practice/Weight-Gain-During-Pregnancy; Mufiza Zia Kapadia et al., "Can We Safely Recommend Gestational Weight Gain Below the 2009 Guidelines in Obese Women? A Systematic Review And Meta-Analysis," *Obesity Reviews* 16, no. 3 (2015): 189–206.

7. American Pregnancy Association, "Mercury Levels in Fish," March 2007, http://www.americanpregnancy.org/pregnancyhealth/fishmercury.htm; American Heart Association, "Fish, Levels of Mercury and Omega-3 Fatty Acids," 2010, http://www.americanheart.org/presenter.jhtml?identifier=3013797; Food and Drug Administration, "Mercury Levels in Commercial Fish and Shellfish," January 2006, http://www.cfsan.fda.gov/~frf/sea-mehg.html; D. G. Andersen, "Omega-3 Fatty Acids in Seafood," 2007, http://www.andersenchiro.com/omega3-fatty-acids-in-seafood-table.shtml.

# Chapter 7: When Pregnancy Becomes Complicated

1. Hien T. Nghiem, "ACOG Guidelines for Treating Nausea and Vomiting in Pregnant Women Reviewed," Medscape, http://www.medscape.org/viewarticle/730520.

2. Patricia Evans and Susan Brunsell, "Uterine Fibroid Tumors: Diagnosis and Treatment," *American Family Physician* 75, no. 10 (2007) 1503–8, http://www.aafp.org/afp/2007/0515/p1503.html.

3. Centers for Disease Control and Prevention, *2010 Guidelines for the Prevention of Perinatal Group B Streptococcal Disease*, November 2010, http://www.cdc.gov/groupbstrep/guidelines/guidelines.html.

4. Susanne Hempel et al., "Probiotics for the Prevention and Treatment of Antibiotic-Associated Diarrhea: A Systematic Review and Meta-analysis," *Journal of the American Medical Association* 307, no. 18 (2012): 1959–69, doi:10.1001/jama.2012.3507.

5. Carla L. DeSisto, Shin Y. Kim, and Andrea J. Sharma, "Prevalence Estimates of Gestational Diabetes Mellitus in the United States, Pregnancy Risk Assessment Monitoring System (PRAMS), 2007–2010," *Preventing Chronic Disease* 11 (2014), http://www.cdc.gov/pcd/issues/2014/13_0415.htm.

6. Lawrence Oppenheimer, "Diagnosis and Management of Placenta Previa," *Journal of Obstetrics and Gynaecology Canada* 29, no. 3 (2007): 261–73, http://sogc.org/wp-content/uploads/2013/01/189E-CPG-March2007.pdf.

7. American Congress of Obstetricians and Gynecologists, *Hypertension in Pregnancy: Report of the American Congress of Obstetricians and Gynecologists' Task Force on Hypertension in Pregnancy* Executive Summary, November 2013, http://www.tsop.org.tw/db/CFile/File/8-1.pdf.

8. Baha M. Sibai, "Diagnosis and Management of Gestational Hypertension and Preeclampsia," *Obstetrics & Gynecology* 102, no. 1 (2003): 181–92.

9. Laurie Barclay, "Preeclampsia: Low-Dose Aspirin May Prevent Poor Outcomes," *Medscape*, April 7, 2014, http://www.medscape.com/viewarticle/823216.

10. Shi Wu Wen et al., "Folic Acid Supplementation in Early Second Trimester and the Risk of Preeclampsia," *American Journal of Obstetrics and Gynecology* 198, no. 1 (2008): 45, e1–7.

11. Sandra A. Founds, "Clinical Implications from an Exploratory Study of Postural Management of Breech Presentation." *Journal of Midwifery & Women's Health* 51, no. 4 (2006): 292–96, doi:10.1016/j.jmwh.2005.11.010.

12. Paul F. Crawford, "Use of External Abdominal Ice to Complete External Cephalic Version in Term Breech Pregnancy," *Journal of the American Board of Family Medicine* 18, no. 4 (2005): 312–13. cold on fundus, doi:10.3122/jabfm.18.4.312.

13. Qin-hong Zhang et al., "Moxibustion for the Correction of Nonvertex Presentation: A Systematic Review and Meta-Analysis of Randomized Controlled Trials," *Evidence-Based Complementary Alternative Medicine* (2013), http://www.hindawi.com/journals/ecam/2013/241027; Meaghan E. Coyle, Caroline A. Smith, and Brian Peat, "Cephalic Version by Moxibustion for Breech Presentation," Cochrane Database of Systematic Reviews, no. 5 (May 2012), doi:10.1002/14651858.CD003928.pub3.

14. Richard A. Pistolese, "The Webster Technique: A Chiropractic Technique with Obstetric Implications," *Journal of Manipulative Physiological Therapeutics* 25, no. 6 (2002): E1–9.

15. G. Justus Hofmeyr, Regina Kulier, and Helen M. West, "External Cephalic Version for Breech Presentation at Term," Cochrane Database of Systematic Reviews, no. 4 (February 2015), doi:10.1002/14651858.CD000083.pub3.

16. Mary E. Hannah et al., "Planned Cesarean Section versus Planned Vaginal Birth for Breech Presentation at Term: A Randomised Multicentre Trial," *The Lancet* 356, no. 9239 (2000): 1375–83.

17. Andrew Kotaska, Savas Menticoglou, and Robert Gagnon, "Vaginal Delivery of Breech Presentation," *Journal of Obstetrics and Gynaecology Canada*, no. 226 (2009): 557–66, http://sogc.org/wp-content/uploads/2013/01/gui226CPG0906.pdf.

# Chapter 8: Planning for Birth and Postpartum

1. Penny Simkin, "Birth Plans: After 25 Years, Women Still Want to Be Heard," *Birth* 34, no. 1 (2007): 49–51; Judith Lothian, "Birth Plans: The Good, the Bad, and the Future," *Journal of Obstetric, Gynecologic & Neonatal Nursing* 35, no. 2 (2006): 295–303; Paulina Perez, "Birth Plans: Are They Really Necessary?" *The American Journal of Maternal/Child Nursing* 30, no. 5 (2005): 288–89; Joanne Motino Bailey, Patricia Crane, and Clark E. Nugent, "Childbirth Education and Birth Plans," *Obstetrics and Gynecology Clinics of North America* 35, no. 3 (2008): 497–509; Shad H. Deering et al., "Patients Presenting with Birth Plans: A Case-Control Study of Delivery Outcomes," *Journal of Reproductive Medicine* 52, no. 10 (2007): 884–87.

2. See note 1 above.

3. See note 1 above.

4. Jacqueline Kelleher, "The Postpartum Plan," *International Doula* 17, no. 4 (2009): 26–28.

# Chapter 9: When and How Labor Begins

1. "Preterm Birth," Centers for Disease Control and Prevention, last updated 2014, http://www.cdc.gov/reproductivehealth/MaternalInfantHealth/PretermBirth.htm.

2. "Fact Sheet: Preterm Birth in Canada: An Environmental Scan," Canadian Premature Babies Foundation, 2014, http://cpbf-fbpc.org/news-and-events-2.

3. Donald Briscoe et al., "Management of Pregnancy Beyond 40 weeks' Gestation," *American Family Physician* 71, no. 10 (2005): 1935–41.

4. Elizabeth R. Cluett et al., "Immersion in Water in Pregnancy, Labour and Birth," Cochrane Database of Systematic Reviews, no. 2 (April 2002), doi:10.1002/14651858.CD000111.pub2.

5. C. Gibbons, C. O'Herlihy, and J.F. Murphy, "Umbilical Cord Prolapse—Changing Patterns and Improved Outcomes: A Retrospective Cohort Study," *BJOG* 121, no. 13 (2014): 1705–8; Glenn Posner et al., *Oxorn-Foote Human Labor and Birth*, 6th ed. (New York: McGraw Hill Medical, 2013).

# Chapter 10: What Childbirth Is Really Like

1. Sarah J. Buckley, *Pathway to a Healthy Birth: How to Help Your Hormones Do Their Wonderful Work* (New York: Childbirth Connection, 2015), http://childbirthconnection.org/pdfs/CC.NPWF.Booklet.Pathway.HealthyBirth.2015.pdf; Sarah J. Buckley, *Gentle Birth, Gentle Mothering: The Wisdom and Science of Gentle Choices in Pregnancy, Birth, and Parenting* (Celestial Arts, 2009).

2. American Congress of Obstetricians and Gynecologists and Society for Maternal-Fetal Medicine, *Obstetric Care Consensus: Safe Prevention of the Primary Cesarean Delivery* (Washington, DC: American Congress of Obstetricians and Gynecologists, 2014), http://

www.acog.org/Resources-And-Publications/Obstetric-Care-Consensus-Series/Safe-Prevention-of-the-Primary-Cesarean-Delivery.

3. See note 1 above.

4. Michel Odent, "Can Water Immersion Stop Labor?" *Journal of Nurse-Midwifery* 42, no. 5 (1997): 414–46.

5. See note 2 above.

6. Emanuel A. Friedman, "Dysfunctional Labor" in *Management of Labor* by Wayne R. Cohen and Emanuel A. Friedman (Baltimore: University Park Press 1983); J. Zhang, J. F. Troendle, and M. K. Yancey, "Reassessing the Labor Curve in Nulliparous Women," *American Journal of Obstetrics and Gynecology* 187, no. 4 (2002): 824–28.

7. See note 2 above.

8. Annemarie Lawrence et al., "Maternal Positions and Mobility during First Stage Labour," Cochrane Database of Systematic Reviews, no. 10 (2013), doi:10.1002/14651858.CD003934.pub4.

9. American Congress of Obstetricians and Gynecologists, *Intrapartum Fetal Heart Rate Monitoring: Nomenclature, Interpretation, and General Management Principles*, ACOG Practice Bulletin No. 106, July 2009, http://www.ncbi.nlm.nih.gov/pubmed/19546798; Robert Liston, Diane Sawchuck, and David Young, "Fetal Health Surveillance: Antepartum and Intrapartum Consensus Guideline," *Journal of Obstetrics and Gynaecology Canada* 29 (2007), S3–56, http://www.sogc.org/guidelines/documents/gui197CPG0709r.pdf; Association of Women's Health Obstetric and Neonatal Nurses, *Fetal Heart Monitoring* (2008), https://www.awhonn.org/awhonn/binary.content.do?name=Resources/Documents/pdf/5_FHM.pdf.

10. Z. Alfirevic, D. Devane, and G. M. Gyte, "Continuous Cardiotocography (CTG) as a Form of Electronic Fetal Monitoring (EFM) for Fetal Assessment during Labour," Cochrane Database of Systematic Reviews, no. 5 (2013), doi:10.1002/14651858.CD006066.pub2; Declan Devane et al., "Cardiotocography versus Intermittent Auscultation of Fetal Heart on Admission to Labour Ward for Assessment of Fetal Wellbeing," Cochrane Database of Systematic Reviews, no. 2 (2012), doi:10.1002/14651858.CD005122.pub4.

11. M. Odent, "The Fetus Ejection Reflex," *Birth* 14 (1987): 104–05; N. Newton, "The Fetus Ejection Reflex Revisited," *Birth* 14 (1987): 106–08; Sarah J. Buckley, *Gentle Birth, Gentle Mothering: The Wisdom and Science of Gentle Choices in Pregnancy, Birth, and Parenting* (Celestial Arts, 2009).

12. M. Prins et al., "Effect of Spontaneous Pushing versus Valsalva Pushing in the Second Stage of Labour on Mother and Fetus: a Systematic Review of Randomised Trials," *British Journal of Obstetrics and Gynecology* 118, no. 6 (2011): 662–70. doi: 10.1111/j.1471-0528.2011.02910.x.

13. William D. Fraser et al., "Multicenter, Randomized, Controlled Trial of Delayed Pushing for Nulliparous Women in the Second Stage of Labor with Continuous Epidural Analgesia," *American Journal of Obstetrics and Gynecology* 182, no. 5 (2000): 1165–72; R. M. Brancato, S. Church, and P. W. Stone, "A Meta-analysis of Passive Descent versus Immediate Pushing in Nulliparous Women with Epidural Analgesia in the Second Stage of Labor," *Journal of Obstetric, Gynecologic, and Neonatal Nursing* 37, no. 1 (2008): 4–12.

14. Joyce Roberts and Lisa Hanson, "Best Practices in Second Stage Labor Care: Maternal Bearing Down and Positioning," *Journal of Midwifery & Women's Health* 52, no. 3 (2007): 238–45; J. I. Schaffer et al., "A Randomized Trial of the Effects of Coached vs. Uncoached Maternal Pushing during the Second Stage of Labor on Postpartum Pelvic Floor Structure and Function," *American Journal of Obstetrics and Gynecology* 192, no. 5 (2005): 1692–96.

15. Joyce Roberts and Lisa Hanson, "Best Practices in Second Stage Labor Care: Maternal Bearing Down and Positioning," *Journal of Midwifery & Women's Health* 52, no. 3 (2007): 238–45.

16. Eugene R. Declercq et al., *Listening to Mothers III: Pregnancy and Birth* (New York: Childbirth Connection, May 2013), http://transform.childbirthconnection.org/wp-content/uploads/2013/06/LTM-III_Pregnancy-and-Birth.pdf; Beverly Chalmers et al., "Use of Routine Interventions in Vaginal Labor and Birth: Findings from the Maternity Experiences Survey," *Birth* 36, no. 1 (2009): 13–25.

17. Vigdis Aasheim et al., "Perineal Techniques during the Second Stage of Labour for Reducing Perineal Trauma," Cochrane Database of Systematic Reviews, no. 12 (2011), doi:10.1002/14651858.CD006672.pub2.

18. See note 17 above.

19. John Kelleher et al., "Oronasopharyngeal Suction versus Wiping of the Mouth and Nose at Birth: a Randomised Equivalency Trial," *The Lancet* 382, no. 9889 (2013): 326–30; Judith Mercer et al., "Evidence-Based Practices for the Fetal to Newborn Transition," *Journal of Midwifery & Women's Health* 52, no. 3 (2007): 262–72.

20. S. J. McDonald et al., "Effect of Timing of Umbilical Cord Clamping of Term Infants on Maternal and Neonatal Outcomes," Cochrane Database of Systematic Reviews, no. 7 (2013), doi:10.1002/14651858.CD004074.pub3.

21. E. R. Moore et al., "Early Skin-to-Skin Contact for Mothers and Their Healthy Newborn Infants," Cochrane Database of Systematic Reviews, no. 5 (2012), doi:10.1002/14651858.CD003519.pub3.

22. S. J. McDonald et al., "Effect of Timing of Umbilical Cord Clamping of Term Infants on Maternal and Neonatal Outcomes," Cochrane Database of Systematic Reviews, no. 7 (2013), doi:10.1002/14651858.CD004074.pub3; International Childbirth Education Association, *Delayed Cord Clamping*, Position Paper, accessed September 20, 2015, http://www.icea.org/sites/default/files/Delayed%20Cord%20Clamping-PP-FINAL.pdf.

23. Eileen Katherine Hutton and Eman S. Hassan, "Late vs Early Clamping of the Umbilical Cord in Full-Term Neonates: Systematic Review and Meta-analysis of Controlled Trials," *Journal of the American Medical Association* 297, no. 11 (2007): 1241–52.

24. See note 23 above.

25. Alice C. Yao, Mahmud Moinian, and John Lind, "Distribution of Blood between Infant and Placenta after Birth," *Lancet* 294, no. 7626 (1969): 871–73; Rebecca J. Palethorpe, Diane Farrar, and Leila Duley, "Alternative Positions for the Baby at Birth before Clamping the Umbilical Cord," Cochrane Database of Systematic Reviews, no. 10 (2010), doi:10.1002/14651858.CD007555.pub2.

26. J. Smith, F. Plaat, and N. M. Fisk, "The Natural Caesarean: A Woman-Centred Technique," *BJOG* 115, no. 8 (2008): 1037–42.

27. H. Rabe et al., "Effect of Timing of Umbilical Cord Clamping and Other Strategies to Influence Placental Transfusion at Preterm Birth on Maternal and Infant Outcomes," Cochrane Database of Systematic Reviews, no. 8 (2012), doi:10.1002/14651858.CD003248.pub3.

28. American Academy of Pediatrics, Section on Hematology/Oncology and Section on Allergy/Immunology, "Cord Blood Banking for Potential Future Transplantation," *Pediatrics* 119, no. 1 (2007): 165–70; M. G. Butler and J. E. Menitove, "Umbilical Cord Blood Banking: An Update," Journal of Assisted Reproduction and Genetics 28, no. 8 (2011): 669–76, doi: 10.1007/s10815-011-9577-x.

29. American Academy of Pediatrics, Section on Hematology/Oncology and Section on Allergy/Immunology, "Cord Blood Banking for Potential Future Transplantation," *Pediatrics* 119, no. 1 (2007): 165–70.

30. See note 1 above.

31. See note 1 above.

## Chapter 11: Labor Pain and Options for Pain Relief

1. S. Kitzinger, "Pain in Childbirth," *Journal of Medical Ethics* 4 (1978): 119–21.

2. Ronald Melzak, "From the Gate to the Neuromatrix," *Pain* 6 (August 1999): S121–26.

3. Nicky Leap and Mary Newburn, "Working with Pain in Labour: An Overview of Evidence," *New Digest* 49 (2010): 22–26.

4. N. Lowe, "The Nature of Labor Pain," *American Journal of Obstetrics and Gynecology* 186 (2002): S16–24.

5. Eugene DeClercq et al., *Listening to Mothers II: Report of the Second National U.S. Survey of Women's Childbearing Experiences* (New York: Childbirth Connection, 2006), http://www.childbirthconnection.org/pdfs/LTMII_report.pdf.

6. R. Melzack and Kenneth Casey, "Sensory, Motivational, and Central Control Determinants of Chronic Pain: A New Conceptual Model," in *The Skin Senses*, ed. Dan R. Kenshalo (Springfield, IL: Charles C. Thomas, 1968), 423–43.

7. N. Chaillet et al., "Nonpharmacologic Approaches for Pain Management during Labor Compared with Usual Care: A Meta-analysis," *Birth* 41, no. 2 (2014): 122–37, http://www.ncbi.nlm.nih.gov/pubmed/24761801.

8. See note 7 above.

9. Ellen D. Hodnett et al., "Continuous Support for Women during Childbirth," Cochrane Database of Systematic Reviews, no. 7 (2013), doi:10.1002/14651858.CD003766.pub5.

10. April Bolding and Penny Simkin, "Supporting the Laboring Woman without Injuring Oneself," *International Journal of Childbirth Education* 22, no. 4 (2008): 17–33.

## Chapter 12: Comfort Techniques for Pain Relief and Labor Progress

1. Penny Simkin and April Bolding, "Update on Nonpharmacologic Approaches to Relieve Pain and Prevent Suffering," *Journal of Midwifery & Women's Health* 49, no. 6 (2004): 489–504; Penny Simkin and Michael Klein, "Nonpharmacologic Approaches to Management of Labor Pain," *UpToDate* (2014), http://www.uptodate.com/contents/nonpharmacologic-approaches-to-management-of-labor-pain.

2. Watty Piper, *The Little Engine That Could* (New York: Platt & Munk, 1930).

3. Gun Ohlsson et al., "Warm Tub Bathing during Labor: Maternal and Neonatal Effects," *Acta Obstetricia et Gynecologica Scandinavica* 80, no. 4 (2001): 311–14, doi:10.1034/j.1600-0412.2001.080004311.x.

4. Elizabeth Cluett et al., "Randomised Controlled Trial of Labouring in Water Compared with Standard of Augmentation for Management of Dystocia in First Stage of Labour," *BMJ* 328 (2004): 314–20; Michel Odent, "Can Water Immersion Stop Labor?" *Journal of Nurse-Midwifery* 42, no. 5 (1997): 414–46.

5. Elizabeth Cluett and Ethel Burns, "Immersion in Water in Labour and Birth," Cochrane Database of Systematic Reviews, no. 2 (2009), doi:10.1002/14651858.CD000111.pub3.

6. Margareta Eriksson et al., "Warm Tub Bath during Labor: A Study of 1385 Women with Prelabor Rupture of the Membranes after 34 weeks of Gestation," *Acta Obstetricia et Gynecologica Scandinavica* 75, no. 7 (1996): 642–44.

7. American Congress of Nurse-Midwives, *Position Statement: Hydrotherapy during Labor and Birth* (Silver Spring, MD: American Congress of Nurse-Midwives, 2014), http://www.midwife.org/acnm/files/ccLibraryFiles/Filename/000000004048/Hydrotherapy-During-Labor-and-Birth-April-2014.pdf; American Congress of Obstetricians and Gynecologists, *Committee Opinion: Immersion in Water during Labor and Delivery* (Washington, DC: American Congress of Obstetricians and Gynecologists, 2014), http://www.acog.org/Resources-And-Publications/Committee-Opinions/Committee-on-Obstetric-Practice/Immersion-in-Water-During-Labor-and-Delivery.

8. American Congress of Obstetricians and Gynecologists, *Committee Opinion: Immersion in Water during Labor and Delivery* (Washington, DC: American Congress of Obstetricians and Gynecologists, 2014), http://www.acog.org/Resources-And-Publications/Committee-Opinions/Committee-on-Obstetric-Practice/Immersion-in-Water-During-Labor-and-Delivery.

9. Mandisa Singata, Joan Tranmer, and Gillian M. L. Gyte, "Restricting Oral Fluid and Food Intake during Labour," Cochrane Database of Systematic Reviews, no. 8 (2013), doi:10.1002/14651858.CD003930.pub3.

10. Andrea Lythgoe, "Peanut Balls for Labor – A Valuable Tool for Promoting Progress?" *Science & Sensibility* (blog), April 8, 2014, http://www.scienceandsensibility.org/?s=peanut.

11. Caroline A. Smith et al., "Acupuncture or Acupressure for Pain Management in Labor," Cochrane Database of Systematic Reviews, no. 7 (2011), doi:10.1002/14651858.CD009232.

12. S. Alehagen et al., "Fear, Pain and Stress Hormones during Childbirth," *Journal of Psychosomatic Obstetrics & Gynecology* 26, no. 3 (September 2005): 153–65; Sarah J. Buckley, *Hormonal Physiology of Childbearing: Evidence and Implications for Women, Babies, and Maternity Care*, Childbirth Connection, January 2015, http://childbirthconnection.org/pdfs/CC.NPWF.HPoC.Report.2015.pdf.

13. Janesh K. Gupta, G. Justus Hofmeyr, and Manjeet Shehmar, "Position in the Second Stage of Labour for Women without Epidural Anaesthesia," Cochrane Database of Systematic Reviews, no. 5 (2012), doi:10.1002/14651858.CD002006.pub3.

14. Michael Beckmann and Owen Stock, "Antenatal Perineal Massage for Reducing Perineal Trauma," Cochrane Database of Systematic Reviews, no. 4 (2013), doi:10.1002/14651858.CD005123.pub3.

## Chapter 13: Medications for Pain Relief during Labor

1. Roz Ullman, Therese Dowswell, and Rintaro Mori, "Parenteral Opioids for Maternal Pain Relief in Labour," Cochrane Database of Systematic Reviews, no. 4 (2008), doi:10.1002/14651858.CD007396.

2. Millicent Anim-Somuah, Rebecca M. D. Smyth, and Leanne Jones, "Epidural versus Non-epidural or No Analgesia in Labour," Cochrane Database of Systematic Reviews, no. 12 (2011), doi:10.1002/14651858.CD000331.pub3.

3. Salvatore Gizzo et al., "Update on Best Available Options in Obstetrics Anaesthesia: Perinatal Outcomes, Side Effects and Maternal Satisfaction, Fifteen Years Systematic Literature Review," *Archives of Gynecology and Obstetrics* 290, no. 1 (2014): 21–34; M. Van de Velde, "Modern Neuraxial Labor Analgesia: Options for Initiation, Maintenance and Drug Selection," *Revista Española de Anestesiología y Reanimación* 56, no. 9 (2009): 546–61; Katherine W. Arendt, Jennifer A. Tessmer-Tuck, and James R. Hebl, "Safe and Individualized Labor Analgesia: A Review of the Current Options," *Minnesota Medicine* (March 2012), http://www.minnesotamedicine.com/Past-Issues/Past-Issues-2012/March-2012/Safe-and-Individualized-Labor-Analgesia; C. Loubert, A. Hinova, and R. Fernando, "Update on Modern Neuraxial

Analgesia in Labour: A Review of the Literature of the Last 5 Years," *Journal of the Association of Anaesthetists of Great Britain and Ireland* 66 (2011): 191–212, http://anaesthetics.ukzn.ac.za/Libraries/Documents2011/Update_on_modern_neuraxial_analgesia_in_labour.sflb.ashx; Millicent Anim-Somuah, Rebecca M. D. Smyth, and Leanne Jones, "Epidural versus Non-epidural or No Analgesia in Labour," Cochrane Database of Systematic Reviews, no. 12 (2011), doi:10.1002/14651858.CD000331.pub3.

4. American Academy of Pediatrics and American Congress of Obstetricians and Gynecologists, *Guidelines for Perinatal Care* (Elk Grove Village, IL: American Academy of Pediatrics, 2012).

5. A. Hager and W. Newton, "Comparing Epidural and Parenteral Opioid Analgesia During Labor," *Journal of Family Practice* 43, no. 3 (1999): 174–5.

6. Katherine W. Arendt, Jennifer A. Tessmer-Tuck, and James R. Hebl, "Safe and Individualized Labor Analgesia: A Review of the Current Options," *Minnesota Medicine* (March 2012), http://www.minnesotamedicine.com/Past-Issues/Past-Issues-2012/March-2012/Safe-and-Individualized-Labor-Analgesia.

7. Kai Wang et al., "The Effects of Epidural/Spinal Opioids in Labour Analgesia on Neonatal Outcomes: A Meta-analysis of Randomized Controlled Trials," *Canadian Journal of Anesthesia* 61, no. 8 (2014): 695–709.

8. Ann M. Dozier et al., "Labor Epidural Anesthesia, Obstetric Factors and Breastfeeding Cessation," Maternal and Child Health Journal 17, no. 4 (2013) 689–98; Siranda Torvaldsen et al., "Intrapartum Epidural Analgesia and Breastfeeding: A Prospective Cohort Study," *International Breastfeeding Journal* 1 (2006): 24; Petri Volmanen, J. Valanne, and S. Alahuhta, "Breast-Feeding Problems after Epidural Analgesia for Labour: A Retrospective Cohort Study of Pain, Obstetrical Procedures and Breast-Feeding Practices," *International Journal of Obstetric Anesthesia*, 13, no. 1 (2004): 25–29.

9. See note 6 above.

10. Andrea Fuller et al., "Obstetric Anesthesia Workforce Survey: Thirty-Year Update," (lecture, American Society of Anesthesiologists Annual Meeting, San Diego, CA, October 14, 2013).

11. M. Van de Velde, "Modern Neuraxial Labor Analgesia: Options for Initiation, Maintenance and Drug Selection," *Revista Española de Anestesiología y Reanimación* 56, no. 9 (2009): 546–61; Mohamed Taha Ismail and Maher Z. Hassanin, "Neuraxial Analgesia versus Intravenous Remifentanil for Pain Relief in Early Labor in Nulliparous Women," *Archives of Gynecology and Obstetrics* 286 (2012): 1375–81.

12. Katherine Arendt and Scott Segal, "Why Epidurals Do Not Always Work," *Reviews in Obstetrics and Gynecology* 1, no. 2 (2008): 49–55; M. Van de Velde, "Modern Neuraxial Labor Analgesia: Options for Initiation, Maintenance and Drug Selection," *Revista Española de Anestesiología y Reanimación* 56, no. 9 (2009): 546–61.

13. Katherine Arendt and Scott Segal, "Why Epidurals Do Not Always Work," *Reviews in Obstetrics and Gynecology* 1, no. 2 (2008): 49–55.

# Chapter 14: When Childbirth Becomes Complicated

1. Stephen T. Chasen and Frank A. Chervenak, "Twin Pregnancy: Labor and Delivery" *UptoDate* (2015), http://www.uptodate.com/contents/twin-pregnancy-labor-and-delivery.

2. F. C. Brownfoot et al., "Different Corticosteroids and Regimens for Accelerating Fetal Lung Maturation for Women at Risk of Preterm Birth," Cochrane Database of Systematic Reviews, no. 8 (2013), doi:10.1002/14651858.CD6764.pubs.

3. J. P. Neilson, H. M West, and T. Dowswell, "Betamimetics for Inhibiting Preterm Labour," Cochrane Database of Systematic Reviews, no. 2 (2014), doi:10.1002/14651858.CD004352.pub3.

4. Vicki Flenady et al., "Calcium Channel Blockers for Inhibiting Preterm Labour and Birth," Cochrane Database of Systematic Reviews, no. 2 (2014), doi:10.1002/14651858.CD002255.pub2.

5. Vicki Flenady et al., "Oxytocin Receptor Antagonists for Inhibiting Preterm Labour," Cochrane Database of Systematic Reviews, no. 6 (2014), doi:10.1002/14651858.CD004452.pub3.

6. American Congress of Obstetricians and Gynecologists and the Society for Maternal-Fetal Medicine, *Obstetric Care Consensus: Safe Prevention of the Primary Cesarean Delivery* (Washington, DC: American Congress of Obstetricians and Gynecologists, 2014), http://www.acog.org/Resources-And-Publications/Obstetric-Care-Consensus-Series/Safe-Prevention-of-the-Primary-Cesarean-Delivery; World Health Organization, *WHO Recommendations for Induction of Labour* (Geneva: World Health Organization, 2011), http://apps.who.int/iris/bitstream/10665/44531/1/9789241501156_eng.pdf.

7. Jennifer M. Walsh and Fionnuala McAuliffe, "Prediction and Prevention of the Macrosomic Fetus," *European Journal of Obstetrics & Gynecology and Reproductive Biology* 162, no. 2 (2012): 125–30; American Congress of Obstetricians and Gynecologists, "Fetal Macrosomia," *Obstetrics & Gynecology* 96, no. 5 (November 2000), reaffirmed 2015, http://www.acog.org/-/media/List-of-Titles/PBListOfTitles.pdf.

8. American Congress of Obstetricians and Gynecologists and the Society for Maternal-Fetal Medicine, *Obstetric Care Consensus: Safe Prevention of the Primary Cesarean Delivery* (Washington, DC: American Congress of Obstetricians and Gynecologists, 2014), http://www.acog.org/Resources-And-Publications/Obstetric-Care-Consensus-Series/Safe-Prevention-of-the-Primary-Cesarean-Delivery.

9. W. Grobman, "Elective Induction: When? Ever?" *Clinical Obstetrics and Gynecology* 50, no. 2 (2007): 537–46; C. Le Ray et al., "Elective Induction of Labor: Failure to Follow Guidelines and Risk of Cesarean Delivery," *Acta Obstetricia et Gynecologica Scandinavica* 86, no. 6 (2007): 657–65.

10. American Congress of Obstetricians and Gynecologists, *Frequently Asked Questions: Elective Delivery before 39 Weeks* (Washington, DC: American Congress of Obstetricians and Gynecologists, June 2013), accessed March 25, 2015, http://www.acog.org/-/media/For-Patients/faq181.pdf; W. Grobman, "Elective Induction: When? Ever?" *Clinical Obstetrics and Gynecology* 50, no. 2 (2007): 537–46.

11. See note 8 above.

12. Joyce A Martin et al., "Births: Final Data for 2013," National Vital Statistics Reports 64, no. 1 (January 2015), http://www.cdc.gov/nchs/data/nvsr/nvsr64/nvsr64_01.pdf.

13. Kelly S. Gibson, Thaddeus P. Waters, and Jennifer L. Bailit, "Maternal and Neonatal Outcomes in Electively Induced Low-Risk Term Deliveries," *American Journal of Obstetrics & Gynecology* 211, no. 3 (2014): 249.e1–16.

14. Anjel Vahratian et al., "Labor Progression and Risk of Cesarean Delivery in Electively Induced Nulliparas," *Obstetrics and Gynecology* 105, no. 4 (2005): 698–704.

15. Anthony J. Kelly, Josephine Kavanagh, and Jane Thomas, "Castor Oil, Bath and/or Enema for Cervical Priming and Induction of Labour," Cochrane Database of Systematic Reviews, no. 7 (July 2013), doi:10.1002/14651858.CD003099.pub2.

16. Josephine Kavanagh, Anthony J. Kelly, and Jane Thomas, "Breast Stimulation for Cervical Ripening and Induction of Labour," Cochrane Database of Systematic Reviews, no. 4 (July 2005), doi:10.1002/14651858.CD003392.pub2 (2005).

17. See note 15 above.

18. Caroline Smith, Caroline Crowther, and Suzanne J. Grant, "Acupuncture for Induction of Labour," Cochrane Database of Systematic Reviews, no. 8 (August 2013), doi:10.1002/14651858. CD002962.pub3.

19. Marta Jozwiak et al., "Mechanical Methods for Induction of Labour," Cochrane Database of Systematic Reviews, no. 3 (March 2012), doi: 10.1002/14651858.CD001233.pub2; C. E. Lim, R. W. Ng, and K. Xu, "Nonhormonal Methods for Induction of Labour," *Current Opinion in Obstetrics and Gynecology* 25, no. 6 (2013): 441–47, doi:10.1097/GCO.0000000000000027.

20. Michel Boulvain , Catalin M. Stan, and Oliver Irion, "Membrane Sweeping for Induction of Labour," Cochrane Database of Systematic Reviews, no. 1 (January 2005), doi:10.1002/14651858. CD000451.pub2 http://www.ncbi.nlm.nih.gov/pubmed/15674873.

21. Rebecca M. D. Smyth, Carolyn Markham, and Therese Dowswell, "Amniotomy for Shortening Spontaneous Labour," Cochrane Database of Systematic Reviews, no. 6 (June 2013), doi:10.1002/14651858.CD006167.pub4.

22. Yvonne W. Cheng, Brian L. Shaffer, and Aaron B. Caughey, "Associated Factors and Outcomes of Persistent Occiput Posterior Position: A Retrospective Cohort Study from 1976 to 2001," *Journal of Maternal-Fetal and Neonatal Medicine* 19, no. 9 (2006): 563–68.

23. G. Justus Hofmeyr, A Metin Gülmezoglu,and Cynthia Pileggi, "Vaginal Misoprostol for Cervical Ripening and Induction of Labour," Cochrane Database of Systematic Reviews, no. 10 (October 2010), doi:10.1002/14651858.CD000941.pub2; Deborah A. Wing et al., "Misoprostol Vaginal Insert for Successful Labor Induction: A Randomized Controlled Trial," Obstetrics & Gynecology 117, no. 3 (2011): 533–41.

24. American Congress of Obstetricians and Gynecologists, "Induction of Labor," *Obstetrics & Gynecology* 114:386–97(August 2009), reaffirmed 2015, http://www.acog.org/-/media/List-of-Titles/PBListOfTitles.pdf.

25. G. Justus Hofmeyr, A Metin Gülmezoglu,and Cynthia Pileggi, "Vaginal Misoprostol for Cervical Ripening and Induction of Labour," Cochrane Database of Systematic Reviews, no. 10 (October 2010), doi:10.1002/14651858.CD000941.pub2; Zarko Alfirevic, Nasreen Aflaifel, and Andrew Weeks, "Oral Misoprostol for Induction of Labour," Cochrane Database of Systematic Reviews, no. 6 (June 2014), doi:10.1002/14651858.CD001338.pub3.

26. Mandisa Singata, Joan Tranmer, and Gillian M. L. Gyte, "Restricting Oral Fluid and Food Intake during Labour," Cochrane Database of Systematic Reviews, no. 8 (2013), doi:10.1002/14651858. CD003930.pub3.

27. Emanuel A. Friedman, "Graphic Analysis of Labor," *Bulletin of the American Congress of Nurse-Midwifery* 4, no. 3–4 (1959): 94–105.

28. Jun Zhang et al., "Contemporary Patterns of Spontaneous Labor with Normal Neonatal Outcomes," *Obstetrics & Gynecology* 116, no. 6 (2010): 1281–87.

29. See note 8 above.

30. Brian L. Shaffer et al., "Manual Rotation to Reduce Caesarean Delivery in Persistent Occiput Posterior or Transverse Position," Journal of Maternal-Fetal and Neonatal Medicine 24, no. 1 (2011): 65–72.

31. Penny Simkin, "The Fetal Occiput Posterior Position: State of the Science and a New Perspective," *Birth* 37, no. 1 (2010): 61–71; Penny Simkin and Ruth Ancheta, *The Labor Progress Handbook: Early Interventions to Prevent and Treat Dystocia*, 3rd ed. (Oxford: Wiley-Blackwell, 2011).

32. Penny Simkin and Michael Klein, "Nonpharmacologic Approaches to Management of Labor Pain," *UpToDate* (2014): http://www. uptodate.com/contents/nonpharmacologic-approaches-to-management-of-labor-pain.

33. J.G.B. Russell, "The Rationale of Primitive Delivery Positions," *British Journal of Obstetrics and Gynaecology* 89, no. 9 (1982): 712–15.

34. Penny Simkin, "The Fetal Occiput Posterior Position: State of the Science and a New Perspective," *Birth* 37, no. 1 (2010): 61–71; Penny Simkin and Ruth Ancheta, *The Labor Progress Handbook: Early Interventions to Prevent and Treat Dystocia*, 3rd ed. (Oxford: Wiley-Blackwell, 2011); D. M. Sherer et al., "Intrapartum Fetal Head Position I: Comparison between Transvaginal Digital Examination and Transabdominal Ultrasound Assessment during the Active Stage of Labor," *Ultrasound in Obstetrics & Gynecology* 19 (2002): 258–63; S. Akmal et al., "Intrapartum Sonography to Determine Fetal Head Position," *Journal of Maternal-Fetal and Neonatal Medicine* 12, no. 3 (2002) 172–77; A. P. Souka et al., "Intrapartum Ultrasound for the Examination of the Fetal Head Position in Normal and Obstructed Labor," *Journal of Maternal-Fetal and Neonatal Medicine* 13, no. 1 (2003) 59–63; S. Akmal et al., "Comparison of Transvaginal Digital Examination with Intrapartum Sonography to Determine Fetal Head Position before Instrumental Delivery," *Ultrasound in Obstetrics & Gynecology* 21, no. 5 (2003): 437–40.

35. See note 8 above.

36. Guillermo Carroli and Luciano Mignini, "Episiotomy for Vaginal Birth." Cochrane Database of Systematic Reviews, no. 1 (January 2009), doi:10.1002/14651858.CD000081.pub2. Review.

37. Joyce A. Martin, "Births: Final Data for 2012," National Vital Statistics Reports 62, no. 9 (December 2013), http://www.cdc.gov/ nchs/data/nvsr/nvsr62/nvsr62_09.pdf.

38. World Health Organization, *WHO Recommendations for the Prevention and Treatment of Postpartum Haemorrhage Guidelines* (Geneva, Switzerland: World Health Organization Press, 2012), http://apps.who.int/iris/bitstream/10665/75411/1/9789241548502_ eng.pdf; American Congress of Obstetricians and Gynecologists, *Optimizing Protocols in Obstetrics: Management of Obstetric Hemorrhage*, Series 2 (Washington, DC: American Congress of Obstetricians and Gynecologists, 2012), http://www.acog.org/ About_ACOG/ACOG_Districts/~/media/Districts/District%20II/ PDFs/Final_Hemorrhage_Web.pdf.

39. Richard G. Lynch, "Surfactant and RDS in Premature Infants," *The FASEB Journal* 18, no. 13 (2004), www.fasebj.org/cgi/content/full/18/13/1624e.

40. Deborah L. Davis and Mara T. Stein, *Parent: You and Your Baby in the NICU*, March of Dimes booklet (2002).

41. S. Ludington-Hoe and S. K. Golant, *Kangaroo Care: The Best You Can Do to Help Your Preterm Infant* (New York: Bantam Books, 1993).

## Chapter 15: All about Cesarean Birth

1. American Congress of Obstetricians and Gynecologists and the Society for Maternal-Fetal Medicine, *Obstetric Care Consensus: Safe Prevention of the Primary Cesarean Delivery* (Washington, DC: American Congress of Obstetricians and Gynecologists, 2014), http://www.acog.org/Resources-And-Publications/Obstet-

ric-Care-Consensus-Series/Safe-Prevention-of-the-Primary-Cesarean-Delivery.

2. José Villar et al., "Maternal and Neonatal Individual Risks and Benefits Associated with Caesarean Delivery: Multicentre Prospective Study," *BMJ* 335 (2007): 1025; Childbirth Connection, *What Every Pregnant Woman Needs to Know about Cesarean Section* (2012), http://www.childbirthconnection.org/pdfs/cesareanbooklet.pdf; National Institutes of Health, "NIH State-of-the-Science Conference on Cesarean Delivery on Maternal Request: NIH Consensus and State-of-the-Science Statements" 23, no. 1 (2006), https://consensus.nih.gov/2006/cesareanstatement.pdf; National Institute for Clinical Excellence, "Cesarean Section," November 2011, https://www.nice.org.uk/guidance/cg132; Marian F. MacDorman et al., "Infant and Neonatal Mortality for Primary Cesarean and Vaginal Births to Women with 'No Indicated Risk,'" *Birth* 33, no. 3 (2006): 175–82; J. Villar et al., "Caesarean Delivery Rates and Pregnancy Outcomes: The 2005 WHO Global Survey on Maternal and Perinatal Health in Latin America," *Lancet* 367, no. 9525 (2006): 1819–29; Shiliang Liu et al., "Maternal Mortality and Severe Morbidity Associated with Low-Risk Planned Cesarean Delivery versus Planned Vaginal Delivery at Term," *CMAJ* 176, no. 4 (2007): 455–60.

3. Shiliang Liu et al., "Maternal Mortality and Severe Morbidity Associated with Low-Risk Planned Cesarean Delivery versus Planned Vaginal Delivery at Term," *CMAJ* 176, no. 4 (2007): 455–60.

4. Marian F. MacDorman et al., "Infant and Neonatal Mortality for Primary Cesarean and Vaginal Births to Women with 'No Indicated Risk,'" *Birth* 33, no. 3 (2006): 175–82.

5. National Institute for Clinical Excellence, "Cesarean Section," November 2011, https://www.nice.org.uk/guidance/cg132.

6. AIDS Info, "Recommendations for Use of Antiretroviral Drugs in Pregnant HIV-1-Infected Women for Maternal Health and Interventions to Reduce Perinatal HIV Transmission in the United States," last updated August 6, 2015, http://aidsinfo.nih.gov/guidelines/html/3/perinatal-guidelines/182/transmission-and-mode-of-delivery.

7. American Congress of Obstetricians, *Obstetric Care Consensus: Cesarean Delivery on Maternal Request* (Washington, DC: American Congress of Obstetricians and Gynecologists, 2013), http://www.acog.org/Resources_And_Publications/Committee_Opinions/Committee_on_Obstetric_Practice/Cesarean_Delivery_on_Maternal_Request.

8. José Villar et al., "Maternal and Neonatal Individual Risks and Benefits Associated with Caesarean Delivery: Multicentre Prospective Study," *BMJ* 335 (2007): 1025.

9. American Congress of Obstetricians and Gynecologists and the Society for Maternal-Fetal Medicine, *Obstetric Care Consensus: Safe Prevention of the Primary Cesarean Delivery* (Washington, DC: American Congress of Obstetricians and Gynecologists, 2014), http://www.acog.org/Resources-And-Publications/Obstetric-Care-Consensus-Series/Safe-Prevention-of-the-Primary-Cesarean-Delivery.

10. American Congress of Obstetricians and Gynecologists, *Intrapartum Fetal Heart Rate Monitoring: Nomenclature, Interpretation, and General Management Principles*, ACOG Practice Bulletin No. 106, July 2009, http://www.ncbi.nlm.nih.gov/pubmed/19546798.

11. José Villar et al., "Maternal and Neonatal Individual Risks and Benefits Associated with Caesarean Delivery: Multicentre Prospective Study," *BMJ* 335 (2007): 1025.

12. Maria Gloria Dominguez-Bello, quoted in "Research: Could Birth-Canal Bacteria Help C-Section Babies?" by Carey Goldberg, WBUR's Common Health Reform and Reality, June 25, 2014, http://commonhealth.wbur.org/2014/06/birth-canal-bacteria-c-section.

13. Mughina Siddiqui et al., "Complications of Exteriorized Compared with In Situ Uterine Repair at Cesarean Delivery Under Spinal Anesthesia," *Obstetrics & Gynecology* 110, no. 3 (2007): 570–75.

14. Deirdre J. Lyell et al., "Peritoneal Closure at Primary Cesarean Delivery and Adhesions," *Obstetrics & Gynecology* 106, no. 2 (2005): 275–80; Kelly J. Hamel, "Incidence of Adhesions at Repeat Cesarean Delivery," *American Journal of Obstetrics and Gynecology* 196, no. 5 (May 2007): e31–32.

15. Dolar S. Patolia et al., "Early Feeding after Cesarean: Randomized Trial," *Obstetrics & Gynecology* 98, no. 1 (2001): 113–16; W. Teoh, M. Shah, C. Mah, "A Randomised Controlled Trial on Beneficial Effects of Early Feeding Post-Cesarean Delivery Under Regional Anesthesia," *Singapore Medical Journal* 48, no. 2 (2007): 152–57.

16. Jan Riordan and Karen Wambach, *Breastfeeding and Human Lactation*, 4th ed. (Sudbury, MA: Jones and Bartlett Publishers, 2005): 204; Gabriel M. Leung, Tai-Ling Lam, and Lai-Ming Ho, "Breast-Feeding and Its Relation to Smoking and Mode of Delivery," *Obstetrics & Gynecology* 99, no. 5, part 1 (2002): 785–94; Kathryn G. Dewey et al., "Risk Factors for Suboptimal Infant Breastfeeding Behavior, Delayed Onset of Lactation, and Excess Neonatal Weight Loss," *Pediatrics* 112, no. 3, part 1 (2003): 607–19; Rafael Pérez-Escamilla, Irene Maulén-Radovan, and Kathryn G. Dewey, "The Association between Cesarean Delivery and Breast-Feeding Outcomes among Mexican Women," *American Journal of Public Health* 86, no. 6 (1996): 832–36; P. Ever-Hadani et al., "Breast Feeding in Israel: Maternal Factors Associated with Choice and Duration," *Journal of Epidemiology Community Health* 48, no. 3 (1994): 281–85.

17. National Institutes of Health, Consensus Development Statement, "NIH Consensus Development Conference Statement on Vaginal Birth after Cesarean: New Insights," vol. 27, no. 3 (March 2010), http://consensus.nih.gov/2010/ images/vbac/vbac_statement.pdf; American Congress of Obstetricians and Gynecologists, *Vaginal Birth after Previous Cesarean Delivery*, ACOG Practice Bulletin No. 115, August 2010, http://www.acog.org/Resources-And-Publications/Practice-Bulletins/Committee-on-Practice-Bulletins-Obstetrics/Vaginal-Birth-After-Previous-Cesarean-Delivery.

18. National Institutes of Health, Consensus Development Statement, "NIH Consensus Development Conference Statement on Vaginal Birth after Cesarean: New Insights," vol. 27, no. 3 (March 2010), http://consensus.nih.gov/2010/ images/vbac/vbac_statement.pdf.

19. See note 18 above.

20. See note 18 above.

21. See note 18 above.

22. Agency for Healthcare Research and Quality, *Vaginal Birth after Cesarean: New Insights*, AHRQ Publication Number 10-E003 (March 2010), http://www.ahrq.gov/sites/default/files/wysiwyg/research/findings/evidence-based-reports/vbacup-evidence-report.pdf; National Institutes of Health, Consensus Development Statement, "NIH Consensus Development Conference Statement on Vaginal Birth after Cesarean: New Insights," vol. 27, no. 3 (March 2010), http://consensus.nih.gov/2010/ images/vbac/vbac_statement.pdf.

23. J. Smith, F. Plaat, and N. M. Fisk, "The Natural Caesarean: A Woman-Centred Technique," *BJOG* 115, no. 8 (2008): 1037–42.

24. Childbirth Connection, "VBAC or Repeat C-Section," last updated November 16, 2012, http://www.childbirthconnection.org/article.asp?ck=10214.

25. International Cesarean Awareness Network, "My Hospital Is Not Allowing VBAC," January 2014, http://www.ican-online.org/wp-content/uploads/2014/06/My-Hospital-Is-Not-Allowing-VBAC.pdf.

26. See note 24 above.

27. American Congress of Obstetricians and Gynecologists, Clinical Management Guidelines for Obstetrician-Gynecologists: Vaginal Birth after Previous Cesarean Delivery, ACOG Practice Bulletin 5, July 1999.

28. Richard G. Roberts et al., "Changing Policies on Vaginal Birth after Cesarean: Impact on Access," *Birth* 34, no. 4 (2007): 316–22; National Institutes of Health, Consensus Development Statement, "NIH Consensus Development Conference Statement on Vaginal Birth after Cesarean: New Insights," vol. 27, no. 3 (March 2010), http://consensus.nih.gov/2010/ images/vbac/vbac_statement.pdf.

29. Eugene DeClercq et al., *Listening to Mothers II: Report of the Second National U.S. Survey of Women's Childbearing Experiences* (New York: Childbirth Connection, 2006), http://www.childbirth-connection.org/pdfs/LTMII_report.pdf.

30. Alan T. N. Tita et al., "Timing of Elective Repeat Cesarean Delivery at Term and Neonatal Outcomes," *New England Journal of Medicine* 360, no. 2 (2009): 111–20.

# Chapter 16: What Life Is Like for a New Parent

1. Centers for Disease Control and Prevention, "Cervical Cancer Screen Guidelines for Average-Risk Women," accessed September 20, 2015, http://www.cdc.gov/cancer/cervical/pdf/guidelines.pdf.

2. American Cancer Society, "American Cancer Society Recommendations for Early Breast Cancer Detection in Women without Breast Symptoms," last revised August 2015, http://www.cancer.org/cancer/breastcancer/moreinformation/breastcancerearlydetection/breast-cancer-early-detection-acs-recs; American Congress of Obstetricians and Gynecologists, *Frequently Asked Questions: Mammography and Other Screening Tests for Breast Problems* (Washington, DC: American Congress of Obstetricians and Gynecologists, April 2015), http://www.acog.org/Patients/FAQs/Mammography-and-Other-Screening-Tests-for-Breast-Problems.

3. US Preventive Services Task Force, "Final Recommendation Statement Breast Cancer: Screening, November 2009," http://www.uspreventiveservicestaskforce.org/Page/Document/RecommendationStatementFinal/breast-cancer-screening.

4. Julie Tupler, *Maternal Fitness: Preparing for a Healthy Pregnancy, an Easier Labor, and a Quick Recovery* (New York: Fireside 1996); Julie Tupler and Jodie Gould, *Lose Your Mummy Tummy* (Boston: Da Capo Press, 2005).

5. Elizabeth Noble, *Essential Exercises for the Childbearing Year: A Guide to Health and Comfort before and after Your Baby Is Born*, 4th ed. (Nottingham, England: New Life Images 1995).

6. See note 5 above.

# Chapter 17: When Postpartum Becomes Complicated

1. Cathryn M. Glazener et al., "Conservative Management of Persistent Postnatal Urinary and Faecal Incontinence: Randomised Controlled Trial," *BMJ* 323 (15 September 2001): 593–96.

2. Cathryn M. Glazener et al., "Conservative Management of Persistent Postnatal Urinary and Faecal Incontinence: Randomised Controlled Trial," *BMJ* 323 (15 September 2001): 593–96; Siv Mørkved and Kari Bø, "Prevalence and Treatment of Post Partum

Urinary Incontinence," *Norsk Epidemiologi* 7, no.1 (1997): 123–27.

3. C. MacArthur, D. E. Bick, and M. R. Keighley, "Faecal Incontinence after Childbirth," *British Journal of Obstetrics and Gynaecology* 104, no. 1 (1997): 46–50.

4. See note 1 above.

5. E. J. Corwin, L. E. Murray-Kolb, and J. L. Beard, "Low Hemoglobin Level Is a Risk Factor for Postpartum Depression," *Journal of Nutrition* 133, no. 12 (2003): 4139–42.

6. Laura A. Matthys et al., "Delayed Postpartum Preeclampsia: An Experience of 151 Cases," *American Journal of Obstetrics and Gynecology* 190, no. 5 (2004): 1464–66.

7. Laura Magee and Peter von Dadelszen, "Prevention and Treatment of Postpartum Hypertension," Cochrane Database of Systematic Reviews, no. 4 (April 2013), doi:10.1002/14651858.CD004351.pub3.

8. Penny Simkin, "Birth Trauma: Definition and Statistics," Prevention and Treatment of Traumatic Childbirth, accessed September 20, 2015, http://pattch.org/resource-guide/traumatic-births-and-ptsd-definition-and-statistics.

9. Pam Belluck, "'Thinking of Ways to Harm Her:' New Findings on Timing and Range of Maternal Mental Illness," *New York Times*, June 16, 2014, http://www.nytimes.com/2014/06/16/health/thinking-of-ways-to-harm-her.html?src=longreads&_r=1.

10. Heather A. Bennett et al., "Depression during Pregnancy," *Clinical Drug Investigation* 24, no. 3 (2004): http://www.medscape.com/viewarticle/474390_3.

11. Rex Gentry, "Psychiatric Complications in Pregnancy and Postpartum," presentation at REACHE conference (November 2002), http://depts.washington.edu/hcsats/FCAP/resources/Psychiatric%20Complications%20of%20Pregnancy%20by%20Rex%20Gentry,%20MD.pdf.

12. See note 5 above.

13. Kathleen Kendall-Tackett, "A New Paradigm for Depression in New Mothers: The Central Role of Inflammation and How Breastfeeding and Anti-inflammatory Treatments Protect Maternal Mental Health," *International Breastfeeding Journal* 2, no. 6 (2007): 1–14, doi:10.1186/1746-4358-2-6.

14. Jean M. Twenge, W. Keith Campbell, and Craig A. Foster, "Parenthood and Marital Satisfaction: A Meta-analysis Review," *Journal of Marriage and Family* 65, no. 3 (2003): 574–83; Philip A. Cowan and Carolyn Pape Cowan, *Normative Family Transitions, Normal Family Process, and Healthy Child Development in Normal Family Processes*, 3rd ed. (New York: Guilford Publications, 2003).

15. Carolyn Pape Cowan and Philip A. Cowan, *When Partners Become Parents: The Big Life Change for Couples*, rev. ed. (London: Routledge 2000); Philip A. Cowan and Carolyn Pape Cowan, *Normative Family Transitions, Normal Family Process, and Healthy Child Development in Normal Family Processes*, 3rd ed. (New York: Guilford Publications, 2003).

16. Carolyn Pape Cowan and Philip A. Cowan, "Interventions to Ease the Transition to Parenthood: Why They Are Needed and What They Can Do," *Family Relations* 44, no. 4 (1995): 412–14; Carolyn Pape Cowan and Philip A. Cowan, *When Partners Become Parents: The Big Life Change for Couples*, rev. ed. (London: Routledge 2000); Martha J. Cox et al., "Marriage, Adult Adjustment, and Early Parenting," *Child Development* 60, no. 5 (1989): 1015–24.

17. National Coalition Against Domestic Violence, "Statistics," accessed September 20, 2015, http://www.ncadv.org/learn/statistics

18. Andrea Carlson Gielen et al., "Interpersonal Conflict and Physical Violence during the Childbearing Year," *Social Science & Medicine* 39, no. 6 (1994): 781–87.

## Chapter 18: Caring for Your Baby

1. Raylene Phillips, "Uninterrupted Skin-to-Skin Contact Immediately after Birth," *Newborn & Infant Nursing Reviews* 13, no. 2 (2013): 67–72.

2. American Academy of Pediatrics, Committee on Fetus and Newborn, "Controversies Concerning Vitamin K and the Newborn," *Pediatrics* 112, no. 1 (2003): 191–92; American Academy of Pediatrics and American Congress of Obstetricians and Gynecologists, *Guidelines for Perinatal Care*, 7th ed., (Elk Grove Village, IL: American Academy of Pediatrics 2012).

3. Dorothy L. Moore et al., "Preventing Opthalmia Neonatorum," *Paediatrics & Child* Health 20, no. 2 (2015): 93–96, http://www.cps.ca/en/documents/position/ophthalmia-neonatorum.

4. See note 3 above.

5. American Academy of Pediatrics, Committee on Genetics, "Newborn Screening Fact Sheet," *Pediatrics* 118, no. 3 (2006): 934–63.

6. Jean H. Dussault, "Screening for Congenital Hypothyroidism," *Clinical Obstetrics and Gynecology* 40, no. 1 (March 1997): 117–23.

7. Maria Owings et al., *Trends in Circumcision for Male Newborns in U.S. Hospitals: 1979–2010*, Centers for Disease Control and Prevention, last updated August 2013, http://www.cdc.gov/nchs/data/hestat/circumcision_2013/Circumcision_2013.htm.

8. American Academy of Pediatrics, Task Force on Circumcision, "Circumcision Policy Statement," *Pediatrics* 130, no. 3 (2012): 585–86.

9. See note 8 above.

10. Centers for Disease Control and Prevention, *Male Circumcision*, accessed September 20, 2015, http://www.cdc.gov/hiv/pdf/prevention_research_malecircumcision.pdf.

11. See note 10 above.

12. See note 10 above.

13. Teresa To et al., "Cohort Study on Circumcision of Newborn Boys and Subsequent Risk of Urinary-Tract Infection," *Lancet* 352, no. 9143 (1998): 1813–16.

14. Alfredo Pisacane et al., "Breast-feeding and Urinary Tract Infection," *Journal of Pediatrics* 120, no. 1 (1992): 87–89.

15. Helen A. Weiss, "Complications of Circumcision in Male Neonates, Infants and Children: A Systematic Review," *BMC Urology* 10, no. 2 (December 2010), doi:10.1186/1471-2490-10-2.

16. American Academy of Pediatrics, Committee on the Fetus and Newborn and Section on Surgery and Canadian Pediatric Society and Fetus and Newborn Committee, "Policy Statement: Prevention and Management of Pain in the Neonate: An Update," *Pediatrics* 118, no. 5 (2006): 2231–41.

17. Barbara Brady-Fryer, Natasha Wiebe, and Janice A. Lander, "Pain Relief for Neonatal Circumcision," Cochrane Database of Systematic Reviews, no. 3 (July 2004), doi:10.1002/14651858.CD004217.pub2.

18. Howard J. Stang, "Beyond Dorsal Penile Nerve Block: A More Humane Circumcision," *Pediatrics* 100, no. 2 (1997): e3, doi:10.1542/peds.100.2.e3.

19. A. Taddio, "Pain Management for Neonatal Circumcision," *Paediatric Drugs* 3, no. 2 (2001): 101–11.

20. Governors Highway Safety Association, "Child Passenger Safety Laws," September 2015, http://www.ghsa.org/html/stateinfo/laws/childsafety_laws.html.

21. Valérie Marchand and the Canadian Paediatric Society, Nutrition and Gastroenterology Committee, "Using probiotics in the paediatric population," *Paediatrics & Child Health* 17, no. 10 (December 2012): 575.

22. T. Penny-MacGillivray, "A Newborn's First Bath," *Journal of Obstetric, Gynecologic and Neonatal Nursing* 25 (1996): 481–87; S. G. Cole et al., "Tub Baths or Sponge Baths for Newborn Infants?" *Mother Baby Journal* 4, no. 3 (1999): 39–43.

23. Harvey Karp, *The Happiest Baby on the Block: The New Way to Calm Crying and Help Your Baby Sleep Longer* (New York: Bantam, 2002).

24. Patricia Franco et al., "Influence of Swaddling on Sleep and Arousal Characteristics of Healthy Infants," *Pediatrics* 115, no. 5 (2005): 1307–11.

25. T. Berry Brazelton, *Touchpoints Birth to 3* (Boston: Da Capo Press, 2006).

26. See note 25 above.

27. Morris A. Wessel et al., "Paroxysmal Fussing in Infancy, Sometimes Called 'Colic,'" *Pediatrics* 14, no.5 (1954): 421–35.

28. See note 21 above.

29. J. N. Critch and the Canadian Paediatric Society, Nutrition and Gastroenterology Committee, "Infantile Colic: Is There a Role for Dietary Interventions?" *Paediatrics & Child Health* 16, no. 1 (2011): 47–49.

30. T. J. Metcalf et al., "Simethicone and the Treatment of Infant Colic: A Randomized, Placebo-Controlled, Multicenter Trial," *Pediatrics* 94, no. 1 (1994): 29–34.

31. Bill Hesselmar et al., "Pacifier Cleaning Practices and Risk of Allergy Development," *Pediatrics* 131, no. 6 (2013): e1829–37.

32. Leo van Vlimmeren et al., "Risk Factors for Deformational Plagiocephaly at Birth and at 7 Weeks of Age: a Prospective Cohort Study," *Pediatrics* 119, no. 2 (2007): e408–18.

33. Marshall H. Klaus and Phyllis Klaus, *Your Amazing Newborn* (Cambridge, MA: Perseus Books, 1998).

34. J. G. Cole, "What Can Babies See at Birth?" *Mother Baby Journal* 2, no. 4 (1997): 45–47.

35. Margaret A. Maglione et al., "Safety of Vaccines Used for Routine Immunization of US Children: A Systematic Review," *Pediatrics*, July 1, 2014, doi:10.1542/peds.2014-1079.

36. Centers for Disease Control and Prevention, *Vaccine Excipient & Media Summary*, last updated February 2015, http://www.cdc.gov/vaccines/pubs/pinkbook/downloads/appendices/B/excipient-table-2.pdf.

37. Centers for Disease Control and Prevention, "Vaccines Do Not Cause Autism," last updated August 28, 2015, http://www.cdc.gov/vaccinesafety/concerns/autism.html.

38. M. Casati et al., "Safety of Use, Efficacy and Degree of Parental Satisfaction with the Nasal Aspirator Narhinel in the Treatment of Nasal Congestion in Babies," *Minerva Pediatrica* 59, no. 4 (2007): 315–25.

39. American Academy of Pediatrics, *SIDS and Other Sleep-Related Infant Deaths: Expansion of Recommendations for a Safe Infant Sleeping Environment, Policy Statement*, 2011, http://pediatrics.aappublications.org/content/early/2011/10/12/peds.2011-2284.full.pdf.

40. See note 39 above.

# Chapter 19: Feeding Your Baby

1. American Academy of Pediatrics, "Breastfeeding and the Use of Human Milk," *Pediatrics* 115, no. 2 (2005): 496–506, doi:10.1542/peds.2011-3552.

2. G. Bauer et al., "Breastfeeding and Cognitive Development of Three-Year-Old Children," *Psychological Reports* 68 (1991): 1281; R. A. Lawrence, "Can We Expect Greater Intelligence from Human Milk Feedings?" *Birth* 19, no. 2 (1992): 105–6; A. Lucas et al., "Randomized Trial of Early Diet in Preterm Babies and Later Intelligence Quotient," *British Medical Journal* 28 (1998): 1481–87; M. C. Temboury et al., "Influence of Breastfeeding on the Infant's Intellectual Development," *Journal of Pediatric Gastroenterology and Nutrition* 18 (1994): 32–36. Erik Lykke Mortenson et al., "The Association between Breastfeeding and Adult Intelligence," *Journal of the American Medical Association* 287, no. 18 (2002): 2365–71.

3. U. M. Saarinen and M. Kajosaari, "Breastfeeding as Prophylaxis against Atopic Disease: Prospective Follow-Up Study until 17 Years Old," *Lancet* 346, no. 8982 (1995): 1065–69; Frank R. Greer, Scott H. Sicherer, A. Wesley Burks, and the Committee on Nutrition and Section on Allergy and Immunology, "Effects of Early Nutritional Interventions on the Development of Atopic Disease in Infants and Children: The Role of Maternal Dietary Restriction, Breastfeeding, Timing of Introduction of Complementary Foods, and Hydrolyzed Formulas," *Pediatrics* 121, no. 1 (2008): 183–91.

4. American Academy of Pediatrics, "Breastfeeding and the Use of Human Milk," *Pediatrics* 115, no. 2 (2005): 496–506, doi:10.1542/peds.2011-3552.; A. Chen and W. J. Rogan, "Breastfeeding and the Risk of Postneonatal Death in the United States," *Pediatrics* 113, no. 5 (2004): e435–39.

5. American Academy of Pediatrics, "Breastfeeding and the Use of Human Milk," *Pediatrics* 115, no. 2 (2005): 496–506, doi:10.1542/peds.2011-3552.; E. A. Mitchell et al., "Results from the First Year of the New Zealand Cot Death Study," *New Zealand Medical Journal* 104 (1991): 71–75; M. Vennemann et al., "Does Breastfeeding Reduce the Risk of Sudden Infant Death Syndrome?" *Pediatrics* 123, no. 3 (2009).

6. American Academy of Pediatrics, "Breastfeeding and the Use of Human Milk," *Pediatrics* 115, no. 2 (2005): 496–506, doi:10.1542/peds.2011-3552.

7. P. A. Newcomb et al., "Lactation and a Reduced Risk of Premenopausal Breast Cancer," *New England Journal of Medicine* 330 (1994): 81–87; National Institutes of Health Consensus Conference, "Ovarian Cancer: Screening, Treatment, and Follow-Up," *Journal of the American Medical Association* 273, no. 6 (1995): 491–47; H. Jernstrom et al., "Breast-Feeding and the Risk of Breast Cancer in BRAC1 and BRAC2 Mutation Carriers," *Journal of National Cancer Institute* 96 (2004): 1094–98.

8. A. Perez et al., "Clinical Study of the Lactational Amenorrhoea Method for Family Planning," *Lancet* 339 (1992): 968–70.

9. P. Erwin, "To Use or Not Use Combined Hormonal Oral Contraceptives during Lactation," *Family Planning Perspectives* 26, no. 1 (1994): 26–33.

10. Geoffrey A. Weinberg, "The Dilemma of Postnatal Mother-to-Child Transmission of HIV: To Breastfeed or Not?" *Birth* 27, no. 3 (2000): 199–205; World Health Organization Collaborative Study Team on the Role of Breastfeeding and the Prevention of Infant Mortality, "Effect of Breastfeeding on Child Mortality Due to Infectious Diseases in Less Developed Countries: A Pooled Analysis," *Lancet* 355 (2000): 450–55; American Academy of Pediatrics, Committee on Infectious Diseases, *Red Book: Report of the Committee on Infectious Disease*, 25th ed., American Academy of Pediatrics (2000) https://www.aap.org/en-us/about-the-aap/Committees-Councils-Sections/Pages/Committee-on-Infectious-Diseases.aspx; Jennifer S. Read and the American Academy of Pediatrics, Committee on Pediatric AIDS, "Human Milk, Breastfeeding, and Transmission of Human Immunodeficiency Virus Type 1 in the United States," *Pediatrics* 112, no. 5 (2003): 1196–205.

11. Jan Riordan and Karen Wambach, *Breastfeeding and Human Lactation*, 4th ed. (Sudbury, MA: Jones and Bartlett Publishers, 2005).

12. Nancy Mohrbacher and Julie Stock, *The Breastfeeding Answer Book* (Schaumburg, IL: La Leche League International, 2003): 470–72.

13. See note 11 above.

14. D. T. Ramsay et al., "Anatomy of the Lactating Human Breast Redefined with Ultrasound Imaging," *Journal of Anatomy* 206, no. 6 (2005): 525–34.

15. Norman A. Grossl, "Supernumerary Breast Tissue: Historical Perspectives and Clinical Features," *Southern Medical Journal* 93, no. 1 (2000): 29–32.

16. D. T. Ramsay et al., "Ultrasound Imaging of Milk Ejection in the Breast of Lactating Women," *Pediatrics* 113, no. 2 (2004): 361–67.

17. C. J. Wilde et al., "Autocrine Regulation of Milk Secretion by a Protein in Milk," *Biochemical Journal* 305 (1995): 51–58.

18. See note 11 above.

19. M. C. Neville, "Studies in Human Lactation; Milk Volumes in Lactating Women during the Onset of Lactation and Full Lactation," *American Journal of Clinical Nutrition* 48, no. 6 (1988): 1375–86.

20. Steven E. Daly et al., "Degree of Breast Emptying Explains Changes in the Fat Content, but Not Fatty Acid Composition, of Human Milk," *Experimental Physiology* 78 (1993): 741–55.

21. See note 11 above.

22. See note 11 above.

23. Laura A. Basile et al., "The Effect of High-Dose Vitamin D Supplementation on Serum Vitamin D Levels and Milk Calcium Concentration in Lactating Women and Their Infants," *Breastfeeding Medicine* 1, no. 1 (2006): 1, 27–35; Bruce W. Hollis and Carol L. Wagner, "Assessment of Dietary Vitamin D Requirements during Pregnancy and Lactation," *American Journal of Clinical Nutrition* 79, no. 5 (2004): 717–26; Carol L. Wagner et al., "High-Dose Vitamin D3 Supplementation in a Cohort of Breastfeeding Mothers and Their Infants: A 6-Month Follow-Up Pilot Study," *Breastfeeding Medicine* 1, no. 2 (2006): 59–70; Carol L. Wagner, Frank R. Greer, and the Section on Breastfeeding and Committee on Nutrition, "Prevention of Rickets and Vitamin D Deficiency in Infants, Children, and Adolescents," *Pediatrics* 122, no. 5 (2008): 1142–52.

24. American Academy of Pediatrics, "Policy Statement: Iodine Deficiency, Pollutant Chemicals, and the Thyroid: New Information on an Old Problem," *Pediatrics* 133, no. 6 (2014): 1163–66; Angela

M. Leung, June 4, 2014, comment on American Academy of Pediatrics, "Policy Statement: Iodine Deficiency, Pollutant Chemicals, and the Thyroid: New Information on an Old Problem," http://pediatrics.aappublications.org/content/133/6/1163/reply#content-block.

25. See note 1 above.

26. American Academy of Pediatric Dentistry, *Policy on Use of Fluoride*, revised 2014, http://www.aapd.org/media/policies_guidelines/p_fluorideuse.pdf.

27. J. Moon and S. Humenick, "Breast Engorgement: Contributing Variables and Variables Amenable to Nursing Intervention," *Journal of Obstetric, Gynecologic, and Neonatal Nursing* 18, no. 4 (1989): 309–15; Y. Yamauchi and H. Yamanouchi, "Breast-Feeding Frequency during the First 24 Hours after Birth in Full-Term Neonates," *Pediatrics* 86 (1990): 171–75.

28. S. Phillips, "When Time Is of the Essence: Establishing Effective Breastfeeding before Early Discharge," *Mother Baby Journal* 1, no. 1 (1996): 15–19.

29. Marianne Neifert et al., "Nipple Confusion: Toward a Formal Definition," *Journal of Pediatrics* 126, no. 6 (1995): S125–29.

30. Betty C. Bowles et al., "Alternate Massage in Breastfeeding," *Genesis* 9 (1988): 5–9.

31. L. Righard and M. O. Alade, "Breastfeeding and the Use of Pacifiers," *Birth* 24, no. 2 (1997): 116–20; Cynthia R. Howard et al., "Randomized Clinical Trial of Pacifier Use and Bottle-Feeding or Cupfeeding and Their Effect on Breastfeeding," *Pediatrics* 111, no. 3: 511–18.

32. Gary Chan, *Lactation: The Breast-Feeding Manual for Health Professionals* (Valley Stream, NY: Precept Press, 1996); Institute of Medicine, *Nutrition during Lactation* (National Academy of Sciences, 1991): 86.

33. Laura A. Basile et al., "The Effect of High-Dose Vitamin D Supplementation on Serum Vitamin D Levels and Milk Calcium Concentration in Lactating Women and Their Infants," *Breastfeeding Medicine* 1, no. 1 (2006): 1, 27–35; Bruce W. Hollis and Carol L. Wagner, "Assessment of Dietary Vitamin D Requirements during Pregnancy and Lactation," *American Journal of Clinical Nutrition* 79, no. 5 (2004): 717–26; Carol L. Wagner et al., "High-Dose Vitamin D3 Supplementation in a Cohort of Breastfeeding Mothers and Their Infants: A 6-Month Follow-Up Pilot Study," *Breastfeeding Medicine* 1, no. 2 (2006): 59–70; Carol L. Wagner, Frank R. Greer, and the Section on Breastfeeding and Committee on Nutrition, "Prevention of Rickets and Vitamin D Deficiency in Infants, Children, and Adolescents," *Pediatrics* 122, no. 5 (2008): 1142–52; E. Reifsnider and S. L. Gill, "Nutrition for the Childbearing Years," *Journal of Obstetric, Gynecologic, and Neonatal Nursing* 29, no. 1 (2000): 50–51.

34. Julie A. Mennella and Gary K. Beauchamp, "Maternal Diet Alters the Sensory Qualities of Human Milk and the Nursling's Behavior," *Pediatrics* 88, no. 4 (1991): 737–44; Julie A. Mennella and Gary K. Beauchamp, "Early Flavor Experiences: Research Update," *Nutrition Reviews* 56, no. 7 (1998): 205–11.

35. See note 34 above.

36. Julie A. Mennella and Gary K. Beauchamp, "Effects of Beer on Breast-Fed Infants," *Journal of the American Medical Association* 269 (1993): 1635–36.

37. Institute of Medicine, *Nutrition during Lactation* (National Academy of Sciences, 1991): 73.

38. Institute of Medicine, *Nutrition during Lactation* (National Academy of Sciences, 1991): 86; Lois B. Duskieder et al., "Is Milk Production Impaired by Dieting during Lactation?" *American Journal of Clinical Nutrition* 59, no. 4 (1994): 833–40; A. Prentice et al., "Energy Requirements of Pregnant and Lactating Women," *European Journal of Clinical Nutrition* 50, no. 1 (1996): S82–111.

39. Mary Ziemer and Joseph Pigeon, "Skin Changes and Pain in the Nipples during the 1st Week of Lactation," *Journal of Obstetric, Gynecologic, and Neonatal Nursing* 22, no. 3 (1993): 247–56.

40. Human Milk Banking Association of North America, *Recommendations for Collection, Storage, and Handling of a Mother's Milk for Her Own Infant in the Hospital Setting* (1993); Academy of Breastfeeding Medicine, "ABM Clinical Protocol Number #8: Human Milk Storage Information for Home Use for Healthy Full-Term Infants" *Breastfeeding Medicine* 5, no. 3 (2010), http://www.bfmed.org/Media/Files/Protocols/Protocol%208%20-%20English%20revised%202010.pdf.

41. ABM Clinical Protocol Number #8: Human Milk Storage Information for Home Use for Healthy Full-Term Infants" *Breastfeeding Medicine* 5, no. 3 (2010), http://www.bfmed.org/Media/Files/Protocols/Protocol%208%20-%20English%20revised%202010.pdf.

42. Soria Eladak et al., "A New Chapter in the Bisphenol A Story: Bisphenol S and Bisphenol F Are Not Safe Alternatives to This Compound," *Fertility and Sterility* 103, no. 1 (2015): 11–21.

43. "How Much and How Often to Feed," Ask Dr. Sears, accessed September 20, 2015, http://www.askdrsears.com/topics/feeding-eating/bottle-feeding/how-much-and-how-often-feed.

44. American Academy of Pediatrics, Committee on Nutrition, *Pediatric Nutrition Handbook*, 6th ed. (American Academy of Pediatrics, 2009).

45. American Academy of Pediatrics, Committee on Nutrition, *Pediatric Nutrition Handbook*, 4th ed. (American Academy of Pediatrics, 1998): 236; Laurie Larson, "Warnings Fail to Slow Low Iron Formula Sales," *AAP News* 11, no. 3 (1995): 1–14; American Academy of Pediatrics, Committee on Nutrition, *Pediatric Nutrition Handbook*, 5th ed. (American Academy of Pediatrics, 2004).

46. American Academy of Pediatrics, Committee on Nutrition, *Pediatric Nutrition Handbook*, 4th ed. (American Academy of Pediatrics, 1998): 36.

47. American Academy of Pediatric Dentistry, Oral Health Policies, "Policy on Use of Fluoride," last updated 2014.

48. Centers for Disease Control and Prevention, "Overview: Infant Formula and Fluorosis," last updated July 31, 2015, http://www.cdc.gov/fluoridation/safety/infant_formula.htm.

# Chapter 20: When Breastfeeding Becomes Challenging

1. V. Cheryl Nicodem et al., "Do Cabbage Leaves Prevent Breast Engorgement? A Randomized, Controlled Study," *Birth* 20, no. 2 (1993): 61–64; K. Roberts, "A Comparison of Chilled Cabbage Leaves and Chilled Gelpaks in Reducing Breast Engorgement," *Journal of Human Lactation* 11, no. 1 (1995): 17–20; K. Roberts et al., "Effects of Cabbage Leaf Extract on Breast Engorgement," *Journal of Human Lactation* 114, no. 3 (1998): 231–36.

2. Jan Riordan and K. G. Auerbach, *Breastfeeding and Human Lactation*, 2nd ed., (Sudbury, MA: Jones and Bartlett, 1998): 294; Penny Simkin, "Intermittent Brachial Plexus Neuropathy Secondary to Breast Engorgement," *Birth* 15, no. 2 (1988): 102–4; Nancy Mohrbacher and Julie Stock, *The Breastfeeding Answer Book* (Schaumburg, IL: La Leche League International, 2003): 492–96.

3. American Academy of Pediatrics, Committee on Drugs, "The Transfer of Drugs and Other Chemicals into Human Milk," *Pediatrics* 108, no. 3 (2001): 776–89.

4. V. Coiro et al., "Inhibition by Ethanol of the Oxytocin Response to Breast Stimulation in Normal Women and the Role of Endogenous Opiods," *Acta Endocrinol* 126, no. 3 (1992): 213–16; C. Berlin et al., "Disposition of Dietary Caffeine in Milk, Saliva, and Plasma of Lactating Women," *Pediatrics* 73, no. 1 (1984): 59–63; A. Dahlstrom et al., "Nicotine and Cotinine Concentrations in the Nursing Mother and Her Infant," *Acta Paediatrica* 79, no. 2 (1990): 142–47.

5. Cheryl Tatano Beck and Sue Watson, "Impact of Birth Trauma on Breast-Feeding: A Tale of Two Pathways," *Nursing Research* 57, no. 4 (2008): 228–36.

6. E. Nissen et al., "Different Patterns of Oxytocin, Prolactin but Not Cortisol Release during Breastfeeding in Women Delivered by Caesarean Section or by the Vaginal Route," *Early Human Development* 45, no. 1–2 (1996): 103–18.

7. C. G. Victora et al., "Caesarean Section and Duration of Breastfeeding among Brazilians," *Archives of Disease in Childhood* 65, no. 6 (1990): 632–34; M. H. Kearney, L. R. Cronenwett, R. Reinhardt, "Cesarean Delivery and Breastfeeding Outcomes," *Birth* 317, no. 2 (1990): 97–103.

8. Annika Karlström et al., "Postoperative Pain after Cesarean Birth Affects Breastfeeding and Infant Care," *Journal of Obstetric, Gynecologic and Neonatal Nursing* 36, no. 5 (2007): 430–40.

9. E. Buescher, "Host Defense Mechanisms of Human Milk and Their Relations to Enteric Infections and Necrotizing Enterocolitis," *Clinical Perinatology* 21, no. 2 (1994): 247–62.

10. A. Lucas et al., "Breast Milk and Subsequent Intelligence Quotient in Children Born Preterm," *Lancet* 339 (1992): 261–64; A. Lucas et al., "Randomized Trial of Early Diet in Preterm Babies and Later Intelligence Quotient," *British Medical Journal* 317, no. 28 (1998): 1481–87.

11. S. Moscone and J. Moore, "Breastfeeding during Pregnancy," *Journal of Human Lactation* 9, no. 2 (1993): 83–88.

12. Centers for Disease Control, "Vaccines for Pregnant Women," last updated October 10, 2014, http://www.cdc.gov/vaccines/adults/rec-vac/pregnant.html.

13. I. Matheson and G. Rivrud, "The Effect of Smoking on Lactation and Infantile Colic," *Journal of the American Medical Association* 261, no. 1 (1989): 42–43.

14. Alistair Woodward et al., "Acute Respiratory Illness in Adelaide Children: Breastfeeding Modifies the Effect of Passive Smoking," *Journal of Epidemiology and Community Health* 44 (1990): 224–30.

# Chapter 21: When You're Pregnant Again

1. Jun Zhang et al., "Contemporary Patterns of Spontaneous Labor with Normal Neonatal Outcomes," Obstetrics & Gynecology 116, no. 6 (2010): 1281–87.

# Glossary

The following are terms that are used to describe pregnancy, childbirth, and newborn care. For further discussion of these terms and their definitions, see the pages noted within the parentheses.

**4-1-1 or 5-1-1 rule**
This rule means that your labor contractions are intense enough to require you to focus and breathe rhythmically through them, and are *four or five* minutes apart with each lasting at least *one minute* for a period of *one hour*. This pattern signals to you that your labor may be progressing and it's time to call your caregiver or birthplace.

**abnormal fetal heart rate**
Term used when your baby's heart rate isn't responding to contractions in a reassuring way. Doesn't necessarily indicate that something is wrong with your baby (there's a high rate of "false positives"); however, it does indicate the need for closer monitoring and a possible need for intervention in labor.

**active labor**
The second phase of the first stage of labor. When your cervix is dilated to 4 to 5 centimeters, your contractions usually reach the 4-1-1 or 5-1-1 pattern. During this phase, dilation usually speeds up, contractions typically become painful (but manageable), and labor progresses with each contraction.

**acupuncture**
An ancient Chinese medicine technique that uses needles placed at strategic points along meridians, or energy flow lines, in your body to guide it toward wellness and balance.

**advanced practice nurse practitioner**
A maternity caregiver who provides prenatal and postpartum care, but doesn't attend women during labor.

**afterpains**
As your uterus contracts after birth to its nonpregnant size (a process called involution), you may experience periods of discomfort or pain. Although this pain is common and isn't nearly as intense as labor contractions, you may need to use slow breathing to help manage it in the first few days.

**alveoli**
Glands in the breast that produce and store milk.

**amniocentesis**
A medical procedure in which a needle is used to withdraw a small amount of amniotic fluid from your uterus. A laboratory analyzes the surfactant levels in the fluid to determine whether your baby's lungs are mature enough to function outside your womb.

**amnioinfusion**
A procedure in which fluids are infused into your uterus to dilute any meconium that was expelled in the amniotic fluid , or to remove pressure on the cord caused by your baby's head or trunk.

**amniotic fluid**
The fluid that surrounds your baby in the amniotic sac. It protects your baby by absorbing bumps from the outside, maintaining an even temperature, providing a medium for easy movement, and allowing your baby to develop her lungs by "breathing" the fluid.

**amniotic sac**
Made up of the membranes (amnion and chorion) that create the sac that surrounds your baby. Also called "bag of waters."

**amniotomy**
See *artificial rupture of membranes (AROM)*.

**analgesia**
Any effect that reduces your perception of pain. In this book, this term is used to refer specifically to medications that act on the brain so you don't recognize pain stimuli or don't interpret them as pain.

**androgens**
Male hormones that signal the development of a baby boy's scrotum and penis.

**anemia**
A condition in which the number of red blood cells is lower than normal, reducing the blood's capacity to carry oxygen.

**anesthesia**
Indicates a loss of sensation, including pain sensation. Anesthetic medications block nerve endings from sending pain impulses to your brain.

**antibodies**
Proteins that protect your body from bacteria and toxins. During pregnancy and breastfeeding, your baby receives antibodies from you, which will protect him against diseases to which you're resistant or immune.

**Apgar score**
Within one minute after your baby's birth and again at five minutes, your caregiver will evaluate your baby's well-being by conducting this routine newborn assessment, which assesses how well she's adapting to life outside your womb.

**areola**
The darker skin surrounding each nipple.

**arrest of labor**
A condition in which labor stops progressing, as measured by cervical dilation.

**artificial rupture of membranes (AROM)**
A procedure in which your caregiver breaks your bag of waters with an amnihook (a long plastic device that resembles a crochet needle) in the attempt to speed up the labor process. Also called *amniotomy*.

**asymmetrical**
One side of your body is doing something different from the other side. For example, the lunge, side-lying, and semi-prone positions are asymmetrical positions.

**asynclitic**
A position in which your baby's head is tilted and the top of it isn't centered on the cervix. Can lead to a prolonged labor.

**augmentation**
Speeding up a slow labor by using self-help methods or interventions such as artificial rupture of membranes (AROM) or Pitocin.

**auscultation**
Listening to sounds inside your womb, such as your baby's heartbeat. In labor, intermittent auscultation describes how your nurse or caregiver listens to your baby's heartbeat during and between contractions with a Doppler ultrasound stethoscope. At the same time, he or she may place a hand on your abdomen to feel your contractions, then count your baby's heartbeats, noting whether they speed up or slow down and recording the findings.

**baby blues**
Emotional changes or mood swings that are common in new parents during the first few weeks after the birth of a baby. For example, going from elation to sadness in a matter of minutes isn't uncommon for new parents.

**benefit-risk analysis**
A process by which your caregiver considers whether treatment will achieve the desired results or create problems, then weighs the treatment's benefits against its risks before forming his or her recommendation for treatment.

**beta-endorphins**
Your body's natural painkillers, these hormones are secreted when you experience pain, stress, and physical exertion. Also called "endorphins."

**birth ball**
A large inflatable plastic physical therapy or fitness ball that provides a soft yet firm place to sit comfortably. Used as a comfort tool in labor to enhance mobility and labor progress.

**birth doula**
Someone (typically a woman) who's trained and experienced in supporting women and their partners during labor and birth.

**birth plan**
A one- to two-page letter to your caregiver and staff that describes your fears and concerns as well as your wishes and priorities for the treatment of you and your baby. Also called a "birth preference list," "wish list," or "goal sheet."

**blastocyst**
After conception, the fertilized egg quickly divides from one cell into two, then four, eight, sixteen, and so on until it becomes a multicellular structure called a blastocyst, which begins to implant in your uterus about five to nine days later. Once it's fully implanted, a blastocyst is called an *embryo*.

**Body Mass Index (BMI)**
A measurement of the relative amounts of fat and muscle in your body. It's calculated by using a ratio of your height to your prepregnancy weight.

**Braxton-Hicks contractions**
Contractions of the uterine muscle that become more frequent and intense in the third trimester, and that make your uterus hard for about a minute but aren't painful. Unlike labor contractions, Braxton-Hicks contractions don't cause changes in your cervix.

**breech presentation**
When your baby is positioned with his buttocks, legs, or feet over your cervix, instead of head down (vertex).

**castor oil**
A strong laxative that causes powerful bowel cramps and contractions, which may initiate uterine contractions to induce labor.

**catecholamines**
Stress hormones, including epinephrine (adrenaline), norepinephrine, and dopamine. High levels of stress hormones can slow labor progress.

**cephalo-pelvic disproportion (CPD)**
A condition in which your baby's head is believed to be too large to fit through your pelvis. This diagnosis may be made by your caregiver based on observations during pregnancy, or may be used as a retrospective diagnosis after a prolonged labor that resulted in the birth of a large baby.

**certified nurse-midwife (CNM)**
A maternity caregiver who has graduated from nursing school, passed an exam to become a registered nurse, and completed one or more years of additional training in midwifery.

**certified professional midwife (CPM)**
A maternity caregiver who has received training from a variety of sources, including apprenticeship, school, and self-study, and has been the primary attendant at twenty or more births. A CPM practices outside hospitals and provides care similar to that of a licensed midwife.

**cervical ripening device**
A silicone catheter that's placed within the cervix, then inflated with saline solution. Used to induce labor by accelerating cervical dilation.

**cervix**
The lower part of the uterus, which protrudes into the vagina.

**certified midwives (CMs)**
Have graduated from a health-related program other than nursing and must complete the same midwifery training and certification exams that CNMs do. They practice in the same settings as CNMs.

**cervical cerclage**
When the cervix is closed with suture thread.

**cesarean birth**
The experience of giving birth by a surgical procedure in which your baby is delivered through incisions in your abdomen and uterus. The procedure is also called a "cesarean section," "C-section," "cesarean delivery," or simply "cesarean."

**circumcision**
The surgical removal of the foreskin covering the glans (tip) of the penis.

**code word**
A word that you choose in advance and share with your caregivers. By saying the word during labor, you communicate that, despite your original plan to birth without pain medications, you now want help getting medicated pain relief.

**colic**
Prolonged crying in a young baby. Typically defined as three or more crying episodes each week for three or more weeks, with each episode lasting three hours or longer.

**colostrum**
The first breast milk: a highly nutritious yellowish fluid that's low in volume, but high in antibodies and the nutrients your baby will need for the first few days of life before your milk supply increases in volume.

**combined spinal-epidural (CSE)**
A method for delivering pain medication. CSE uses a spinal narcotic in early labor (which may allow for more mobility), then an epidural anesthetic later in labor, when you need more pain relief.

**complicated labor**
A labor that is longer, more painful, or more difficult than a normal labor, and may require medical help to ensure the well-being of you and your baby.

**conception**
Occurs when a sperm fertilizes an egg. The beginning of pregnancy.

**contraction**
Tightening of the uterine muscle. During labor, these muscle contractions help open your ripe, effaced cervix and help your baby descend. Contractions become more frequent and more intense as labor progresses.

**corticosteroids**
Medications that may be given to speed up the maturation of your baby's lungs if a preterm birth can't be prevented.

**corticotropin-releasing hormone (CRH)**
Comes from your baby, the placenta, and tissues within your uterus. Increased levels of CRH in late pregnancy may help initiate labor.

**crowning**
The third phase of the second stage of labor. It begins when the widest part of your baby's head is visible at the vaginal opening and no longer retreats between pushes, and it ends with her birth.

**delayed pushing**
An option for the second stage of labor, in which a woman who doesn't have an urge to push (such as after receiving an epidural) may wait an hour or two, or until her baby's head crowns, before pushing actively. Also called *passive descent*.

**descent**
The downward movement of your baby into your pelvis.

**diagnostic test**
Term used to describe a test that is more specific and more reliable than a screening test in identifying a woman with a pregnancy complication or a baby with a problem.

**dilation**
The opening of the cervix, which allows your baby to pass through for birth.

**directed pushing**
An option for the second stage of labor, in which your caregiver tells you how long and how hard to push. This method is used if you can't feel your contractions and delayed pushing isn't an option or if spontaneous pushing isn't effective.

**Doppler ultrasound**
A device that uses sound waves to monitor your baby's heart rate. Typically used at prenatal visits as well as during labor and birth.

**due date**
An estimate of when your baby will be born. The majority of babies are born in the period from two weeks before their due dates to two weeks after their due dates.

**early labor**
Usually the longest phase of the first stage of labor, often because contractions are further apart, shorter, and less intense than they'll be later in labor. Contractions are generally more than five minutes apart, and you can walk and talk during them. Also called the *latent phase*.

**ectopic**
An ectopic pregnancy occurs when the fertilized egg implants itself outside the uterus, usually in the wall of a fallopian tube (called a tubal pregnancy) but sometimes in the cervix, ovary, or abdomen. Most ectopic pregnancies can't develop into a live birth and typically require medical intervention to manage.

**effacement**
The thinning and shortening of the cervix in preparation for birth.

**elective induction**
An induction done without a medical reason, either because a woman requested induction or because her caregiver recommended it. Also called a "social induction."

**electronic fetal monitoring (EFM)**
Used to monitor your baby's heart rate and your contractions, to assess how your baby is responding to labor. There are two types of EFM. External EFM uses belts to hold two sensors on your abdomen, and the less commonly used internal EFM uses two sensors placed inside your uterus.

**embryo**
By two weeks after conception, your baby is called an embryo.

**engagement**
About two weeks before the birth, your baby descends deeper into your pelvis. You may feel less pressure on your diaphragm and find breathing and eating easier. Also called *lightening* or "dropping."

**engorgement**
Painful swelling of the breasts.

**epidural catheter**
A tube inserted into the epidural space near the spinal nerves and used to deliver pain medication.

**episiotomy**
A surgical incision of the perineum that enlarges the vaginal outlet. Once common practice, now the majority of caregivers use it only when medically necessary to deliver the baby quickly.

**estrogen**
A hormone that promotes the growth of the uterine muscles and their blood supply, encourages production of vaginal mucus, and stimulates the development of the ductal system and blood supply in the breasts. In late pregnancy, rising estrogen levels increase the uterus's sensitivity to oxytocin and help start labor.

**evert**
To draw out your nipple to allow your baby to latch on well for nursing. Typically occurs when your baby suckles.

**expression**
Removing milk from the breast by hand or by using a pump. May be used to relieve fullness, maintain milk supply, or store milk for your baby's consumption.

**expulsion breathing**
A way to breathe during spontaneous bearing down. During the pushing stage, use relaxed breathing when you don't have the urge to push. When you have an urge to push, you may briefly hold your breath and bear down, or you may exhale with an open throat while pushing.

**external version**
A procedure used to attempt to manually turn a baby from a breech or transverse position to a head-down position (vertex).

**failure to progress**
Term used either to describe a labor that's taking longer than expected for the cervix to dilate to 10 centimeters, or to describe a pushing stage that's taking longer than expected. May be treated with augmentation or cesarean delivery; however, if your baby is handling labor well, you may also ask whether self-help measures can effectively help with labor progress.

**fallopian tubes**
Provide the path for an egg to travel from your ovaries to your uterus.

**false positives**
Describes situations in which test results for a condition are positive, but the condition isn't present (for example, the fetal heart rate pattern indicates distress, but your baby turns out to be fine).

**family physician**
A physician who has graduated from medical school or a school of osteopathic medicine and has completed two or more years of additional training in family medicine, including maternity and pediatric care.

**feeding cues**
How your baby shows he's hungry. Include rooting, mouthing, tongue thrusts, sucking, and increased activity levels. Crying is a late feeding cue, used when the other cues have gone unnoticed.

**fetal intolerance of labor**
See *abnormal fetal heart rate*. Also called "fetal distress."

**first stage of labor**
The period that begins when contractions are becoming longer, stronger, and closer together (progressing) and ends when your cervix is completely dilated.

**forceps**
A tool (steel tongs) that's used to assist with a vaginal birth.

**foremilk**
Breast milk produced early in the feeding. Foremilk is lower in fat and higher in sugar than hindmilk.

**fourth stage of labor**
Begins after the placenta is delivered and ends one to several hours later, when your and your baby's conditions have stabilized.

**freestanding birth center**
A birth center unaffiliated with a hospital.

**fundus**
The top of your uterus.

**general anesthesia**
A systemic medication that causes a total loss of sensation and consciousness.

**gestation**
Another term for pregnancy, which lasts an average of 280 days or forty weeks after the first day of your last menstrual period.

**gestational age**
The age of your baby from the first day of your last menstrual period. Note that conception occurs within twelve to twenty-four hours after ovulation, which typically occurs fourteen days after the beginning of your last period. So, two weeks after conception your baby's gestational age is four weeks.

**gestational hypertension**
High blood pressure that develops during pregnancy, defined as at least two consecutive readings that are over 140/90. This condition affects 10 percent of pregnant women in the United States. Also called *pregnancy-induced hypertension (PIH)*.

**glycemic index**
An index that ranks foods according to how quickly and significantly they elevate your blood sugar.

**Group B streptococcus (GBS)**
A type of bacteria. If you test positive for GBS in pregnancy, you may be given antibiotics during labor.

**hemorrhoids**
Swollen varicose veins in the rectal area that may be as small as a pea or as large as a grape.

**Heparin Lock**
Involves inserting an intravenous (IV) catheter, but doesn't require hooking it to an IV bag and pole until IV fluids are needed. Also called "Hep-Lock."

**hindmilk**
Breast milk produced later in a feeding session, released with the let-down reflex. This milk provides most of the calories and contains more fat and protein than foremilk.

**homeopathy**
A complementary medicine technique that uses diluted derivatives of natural substances to stimulate your body to respond in a way that heals or corrects a specific problem, such as a labor that won't start.

**human chorionic gonadotropin (hCG)**
A hormone produced only during pregnancy. It ensures that your ovaries produce estrogen and progesterone for the first two to three months of your pregnancy, until your placenta matures and produces the appropriate amount.

**hyperventilation**
Overbreathing. If you find yourself feeling lightheaded or dizzy while using a breathing technique, try either slowing down your breathing, focusing on the exhalation rather than the inhalation, or breathing into your cupped hands.

**immunization**
See *vaccination*.

**incompetent cervix**
A cervix that shortens and opens in midpregnancy without preterm labor contractions.

**incontinence**
A condition that causes you to leak urine when you have a full bladder, exercise, cough, or sneeze (urinary incontinence) or uncontrollably pass gas or leak stool (fecal incontinence).

**induction**
An intervention used to start labor.

**infant cues**
Your baby's nonverbal communication. For example, when she's overstimulated, she may close his eyes, yawn, get glassy—eyed, turn away, or stiffen. If you miss these cues and continue to stimulate her, she may begin a prolonged bout of crying.

**informed choice**
See *informed decision*.

**informed consent**
After becoming informed about an option or treatment, you agree to it.

**informed decision**
The decision you make to refuse or consent to a health care option or medical treatment, after becoming informed about it through research and consultation with your caregiver and other knowledgeable medical professionals, as well as with supportive friends and family. Also called *informed choice*.

**informed refusal**
After becoming informed about an option or treatment, you refuse it.

**inhalation medication**
A gas you breathe to receive pain medication.

**intervention**
A medical procedure used to intervene in the natural labor process, such as induction, augmentation, episiotomy, or cesarean surgery.

**intramuscular (IM) medication**
A shot given into a muscle to deliver medication.

**intrathecal space**
The space inside the dura (the membrane that surrounds your spinal cord) that's filled with cerebrospinal fluid. It's where spinal medications are injected.

**intravenous (IV) catheter**
A tube that's inserted into a vein through a needle, allowing fluids and medications to be given directly into your circulatory system.

**intravenous (IV) medication**
An injection into a vein, often through an IV catheter, to deliver medication.

**involution**
After the birth, your uterus begins the six-week process of contracting to its nonpregnant size.

**jaundice**
An excess of bilirubin that causes your baby's skin or the whites of his eyes to become yellow by the third or fourth day after the birth.

**Kegel**
An exercise used to maintain the tone of your pelvic floor muscles, improve blood circulation in that area, decrease the incidence and severity of hemorrhoids and incontinence, and support your uterus and other pelvic organs.

**lactation consultant**
A breastfeeding expert.

**lanugo**
Fine, downy hair that develops on your baby's arms, legs, and back while in the womb.

**latch**
Your baby's connection with the breast to feed. A good latch permits your baby to nurse effectively.

**latent phase**
See *early labor*.

**lay midwife**
A maternity caregiver who might or might not be legally registered with the state or province, and whose qualifications and standards of care might or might not meet state or provincial standards. Also called "empirical midwife."

**Leopold's maneuvers**
The technique your caregiver uses to determine the baby's position by feeling your abdomen.

**let-down reflex**
When your baby nurses, the suckling stimulates your pituitary gland to release oxytocin, which makes your milk-producing cells contract and release (let down) milk for your baby to drink.

**leukorrhea**
A thin, liquid mucus discharge from the vagina.

**licensed midwife (LM)**
A maternity caregiver who has completed up to three years of formal midwifery training according to state requirements.

**lightening**
See *engagement*.

**local anesthetic**
Injection or application of pain medication that affects a specific, relatively small part of your body.

**lochia**
The heavy red discharge that flows from your vagina in the six weeks after the birth. It's made of the extra blood and fluid that supported your pregnancy and the uterine lining that sustained your baby.

**malposition**
When your baby is in an unfavorable position in the womb, which may lead to a prolonged labor. Can often be corrected by changing positions frequently.

**mastitis**
An infection of the breast.

**meconium**
Your baby's first bowel movements, a collection of digestive enzymes and residue from swallowed amniotic fluid. Appears as a sticky, greenish-black substance.

**membranes**
The amnion and chorion membranes create the amniotic sac that surrounds your baby in your uterus.

**miscarriage**
The unexpected death and delivery of a baby before the twentieth week of pregnancy. Also called "spontaneous abortion."

**misoprostol (Cytotec)**
A medication used to induce labor.

**Montgomery glands**
Small bumps on your areolae that secrete a lubricating substance that keeps the nipple supple and prevents infection.

**morning sickness**
Nausea and vomiting in the early months of pregnancy. Despite its name, morning sickness can occur at any time of day.

**moxibustion**
A version of acupuncture that doesn't use needles but instead uses burning herbs placed close to the acupuncture points.

**mucous plug**
Mucus that fills the cervical opening during pregnancy to provide a barrier to help protect your baby.

**multipara**
A woman who has given birth more than once.

**multiples**
Two or more babies gestating in the same womb.

**narcotics and narcotic-like drugs**
Medications that reduce the transmission of pain messages to the pain receptors in your brain.

**naturopathic doctor (ND)**
A health care provider who has completed three to four years of postgraduate training in natural medicine. May also have taken an additional year of midwifery training to be able to provide prenatal care and attend births.

**neonatal intensive care unit (NICU)**
A hospital unit where medically challenged newborns stay for monitoring and treatment until they can breathe on their own, stay warm at room temperature, and breastfeed or take a bottle.

**neuraxial medications**
Drugs that are injected into the space surrounding the spinal cord (neuraxis), such as epidurals and spinal blocks.

**nipple confusion**
A condition experienced by some babies who have difficulty adapting to different sucking patterns and flows of liquid, when they're fed alternately by a bottle and at the breast.

**nullipara**
A woman who has never given birth.

**obstetrician/gynecologist (OB-GYN)**
A physician who has graduated from medical school or a school of osteopathic medicine and has had three or more years of additional training in obstetrics and gynecology.

**occiput anterior**
The back of baby's head (occiput) is toward the front of your body.

**occiput posterior**
The back of baby's head (occiput) is toward your back.

**occiput transverse (ROT or LOT)**
The back of your baby's head is toward your right (or left) side.

**oral medication**
A pill or liquid you swallow to receive a medication.

**ovaries**
Female sex glands where eggs are produced.

**ovulation**
When a ripened egg is released into your fallopian tubes. On average, this happens fourteen days after the first day of your last menstrual period. If you have intercourse between four days before and one day after ovulation, there's a chance of conception.

**ovum**
An egg produced by a woman. When an egg is fertilized by a sperm, conception occurs.

**oxytocin**
A hormone produced in your pituitary gland, which stimulates uterine contractions to help trigger the onset of labor and promote labor progress. Also present during orgasm and during breastfeeding, it's often called "the love hormone."

**pain modifiers**
External stimuli that affect your awareness and perception of pain.

**parity**
Describes the condition of having given birth.

**passive descent**
See *delayed pushing*.

**patient-controlled epidural analgesia (PCEA)**
A device that allows you to increase your epidural dosage when you need more pain relief.

**pediatric and family nurse practitioner**
A registered nurse who has additional training in pediatrics or family health. Provides well-child care and treats common illnesses.

**pediatrician**
A physician who specializes in children's health care.

**pelvic floor muscles**
Muscles attached to the pelvis that support your abdominal and pelvic organs. These muscles form a figure-eight around your urethra, vagina, and anus.

**perinatologist**
An obstetrician/gynecologist (OB-GYN) who has received further training and certification in managing very high-risk pregnancies and births.

**perineal massage**
A massage that stretches the inner tissue of your lower vagina. Can be used during pregnancy or the second stage of labor to relax the tissue so it will stretch around your baby's head.

**perineum**
The external genitals (labia, urethra, clitoris, vaginal opening) and anus.

**phototherapy**
A medical procedure used to treat jaundice that shines a special type of cool light on your baby's skin, causing the bilirubin level to drop.

**Pitocin**
Commonly referred to as "Pit," this is a synthetic version of oxytocin.

**placenta**
An organ that develops in pregnancy, the placenta produces hormones and exchanges oxygen, nutrients, and waste products for your developing baby. It's released and delivered shortly after your baby's birth.

**position**
Refers to where the back of your baby's head (occiput) is in relation to your body.

**positive signs of labor**
Include contractions that become longer, stronger, and more frequent (progressing) and the rupture of membranes in a gush of amniotic fluid. These are the only reliable signs that labor has begun and your cervix is dilating.

**possible signs of labor**
Occur in late pregnancy and may indicate that hormonal changes are underway but cervical changes aren't yet occurring. These signs occur intermittently for days or weeks, but they don't indicate labor.

**post-date pregnancy**
A pregnancy that has lasted to at least forty-two weeks. Although the average length of pregnancy is forty weeks, many pregnancies last longer. Caregivers may misuse the term "post-date" as early as forty weeks.

**postmaturity**
A condition in which the placenta stops functioning well, the baby's growth slows or stops, and the risk of stillbirth increases. True postmaturity is rare even in babies born two weeks after their due dates. "Postmature babies" at birth have an absence of lanugo, scant vernix caseosa; long fingernails and toenails; and dry, peeling, or cracked skin.

**postpartum depression**
A condition that generally presents itself between two weeks to one year after the birth. Symptoms vary in severity among women.

**postpartum doula**
Someone (typically a woman) who's trained and experienced with helping a woman and her family adjust to postpartum life by teaching them about newborns' needs and abilities, and about infant feeding, sleep, and cues, while providing assistance with household tasks.

**postpartum hemorrhage**
The excessive loss of blood (more than 500 milliliters or 2 cups) during the first twenty-four hours after the birth.

**postpartum mood disorders (PPMD)**
Emotional conditions that can develop in the first year after birth, such as anxiety and panic disorder, obsessive-compulsive disorder, postpartum depression, bipolar disorder, and post-traumatic stress disorder.

**postpartum psychosis**
A rare condition that occurs in women after the birth and requires immediate care and psychiatric treatment. Symptoms include severe agitation, mood swings, depression, and delusions.

**precipitate birth**
A birth that results from a very fast labor. For a first-time mother, may be defined as an entire labor that lasts six hours or less, but it's more often applied to a labor that is three hours or less. For a woman who has previously given birth, it's one hour or less.

**preeclampsia**
High blood pressure and protein in the urine. A multi-organ condition with mild to severe symptoms that affects 5 to 8 percent of pregnancies. Previously called "toxemia."

**pregnancy-induced hypertension (PIH)**
See *gestational hypertension*.

**prelabor signs of labor**
Indicate that your cervix is probably moving forward, ripening, or effacing. These signs may progress into positive labor signs the same day they begin, or they may simply alert you that labor will begin in a few days or weeks.

**prelabor**
A period of hours or days in which you experience contractions, but your cervix isn't actively dilating. It's likely that these contractions are getting your cervix ready to dilate by moving it forward and helping it ripen and efface. Prelabor contractions may range from as little as thirty seconds long and twenty minutes apart, to as much as one or two minutes long and five to eight minutes apart. However, the contractions change very little in length, frequency, and intensity over time (nonprogressing).

**premature**
A baby that's born before the thirty-seventh week of pregnancy.

**presentation**
Describes the part of your baby that's lying over your cervix and will emerge from your body first. Also called *presenting part*.

**presenting part**
See *presentation*.

**preterm labor**
A labor that begins before the thirty-seventh week of pregnancy.

**primigravida**
A woman who is pregnant for the first time.

**primipara**
A woman who has given birth once.

**progesterone**
A hormone that relaxes your uterus during pregnancy, keeping it from contracting too much. It also relaxes the walls of blood vessels (helping you maintain a healthy blood pressure) and the walls of your stomach and bowels (allowing for greater absorption of nutrients).

**progressing contractions**
Contractions that become longer, stronger, and more frequent over time.

**prolactin**
A hormone that's produced after the birth and stimulates the production of breast milk.

**prolapsed cord**
A rare condition that occurs when the water breaks and the umbilical cord slips below the baby so it's either in the vagina or lying between the baby and the cervix. Requires a call to 911 and transport to the hospital for an immediate cesarean.

**prolonged labor**
A labor that progresses more slowly than expected. Diagnosis is somewhat subjective.

**prolonged prelabor**
Prelabor that lasts longer than a day.

**prostaglandin**
A hormone produced in your amniotic membrane. Increased levels in late pregnancy ripen your cervix in preparation for labor and stimulate muscles in your uterus and bowels to begin labor.

**quickening**
Describes the moment when you feel your baby's movements for the first time, during the second trimester.

**regional anesthetic**
Pain medication that affects a large area of your body.

**relaxin**
A hormone from your ovaries that relaxes and softens your ligaments, cartilage, and cervix, making these tissues more stretchable during pregnancy and letting your pelvic joints spread during birth.

**respiratory distress syndrome (RDS)**
A condition in which a newborn infant has difficulty breathing and is unable to get sufficient oxygen due to immature lungs. The most common complication of premature birth, it requires immediate medical treatment.

**rhythm**
Women who cope well in labor rely on rhythm in various forms. Rhythmic activity calms the mind and lets a woman work well with her body.

**ripening**
The softening of the cervix.

**ritual**
The repetition of a meaningful rhythmic activity during contractions to increase your ability to cope.

**routine**
Procedures or treatment that's offered to all pregnant women and their newborns, regardless of medical status.

**rupture of membranes**
Breaking of the bag of waters that may manifest itself either as the leaking of a small amount of amniotic fluid from the vagina, or as a gush of fluids. Rupture may happen before labor or may signal the onset of labor, or it can happen at any point during labor and birth.

**screening test**
A medical test that can rule out a particular condition or may indicate an increased chance that the condition is present. In the latter case, a diagnostic test confirms the condition.

**second stage of labor**
The birth of your baby. This stage begins when your cervix is fully dilated and ends when your baby is born.

**serial induction**
Medication to induce labor is given during the day, but is discontinued at night to allow you to eat and sleep.

**shared decision making**
A collaborative approach to making an informed decision, in which you and your caregiver discuss the medical risks and benefits of treatment and any possible alternatives.

**special care nursery**
A hospital unit for newborns who need extra medical monitoring or support, but don't need the intensive care of a NICU.

**spinal block**
An injection of anesthetic near the spinal nerves that takes effect quickly and lasts for an hour or two.

**spit up**
When a baby expels a dribble or more of milk (up to 2 to 3 tablespoons is common) after a feeding.

**spontaneous bearing down**
An option for the second stage of labor, in which you naturally bear down or strain for five to six seconds at a time and take several breaths between efforts. This type of pushing makes more oxygen available to your baby than if you hold your breath and bear down for as long as possible.

**spontaneous rituals**
Methods of coping invented by you over the course of your labor and reinforced by your support team. May include positions, movement, repeated words or sounds, specific kinds of touch, and so on.

**station**
Refers to the location of the top of your baby's head (or other presenting part) within your pelvis. Descent is measured by station.

**sterile water block**
An alternative option for relief of back pain during labor. A caregiver or nurse injects tiny amounts of sterile water into four places on your lower back. The injections cause severe stinging for a minute or more, but then provide pain relief by rapidly increasing endorphin production.

**sudden infant death syndrome (SIDS)**
The sudden death of a baby younger than one year that remains unexplained after a thorough investigation. There are steps that can be taken to further reduce the rare chance of SIDS; however, for about 1 in 2,000 babies, it appears to be impossible to predict or prevent.

**supine hypotension**
When lying on your back makes your uterus press on the abdominal vein that carries blood from your legs to your heart (inferior vena cava), causing a drop in blood pressure.

**surfactant**
A substance that allows your baby's lungs to expand during an inhalation and remain partially inflated during an exhalation.

**synthetic prostaglandins**
Medications that mimic the hormone prostaglandin.

**systemic**
Describes a medication that affects your entire body.

**tandem nursing**
Breastfeeding two children at the same time (such as twins or your baby and toddler).

**tension spots**
Body areas that you habitually tense when stressed. For example, your shoulders, forehead, mouth, jaw, or fists.

**third stage of labor**
Begins with the birth of your baby and ends with the delivery of the placenta.

**Three Rs: relaxation, rhythm, and ritual**
A theory about how women cope with labor when given support and freedom to explore coping options. You stay as relaxed as possible throughout labor, until you discover your coping rhythm. Your partner's role is to reinforce this ritual for as long as it continues to help you.

**tocolytic medication**
A drug used to slow or stop contractions; for example, during preterm labor.

**transition**
Final phase of the first stage of labor, which serves as the transition to the second stage of labor. Your cervix is reaching complete dilation, and your baby is beginning to descend into your birth canal. Contractions are ninety seconds to two minutes long and two to three minutes apart.

**transverse incision**
The most common incision (cut) for a cesarean birth. Horizontal incision on the lower abdomen (at the "bikini line") through the bottom of the uterus.

**transverse lie**
When your baby is positioned sideways in the uterus, with his back or shoulder closest to the cervix. Only occurs in 1 in 2,500 births. Your caregiver will attempt an external version to turn your baby, and if unsuccessful, your baby will be delivered by cesarean.

**triage**
Observation area in the hospital, where an admitting nurse assesses your condition, your pattern of contractions, your dilation (with a vaginal exam), and your baby's well-being, in order to determine whether you're ready to be admitted to the hospital, or whether you should return home with instructions on when to return.

**trial of labor after cesarean (TOLAC)**
When a woman with a prior cesarean chooses to let labor begin and progress, with the hope of having a vaginal birth after cesarean (VBAC).

**trimesters**
Pregnancy is divided into three trimesters, each one lasting about three months.

**ultrasound**
See *Doppler ultrasound* and *ultrasound scan*.

**ultrasound scan**
Equipment that uses intermittent transmission of sound waves to help your caregiver "see" inside the uterus. Can be used as a screening test or a diagnostic test for evaluating your baby's development.

**umbilical cord**
Links the placenta to your baby's navel, and together the umbilical cord and placenta pass oxygen and nutrients from you to your baby. While the placenta provides a barrier against most (but not all) bacteria in your bloodstream, most viruses and drugs cross to your baby. The placenta also exchanges waste products from your baby, which your blood then carries to your kidneys and lungs for excretion.

**urge to push**
The most significant sign of the second stage of labor. You may find yourself holding your breath and straining or grunting during each contraction.

**uterine atony**
Poor uterine muscle tone. The most frequent cause of postpartum hemorrhage.

**uterine rupture**
The separation of a uterine incision from a previous cesarean or uterine surgery.

**uterus**
A hollow, muscular organ the size and shape of a pear in which a baby develops.

**vaccination**
An administration of a vaccine to prevent illness. Also called *immunization*.

**vacuum extractor**
A tool (silicone suction cup) that's used to assist with a vaginal delivery.

**vaginal birth after cesarean (VBAC)**
A vaginal birth after a previous cesarean, as a result of a successful trial of labor after cesarean (TOLAC).

**vernix caseosa**
A white, creamy substance that protected your baby's skin in your womb.

**vertex**
Presentation in which the top of your baby's head is down over your cervix.

**wireless (or telemetry) monitoring**
Wireless electronic fetal monitoring, which allows you to walk and use the shower or bath.

# Index